BRADY

From Nursing Assistant To Clinical Care Associate

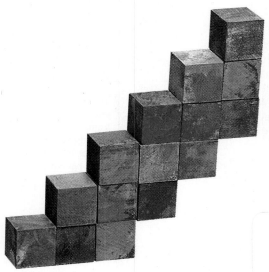

Carole Miele

Teresa England

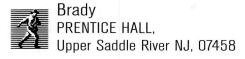

Brady
PRENTICE HALL,
Upper Saddle River NJ, 07458

Library of Congress Cataloging-in-Publication Data

Miele, Carole.
  From nursing assistant to clinical care associate /
Carole Miele, Teresa England.
    p.   cm.
  Includes index.
  ISBN 0-8359-5108-1
  1. Nurses' aides.   I. England, Teresa. II. Title.
    [DNLM: 1. Nurses' Aides.   2. Clinical Competence
programmed instruction. 3. Anatomy programmed instruction. 4. Physiology programmed instruction. WY
18.2 M631f 1999]
RT84.M54 1999
610.73'06'98—dc21
DNLM/DLC
for Library of Congress   98-23249
                                                  CIP

Publisher: Susan Katz
Marketing Manager: Tiffany Price
Acquisitions Editor: Barbara Krawiec
Managing Development Editor: Marilyn Meserve
Project Development Editor: Elizabeth Egan-Rivera
Editorial Assistant: Stephanie Camangian
Director of Manufacturing & Production: Bruce Johnson
Managing Production Editor: Patrick Walsh
Senior Production Manager: Ilene Sanford
Production Editor: Janet McGillicuddy
Art Director: Marianne Frasco
Interior Design: Amy Rosen
Cover Design: Joe Sengotta
Cover Photo: Yoshiki Komai
Managing Photography Editor: Michal Heron
Composition: TSI Graphics
Printing & Binding: Webcrafters

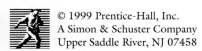

Printed in the United States of America
10 9 8 7 6 5 4 3 2 1

ISBN 0-8359-5108-1

Prentice-Hall International (UL) Limited, *London*
Prentice-Hall of Australia Pty. Limited, *Sydney*
Prentice-Hall Canada Inc., *Toronto*
Prentice-Hall Hispanoamericana, S.A., *Mexico*
Prentice-Hall of India Private Limited, *New Delhi*
Prentice-Hall of Japan, Inc., *Tokyo*
Simon & Schuster Asia Pte. Ltd., *Singapore*
Editora Prentice-Hall do Brasil, Ltda., *Rio de Janeiro*

To our parents, family, friends, and students for their encouragement, support, sacrifice, and understanding of our marriage to this project.

NOTICE

The procedures described in this textbook are based on consultation with nursing authorities. The author and publisher have taken care to make certain that these procedures reflect currently accepted clinical practice; however, they cannot be considered absolute recommendations.

The material in this textbook contains the most current information available at the time of publication. However, federal, state and local guidelines concerning clinical practices, including without limitation, those governing infection control and standard precautions, change rapidly. The reader should note, therefore, that new regulations may require changes in some procedures.

It is the responsibility of the reader to familiarize himself or herself with the policies and procedures set by federal, state and local agencies, as well as the institution or agency where the reader is employed. The authors and the publishers of this textbook, and the supplements written to accompany it, disclaim any liability, loss or risk resulting directly or indirectly from the suggested procedures and theory, from any undetected errors, or from the reader's misunderstanding of the text. It is the reader's responsibility to stay informed of any new changes or recommendations made by any federal, state and local agency as well as by his or her employing health care institution or agency.

NOTE ON GENDER USAGE

The English language has historically given preference to the male gender. Among many words, the pronouns, "he" and "his" are commonly used to describe both genders. The male pronouns still predominate our speech, however, in this text "he" and "she" have been used interchangeably when referring to the Nursing Assistant and/or the patient. The repeated use of "he or she" is not proper in long manuscript, and the use of "he or she" is not correct in all cases. The authors have made great effort to treat the two genders equally. Throughout the text, solely for the purpose of brevity, male pronouns and female pronouns are often used to describe both males and females. This is not intended to offend any reader of the female or male gender.

NOTICE: APPLICATION TO PRACTICE

The names used in the case studies throughout this text are fictitious.

TO THE STUDENT

A self-instructional workbook for this text is available through a college bookstore under the title, Workbook, From Nursing Assistant to Clinical Care Associate [ISBN #0-8359-5117-0]. If not in stock, ask the bookstore manager to order a copy for you. If your course is being offered off-campus, ask your instructor where to obtain a copy. The workbook can help you with course material by acting as a tutorial review and study aid.

Brief Contents

unit 1   The Health Care Industry   1

Chapter 1   *The Health Care Environment*   3
Chapter 2   *Care Delivery Alternatives*   13

unit 2   Employment of Clinical Care Associates   25

Chapter 3   *Emerging Health Care Roles*   27
Chapter 4   *Health Care Employment*   35

unit 3   The Language of Medicine   47

Chapter 5   *Medical Terms and Abbreviations*   49

unit 4   The Human Body   67

Chapter 6   *The Body as a Whole*   69
Chapter 7   *The Skin*   79
Chapter 8   *The Skeletal System*   87
Chapter 9   *The Muscular System*   95
Chapter 10   *The Nervous System*   105
Chapter 11   *The Cardiovascular System*   119
Chapter 12   *The Respiratory System*   135
Chapter 13   *The Digestive System*   145
Chapter 14   *The Urinary System*   159
Chapter 15   *The Reproductive System*   169
Chapter 16   *The Endocrine System*   183

unit 5   Problem Solving and the Fundamentals of Patient Care   195

Chapter 17   *A Nursing-Process Approach to Care Delivery*   197

unit 6   Nutrition   223

Chapter 18   *Elementary Nutrition*   225

unit 7   The Human Person   241

Chapter 19   *Care Delivery for the Whole Person*   243
Chapter 20   *Care Delivery for the Dying Patient*   261

unit 8   Mental Health Needs   273

Chapter 21   *Understanding Mental Illness*   275
Chapter 22   *Treating Mental Illness*   293

unit 9   The Environment of Care   311

Chapter 23   *Safety and Security Issues in Health Care*   313
Chapter 24   *The Client's Care Environment*   323

unit 10   Essential Procedures and Tasks: Critical Elements and Problem-Solving Tools   335

Chapter 25   *Essential Procedures and Tasks*   337

unit 11   Advanced or Expanded Procedures and Tasks: Critical Elements and Problem-Solving Tools   399

Chapter 26   *Advanced or Expanded Procedures and Tasks*   401

unit 12   Emergency Preparedness   447

Chapter 27   *Clinical and Environmental Emergencies*   449

Contents

Procedures   xviii
Guidelines   xix
Preface   xxi
About the Authors   xxii
Acknowledgments   xxiii
Introduction   xxv

u n i t   1   The Health Care Industry   1

C h a p t e r   1   *The Health Care Environment*   3
Defining Health Care   4
Hospitals   5
   Employees   5
   Consumers   5
   Payers   6
   Regulatory Agencies   7
   Reengineering Health Care in Hospitals   9
   Nursing Models   9
Application to Practice   10
Examination Review Questions   11

C h a p t e r   2   *Care Delivery Alternatives*   13
Long-Term Care Facilities   14
   Employees   14
   Consumers   14
   Regulatory Agencies   15
   Payers   18
Community and Ambulatory Care   18
Community Mental Health and Mental Retardation Agencies   19
   Consumers   19
   Employees   19
   Payers   20
   Regulatory Agencies   20
Home Care   20
   Facilities   20
   Employees   21
   Consumers   21
   Regulatory Agencies   21
Application to Practice   21
Examination Review Questions   23

u n i t   2   Employment of Clinical Care Associates   25

C h a p t e r   3   *Emerging Health Care Roles*   27
The Role of the Multiskilled Worker   28
   "Ready-to-Work" Time   28
   Standard Skill Sets   29

The Health Care Team   30
   Licensed Team Members   31
   Unlicensed Team Members   31
Principles of Computers and Data Entry   32
Application to Practice   33
Examination Review Questions   33

C h a p t e r   4   *Health Care Employment*   35
Employability of Multiskilled Assistive Personnel   36
   Résumés   38
   Knowing Yourself   38
   Interviews   38
   Job Search   39
Employment Opportunities for Assistive Personnel   41
   Hospitals   41
   Long-Term Care Facilities   41
   Community Mental Health and Mental Retardation Agencies   42
   Home Care Agencies   43
Application to Practice   44
Examination Review Questions   45

u n i t   3   The Language of Medicine   47

C h a p t e r   5   *Medical Terms and Abbreviations*   49
Rules for Pronouncing and Spelling Medical Terms   50
Understanding Word Parts   51
Building and Defining Medical Terms   51
   Analyzing Terms to Define Them   54
Medical Abbreviations   55
   Practice Reading Terms   61
Application to Practice   63
Examination Review Questions   65

u n i t   4   The Body Human   67

C h a p t e r   6   *The Body as a Whole*   69
Structural Units   70
   Cells   70
   Tissues   73
   Organs   73
   Systems   73
Anatomical Systems of Reference   75
   Anatomical Directions   76
   Reference Cavities   76
   Quadrants   77
Application to Practice   77
Examination Review Questions   78

C h a p t e r   7   *The Skin*   79

Structures of the Skin   80
    Epidermis   80
    Dermis   80
Functions of the Skin   80
Common Conditions and Diseases of the Skin   81
Application to Practice   82
Examination Review Questions   86

C h a p t e r   8   *The Skeletal System*   87

Structures of the Skeletal System   88
    Appearance and Structures of Long Bones   88
    Divisions of the Skeletal System   88
    The Vertebral Column   88
    Articulations   90
    Ligaments   90
Functions of the Skeletal System   90
Conditions and Diseases of the Skeletal System   91
Application to Practice   92
Examination Review Questions   93

C h a p t e r   9   *The Muscular System*   95

Skeletal Muscle: Structure and Function   96
    Movement of Skeletal Muscles   96
    Types of Skeletal Muscle Movements   96
    Skeletal Muscles Used for Intramuscular Injections   99
Smooth Muscle: Structure and Function   99
Cardiac Muscle: Structure and Function   99
Muscle Tone   100
    Exercise and Its Benefits   100
Conditions and Diseases of the Muscular System   100
Application to Practice   101
Examination Review Questions   103

C h a p t e r   1 0   *The Nervous System*   105

The Basic Unit of the Nervous System   106
    Types of Neurons   106
    Transmission of Signals   108
Divisions of the Nervous System   108
    The Central Nervous System: Structures and Functions   108
    The Peripheral Nervous System: Structures and Functions   110
Special Sense Organs: Structures and Functions   111
    The Eye   111
    The Ear   112
Conditions and Diseases of the Nervous System   113
Application to Practice   115
Examination Review Questions   116

C h a p t e r   1 1   *The Cardiovascular System*   *119*
The Circulatory System: Structures and Functions   120
   The Heart   120
   Blood Vessels   123
   Blood   125
   The Lymphatic System   128
Conditions and Diseases of the Circulatory System   129
Application to Practice   131
Examination Review Questions   133

C h a p t e r   1 2   *The Respiratory System*   *135*
Functions of the Respiratory System   136
Structures of the Respiratory System   136
   The Thoracic Cavity   137
   The Nose   137
   The Pharynx   138
   The Larynx   138
   The Trachea   139
   The Bronchi   139
   The Lungs   139
Respiration   139
Conditions and Diseases of the Respiratory System   140
Application to Practice   142
Examination Review Questions   143

C h a p t e r   1 3   *The Digestive System*   *145*
Functions of the Digestive System   146
   Metabolism   147
Structures of the Alimentary Canal   147
   The Mouth   147
   The Tongue   147
   The Teeth   147
   The Salivary Glands   147
   The Pharynx   147
   The Esophagus   148
   The Stomach   148
   The Small Intestine   149
   The Large Intestine (Colon)   149
The Protective Membrane of the Abdominal Cavity   150
Accessory Organs of the Gastrointestinal System   150
   The Liver   150
   The Gallbladder   150
   The Pancreas   150
Conditions and Diseases of the Digestive System   151
   Surgical Treatments   152
   Tumors of the GI System   153
   Hepatitis   153
   Diabetes Mellitus   154

Application to Practice   154
Examination Review Questions   157

C h a p t e r   1 4   *The Urinary System*   *159*
Functions of the Urinary System   160
Structures of the Urinary System   160
   The Kidneys   160
   The Ureters   163
   The Bladder   163
   The Urethra   163
Conditions and Diseases of the Urinary System   163
   Infections of the Urinary System   164
Surgical Procedures for Urinary Diversion   165
Application to Practice   165
Examination Review Questions   168

C h a p t e r   1 5   *The Reproductive System*   *169*
The Male Reproductive System   170
   The Scrotum   170
   The Penis   170
   The Testes: The Male Gonads   171
   The Ducts   171
   The Glands   171
Conditions and Diseases of the Male Reproductive System   172
   Testicular Exams   172
   Infertility   172
The Female Reproductive System   172
   The Vulva   173
   The Ovaries   174
   The Fallopian Tubes   174
   The Uterus   175
   The Vagina   175
   The Mammary Glands   175
   The Menstrual Cycle   175
   Pregnancy   175
Conditions and Diseases of the Female Reproductive System   176
   Tumors of the Female Reproductive Organs   177
   Breast Self-Examination   178
Application to Practice   178
Examination Review Questions   182

C h a p t e r   1 6   *The Endocrine System*   *183*
The Endocrine Glands and Their Hormones   184
   Classes of Hormones   185
   The Pituitary Gland   185
   The Thyroid Gland   187
   The Parathyroid Glands   187
   The Adrenal Glands   187
   The Pancreas   188

The Ovaries   188
The Testes   189
Conditions and Diseases of the Endocrine System   189
Disorders of the Thyroid Gland   189
Disorders of the Parathyroid Gland   189
Disorders of the Adrenal Glands   190
Disorders of the Pituitary Gland   190
Diabetes Mellitus   190
Application to Practice   191
Examination Review Questions   193

u n i t   5   Problem Solving and the Fundamentals of Patient Care   195

C h a p t e r   1 7   *A Nursing-Process Approach to Care Delivery*   197
Problem Solving   198
The Nursing Process   198
Scope of Practice   199
Licensure   201
Fundamentals of Patient Care   202
Ethics   202
Teamwork   205
Patient-Centered Care   212
Clients'/Patients' Rights   213
Guidelines: To Protect Patient Privacy and Confidentiality   214
Application to Practice   218
Examination Review Questions   221

u n i t   6   Nutrition   223

C h a p t e r   1 8   *Elementary Nutrition*   225
The Process of Nutrition   226
Seven Essential Nutrients   226
The Food Pyramid   230
Calories   230
Therapeutic Diets   231
Life-Span Nutritional Needs   233
Age-Specific Requirements   233
Alternative Nutritional Support   235
Parenteral Nutrition   235
Tube Feedings   235
The Cultural and Social Importance of Food   236
Application to Practice   237
Examination Review Questions   239

u n i t   7   The Human Person   241

C h a p t e r   1 9   *Care Delivery for the Whole Person*   243
The Basic Needs of Humans   244
Maslow's Hierarchy of Needs   244

Erikson's Eight Stages of Man   245
Age-Specific Competencies   250
Human Sexual Behavior   253
Sexual Behavior Research   253
Sexual Behavior and Patient Care   253
Growth and Development and Sexuality   254
Care Delivery and Patients' Sexuality   255
The Spiritual Needs of Patients   256
Cultural Diversity   257
Application to Practice   257
Examination Review Questions   259

Chapter 20 *Care Delivery for the Dying Patient*   261
The Stages of Death and Dying   262
Hospice   262
Decisions at the End of Life   263
Types of Written, Advanced Directives   263
Advanced Directives   263
Living Wills   263
Durable Power of Attorney for Health Care   264
Death with Dignity   266
Ethical Dilemmas   266
A Case in Point   267
Application to Practice   269
Examination Review Questions   272

unit 8   Mental Health Needs   273

Chapter 21 *Understanding Mental Illness*   275
Mental Health   276
Diagnostic Categories of Mental Health   277
Psychotic Disorders   277
Thought Disorders   277
Personality Disorders   279
Mood Disorders   281
Neurotic Disorders   282
Defense Mechanisms   282
Anxiety Disorders   283
Addictive Disorders   284
Cognitive Disorders   286
Mental Retardation   288
Causes of Mental Retardation   290
Application to Practice   290
Examination Review Questions   291

Chapter 22 *Treating Mental Illness*   293
General Guidelines   294
Managing Behavior: Guidelines and Therapeutic Approaches   294
Anxious Behavior   294

Angry, Demanding, and Verbally Abusive Behavior   295

Depressed Behavior   296

Hallucinations or Delusions   298

Behavior Modification   298

Types of Reinforcement   302

Scheduling Reinforcement   303

Understanding Behavior   303

Using Behavior Modification to Teach   304

Mini-Mental State Examination   304

Application to Practice   304

Examination Review Questions   310

u n i t   9   The Environment of Care   311

C h a p t e r   2 3   *Safety and Security Issues in Health Care*   313

The Environment of Care   314

Body Mechanics   314

The Cycle of Infection   315

The Autoclave   317

Aseptic Technique   317

CDC Guidelines for Isolation   318

Standard Precautions   318

Guidelines: Standard Precautions   318

Isolation Precautions   318

Guidelines: Airborne Isolation Precautions   319

Guidelines: Droplet Isolation Precautions   319

Guidelines: Contact Isolation Precautions   319

The Care Environment and Personal Security   320

Guidelines: Basic Security   320

Guidelines: Personal Security   321

Application to Practice   321

Examination Review Questions   322

C h a p t e r   2 4   *The Client's Care Environment*   323

The Nursing Home as the Care Environment   324

Personal Space in the Nursing Home   324

Helping the Resident Adapt   325

Special Safety Issues in the Nursing Home   325

Guidelines: To Reduce the Risk of Falls   326

Guidelines: Techniques to Respond to Wandering   329

The Home as the Care Environment   329

Safety Issues in the Home Care Environment   329

The Hospital as the Care Environment   330

The Hospital Experience   331

Personal Space and Safety in the Hospital   331

Application to Practice   332

Examination Review Questions   333

u n i t   1 0   Essential Procedures and Tasks: Critical Elements and Problem-Solving Tools   335

C h a p t e r   2 5   *Essential Procedures and Tasks*   *337*

Major Principles for the Implementation of Procedures   338

    Time Management   338

    Safety   339

    Patients' Rights   340

    Outcome-Based Goal Setting   340

    Competence   340

    Comfort   340

Basic Hygiene   341

    Handwashing   341

    procedure   Handwashing   341

    Bedmaking   341

    procedure   Bedmaking   342

    Bathing   345

    procedure   Bathing   345

    Mouth Care   345

    procedure   Mouth Care   346

    Hair Care   348

    procedure   Hair Care   348

    Nail Care   349

    procedure   Nail Care   349

    Shaving   349

    procedure   Shaving   349

    Changing a Patient's Clothing   350

    Skin Care   350

    Massage   352

    procedure   Massage   352

Measuring Skills   352

    Vital Signs   352

    Temperature   352

    procedure   Measuring Oral Temperature Using a Glass Thermometer   355

    procedure   Measuring Aural Temperature Using a Tympanic Thermometer   355

    procedure   Measuring Axillary Temperature Using a Glass Thermometer   356

    procedure   Measuring Rectal Temperature Using a Glass Thermometer   356

    Pulse   356

    procedure   Measuring Pulse   357

    Respirations   357

    procedure   Measuring Respirations   358

    Blood Pressure   358

    procedure   Measuring Blood Pressure   359

Intake and Output   359

p r o c e d u r e   Measuring Intake and Output   361

Height   362
p r o c e d u r e   Measuring Height   362

Weight   362
p r o c e d u r e   Measuring Weight   363

Restorative Care Skills   363

Body Alignment   365
Turning and Moving a Patient   365
Range-of-Motion Exercises   366
p r o c e d u r e   Performing Range-of-Motion Exercises   367

Ambulation with Assistive Devices   372
p r o c e d u r e   Ambulation with Crutches   373
p r o c e d u r e   Ambulation with a Quad Cane   375

Transfers   374
p r o c e d u r e   Transfers   375
p r o c e d u r e   Transfer with a Mechanical Lift   377

Specimen-Collection Skills   377

Urine Specimens   377
p r o c e d u r e   Collecting a Urine Specimen   378
p r o c e d u r e   Collecting an Infant Urine Specimen   379
p r o c e d u r e   Collecting a 24-Hour Urine Specimen   380

Straining Urine   380
Collecting Stool Specimens   380
p r o c e d u r e   Straining Urine   381
p r o c e d u r e   Collecting a Stool Specimen for Occult Blood   381
p r o c e d u r e   Collecting a Stool Specimen for Ova and Parasites Test   382

Collecting Sputum Specimens   382
p r o c e d u r e   Collecting a Sputum Specimen   383

Collecting Throat Cultures   383
p r o c e d u r e   Collecting a Throat Culture   383

Nutrition Skills   384

Feeding a Patient   384
p r o c e d u r e   Feeding a Patient   384

Basic Elimination Skills   385

Assisting with a Bedpan   385
p r o c e d u r e   Assisting with a Bedpan   385

Assisting with an Enema   386
p r o c e d u r e   Assisting with an Enema   387

Catheter Care   388
p r o c e d u r e   Catheter Care   389

Special Applications and Preps   389
   Heat and Cold Applications   389
   Sitz Baths   389
   procedure   Sitz Bath   390

   Preparing a Patient for an Exam   390
   procedure   Preparing a Patient for an Exam   391

   Applying Support/Therapeutic Hose   392
   procedure   Applying Elastic Support Hose   393

   Applying Ace Bandages   393
   procedure   Applying Ace Bandages   394

   Preoperative Shaving   394
   procedure   Preoperative Shaving   396

Application to Practice   396
Examination Review Questions   397

unit 11   Advanced or Expanded Procedures and Tasks: Critical Elements and Problem-Solving Tools   399

Chapter 26   *Advanced or Expanded Procedures and Tasks*   401
Catheterization of the Urinary Bladder   402
   Inserting a Catheter   402
   procedure   Inserting a Catheter   403

   Removing an Indwelling Catheter   406
   procedure   Removing an Indwelling Catheter   407

Gastrostomy Tubes: Tube Feedings, Irrigation, and Aspiration of Residual Feeding   407
   procedure   Aspiration of Residual Stomach Contents   409
   procedure   Bolus PEG Feeding   410
   procedure   Continuous Gastrostomy Feeding with a Pump   411

   A Note about Feeding Pumps   412
The Twelve-Lead Electrocardiogram   412
   ECG Machines   413
   Limb Lead Placement   414
   Chest Lead Placement   414
   Entering Patient Information   415
   procedure   Twelve-Lead ECG   416

   Technical Quality of the ECG Tracing   416
   Troubleshooting the ECG Machine   417
Dressings   419
   Tegaderm Dressings   419
   procedure   Applying a Tegaderm Dressing   420

   Duoderm Dressings   420
   procedure   Applying a Duoderm Dressing   420

Wet-to-Dry Dressings   421
  procedure   Applying a Wet-to-Dry Dressing   422

Ostomy Care   422
  procedure   Emptying the Ostomy Appliance   424
  procedure   Changing the Ostomy Appliance   424

Respiratory Care   425
  Oxygen Therapy   425
  procedure   Applying a Nasal Cannula   426
  procedure   Applying a Face Mask   427

  Pulse Oximetry   427
  procedure   Measuring SaO$_2$ Using a Pulse Oximeter   428

  Incentive Spirometry   428
  procedure   Assisting with an Incentive Spirometry   429

  Oral Suctioning   429
  procedure   Performing Oral Suctioning   430

  Percussion   431
  procedure   Performing Percussion   432

Phlebotomy   432
  Types of Specimens   432
  Phlebotomy Needles   433
  Vacutainer Tubes   433
  Labeling Blood Specimens   434
  Blood Bank Specimens   434
  Approaching the Patient   434
  Performing the Venipuncture   435
  procedure   Performing Venipuncture to Obtain a Venous Blood Sample   438

Capillary Blood Glucose Measurements   440
  Principles of Glucose Meters   440
  Asepsis   440
  Quality Control   441
  Operating a Glucose Meter   441
Capillary Blood Specimens   441
  procedure   Obtaining a Capillary Blood Specimen   441

Pneumatic Hose   442
  procedure   Applying Pneumatic Hose   443

Application to Practice   443
Examination Review Questions   445

unit 12   Emergency Preparedness   447

Chapter 27   *Clinical and Environmental Emergencies*   *449*
Seizures   450
  Petit Mal Seizures   450
  Grand Mal Seizures   450

Shock   451

Loss of Consciousness   452

Cardiopulmonary Resuscitation (CPR)   452

    Airway   452

    Breathing   452

    Circulation   453

Choking   454

    The Heimlich Maneuver   455

    Obstructed Airway—Unconscious Adult   455

Cardiac Arrest   455

Fire Safety   456

    Fire Extinguishers   457

    RACE   457

Electrical Safety   458

Disaster Plans   459

Bomb Threats   459

Biohazardous Wastes   459

Hazardous Materials   460

Application to Practice   464

Examination Review Questions   465

Index   *467*

- Handwashing*
- Bedmaking*
- Bathing*
- Mouth Care*
- Hair Care*
- Nail Care*
- Shaving*
- Massage*
- Measuring Oral Temperature Using a Glass Thermometer*
- Measuring Aural Temperature Using a Tympanic Thermometer
- Measuring Axillary Temperature Using a Glass Thermometer*
- Measuring Rectal Temperature Using a Glass Thermometer*
- Measuring Pulse*
- Measuring Respirations*
- Measuring Blood Pressure
- Measuring Intake and Output*
- Measuring Height*
- Measuring Weight*
- Performing Range-of-Motion Exercises*
- Ambulation with Crutches
- Ambulation with a Quad Cane
- Transfers*
- Transfer with a Mechanical Lift
- Collecting a Urine Specimen
- Collecting an Infant Urine Specimen
- Collecting a 24-Hour Urine Specimen
- Straining Urine
- Collecting a Stool Specimen for Occult Blood
- Collecting a Stool Specimen for Ova and Parasites Test

- Collecting a Sputum Specimen
- Collecting a Throat Culture
- Feeding a Patient*
- Assisting with a Bedpan*
- Assisting with an Enema
- Catheter Care
- Sitz Bath
- Preparing a Patient for an Exam
- Applying Elastic Support Hose
- Applying Ace Bandages
- Preoperative Shaving
- Inserting a Catheter
- Removing an Indwelling Catheter
- Aspiration of Residual Stomach Contents
- Bolus PEG Feeding
- Continuous Gastrostomy Feeding with a Pump
- Twelve-Lead ECG
- Applying a Tegaderm Dressing
- Applying a Duoderm Dressing
- Applying a Wet-to-Dry Dressing
- Emptying the Ostomy Appliance
- Changing the Ostomy Appliance
- Applying a Nasal Cannula
- Applying a Face Mask
- Measuring SaO_2 Using a Pulse Oximeter
- Assisting with an Incentive Spirometry
- Performing Oral Suctioning
- Performing Percussion
- Performing Venipuncture to Obtain a Venous Blood Sample
- Obtaining a Capillary Blood Specimen
- Applying Pneumatic Hose

indicate mandatory OBRA content.

Guidelines:

- To Protect Patient Privacy and Confidentiality*
- Standard Precautions*
- Airborne Isolation Precautions*
- Droplet Isolation Precautions*
- Contact Isolation Precautions*

- Basic Security*
- Personal Security
- To Reduce the Risk of Falls*
- Techniques to Respond to Wandering*

* indicate mandatory OBRA content.

Preface

The health care industry has become an ever-changing market place for consumers, employers, and employees. Today's nursing assistant and all unlicensed care providers must be equipped with precise technical skills, sound principles, keen critical thinking abilities and flexible interpersonal skills. The assistant in health care should be prepared to function in a wide array of health environments. Individuals who possess a solid foundation of core nursing assistant skills may build upon these skills and expand the horizons of their employability. This textbook provides the reader with current information applicable to the variety of health care settings that use the standard skill sets. Employment roles and requirements in a hospital long-term care facility, home care agency or a community mental health and mental retardation residential care setting are explored.

The textbook uses a holistic approach to client care. The human experience is examined in body, mind, and spirit from birth until death. Each chapter is complete with case studies. The exercises prepare the learner for realistic "what if" situations. The concepts are written across the curriculum and address all learning styles. The curriculum is built for partners, small group learning, teamwork, and collaborative efforts—all necessary proponents of the interdisciplinary health care team. The text is culturally sensitive. Case studies and learning activities involve the reader. Comprehensive answers provide immediate feedback of knowledge acquisition and assessment of learning.

The nursing skills are taught using the nursing process methodology. This method of instruction guides the learner with an analytical approach to skill acquisition. Further, the text emphasizes the scope of practice of the unlicensed assistant and delineates the role as a patient care technician. Essential nursing assistant skills, as well as expanded skills of the multi-skilled worker are fully discussed in a unique format based on fundamental principles of care.

The unit, The Body Human, is an ideal study of anatomy and physiology. Common conditions and diseases and applicability to the nursing assistant are included for each body system. A comprehensive guide to master the language of medicine is complete with recipes for easy learning. Up-to-date information on OBRA, OSHA, and JCAHO standards, safety, and personal security, CDC guidelines, age specific competencies, ethical dilemmas and advanced technical skills are included.

The unit on mental health needs provides guidelines for managing behavior, DSM IV diagnostic criteria, and behavior modification techniques. Human growth and development is approached using *Erikson's Eight Stages of Man*. Incorporated are age-specific needs and sexual development. Basic nutrition and nutritional needs throughout life stages are examined.

This is the textbook that instructors, students and employers have been awaiting. It is an essential guide to the cross-trained, multi-skilled unlicensed caregiver.

About the Authors

Carole Miele
RN, MEd

Carole is a nurse educator for the University of Pennsylvania Health System. She has had a long career in nursing and in education. She developed the curriculum for the redesign of patient care delivery at Presbyterian Medical Center and designed and taught a nurse extender program. She has worked clinically in acute care and long-term care—her area of specialty is psychiatry. She has taught the range from high school to graduate school programs. Her expertise in education is curriculum redesign.

Teresa England
RN, MSN

Teresa is a secondary vocational instructor for North Montco Technical Career Center. Her extensive nursing career has spanned from dialysis to home care. Her area of specialty is gerontology. Since 1983, she has developed and implemented curricula in health occupations for secondary and adult vocational education, and has taught the range from secondary to graduate education students. She has been actively involved in reviewing health occupations texts and has contributed to several published texts in the past ten years.

Acknowledgments

This text has been carefully written by Carole Miele and Teresa England. Individually, they worked with extraordinary commitment on the project. Together, they are a dedicated, professional team with the highest standards of current instruction for Clinical Care Assistants.

In addition, the authors would like to acknowledge and thank the following organizations and individuals for contributing immeasurably to the development of this text.

Editorial Development

Kristin Kiefer for her assistance and review of the original manuscript.

Marti Burton for her contributions and assistance with the writing and editing of Chapters 25 and 26.

Brady/Prentice Hall

Susan Katz, Publisher, for her support of this project.

Barbara Krawiec, Acquisitions Editor, for her belief in the authors and our ideas, for her vision and zeal.

Marilyn C. Meserve, Development Managing Editor, for her commitment, efficiency, and empathy.

Janet McGillicuddy, Production Editor, for her attention to important details.

Stephanie Camangian, Editorial Assistant, provided editorial support and assistance throughout the project.

Elizabeth Egan-Rivera, Project Editor, for her commitment to the integrity of the text.

Pat Walsh, Production Managing Editor, and additional production team members including Ilene Sanford, Manufacturing buyer, Marianne Frasco, Creative Director, and Larry Hayden, Production Editor for their knowledge, skill, patience, and competency in driving the book through the production process.

Judy Stamm, Brady Sales Manager and the Brady Sales Team for their support, suggestions, and resources.

Tiffany Price, Marketing Manager, for her energy and marketing support.

Cindy Frederick, Marketing Coordinator, for her ability to envision our product.

Judith Mara Riotto, Copyeditor, for her attention to consistency and details.

Organizations

Our very special thanks to North Penn Hospital, Lansdale, PA and COMHAR, Inc., Philadelphia, PA for the gracious use of their facilities.

Thanks to the clients of COMHAR, Inc. for their participation in the photographs.

Thanks to the North Montco Health Occupations Students for their enthusiasm and willingness to participate in pilot studies.

Photography Team

Michal Heron, Photography Managing Editor, for her precision and artistry, tenacity and professional dedication.

Kelly Dillon, Photo Assistant, for her flexibility and creative contributions

The authors give a special thanks to volunteer models for their patience in the long hours of photo shoots and for their desire to recreate realistic scenes: Chris Miller, Ross Hancock, Carolyn Hayward, Cecelia Fiorillo, Debbie Sherman, Jose Enrique Rivera, Tanny McKnight, Larry Dang, and Richard Lewis.

Reviewers

The following reviewers provided invaluable feedback and suggestions. We wish to thank each of these professionals for their contributions.

Barbara E. McQuade, QAI Coordinator / Inservice Educator, Nursing Staff Development / QA, University Hospital at Stonybrook, Stonybrook, NY

Judie T. Kautz, MS, RN, Education Director, Department. of Education, Pima Medical Institute, Tucson, AZ

M. Donna House, Ph.D., Instructional Dean, Health Occupations, Emily Griffith Opportunity School, Denver, CO

Ruth S. Campbell, RN, Nursing Assistant. Program Coordinator, Human Services Division, Nursing Department, Alamance Community College, Graham, NC

Barbara Prickett Ramutkowski, RN, BSN, Pima Medical Institute, Tucson, AZ

Joyce F. Smith, RN, MN, Instructor, New Orleans Public Schools, Nursing Department, N.O. Center for Health Careers, New Orleans, LA

J. Gaynelle Rogers, Coordinator, Health Occupations, Continuing Education Department, Asheville-Buncombe Technical CC, Asheville, NC

Carol B. Bartolotti, RN, C, MPA, Coordinator of Nursing Staff Development, Nyack Hospital, Nyack, NY

Julie Capriola, Coordinator Nurse Aide Program, Vance Granville Community College, Henderson, NC

Jillian Ashmen, MS, CHES, Nursing/Allied Health Administrator, Community Education Department, Ocean County College, Toms River, NJ

Robert DeJoy, Executive Director / President, Department of Education, Medical Career College, Phoenix, AZ

Introduction

From Nursing Assistant to Clinical Care Associate is a text designed to meet your learning needs. If you are beginning your career as a nursing assistant, this text offers the core skills necessary to complete a state-certified CNA program. If you are employed as an assistant and you are expanding your skills, this text strengthens your skills by challenging you to approach these skills in a critical thinking style. In addition, this text demonstrates opportunities to transfer these skills as an unlicensed assistant in a variety of care settings, including a hospital, community residential setting, long-term care setting, or home care setting. The text will open your eyes to the employment opportunities available to you as a multi-skilled worker. The health care industry is in a constant state of change and guaranteed employment is not a reality. However, employability is achievable.

The authors have included information shaping today's health care marketplace. Employers are seeking individuals who can think critically, adapt to change, communicate effectively, and identify problems that affect quality and performance.

The most dynamic feature of this text is that the information is presented in an interesting and thought-provoking manner, never separating the person from the patient. Patient care will come alive for you as you discover the reasons for your actions and discover the value of your position.

Your study of this textbook will present you with fundamental principles and problem-solving skills that will guide you to be successful as a student, a worker, and an individual.

The information below will highlight some key features of this book.

Contents

All chapters and main headings, as well as procedures and guidelines that appear in the chapters, are listed in the Contents.

Introduction

Each unit begins with an introduction demonstrating the importance of the material discussed in the associated chapters. The introduction will spark your interest and engage you in wanting to read about the topics.

Key Terms

Key terms are listed at the beginning of each chapter and are indicated in bold in the chapter location where their definitions may be found.

Objectives

The objectives listed for each chapter summarize the important concepts in each chapter. Read the objectives before reading the chapter. These are measurable and attainable goals to be achieved through chapter study. Reread the objectives upon chapter completion. View the objectives as test questions. If you answer the objectives upon chapter completion, you have mastered the chapter concepts.

Examination Review Questions

For each chapter, there are ten multiple-choice questions for self-examination. These questions prepare you to sit for certifying examinations.

Learning Activities

After completion of the chapter readings, you are asked to apply the knowledge you have gained to solving problems. The case scenarios provide a realistic picture of applying your skills in the workplace. The authors provide comprehensive answers to guide you through and assure your success. You will find that the learning activities are an enjoyable way to learn.

Procedures

All procedures are approached using the nursing process, and the fundamental principles of care. Role delineation is clearly defined. This method of skill delivery is more effective than rote learning in which tasks are memorized. The cumbersome number of steps in the standard skill sets frightens the learner. In actual care delivery, the environment is never conducive to executing skills in this way. Modifications are generally necessary. As long as the principles of care are mastered and the critical elements of a skill are understood, the skill can be thought through and delivered safely.

If you are preparing for entry-level CNA, this will be an easier way of mastering the many care skills required for certification. If you are currently employed as a CNA, this text will reveal the "why" of the skills you perform. Your job performance will improve, and, ultimately, delivery of patient care will be enhanced.

The Health Care Industry

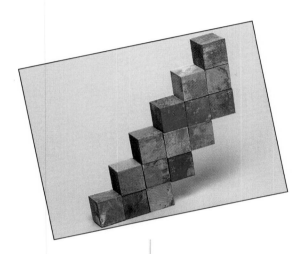

In this unit, you will be introduced to the health care industry. You will learn about traditional care-delivery environments including hospitals, long-term care facilities, and the home, as well as alternative care-delivery environments. Major changes are taking place in the industry, among the insurers of health care, and among the consumers of health care. These changes are discussed, along with the concepts—diagnostic related groups, critical pathways, patients' rights—and regulatory agencies that have initiated or formulated these changes.

Chapter 1

The Health Care Environment

As you explore this chapter, you will see that today's health care industry is shaped by the need to deliver personalized (patient-focused), quality care in a cost-effective and timely manner and by the need to protect the rights of the individuals for whom care is provided. The *reengineering* of care, as it has been termed, has reshaped the job descriptions of care providers. To function well at your job and to contribute to the health care environment, you need to understand care delivery and the participants who shape an efficient and well-run work environment. The concepts introduced in this chapter include the three levels of care, diagnostic related groups, critical pathways, quality assurance, nursing models, and regulatory agencies.

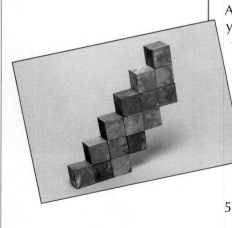

OBJECTIVES

After completing this chapter, you will be able to

1. List and describe the three levels of health care

2. Name some types of health care facilities

3. Describe the reasons for changes in the delivery of health care

4. Identify the customers you will serve

5. List ways *diagnostic related groups* have revolutionized hospital care and cost

6. Discuss the types of external regulatory agencies that affect the health care industry

7. Describe what is meant by reengineering health care in hospitals

8. Name some qualities of the *patient-focused care* delivery model

9. Define and spell all key terms correctly

key terms

consumers	Joint Commission on Accreditation	Occupational Safety and Health
critical pathway	of Healthcare Organizations	Administration (OSHA)
diagnostic related groups	(JCAHO)	patients
(DRGs)	medical diagnosis	primary care
for-profit	nonprofit	primary nursing model
health care	Nuclear Regulatory Commission	quality assurance
health maintenance organizations	(NRC)	secondary care
(HMOs)	nurse extenders	team nursing models
JCAHO accreditation	nursing process	tertiary care

Defining Health Care

In some respects, the term **health care** is misleading because it is used to describe institutions that primarily treat people who are ill, rather than people who are well. There are three levels of health care. They are categorized as *primary care*, *secondary care*, and *tertiary care*. Primary care can be seen in today's health care industry as providing op-portunities for health maintenance and health education programs for people who are well. The purpose of a primary-care physician is to prevent and to treat illness as well as to provide education and resources to maintain a state of wellness (optimal health).

Primary care measures and interventions are aimed at preventing illness and maintaining wellness (Figure 1-1A). Americans are introduced to education and prevention of disease in television advertise-

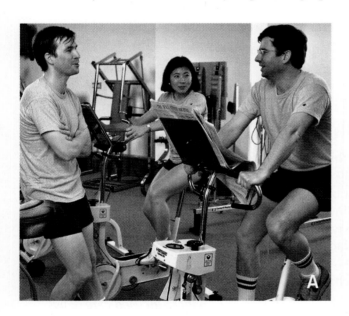

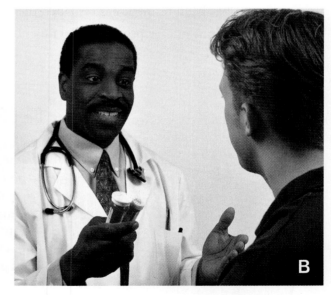

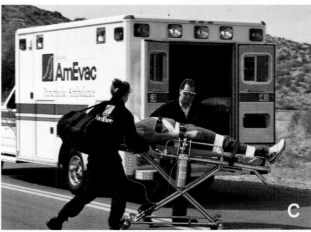

FIGURE 1-1   Continuum of health care.

ments and news programs, in newspapers, magazines, and schools. Health classes in schools provide primary (first-line) health care interventions through education about the benefits of exercise and a well-balanced diet. School health programs also check children's immunization records and provide education about disease, the health hazards of smoking and high-fat diets, drug abuse, sex education, and life safety. Nonetheless, most Americans visit a health care facility when they are ill, not when they are well.

Secondary care measures and interventions are aimed at treating illnesses before they necessitate hospital treatment. Preventing high blood pressure through exercise, diet, and blood pressure checks is a primary measure (Figure 1-1B). Receiving blood pressure medication from a family physician is a secondary measure aimed at reducing blood pressure before it leads to heart, vascular, or kidney disease.

Tertiary care measures and interventions refer to care that would be implemented if someone, for example, has a stroke because of dangerously high blood pressure and is admitted to a hospital for treatment of the stroke (Figure 1-1C).

Because there is a vast amount of knowledge about health and the causes of diseases, the aim of health care today is to prevent illness. Educating people about the effects of diet, exercise, and lifestyle is an essential or primary measure of health care. It is certainly prudent (smart) and less costly to prevent illness than it is to treat illness that could have been prevented. Consider the importance of childhood immunizations, such as the diphtheria, pertussis, and tetanus (DPT) vaccine. This immunization helps to prevent infectious diseases that once took the lives of children and adults. Childhood immunizations and other primary measures are not only prudent because they cost less than treating diseases, but they reduce human suffering and the loss of human lives.

Hospitals

Most of us think of hospitals as the main type of health care facility. Hospitals can be connected to a university, to a health system, or to a system of merged health care facilities (Figure 1-2). Hospital care also can be community-based and county-funded. The types of services provided by hospitals vary. The services hospitals offer vary according to the health care needs of the community, the nature of the research conducted at the hospital, and the grants that fund particular hospital services. Some hospitals that are part of a larger health system offer specialized services for that system. For example, one hospital in a health system may specialize in the treatment of musculoskeletal disorders, and another hospital in the sys-

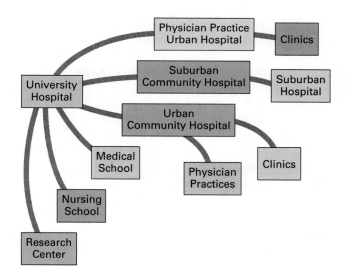

FIGURE 1-2　Hospitals are frequently part of large health systems.

tem may specialize in diseases of the cardiovascular system. All hospitals have some type of emergency department, and some may have a trauma center.

Today, many hospitals are part of a larger health care system. A hospital that is part of a health system is one facility that the health system owns and operates. Health systems may operate and affiliate with several hospitals, physician group practices, community-based primary care, and mental health care agencies. Some health systems are spread throughout a city, some are located throughout a state, and others cross state lines. We discuss this further in the section "Reengineering Health Care in Hospitals" later in this chapter. Hospitals generally provide emergency care, medical care, and surgical services.

Employees

Hospitals require the services of many professional and nonprofessional individuals. In essence, hospitals are like little cities. They need the services of housekeepers, plumbers, electricians, carpenters, lawyers, accountants, secretaries, nurses, doctors, technicians, nutritionists, chefs, nursing care associates, telephone operators, security guards, computer experts, and so on. Hospitals operate 24 hours a day, 7 days a week. When you are hired by a hospital as a clinical care associate, you will work under the direct supervision of a registered or professional nurse. The nature of your work is discussed in Unit 2, "Employment of Clinical Care Associates."

Consumers

The primary **consumers** (customers) of hospitals are patients. Yes, **patients** are our customers in the business of hospital services. Other customers of hospitals include the visitors of hospitalized patients, the doctors who admit patients to that hospital, the vendors who supply goods and services to the hospital, and the staff who work in the hospital. It is important to recognize the importance of customer service and satisfaction when you work in any industry. It is especially important to recognize that patients are the reason hospitals are in business. Patients need to be treated well, and the staff of the hospital should treat patients with customer service in mind.

If you go to a restaurant and the food is terrific but the service staff are not friendly or are not responsive to your needs, you would probably not return to that restaurant. In fact, you would probably tell ten other people about the lack of good service. This holds true for hospitals and all health care services. Consumers of health care expect excellence in service, and although hospitals are not hotels or restaurants, they provide services to customers who either will return or will choose another health care service if they are dissatisfied. Every patient needs to feel first in importance by the people providing care.

Payers

Hospitals are funded by a variety of sources, including direct payment by patients, health care insurance payments (including Medicare), grants for research, endowments from philanthropists, and city and state funds. The third-party payers (insurance companies) pay for a large percentage of hospital costs. Today, insurance companies are generally **health maintenance organizations (HMOs)**. HMOs may pay for services at specific hospitals in a geographic area. Not every insurance company will provide for the cost of care at all hospitals or for any physician that the patient chooses. When choosing an HMO, it is important to check the listing of insurance companies and their specific payment plans to particular hospitals, physicians, and community health and mental health agencies.

Nonprofit and For-Profit Organizations

Many hospitals are **nonprofit** organizations, which means that they do not provide services for a profit. Other hospitals are owned and operated by **for-profit** organizations. This means that the revenue or money generated by the hospital is invested and reinvested by companies that use the profit (money made) for other money-making endeavors. Whether hospitals are for-profit or nonprofit corporations, they must stay out of debt to continue to provide services to the public. Even nonprofit organizations that are funded heavily by state and federal money

must continue to break even (not lose money). State and federal money must be accounted for by demonstrating appropriate and nonwasteful use of the funds provided. In other words, a hospital cannot use the Medicare dollars provided for direct patient services to pay for services that were not related to providing patient care. State and federal funds cannot be used for services or facilities that are not traced directly to the cost of a patient's care.

Medicare

Let's imagine that your father has surgery in a nonprofit hospital to remove his gallbladder. He is sixty-seven years old and is covered by Medicare. His gallbladder surgery requires 3 days of hospitalization, plus the costs of the surgeon, anesthesiologist, nursing care, medications, housekeeping, food, and billing, which total $10,000. Medicare expects that the $10,000 will be used to cover *only* these costs. Medicare is not interested in paying for the hospital's plan to, for example, build a new employee parking lot. Similarly, in a for-profit hospital, Medicare would expect the same accounting practices for the funds it provided. However, the hospital could use the additional money charged to the patient that Medicare does not pay to help pay for a new employee parking lot.

Diagnostic Related Groups (DRGs)

In the initial years of Medicare, the federal funds obtained through Medicare would pay whatever the hospital charged for the gallbladder surgery. Furthermore, hospitals charged for treatment based on the needs of the hospital, not on the actual cost of a particular treatment. Now, the emergence of **diagnostic related groups (DRGs)** has changed Medicare funding for hospital treatment. To form these related groups, researchers gathered statistics and grouped related or similar diagnoses so that the average length of hospital stay and costs for treatments would be standardized. A **medical diagnosis** is a classification for a disease or a condition. Physicians establish a medical diagnosis by investigating the patient's symptoms and signs of illness. Through diagnostic procedures (blood tests, x-rays, computerized axial tomography [CAT] scans, and so on), they confirm the diagnosis (*dia-* means "through," and *gnosia* means "knowing"). Physicians diagnose the signs and symptoms of the patient and determine the type or cause of a health condition. The emergence of DRGs essentially revolutionized hospitals and all health facilities.

In the late 1970s, Medicare and insurance companies began to look at the fees physicians and hospitals charged for services, and by 1983, DRGs became the basis for Medicare payment. This was the first concerted effort to limit the escalating cost of health care, and it drastically changed the way insurance companies determine the amount they will pay for a particular service. Before the early 1980s, hospitals and physicians were paid the amount they charged for services provided. The cost of care, then as now, varied greatly from circumstance to circumstance.

Rates Based on DRGs   Let's assume that a patient had open-heart surgery at one hospital and it cost the patient and the insurance company $25,000. At another hospital it cost $18,000. Each physician who treated the patient decided on the cost of this care. The hospital also determined the payment it sought for services. Also, the length of stay (the amount of time the patient spent inpatient) for this open-heart surgery varied as much as the cost. At Hospital A, the patient stayed 12 days, and at Hospital B, the patient stayed 8 days. The outcomes (the survival rates) and improvement or lack of complications for the treatment of the specific DRG were compared from one hospital to the next. If Hospital A had more incidents of infection post-operatively or more incidents of death post-op than Hospital B, these data would be evaluated to determine the best method of treatment and practice for a specific diagnosis.

Today, hospitals still charge variable rates, as do physicians. However, insurance companies will pay only the standard and customary rate for treatment of a specific DRG. Costs are adjusted for the geographic location and the cost of living in a particular region. A patient choosing to go to Hospital A instead of Hospital B will be required to pay the additional costs of the open-heart surgery beyond what is customary for that geographic area.

Critical Pathways of Care   Today, the DRGs have generated the emergence of critical (or clinical) pathways of care. A **critical pathway** is a written document that outlines for the physician, nurse, and patient the expected or usual course of treatment for a specific DRG. In this pathway, the expected course of treatments, diagnostic tests, and outcome measures (results of diagnostic tests) are detailed. The physician, nurse, and patient know the expected or usual course of care for a specific diagnosis. Figure 1-3 pictures a registered nurse using a critical pathway to explain the patient's plan of care. At this time, not every hospital uses pathways, nor does every DRG have an established pathway. Nonetheless, these critical pathways are the wave of the future in health care. Sometimes, patients have complications or unexpected outcomes (results) that must be documented and accounted for by the doctor and nurse. Complications

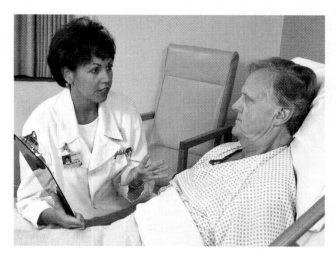

FIGURE 1-3   A critical pathway is used to discuss the patient's plan of care.

arise, or the patient has other conditions that cause a deviation in the expected path of the DRG category and treatment.

Without a doubt, DRGs have revolutionized hospital care and cost. Patients are staying in the hospital for shorter periods of time than ever before. For example, in the 1970s, when total hip replacements were a new procedure, a patient may have spent 14 days inpatient for treatment post-op. In the 1990s, the typical length of stay for a total hip replacement is about 7 days. The rehabilitation of this patient for walking and self-care maintenance is no longer extended in the hospital. Patients rehabilitate in the home. Home care services for physical therapy and nursing care, or a rehabilitation center for continued care, may be ordered.

Health care is one of the leading costs of the federal government. Controlling costs and ensuring health care for all citizens is a major initiative of the U.S. government.

Regulatory Agencies

Hospitals are regulated by many external agencies. One such organization is the **Joint Commission on Accreditation of Healthcare Organizations (JCAHO)**. Hospitals must be accredited by JCAHO to receive federal funds or Medicare. **JCAHO accreditation** means that a health care facility has conformed with established standards and has gained official approval by the JCAHO. An external organization that accredits hospitals and long-term care facilities, JCAHO also accredits ambulatory care or physician's practices of a health system. The Joint Commission was established to set the standards of care that must be assured to the consumers of that institution's services. JCAHO inspectors visit and survey a hospital or health system to measure compliance with their standards. The functions of hospital operations and practices measured according to JCAHO standards are given in Table 1-1.

If a hospital is not accredited by JCAHO, it will not be able to receive Medicare funds. Most hospitals could not survive financially without this funding.

Hospitals are also regulated by the state in which they operate. State surveyors visit hospital facilities to ensure compliance with fire, sanitation, and safety and security codes. The state surveyors also review the quality of care, the credentials of the staff, the hospital's accounting practices, and its compliance with federal and state laws established to protect patients and staff.

The **Occupational Safety and Health Administration (OSHA)** also surveys or visits hospitals to ensure the hospital's compliance with safety and

TABLE 1-1 Functions Surveyed for JCAHO Accreditation

Patient-Focused Functions

- Patients' rights
- Organization ethics
- Assessment of patients
- Care of patients
- Education of patients and significant others
- Continuum of care

Organizational Functions

- Improving organizational performance
- Leadership: planning, directing, and integrating services
- Management of the environment of care
- Management of human resources: orientation, training, competence assessment, and staff rights
- Management of information
- Surveillance, prevention, and control of infection
- Governance of the facility
- Management
- Credentialing of medical and nursing staff

health codes established by OSHA. Through its regulations, OSHA ensures the safety of workers in the workplace. The JCAHO and OSHA survey the hospital to make sure that the hospital trains employees on fire safety, disaster preparedness, back safety, hazardous materials safety, radiation safety, electrical and biomedical equipment safety, and standards of infection control. When you are hired by a hospital, you must be trained in the hospital's plans for fire and disaster preparedness as well as the topics mentioned above. Annually, you will be retrained and tested in these areas. The purpose of training is to update you on changes. The testing ensures that you are competent and safe in these areas.

When the state or JCAHO surveys or visits the hospital, they inspect employee files, inpatient and discharged patient records, the physical environment, and every department in the facility. The surveyors will talk to administrators, staff, and patients to determine compliance with codes and standards. Hospitals can lose funding, receive monetary fines, or lose their accreditation if they do not comply with standards and codes. Let's assume that a hospital employs a nurse whose license has expired; the hospital could lose its accreditation, receive a fine, or both for failing to check the credentials of the nurse. Hospitals are also surveyed by Medicare to ensure that hospitals that receive federal Medicare or Medicaid funding use these government funds appropriately.

The **Nuclear Regulatory Commission (NRC)** also inspects hospitals to ensure that radiation and radioactive materials used in medical imaging departments and in the treatment of patients are safe for the patient and the employees. Have you ever seen the little badges that technologists and technicians in an x-ray department wear on their uniforms? These badges measure the amount of radiation exposure. Monthly, these badges are read to determine the amount of radiation to which the employees have been exposed. The NRC also inspects the equipment and the containment of radioactive materials.

Quality Assurance and Improvement

If you work for any health care agency, but especially a hospital, you have heard the term **quality assurance**, *performance improvement*, or *continuous quality improvement* used. Whatever the hospital calls this function, the goals of quality measurement and improvement are essential to the institution, the employees, and the patients. Hospitals and all health care facilities must measure and improve the quality of care provided. Usually, there is a department of quality or performance improvement in the hospital. Most institutions use this method of problem solving for quality or performance improvement:

Design—examine a process and decide how to monitor it.

Measure—collect information or data to determine the current level of performance.

Assess—evaluate the data or information gathered.

Improve—institute interventions or methods to improve the current status.

Reassess—determine the effectiveness of the interventions or methods used.

This is the performance-improvement method of problem solving that is traditionally used by health care facilities. You may be involved in data collection in a quality-improvement study. It is important for you to understand the process and the role you play in accurate data collection. In Unit 5, you will be introduced to the **nursing process**, which is another method of problem solving.

Reengineering Health Care in Hospitals

The trend of the 1990s is to examine the efficiency of hospital care. Much of the cost of operating a hospital results from providing nursing and hospital support services. Hospitals have been forced to look at the way they conduct business; patient satisfaction and rising costs of providing the services that patients need and require are only two factors, among many, that are influencing this action. Most hospitals are examining their efficiency in delivering care and services to patients. Hospitals across the country have studied the ways in which patient care and services are provided. Hospitals have also studied patient satisfaction with hospital care. Two important facts learned from the research have influenced the reengineering and redesigning of patient care delivery models:

- Patients have reported dissatisfaction with the large number of care and service providers that they encounter during one short hospital stay. In one hospital day, a patient might encounter sixty hospital staff.
- Staff who do not work on the nursing or patient care units or who operate from a central location in the hospital spend about 40 percent of the workday "ready to work." This means that the technical staff (for example, phlebotomist, electrocardiogram [ECG] technician, respiratory therapist) who traditionally see patients to conduct a single diagnostic test or treatment spend 40 percent of their day waiting or traveling to perform one specific test or treatment.

In upcoming chapters, you will learn more about the concept of redesigning patient care delivery mod-els. These chapters will help you to understand the inefficiency of single-task care providers who are located in a centralized department away from the patient care units. In these chapters, you will also learn more about the emergence of what are now called the *multiskilled worker* and the *patient-focused care delivery model*. These reengineering and redesign efforts are helping hospitals to provide more efficient, patient-centered, quality care for their patients. Patient-focused care delivery models reduce the "ready-to-work" time and the number of unfamiliar staff that patients encounter. There is controversy about the use of unlicensed multiskilled care providers. The nursing and allied health academic and professional communities are concerned with the type of supervision and the education of unlicensed care providers in acute-care settings. What is foremost in their concerns is the quality of patient care that will be provided by reducing the number of licensed professionals, primarily registered nurses (RNs), at the patient's bedside.

Nursing Models

Nursing has undergone many changes since the profession began. Models for the delivery of nursing care have changed many times. Some of the changes have been based on the availability of other care providers at the patient's bedside, the availability of professional nurses, the business trends of the health care industry, and the needs of patients in specific patient care settings. One model that has been the most desirable to the profession of nursing is the **primary nursing model**. Primary nursing is based on the premise that a professional nurse provides all the care to assigned patients from the day of admission to the day of discharge. In the primary nursing model, only professional nurses (RNs) care for patients at the bedside. The RN manages the care of a specific number of hospitalized patients and provides all the required care without the assistance of nursing assistants or clinical care associates. Throughout the 1980s and early 1990s, this was the most prominent model of nursing in hospital care. In the 1980s, hospitals experienced a shortage of RNs for primary nursing. Nursing salaries were raised, and many efforts were made to attract nurses to work in hospitals. As the shortage of nurses for primary nursing models became more severe and the costs of hospital care soared, hospitals began to redesign the delivery of nursing care.

Many hospitals introduced the role of the nurse extender. **Nurse extenders** were the forerunners of today's multiskilled workers. For many nursing leaders, the use of unlicensed care providers (nursing assistants or clinical care associates) represents a return to former models of nursing care delivery, such as team nursing. **Team nursing models** used licensed practical nurses (LPNs) and nursing assistants to perform nursing care tasks (Figure 1-4). The RN served as team leader, identified the nursing care that needed to be provided, and delegated care activities to other nursing associates. Today, the team nursing model raises concern among nursing leaders because hospitalized patients in the 1990s require high-tech care during their shorter stays. There is no doubt that professional nursing supervision and judgment are required for today's hospitalized patients. Nonetheless, many tasks that the professional nurse would provide in a primary nursing model can be performed by associates in care who are not RNs. Why should the professional nurse give a bed bath or measure fluid intake and output for patients who do not need the RN to perform these tasks? There are patients for whom the RN should provide all activities of care, and others who can have other nursing associates involved in the process of providing nursing care. The professional nurse needs to employ his or her professional knowledge, skill, and judgment in determining the tasks that can be delegated based

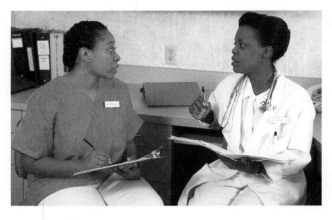

FIGURE 1-4 In a team nursing model, the RN identifies and assigns tasks.

on the needs of the patient. Unit 5 explains more fully the concepts of scope of practice and the art of delegation that describe the role of the RN in the use of clinical care associates.

application to practice

Knowledge of what health care is, the facilities in which it is provided, and the regulatory agencies that govern health care is essential for health care consumers as well as the providers of care. Apply the information you have gained from this chapter to the following learning situations.

Learning Activities

Situation 1: What are some primary care measures that you are using to improve or maintain your state of wellness?

Author's Explanation: If you quit smoking recently, you implemented one measure of disease prevention and a way to maintain wellness. An aerobic exercise routine, such as walking, is another primary or preventive measure. Did you get a flu shot this year? For each of us, there are different measures that we use to prevent illness and to stay well. List some other measures that you are currently taking.

Situation 2: What are some primary or preventive measures that you want to begin taking to improve your current state of wellness?

Author's Explanation: Take some time to consider your response. We are not all trying to achieve the same health goals, but each of us could probably do something else to improve or maintain our

current state of wellness. It may be that you want to improve your state of emotional well-being. What could you do to feel more relaxed and confident?

Situation 3: Is taking a medication for high blood pressure a secondary or a tertiary care measure?

Author's Explanation: Taking prescribed medication to treat high blood pressure is a secondary measure of care.

Situation 4: (Use the Quality Assurance and Improvement problem-solving method presented in this chapter to resolve the situations that follow.) Imagine that you work on a surgical floor in a hospital. Postoperatively (after surgery), some patients who have had a hysterectomy (removal of the uterus, or womb) are beginning to develop infection of the surgical incision. This is certainly not a desirable situation! What do you think your surgical patient care unit should do?

Author's Explanation: The unit should design a quality measure to examine the process. The unit surgeons, nurses, and manager should monitor the postoperative care of women who have hysterectomies.

Situation 5: What should they measure? What data or information should be collected? What information is needed to investigate and then solve this problem?

Author's Explanation: Hysterectomy patients should be monitored in the hospital for a specific period of time—let's say 6 months. For the next 6 months, then, every woman who has a hysterectomy will be monitored for infection. The surgeon who performed the surgery should be noted for every patient in the study. The post-operative care should be studied. A list of questions should be answered to provide the data or information that needs to be studied. Some of the data collection will include the antibiotics that are given post-operatively, the schedule for dressing changes, and the type of dressings used. The sterile technique of the nurses or surgeons who change the dressings should also be examined. The sterile technique in the operative procedure could also be reviewed.

Situation 6: Suppose that the data for the above items have been collected for six months. The data must now be assessed. How would you assess the data? In other words, what data should be collected and how should the data be compared?

Author's Explanation: The surgeon, the type of antibiotic used, the dressing schedule, the type of dressing, and the surgeon's and nurse's sterile technique during dressing changes would be collected and compared.

Situation 7: Let's imagine that there are two surgeons who admit patients and perform the hysterectomies. One surgeon uses Antibiotic A, and the other uses Antibiotic B. Both surgeons permit the nurse to change the first dressing. Both sur-geons order dry sterile dressings. The surgeons and nurses use proper sterile technique. Both surgeons order dressing changes on the same schedule. What do you think the data might show? Do you think that the type of antibiotic makes the difference in the rate of infection? Do you think the antibiotic ointment at the incision site makes a difference? Do you think whether a surgeon or nurse changes the first dressing will determine the rate of infection?

Author's Explanation: Only an analysis of the data will identify the differences in treatment that resulted in post-operative infections.

Situation 8: Let's assume now that the only difference noted was the type of antibiotic used post-operatively. What measures do you think could be used to improve the rate of infection after a hysterectomy?

Author's Explanation: The antibiotic that was most effective in controlling post-operative infection was Antibiotic A. This would be the antibiotic used to prevent infections in the post-operative care of women who have a hysterectomy.

Situation 9: Describe the meaning of the term *reengineering of health care*. What is the reason for changing the way hospitals deliver health care?

Author's Explanation: Return to the section "Reengineering Health Care in Hospitals" and review the two main reasons for redesigning or reengineering patient care delivery in hospitals.

Examination Review Questions

1. If the physician orders an antibiotic for urinary tract infection, what type of health care is this?
   a. primary
   b. reengineered
   c. secondary
   d. tertiary

2. What is the term for a written document outlining the expected course of treatment for a specific DRG?
   a. team model
   b. managed care
   c. critical pathway
   d. quality assurance

3. Which is the external regulatory agency that accredits hospitals for receipt of federal funds?
   a. HMO
   b. DRG
   c. JCAHO
   d. OSHA

4. Regulation of hospital safety and health codes is governed by
   a. OSHA
   b. NRG
   c. HMO
   d. OBRA

5. The model of delivery in which one nurse provides all the care from admission to discharge is called
   a. LTN
   b. team nursing
   c. primary nursing
   d. nurse extending

6. The performance improvement method of problem solving includes which of the following steps
   a. design
   b. measure
   c. assess
   d. all of the above

7. The term used to describe hospital health care workers who perform multiple patient care tasks is
   a. ECG technician
   b. phlebotomist
   c. multi-skilled worker
   d. environmental service technician

8. A document that outlines for the physician, nurse and patient the expected or usual course of treatment for a specific DRG is called
   a. critical pathway
   b. nursing care plan
   c. physician summary
   d. diagnostic related group

9. What credential does a professional nurse possess?
   a. LPN
   b. CNA
   c. MD
   d. RN

10. Primary Care Measures are aimed to
    a. prevent illness
    b. treat illness
    c. cause illness
    d. raise health care costs

Chapter 2

Care Delivery Alternatives

In this chapter, you will learn that employment in the health care industry reaches far beyond the walls of the hospital. Alternative health care environments are practical solutions for providing quality care and reducing the overhead costs incurred by large institutions. Long-term care facilities, home care, and community agencies offer consumers choices for personalized care based on specific needs. For example, one-to-one home care delivery or small group living arrangements integrate and maintain the individual in a natural living environment while reducing the cost of care per client. The major participants and the environments of alternative systems are presented here.

OBJECTIVES

After completing this chapter, you will be able to

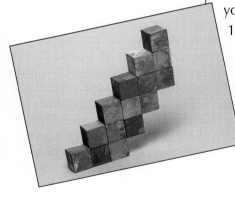

1. List the alternative types of working environments in which the clinical care associate can find employment
2. Describe the consumers who utilize long-term, ambulatory, and home care
3. Describe the services included in ambulatory care
4. Describe the consumers who utilize community mental health and retardation agencies
5. Define and spell all key terms correctly

key terms

ambulatory	mental health and mental	prn
ambulatory care services	retardation (MH/MR)	residents
certified nurse practitioner	Mental Health Law of 1979	visiting nurses association (VNA)
clients	Minimum Data Set (MDS)	wellness
contractual basis	Omnibus Budget Reconciliation	
home care departments	Act (OBRA)	
long-term care	physician assistant	

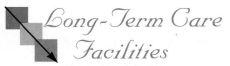

Long-Term Care Facilities

Long-term care facilities include nursing homes, convalescent homes, and rehabilitation centers. **Long-term care** essentially means that people treated in this type of facility will remain there for a long period of time. Patients may stay for weeks, months, or years. Nursing homes are also called skilled nursing facilities (SNFs). Hospitals may have an SNF within the hospital. The SNF is then regulated by hospital standards and long-term care facility standards. Some nursing homes are part of a retirement village. Residents may live in an individual cottage, a condominium, or an apartment on the grounds of the retirement community (Figure 2-1). When the individual needs nursing home care, the person is guaranteed admission to the skilled nursing facility. These retirement communities are costly, and couples or individuals who decide to live in a retirement village pay all the costs up front. It can cost $50,000 to several hundred thousand dollars, and the apartment or cottage is not purchased and cannot be sold. These retirement communities offer many services and activities for older adults who want the assurance of nursing home care should they need it.

Employees

Long-term care facilities employ many of the same types of personnel as hospitals. The environmental needs of long-term care (LTC) facilities are the same as those of hospitals, and the care of LTC residents require the same care providers. The difference between LTC facilities and hospitals is that LTC facilities generally have a nursing staff mix of licensed practical nurses (LPNs) and nursing assistants. Hospitals have a nursing staff mix of registered nurses (RNs) and nursing assistants or clinical care associates. Some hospitals do not employ LPNs. Nursing homes are only required to have one registered nurse on duty for 8 hours per day. An RN must be *on call* 24 hours a day but is required by law to be *on site* for only 8 hours. In hospitals, RNs are required to be on duty 24 hours a day.

Long-term care facilities employ physical and occupational therapists, recreational or activities therapists, social workers, dietitians or nutritionists, and clerical and administrative personnel. Most LTC facilities contract the services of laboratories, respiratory therapists, and psychologists. This means that these services are provided on a **prn** (as needed) basis by an outside agency. The charge nurses are generally LPNs, and the majority of nursing employees are nursing assistants. Some nursing homes employ a physician, but most physicians are contract employees. Some residents are seen by their personal physician. Diagnostic and treatment services are usually provided by a hospital located in the same city or county as the long-term care facility. It is not necessary to have an x-ray or laboratory department in an LTC facility. Residents are transported via ambulance or paratransit services to nearby hospitals or ambulatory care facilities for diagnostic and treatment services.

Consumers

When most people think about long-term care, they think about the care of elders in nursing homes.

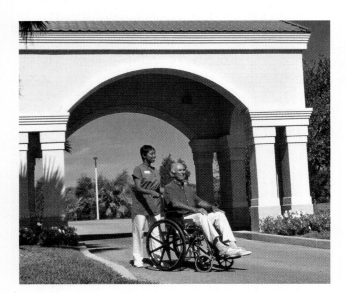

FIGURE 2-1 Retirement community.

Nonetheless, people of all ages sometimes require extended care when their conditions are not completely treatable or when their conditions require an acute-care setting or a hospital. Young people who have conditions or injuries that require around-the-clock nursing interventions or extensive physical or occupational therapy are treated in a long-term care setting. Long-term care facilities have traditionally been nursing homes.

Consumers of long-term care facilities are called **residents**, not *patients*. A nursing home is considered to be the residents' home, just as your home is your residence.

Regulatory Agencies

For many years in the United States, nursing homes were family-operated businesses that provided nursing care for elders who needed close supervision and nursing care. Because many nursing homes were operated as a family business, they were regulated as small, private corporations or businesses and were not regulated in the same way as acute-care settings or hospitals. Unfortunately, some nursing homes were not in the business of providing quality care. Some nursing homes had business and resident care practices that were unlawful, unscrupulous, and unethical. As public need and interest in nursing home care increased in the early 1980s, nursing homes came under scrutiny by the federal government and the public. The number of people who were surviving into "old age" rose sharply, and the number of new nursing homes soared. Nursing homes became big business, and opportunities for long-term care entrepreneurs increased. This meant that any businessperson could buy a nursing home. Unfortunately, not all nursing home proprietors were ethical business leaders or health care providers. Residents of some nursing homes were charged unfairly for services and treated unethically by care providers. The federal government began an investigation of nursing homes around the country, only to find that unethical and uncaring situations existed in many nursing homes. Nursing homes were receiving government Medicare and Medicaid funding for resident care, and these funds were not monitored by a federal oversight agency. Many people who worked in nursing homes were not educated, nor were they trained; admission policies and charges for services were not controlled, and residents of these facilities were not informed of or aware of their rights. Adequate care was not provided to many people who resided in nursing homes across the country. No standards of care or standards of business practices could be measured because the federal government had not established any minimum standards for this division of health care.

In 1987, the **Omnibus Budget Reconciliation Act (OBRA)** was enacted. Long-term care facilities have changed dramatically since 1987. In 1987, the federal government began to enact a law that would regulate the business practices and care activities of the long-term care industry. Until OBRA was passed, the LTC portion of health care was essentially unregulated by law. The regulations of OBRA brought about great change in the provisions of care in long-term care facilities. Now, every unlicensed care provider, nursing aide, and assistant must receive a minimum of 75 hours of training before being employed in a nursing home or LTC facility.

Before OBRA, nursing homes could employ anyone to serve as caregivers for those who needed long-term care. In addition to this, many people could be indiscriminately placed in an LTC at any age because of a mental illness or mental retardation. Imagine that no one would regulate the admission of individuals who would have been better served in a facility that treated their condition outside of an LTC. For example, before OBRA, your parents could have decided that you needed long-term care because you had an alcoholism problem even though you were only forty-five years old. Because your parents could pay a private facility to "care" for your needs, you could have been admitted and could have resided there for the rest of your life. Today, because of OBRA, you would not be able to reside in a nursing home for life because of alcoholism. Or, at least, you could not live in a nursing home without treatment for this condition. Table 2-1 lists the provisions of care regulated by OBRA in long-term care facilities.

Providers of long-term care consider their industry to be the most highly regulated of any industry in American society. Long-term care facilities are said to be as highly regulated as the nuclear industry. In 1989, the federal government turned over to the states the oversight of OBRA. Each state is responsible for ensuring that the federal regulations are followed. As a result of this measure, each state ensures compliance with OBRA requirements for LTC facilities in that state. Annually, each LTC facility is surveyed by the state's site visitor under the auspices of the federal regulations of OBRA. If the LTC facility is also accredited by the Joint Commission on Accreditation of Healthcare Organizations (JCAHO), then the facility is also surveyed every three years by the Joint Commission's site visitors. Residents' records, administrative practices, standards of care, and infection control are reviewed. Nutritional and environmental housekeeping and maintenance are examined. Residents, staff, and administrators are questioned about the care and operations of the facility. The credentials of the staff are reviewed for

TABLE 2-1 Primary Areas of OBRA Legislation

Area	Description
Resident Rights	• Resolution of grievances • Freedom of visitation • Notification of room or roommate changes • Access to a telephone • Retention of personal property • Privacy and confidentiality • Notification of changes in treatment • Freedom from verbal, sexual, physical, and mental abuse and freedom from restraints and seclusion
Nurse Aide Training, Testing, and Registration	Nurse aides must receive a minimum of 80 hours of training before they can work in a long-term care facility. The state must provide a system of registration of nurse aides and must provide a system of testing competence before the nurse aide can be registered in the state. Yearly, the nurse aide must receive at least 12 hours of in-service education.
Quality of Life	Facilities must provide recreational and social activities and a clean, safe, comfortable, and homelike environment.
Classification of Facilities and Nurse Staffing	OBRA eliminated the separate classification of nursing homes. Formerly, facilities were designated as skilled nursing facilities or intermediate care facilities. Now the requirements for nursing staff are the same for both. The requirements are the same as they were for skilled nursing facilities.
Resident Assessment	The goal of OBRA has been to assure every nursing home resident throughout the country assessment in the same areas. This standardized assessment is called the **Minimum Data Set (MDS)**. Refer to Table 2-2 for a list of the areas assessed in the Resident Assessment Protocol Summary, a key section of the Minimum Data Set. This assessment is key in creating the resident's plan of care.
Quality of Care	Another goal of OBRA is to ensure that all residents receive the "necessary care and services to attain or maintain the highest practical physical, mental and psychosocial well-being." Areas needed to meet this goal include: • Activities of daily living (ADLs) • Pressure sores • Range of motion • Mental and psychological functioning • Accident prevention • Readmission assessment and screening • Incontinence care • Vision and hearing testing • Rehabilitation services
Quality of Assessment and Assurance	Every nursing home must have a quality-assurance program that is conducted in every department on a regular basis to determine if there are any problems, including problems with provision of care. When a problem is identified, the solutions must be identified and put into action.

TABLE 2-1   Primary Areas of OBRA Legislation (continued)

Area	Description
Other Areas of Concern	
Infection control	Infection control standards must be ensured. Linens must be stored, processed, and transported to ensure that they do not become contaminated.
Nutrition and special diets	Meals must be attractive, contain proper nutrients, and be served at proper temperatures. Special diets must be provided, and resident food likes and dislikes must be observed.
Ancillary services	Laboratory, dental, radiology, pharmacy, x-ray, and other diagnostic services must be available for residents.
Survey and enforcement	To ensure that these regulations are enforced, surveyors will list any deficiencies they find. Minor deficiencies can usually be corrected quickly. If serious problems are found, enforcement penalties are imposed. These penalties might be fines, denial of payment, temporary admission freezes, appointment of temporary management, or closing of the facility.

TABLE 2-2   Assessment Areas from the MDS

Resident Assessment Area	
1. Delirium	10. Activities
2. Cognitive loss	11. Falls
3. Visual function	12. Nutritional status
4. Communication	13. Feeding tubes
5. ADL functional/rehabilitation potential	14. Dehydration/fluid maintenance
6. Urinary incontinence and indwelling catheter	15. Oral/dental care
7. Psychosocial well-being	16. Pressure ulcers
8. Mood state	17. Psychotropic drug use
9. Behavioral symptoms	18. Physical restraints

compliance with OBRA regulations. The appropriate number of professional and practical nurses must staff the facility. The administrator must be certified as a nursing home administrator. For this position, specific requirements of education, supervised practice, and examination are mandated by each state.

If the facility is surveyed and found to be deficient in compliance with state and OBRA regulations, the facility can be fined and placed under new management until it is in compliance with all regulations. A LTC facility can be closed if the standards of care and environmental standards are determined unfit for resident care. If you are employed by an LTC facility, you should be aware of the regulations so that you will uphold your responsibilities to the established standards and regulations of the long-term care industry.

Payers

A variety of payers support the cost of long-term care. A number of factors determine the source of payment for long-term care. The long-term care facility establishes the charges for resident care and determines the sources of payment that it will accept. The financial resources of the resident also determine the sources of payment. If the person seeking admission has financial resources, such as money saved, a house, car, stocks, or Social Security or retirement benefits, all of these resources must be used first to pay for admission. After these financial resources have been exhausted, then Medicaid funds generated by the state continue the payment. Medicaid pays a set fee for long-term care. On the average, the yearly fee for nursing home care is $30,000. If the resident has a living spouse, the spouse is allowed to keep a portion of the couple's financial assets and receives a monthly stipend. This monthly check from Social Security is provided for the spouse who resides outside of the nursing home.

Today, there is insurance available for long-term care. The cost for this insurance depends on the age of the person who begins to invest in the long-term care insurance policy. The monthly cost can be hundreds of dollars; the older the person is when long-term care insurance payments are initiated, the higher the cost.

Medicare will pay initial charges for admission to a nursing home when the resident is admitted following hospitalization and when the resident requires skilled nursing care. After a period of 90 days, Medicaid funding is initiated to pay the nursing home. Some nursing homes are funded primarily by Medicaid, and others only take a small percentage of Medicaid-funded residents.

The long-term care industry is a growing marketplace for employment of associates or assistants in nursing care. The largest growing segment of the U.S. population is people age sixty-five and older. This segment of the population will boom in the next 20 years as the "baby boomers" reach age sixty-five. The demand for care of elders and those who need continual assistance with self-maintenance or management of personal care needs will continue to grow in the next century. Employment opportunities in long-term care for nursing associates or assistants will continue to increase as the number of people reaching "old age" rises.

Community and Ambulatory Care

Community care facilities include physician's offices, health maintenance group practices, community health services, and community mental health and mental retardation settings. The range of community or ambulatory care services is large.

Patients are treated in the community by primary doctors in private practices, in group practices that are not associated with a hospital, or in private practices that are associated with a hospital or health maintenance organization. These are often referred to as **ambulatory care services**. The term **ambulatory** refers to the ability to ambulate (walk). *Ambulatory care*, therefore, refers to services for which an individual can "walk in" (Figure 2-2). Needless to say, people do not necessarily walk into the doctor's office. Some ambulatory care services include public welfare clinics and outpatient diagnostic centers.

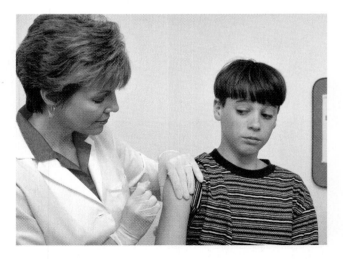

FIGURE 2-2 Immunizations are administered as part of wellness care in walk-in clinics.

Community Mental Health and Mental Retardation Agencies

Community **mental health and mental retardation (MH/MR)** facilities are funded by the county, Medicaid, private insurance, or managed care facilities that treat patients with mental health or mental retardation diagnoses. These community MH/MR facilities provide services in outpatient or day treatment facilities, residential or group homes, or vocational workshops that are located in counties throughout a state (Figure 2-3). Many community MH/MR facilities were developed as a result of the closure of state mental health and retardation hospitals.

The **Mental Health Law of 1979** stimulated the closure of state hospital facilities throughout the United States. The movement through the 1980s was to release patients from long-term care state facilities for the treatment of mental health and mental retardation conditions. It was determined that inpatient treatment in state mental hospitals was not productive or efficient for patients with mental conditions. Some patients lived in state hospitals for many years and did not improve or return to the community. It was not effective or humane to keep people locked in state hospitals for "care." The number of community MH/MR agencies grew sharply in the 1980s as many state facilities closed. People who have mental health conditions or mental retardation improve their adaptability by remaining in the community for care. Today, community MH/MR agencies, which were once funded by the county office of mental health and retardation, are facing the financial crisis of a managed care marketplace for health care. Physicians

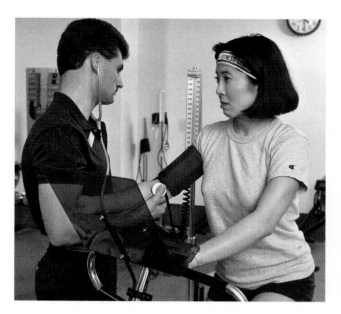

FIGURE 2-4   An example of a wellness activity.

who have private ambulatory care practices in the community are also confronted with the need to associate and accept health maintenance organization insurance funds for services provided to patients.

Consumers

The consumers of ambulatory care practices and centers are called patients or clients. Those who are treated in community MH/MR agencies are called **clients** in outpatient settings and residents in residential or group home settings. The term *patient* is avoided in community MH/MR agencies because this term implies "sickness," not wellness. Most people who have a mental health or mental retardation condition do not want to be seen as "sick." This stigmatizes or labels the person with such a condition. The movement is to focus on the person's state of health or **wellness**, not to focus on the disability. Figure 2-4 is an example of a wellness activity.

Employees

In an ambulatory care setting, those who are employed by an outpatient diagnostic center are usually technicians in a specialty field. Examples include laboratory technicians, radiology (x-ray) technologists, electroencephalograph (brain wave) technicians, and other technical experts who perform diagnostic tests. Individuals employed by physician groups or private practices are employed by the physician in private practice or by the health maintenance organization. Medical assistants are often employed in these settings. Medical assistants (MAs) are educated

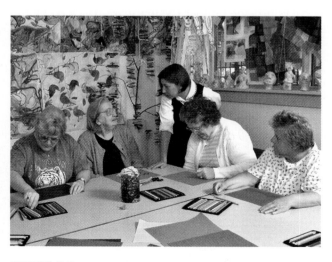

FIGURE 2-3   Clients of group homes or day hospitals interact regularly as part of a treatment program.

to perform clinical, laboratory, and clerical duties. An MA may work for a physician or group of physicians to schedule and bill patients, perform laboratory studies in the office, measure vital signs, assist with physical examinations, draw blood samples, perform electrocardiograms (ECGs), and generally assist the doctor with all clinical and clerical office work. The specialty of the doctor will determine the clinical duties of the MA.

A clinical care associate can perform the same clinical tasks as a medical assistant. If the clinical care associate is also skilled in clerical tasks (filing, typing, and billing), employment in an ambulatory care setting can be sought. Physicians may also employ certified nurse practitioners or physician assistants. A **certified nurse practitioner** is a registered nurse who has a master's degree in this field of nursing and also has a specialty area of practice, such as pediatrics, women's health, or geriatrics. A **physician assistant** usually holds a bachelor's degree in this field and is licensed in the state to perform as a physician assistant. A physician assistant (PA) is not a nurse; the role of the PA is to perform physical examinations and to work with the doctor to treat patients. Certified nurse practitioners are able to practice in some states in the United States without a physician's signature for prescribing medications.

In community mental health and retardation agencies, employees usually have bachelor's or advanced degrees in a specialty field, such as social work, psychology, or creative arts (music or art therapy). These agencies also employ people with basic nursing assistant skills to work in group home settings. Of course, community and ambulatory care settings employ administrative and clerical staff. Maintenance and housekeeping workers are either contracted employees or, in large agencies, direct employees of the facility.

Payers

The cost of ambulatory or community care is funded by a variety of payment sources: health care insurance providers, county funds, medical assistance, Medicare and Medicaid, and self-paying customers (patients or clients). Most insurance companies and health maintenance organizations (HMOs) have an established fee for services they will pay to providers. Individuals who receive the services have to assume the additional costs. Medicare or Medicaid assumes the cost depending on the person's age and financial or welfare status. Community mental health and mental retardation agencies once were supported totally by state and county grants or block funds and medical assistance. Many people who are treated in community MH/MR agencies have had medical assistance, and Medicare pays for individual and group treatment. Today, medical assistance is being assumed by managed care insurers. The cost for services is billed to the managed care insurer, who refunds the agency with the established fee allotted for a specific treatment.

Regulatory Agencies

Ambulatory care settings are not regulated by a specific agency unless they are diagnostic centers. Diagnostic centers are regulated by the laboratory accreditation commissions and the state in which they operate. Radiology and medical imaging services are regulated by the Nuclear Regulatory Commission (NRC) and the state. These types of outpatient diagnostic centers are licensed by the state. The state surveys these facilities to examine their compliance with standards and regulations of the industry for safe practice.

Physicians' private offices are not regulated by a specific agency or accreditation commission. It is the physician's license that permits the operation of a medical practice. Ambulatory care settings that are attached to or that are operated by a hospital or health system are surveyed by the state. If the health system or hospital owns and operates these practices, they will be surveyed by the JCAHO when the accreditation commission surveys the hospital or health system.

Community mental health and mental retardation agencies are usually licensed by the state. Annually, the state will survey all of the facilities that the community MH/MR agency operates. The survey includes all of the same examination of practices that the state performs in hospitals and long-term care facilities. Some community agencies have sought accreditation from the JCAHO or other accreditation commissions. These accreditation commissions survey and review compliance with their standards. If community agencies have grants from the National Institute of Mental Health or from a Charitable Trust, then the specific services provided under the grant are reviewed by the granter. This review is to determine if the agency is using the grant funds to provide the services that the grant proposal stated. The results or outcomes of the services provided by the grant money are reviewed to determine if indeed the results are measured and the measured outcomes are valid and reliable.

Home Care
Facilities

Home care agencies include community **visiting nurse associations (VNAs)**, **home care departments** in hospitals, and independent nonprofit and profit-making agencies (Figure 2-5).

The original nursing model, theorized and implemented by Florence Nightingale in England in

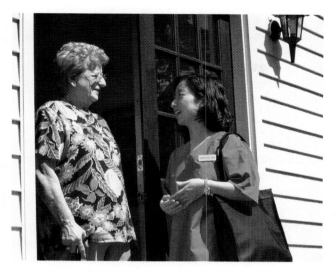

FIGURE 2-5 Home health aide visiting client at home.

the late 1800s, was a public health model where nurses visited the homes and cared for the health needs of the community. Because nursing originated as primarily a female role, the nurse would visit the home and tend the sick by providing nutritious meals and teaching the importance of sunlight, ventilation, nutrition, and asepsis. Her role was primary intervention, with secondary measures when necessary. Sometimes, she functioned as a nurse midwife and at other times as a homemaker, when, for example, the mother of the household was ill. This model continued to evolve in the United States with the establishment of the VNA, whose role was to care for the public health of the community.

In the early to mid-1970s, a push for cost containment created a need for more home care management, especially in the elderly population. Studies proved that it was far cheaper to provide rehabilitation services in the home of an elderly client than in a facility. Under Part A of Medicare benefits, patients were allotted one hundred visits of professional and ancillary staff per calendar year per illness. Part B of Medicare also made provisions for up to one hundred home care visits. Later, private third-party insurance, such as HMOs, looked at the Medicare model and agreed that home care was an effective alternative to lengthy hospital recuperative stays or SNF placement for rehabilitation.

Employees

The primary full-time employees of a home care agency are registered nurses and home health aides. Nurses act as the coordinator of services in the home under the orders of a primary physician. The nurse evaluates the needs of the client in an initial assessment, the physician is called, and the services are activated. The home health aide works under the supervision of the nurse, providing personal care and ADL assistance. In addition, physical therapists (PTs), speech therapists (STs), occupational therapists (OTs), and medical social workers (MSWs) may be employed on a **contractual basis** (fee for services).

Consumers

Consumers for home care are generally those with rehabilitation potential who have been discharged from a hospital or nursing home. In addition, home care may be activated to prevent hospitalization, to assist with dying at home, or to prevent SNF placement.

A candidate for home care is one who is homebound, who requires acute intervention with rehab potential, or who can eventually be taught directly or through family members to take over the care that has been delivered on a short-term basis. It is rarely a long-term situation. Visits are intermittent and for a short duration. Home care services may also be private-pay cases that are long term. The visit of a home health aide generally is not longer than 2 hours. Cases can range from someone receiving intravenous (IV) antibiotic therapy to a ventilator-dependent client. Wound care, diabetic instruction, post-myocardial-infarction (MI) monitoring, postpartum care, and respiratory, urologic, and cancer clients are among the most common cases.

Regulatory Agencies

In essence, the payers are the regulatory agencies for home care. Medicare established the model that other third-party payers have adopted with some modifications.

application to practice

Your knowledge and understanding of the various types of care delivery alternatives, the way they function, and the regulatory agencies that govern them will form the basis for your interactions with staff and clients. Awareness of and adherence to specific state and facility- or agency-based procedures regarding client or patient care are your personal responsibility. Use the information that you learned in this chapter to respond to the following situations.

Learning Activities

Situation 1: What motivated the legal enforcement of OBRA in the U.S. long-term care industry? Why would *you* want to see the regulations of OBRA enforced for yourself or a person that you love?

Author's Explanation: The purpose of OBRA is discussed in the section "Long-Term Care Facilities." If you do not know this answer, reread the section and the OBRA regulations. We believe that this legislation is enormously important to the safety and quality care of our elders and those family members who may require long-term care. We would not feel assured that our mothers, fathers, sisters, and brothers were guaranteed safe and quality care by trained professional and nonprofessional staff unless LTC facilities were measured against a standard of expected care and quality of life. We would never want to admit a family member to an LTC facility that failed to comply with OBRA regulations. Would you?

Situation 2: How would you explain the purpose of regulations, standards of care, and laws in the health care industry? Why do you think it is necessary for you to understand this information in your role as a clinical care associate?

Author's Explanation: As a clinical care associate, you will be prepared to work in a variety of health care settings. You will need to know the requirements and purpose of your educational preparation and ongoing educational requirements for safe practice. When you work in a highly regulated industry such as health care, it is important to understand the regulations and standards. Otherwise, you will not recognize the reasons for employer expectations of your compliance with certain rules and policies. Your employer will expect you to participate and prepare for state and accreditation commission surveys. Your employer will require annual updates of safety training and proof of competence in the areas of fire safety, infection control standards, disaster preparedness, and electrical and other safety issues. You must recognize the significance of your role in the monitoring of safe patient, client, and resident care and the assurance of consumer rights and satisfaction. You will work as part of a team of the entire health care facility, and all members of the team must work to achieve safe and effective care practices. Each health care team member should understand his or her personal responsibility in achieving the organization's mission for continued existence and success.

Situation 3: Since you are not paid directly by the consumer or the insurance companies, why should you know and care about who pays and what the costs of health care are?

Author's Explanation: Every person who works in health care should recognize that it is a business that must charge for services and that the amount of money received is limited by many factors. It is the responsibility of all health care workers to consider the efficient use of limited money. If you think that health care industry employers have unlimited money, then you will not appreciate the need to be responsible for cost containment and time-efficient practice. Sometimes, it is hard to understand why a patient is being discharged from the hospital when the patient is still in pain or why home care is not being provided to some individual who seems to need it. If you work in a nursing home, you may at times be frustrated by the limitations of supplies of linen and personal grooming items. You might feel that there is no reason for limits on such supplies. It is important to understand the reimbursement of money that is controlled by Medicare, Medicaid, and the HMOs.

Situation 4: Why do you think that patients, clients, and residents are called *customers* or *consumers*?

Author's Explanation: People who receive health care are purchasing a service. When you purchase a service or item, you are a customer or a consumer. Health care has become a competitive industry. All business is competitive, and if a customer is dissatisfied with the service or goods of one company, he or she will switch to another company that provides or sells the same goods or services. People who purchase the services of health care will change doctors, hospitals, clinics, or long-term care facilities if they are not satisfied with the care and treatment they receive. To stay in business, hospitals and other health care agencies must treat the consumer of their services as a customer. Customers should get what they pay for, and customers should be given respect and fair treatment in any business.

Examination Review Questions

1. Care services in which an individual can "walk in" are termed
   a. skilled nursing facilities
   b. ambulatory care services
   c. alternative health services
   d. one-day inpatient facilities

2. People treated in MH/MR agencies are called
   a. patients
   b. consumers
   c. clients or residents
   d. buyers

3. Community health care facilities do *not* include
   a. physicians' offices
   b. skilled facilities
   c. day care
   d. welfare clinics

4. The original Florence Nightingale model evolved into today's
   a. CLA
   b. MRR
   c. VNA
   d. SNF

5. The following federal law regulates business and care in LTC facilities
   a. MDS
   b. ADL
   c. OSHA
   d. OBRA

6. Managed care insurers have assumed which state funding?
   a. medical assistance
   b. Medicare
   c. private pay
   d. HMOs

7. Medicare Part A allots how many home care visits per year?
   a. 200
   b. 100
   c. 50
   d. unlimited

8. Home health aides work under the supervising license of the
   a. physician
   b. nurse
   c. agency
   d. professional

9. Home care services are generally
   a. short term
   b. long term
   c. for life
   d. nonnegotiable

10. The facilities for home care services are
    a. clinics
    b. offices
    c. hospitals
    d. residences

Employment of Clinical Care Associates

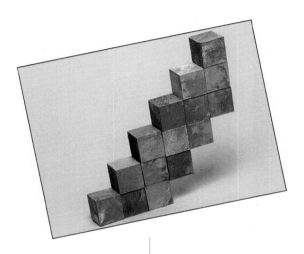

The twenty-first century brings changes to the world and to the job market. Technology has replaced many entry-level, unskilled positions. This is true in health care. Entry-level positions in health care require the same important elements that shape jobs in all fields. New roles for unlicensed multi-skilled workers are emerging in health care. The clinical care associate can compete in the job market of today and tomorrow with critical-thinking and problem-solving skills, the ability to work as part of a team, the desire to learn, and knowledge of computers.

The skills and knowledge you will acquire from your training program and from the study of this textbook are just the beginning. The competence that you will gain through your work experience will be transferable from one position in the health care industry to another. Of course, as with any job, you will need to learn the expectations of your superiors and the specific competencies that you must possess to perform successfully in each new role.

Emerging Health Care Roles

In this chapter, the concept of the multi-skilled worker is developed, and you will be introduced to the variety of health care settings in which you may find employment. Each setting uses the clinical care associate in a specific role. A competent care associate brings to each of these roles a standard set of skills that can be used to fulfill the requirements of each position. You will be introduced to the varied roles of the clinical care associate in a hospital, in a long-term care agency, in home care, and in community mental health and retardation agencies.

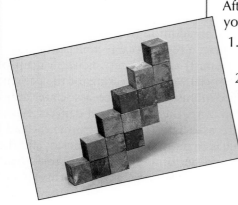

OBJECTIVES

After completing this chapter, you will be able to

1. Define the term *multiskilled worker*
2. Describe what is meant by "*ready-to-work*" time
3. List at least fifteen tasks outlined in the Standard Skill Set
4. Explain the difference between *license* and *certification*
5. Define and spell all key terms correctly

key terms

booting up the system	hard drive	neurologist
CD-ROM drive	hematologist	oncology
central processing unit (CPU)	keyboard	orthopedist
certificate	license	physiatrist
clinical care associate (CCA)	monitor	random-access memory (RAM)
data entry	mouse	read-only memory (ROM)
diskette	multiskilled worker	service associate
electrocardiogram (ECG)	network	unlicensed

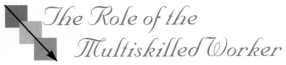

The Role of the Multiskilled Worker

As we discussed in Chapter 1, the term **multiskilled worker** has become popular for describing the expanded role of unlicensed care providers. Employers are retraining unlicensed personnel to perform new tasks in their traditional roles. This is most prevalent in the hospital setting because care must be delivered in a timely fashion to acutely ill patients who have limited lengths of stay in the hospital. Hospitals want to be able to deliver the needed services to patients and families in an efficient, competent, and cost-effective fashion. Patients must have tests and procedures performed when they need them, not when the technician is available. Many of the technical staff who formerly performed one task in their job have been retrained to perform additional tasks. This has happened for many reasons. One reason is the amount of time some technical staff spent "ready to work" but unable to perform their task because of travel time to the patient or waiting time for the patient to become available for the test or procedure.

"Ready-to-Work" Time

Imagine that you are an **electrocardiogram (ECG)** technician and that you have ten ECGs to perform on Unit 3 North. You must travel from the heart station to 3 North, which takes about 10 minutes. When you arrive at 3 North, you go from room to room, performing the ECGs. After performing three ECGs, you have a stat page directing you to go to 3 South to do an ECG, so you travel there. You perform the stat on 3 South, and return to 3 North 10 minutes later. You arrive at the fourth patient's room to discover that the patient is receiving personal hygiene assistance, so you travel to the fifth room. This patient is having blood drawn by the phlebotomist. Patient number six is on neutropenic precautions, so you must don a gown, mask, and gloves before you enter the room. When you enter the isolation room, the patient's husband tells you that the patient has not slept all night and requests that you not awaken

her now; you agree to return in an hour. In the end, you have spent about 40 percent of your time "ready to work" but unable to work.

Now, imagine that you and all of the other clinical care associates and nurses in the hospital can perform ECGs. You are stationed to work on a patient care unit and have assigned patients. You know who has not slept and who needs a bath. You can also perform the phlebotomy. As a result, your patients receive more timely services, and you are able to manage your assigned patient care tasks more efficiently. This is the primary reason for a multiskilled patient care team.

Under the former system, patients who stayed in the hospital for 5 days were seen on the average by sixty different staff members who provided some service to them. Think about sixty different strangers touching you, entering your room, and asking you questions. Before hospitals restructured care delivery, a patient would have had a housekeeper to clean the room, a dietary aide to deliver meals, and a transporter to take the patient to different areas for tests and procedures, in addition to a nursing assistant, a professional nurse, a respiratory technician or therapist, a phlebotomist, an ECG technician, a team of doctors, and a social worker all caring for the patient.

Today, one multiskilled **service associate** cleans the room, transports the patient, and delivers meals. A **clinical care associate (CCA)** performs the tasks of the nursing assistant, the ECG technician, and the phlebotomist and performs simple respiratory treatments. The professional nurse also performs ECGs, phlebotomy, and more invasive respiratory treatments, and most important, he or she directs the delivery of patient care. Respiratory therapists and technicians also perform ECGs and phlebotomy. Many hospitals have decentralized these services, which means, for example, that respiratory therapy, physical therapy, and pharmacy departments that once operated from a central office are now located right on the patient care units. While these departments still exist, the staff and equipment are located on the patient care units to make services more readily available and to allow these staff members to assist in other patient care tasks. For example, a respiratory therapist who is performing a nebulizer treatment might see that the patient needs to get out of bed and use the bathroom. The therapist can help the patient to the bathroom without the patient's having to wait until the nursing assistant is available.

The term *multiskilled worker* is used generically to refer to a variety of unlicensed service staff and clinical staff positions. Health care employers are no longer seeking to employ the one-task employee; they are searching for the employee who can perform multiple tasks competently. Parts A to D of Figure 3-1 depict the many roles open to multiskilled care deliverers, and Part E shows an individual reflecting on these possible career path options.

Standard Skill Sets

The **unlicensed** care providers or unlicensed assistive personnel are the care providers who are not licensed by a state board or state registry. Clinical care associates are unlicensed personnel. Generally, hospitals and other health care agencies employ unlicensed caregivers to work under the supervision of licensed personnel. We will discuss these roles in the next section. Let's now examine the standard set of skills that an unlicensed care provider brings to hospitals and other health care agencies. The tasks that you will use

in a particular job will vary, depending on the environment of care, the availability of supervision by licensed staff, and the regulations of the accrediting agencies and state regulatory bodies. In a long-term care environment, the unlicensed care provider is permitted to perform nursing assistant tasks sanctioned by the state nurse aide registry. In a hospital, you may perform these tasks and additional expanded duty tasks under the supervision of a professional nurse. In all health care environments, employers seek individuals with skills in communication, interpersonal relations, critical thinking, problem solving, and technology.

Basic Nursing Assistant/Nurse Aide Skills

The knowledge and skills of the nursing assistant are the foundation of the standard skills of multiskilled workers. These skills are needed to perform tasks that are noninvasive, such as

- Bathing
- Feeding
- Bedmaking
- Measuring vital signs
- Measuring height and weight

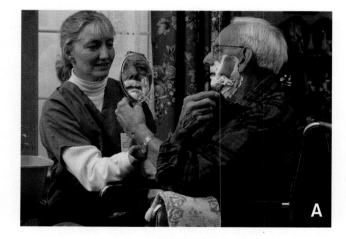

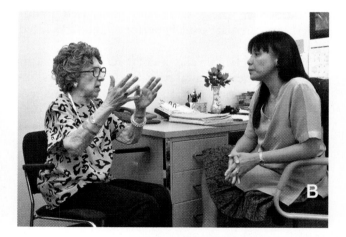

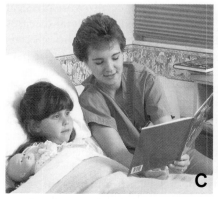

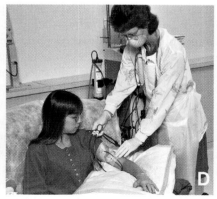

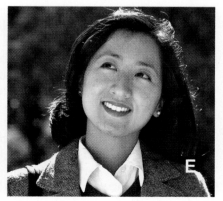

FIGURE 3-1 There are many roles for the multiskilled worker.

- Measuring intake and output
- Ambulating patients
- Assisting with dressing and grooming
- Assisting with skin, hair, mouth, and nail care
- Transporting patients (wheelchair, stretcher)
- Positioning and transferring patients
- Applying hot and cold applications
- Assisting with range-of-motion exercises
- Doing skin preps for surgery
- Collecting urine specimens
- Collecting stool and sputum specimens
- Applying TED hose stockings and dry dressings
- Applying nonsterile dressings

Other standard skills essential to the multiskilled worker include

- Knowledge of the human body
- Knowledge of medical terminology
- Verbal and written communication skills
- Fire safety
- Electrical and hazardous material safety
- Infection control and disaster preparedness

Expanded Skills for the Multiskilled Care Associate

In addition to these skills, the unlicensed multi-skilled care associate usually performs the tasks listed in Table 3-1.

In mental health and mental retardation facilities, knowledge of mental retardation and mental illness and basic counseling and teaching skills are necessary to fulfill position requirements. In home care agencies, the assistant must be able to adapt tasks and care to the home, to the client, and to the family's needs. Knowledge of basic housekeeping and cooking are necessary for successful employment.

The Health Care Team

The composition of the health care team varies according to the health care facility. Hospitals have the largest and most diverse health care teams. Hospital patient care units have team members representing specialties of care. For example, an **oncology** unit (for the care of patients with cancer) will have professional nurses who are certified to give chemotherapy, an oncology physician, maybe a **hematologist** (a doctor who specializes in blood cell diseases), and a nurse clinical specialist in oncology.

In long-term care (LTC) facilities, the team members will vary, depending on the nature of the residents in the facility. If the LTC facility has a reha-

TABLE 3-1   Tasks Performed by Unlicensed Multiskilled Care Associates[a]

Expanded Tasks

1. Twelve-lead ECG
2. Phlebotomy
3. Blood glucose monitoring
4. Application of dressings
5. Specimen collection from Foley catheters
6. Gastrostomy tube feedings
7. Computer entry of patient data
8. Pulse oximetry
9. Insertion and removal of Foley catheters
10. Measurement of drainage from multiple collection devices
11. Application of pneumatic pressure stockings
12. Administration of enemas
13. Preparation of oxygen setups
14. Incentive spirometry
15. Oral suctioning
16. Stoma care and application of ostomy appliances

[a]Tasks will vary from state to state and from facility to facility.

bilitation unit, for example, the team will include a **physiatrist** (a physician who specializes in physical rehab medicine), an **orthopedist** (a skeletal diseases specialist), a **neurologist** (a physician who specializes in neurological disorders), a psychiatrist or psychologist, a professional nurse, a social worker, nursing assistants, a nutritionist, occupational and speech therapists, a physical therapist, on so on. And if this rehabilitation facility has children, there will also be a pediatrician and a pediatric nurse specialist. The other physicians may also have a dual specialty in pediatrics, such as a pediatric neurologist.

In community mental health and mental retardation facilities, there will be fewer professional nurses on the team and more social workers, counselors, psychologists, psychiatrists, client care workers, vocational counselors, and perhaps occupational and physical therapists.

Licensed Team Members

Licensed team members have attended an educational program with specific academic courses and clinical preparation. Upon completion of all required education and clinical practice, these individuals are eligible to take the required examination. A **license** is awarded by the state board of examiners after successfully passing the examination. A license indicates that the individual has met the minimal requirements to prove competence in the field. Licenses are designed to ensure the safety of those who receive services from these individuals. Nurses must be licensed by the state to practice nursing in that particular state. A professional nursing license (RN) and a practical or vocational nursing license (LPN or LVN) are distinct and permit the nurse to practice within the respective guidelines of the state's nurse practice laws. The following descriptions of licensed health care practitioners will provide you with an understanding of the licensed team members.

Licensed Practitioners

Some of the licensed personnel who are members of the health care team are listed in Table 3-2. The type of health care setting, the acute needs of the pa-

tients, and the requirements of the state or accrediting body will determine the type and number of licensed practitioners employed. The table lists some of the licensed practitioners that might be staff members in various health care settings.

Unlicensed Team Members

Members of the health care team who do not require a license to provide care to clients, patients, or residents generally work under the direct supervision of individuals on the team who have a license. Nurse aides in a nursing home work under the supervision of an LPN or an RN. In a hospital setting, the nursing assistant or multiskilled worker works under the supervision of an RN. In a physician's office, the medical assistant works under the supervision of the physician. Unlicensed assistive personnel are permitted to provide care under the supervision of a licensed practitioner. Unlicensed care providers do not attend a prescribed academic and clinical education program and do not take an examination that awards a license to practice.

Nursing assistants in long-term care facilities must attend a nurse aide program that is certified by the state to provide instruction for the nurse aide. The nurse aide who works in long-term care must successfully complete or pass the nurse aide competency examinations. This does not award a license. After passing the examination, the nurse aide will be listed on the state's nurse aide registry. This ensures minimum competence to work in an LTC facility.

TABLE 3-2 Licensed Practitioners

Practitioner	Academic Degree or Professional Title
Physician (licensed to practice medicine and board-certified in specialty area)	Doctor of medicine (MD) Doctor of osteopathy (DO) Doctor of podiatric medicine (DPM)
Dentist	Doctor of medical dentistry (DMD) Doctor of surgical dentistry (DDS)
Nurse	Registered nurse or professional nurse (RN) Licensed practical nurse (LPN) Licensed vocational nurse (LVN) Certified registered nurse practitioner (CRNP)
Other	Physical therapist (PT) Occupational therapist (OT) Registered pharmacist (RPh) Medical social worker (MSW) Psychologist (PhD) Registered dietitian (RD)

This is discussed in the section on long-term care facilities in Chapter 2.

The titles for unlicensed assistive personnel are numerous. They vary according to the health care environment, and they may be different from one facility to the next. Some unlicensed assistive personnel have attended a specific educational program that permits them to sit for examinations that provide certification. This certification examination does not lead to a license, and it is not administered by a state board or government regulatory agency. Some unlicensed health care workers have a representative organization or association that accredits educational programs and may administer examinations for certification in an unlicensed specialty field. Dental assistants, medical assistants, and unit clerks/secretaries have organizations that provide certification examinations. This certification tells employers that the individual has passed the association's certification examination. These certifications add credibility to the title and generally tell employers that the person has the minimum competence expected by the association and has the association's "stamp of approval." A **certificate**, not a license, is issued to such individuals by these associations. In many situations, the certified medical assistant, for example, is sought by the employer; therefore, it is beneficial for those who are eligible to take certification examinations to do so. Dentists and physicians advertise for certified assistants because they know that the person they will hire has attended an educational program and has the knowledge and skills that they desire in an unlicensed assistant.

Principles of Computers and Data Entry

Not only have computers revolutionized our society, they have redefined health care. From medical records to diagnostic imaging, computers have improved care delivery. How does that compute for the multiskilled worker? Because of the legal ramifications, precise charting has become essential to all health care institutions. Therefore, it is imperative to understand the basic computer and its health care applications. Figure 3-2 shows the basic components of a computer system.

The computer has several major parts:

■ The **central processing unit (CPU)** is the computer's brain.
■ **Read-only memory (ROM)** is the permanent data saved as special programs that permit the computer to operate.

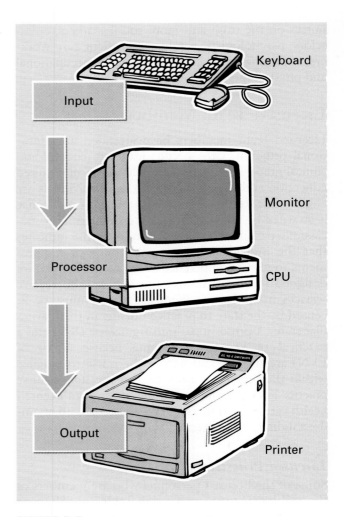

FIGURE 3-2   Basic components of a computer system.

■ **Random-access memory (RAM)** is the memory to which you have access. This is the temporary work space memory.
■ The **hard drive** is a device that stores files within the computer.
■ The **monitor** is the visual screen that displays the work.
■ The **diskette** is a small plastic wafer that permits portable storage.
■ The **CD-ROM drive** is the port where CDs are inserted, just like a CD player.
■ The **mouse** is a handheld device that rolls on a hard surface and enables control of computer functions.
■ The **keyboard** is similar to a typewriter with added function keys.

Each institution has a software program that has been installed on the hard drive. This facilitates data entry because charts, graphs, and tables are preset.

Data entry means entering the information into the special program.

Here is some additional computer language that you need to know:

- **Booting up the system** is the process of turning on the computer.
- A **network** is a series of computers linked together to share information and programs.

Here are some diskette do's and don'ts:

- Do store the diskette in a dry area away from heat and dust.
- Do keep the diskette away from magnets.
- Do lock the diskette when not in use to prevent overwriting it.
- Don't drop or mutilate the diskette.

application to practice

Use what you have learned in this chapter about health care workers to respond to the situations that follow. Understanding the current roles and fundamental skills of a clinical care associate will serve to distinguish the roles of licensed and unlicensed caregivers.

Learning Activities

Situation 1: What are some reasons for the development of multiskilled workers?

Author's Explanation: Multiskilled workers developed as the result of efforts to reduce the number of care providers seen by the patient, to decrease the amount of time spent "ready to work," to provide more personalized care based on better knowledge of the patient's needs, and to increase patient satisfaction with care delivery.

Situation 2: Which holds more weight, a license or a certificate?

Author's Explanation: If you said license, you are correct. If you did not, reread the section "The Health Care Team."

Situation 3: Can a health care provider hold a license and a certificate at the same time?

Author's Explanation: Yes. For example, an RN is licensed and can also hold a certificate in a specialty field of nursing, such as oncology.

Situation 4: List some job titles of unlicensed care providers.

Author's Explanation: Nursing assistant, patient care technician, medical assistant, and mental health technician are some examples of titles of unlicensed care providers.

Situation 5: What data might a clinical care associate need to enter into a computer?

Author's Explanation: A care associate might enter the patient's height, weight, and vital signs and might indicate the completion or cancellation of a test such as an electrocardiogram.

Examination Review Questions

1. The multiskilled worker is
   - a. unlicensed
   - b. licensed
   - c. noncertified
   - d. registered

2. The scope of the clinical care associate does *not* include
   - a. noninvasive testing
   - b. theoretical knowledge
   - c. prescription of medications
   - d. delegated tasks

3. Nurses can practice in
   - a. any state
   - b. most states
   - c. their licensing state
   - d. any country

4. A DO practices _____ medicine.
   - a. pediatric
   - b. diabetic
   - c. dental
   - d. osteopathic

5. An LPN is a licensed practical
   - a. nutritionist
   - b. naturopath
   - c. neurologist
   - d. nurse

6. Downtime for "ready-to-work" technical staff occurred because of
   - a. contract disputes
   - b. scope limitations
   - c. staffing numbers
   - d. wait time

7. Which type of health care facility employs the most diverse and numerous health team members?
   a. skilled nursing facilities
   b. hospitals
   c. home health care agencies
   d. clinics

8. Which of the following is *not* a licensed health care team member?
   a. physician
   b. nurse aide
   c. dentist
   d. dietitian

9. Unlicensed assistive personnel do *not* include
   a. dental hygienists
   b. medical assistants
   c. unit clerks
   d. first responders

10. The Standard Skill Set includes tasks that vary, depending on all of the following *except*
    a. environment of care
    b. availability of supervision
    c. state regulations
    d. third-party payers

Chapter 4

Health Care Employment

Being a multiskilled care provider will be an advantage in the health care employment scene of tomorrow. A multiskilled worker is one who can perform the functions of a health assistant. In addition, the multiskilled worker is competent to perform some expanded skills of allied health technicians. But the most important skills a multiskilled health care worker must possess are critical thinking, problem solving, and team playing. With all of this in place, the clinical care associate will have many employment opportunities from which to choose.

In this chapter, you will learn how to prepare a résumé, to seek out a position in which you are interested, and to interview for that position.

OBJECTIVES

After completing this chapter, you will be able to

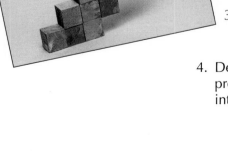

1. Describe the process of marketing yourself for employment

2. Discuss the ways in which you can search for a job

3. Prepare a résumé and cover letter as part of a job search

4. Describe the interview process and role-play an interview

5. List health care agencies that might employ multiskilled workers

6. List the job titles for which you might seek employment and identify the major responsibilities for each title

7. Define and spell all key terms correctly

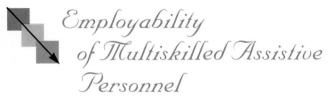

Employability of Multiskilled Assistive Personnel

To successfully gain employment, you must **market** yourself and your "wares." In essence, you are a salesperson selling your talents and abilities. Marketing requires some work, but doesn't everything? Before you can begin to "sell your wares," you need a "brochure" that lists your talents and abilities. This brochure is called a *résumé*. There are many ways to format this résumé. Personnel departments, or the employees of institutions responsible for interviewing and hiring, must find top-notch employees who meet the job requirements for available positions. Most personnel departments use computers to scan résumés for key words so they can "weed out" those résumés that do not contain the key words. This eliminates needless time in lengthy interviews, reduces the flood of applications for a position, and singles out the best possible candidates. Do you know what this means? It means that your résumé can make or break a chance for an interview. What else does this mean? It means that your résumé is possibly the only chance of gaining employment since you may be eliminated before you have the opportunity to sell your wares in a personal interview. With all that said, you now must understand the importance of developing a leading-edge résumé. Figure 4-1 shows a sample résumé.

Notice that the résumé is only one page. This took some work. It was thought out carefully. It is not wordy. It was word-processed and spell-checked. It was printed on quality résumé paper. Most important, however, it contains the "buzz words" that institutions look for in the selection process. Notice the categories of the résumé. A résumé always begins with your name, address, and phone number. Under that is the objective. The objective reflects your employment goal. It can be general or more specific—for example, "An entry-level home health aide position for Medicare clients." Think of one job objective for a clinical care associate (CCA).

A summary of the special abilities or traits that are desirable in a CCA follows. What are special abilities? Special abilities are those strengths unique to you. Are you organized, dependable, and analytical?

Do you have excellent follow-through? Read the list of special abilities below, and then list the qualities or special abilities you believe you possess. Go over your list with a close friend, with your spouse, or with family members to see if they agree with the list you made.

List of Special Abilities or Traits

1. I deal honestly and fairly with myself and others.
2. I try to solve problems encountered each day.
3. I adapt to new situations.
4. I am reliable.
5. I am thoughtful of others' feelings.
6. I get along well with others.
7. I remember names and faces.
8. I am enthusiastic.
9. I am a good listener.
10. I try to understand the other person's point of view.
11. I can take constructive criticism.
12. I am neat and clean in my work.
13. I can set goals and meet them.
14. I am interested in other people.
15. I strive to be on time.

Once you have chosen and written out your special abilities, you may wish to list them under a category called *special abilities*. Use bullets (→, *, and • are a few samples) to highlight each item. For example,

Dependable
Organized

The next category should be *work history*. Work history should begin with your present or most recent position and should work backward chronologically. For example,

1985–present
1983–1985
1981–1983

Include dates or years of your employment, the company's name and address, the position you held, and a brief summary of your duties. In this area, use action words to describe the duties you performed.

PAULA SMITH

555 Knox Street
Collegeville, PA 10001
717-555-5555 Home
717-555-0000 Office

OBJECTIVE	Seeking an entry level position as a nursing assistant.
STRENGTHS	Results oriented; Adaptable to challenges; Establishment of excellent patient relations.
EXPERIENCE	
Nursing Assistant	Nursing Assistant for 32 bed dementia unit, Lansdale Convalescent Home, Lansdale, PA 20002; 19xx–19xx.
Intern	One Year ICU Unit Intern, Sacred Heart Hospital, 103 Main Street, Norristown, PA 30003; 19xx–19xx.
EDUCATION	
Nursing Assistant Certification	North Montco Technical Career Center, Lansdale, PA 20002
ORGANIZATIONS	National Honor Society; Health Occupations Students of America; Vocational Student Organization.
CONFERENCES	Vocational Student Organization Conference 19xx.
AWARDS AND ACHIEVEMENTS	First Place Award in State Competition for Nursing Assistants; Leadership Certificate for demonstration of skills;
SPECIAL COMPETENCIES	Fluent in Spanish.
REFERENCES	Furnished upon request.

FIGURE 4-1   Sample résumé.

Below are just a few of the action words you might use:

Planned	Followed
Implemented	Handled
Administered	Designed
Organized	Generated
Started	Initiated
Managed	Supervised
Identified	Coordinated

Beneath work history is *education*. Obviously, you will want to begin this section with your current course program. If you've had previous health care education, include it in this section.

The next section is *community service and achievements*. This section is very valuable, especially if you've had little or no work history. Include here such things as church work, volunteer work, self-help seminars attended, and awards received.

The last section is the *reference* section. References should be selected carefully. They can increase or decrease your chances for employment. You should secure the names, addresses, and phone numbers of two professional and two personal references. Make a list of all the people you might use. Contact them, and ask them if you may use them as references. Professional references include your previous supervisors, or those for whom you have demonstrated a positive work history. If you have never held gainful employment, you could use a minister or perhaps a neighbor for whom you provided child care. Your two personal references should be chosen among those who can testify to all the special qualities and abilities you have listed on your résumé. Never use a relative. This includes all in-laws. If the response from your contacts is positive, alert them that you are actively seeking employment and that they may be contacted in the near future.

Résumés

A **résumé** is a brief overview of your work history, education, and skills or talents. There are many résumé formats from which to choose, but here are some basic guidelines.

Résumés should

- Be no longer than one page
- Include work experience in reverse chronological order (from present to past)
- Include education, community service, and highlights of skills and qualities

References should include two professional and two personal names, addresses, and phone numbers, including area codes. If you have no work history, you can use your pastor, rabbi, or other religious leader where you worship or a community agency representative who supervised your volunteer services. Never use a relative, including an in-law, unless you were a paid employee.

Knowing Yourself

To find the "right job," you have to be in tune with *you*. So let's step back for a minute to evaluate who you are. If you feel comfortable, ask your lab partner or a friend to assist you with this inventory.

Answer yes or no to the following statements:

1. I like having several projects at the same time. _____

2. I like a workplace in which my superior is there in a crisis. _____

3. I like to know my coworkers and work closely with them. _____

4. I like different tasks with a change of scenery each day. _____

5. I like to work independently. _____

6. I like to care for the physical needs of clients. _____

7. I like to care for the mental needs of clients. _____

8. I enjoy running a household. _____

9. I am an excellent manager of my home. _____

Check your preferences:

- If you answered yes to 1, 2, and 3, you probably would work well in a nursing home or hospital.
- If you answered yes to 4, 5, and 6, you probably would work well in home care.
- If you answered yes to 7, 8, and 9, you probably would work well in the community mental health setting.

Interviews

Why should I hire you? That's the underlying question every employer is asking when you are being interviewed. Therefore, with every question you answer, respond with information that shows your value to the employer.

An interview between Inez and Mrs. Potts is given in Table 4-1. Inez just completed a certified nursing assistant (CNA) course and is being interviewed for full-time employment at a skilled nursing facility. Inez has no work history but has successfully raised two children, and she took care of her mother who recently died of terminal cancer. Mrs. Potts, the director of nursing, is conducting the interview.

Remember, the interview is an opportunity for you to get answers to your questions about the organization, facility, or agency in which you are seeking employment. Here are some questions you might ask during an interview:

- What kind of orientation program does your organization offer?
- What are the uniform requirements of this position?
- How long will my résumé remain in the active file?

What kinds of information are important to gather at the time of the interview? Following is a list of the kind of information you might want to secure during an interview:

- Type of patients
- Openings: full- or part-time
- Shifts available
- Weekend rotation expected
- Status of résumé if not hired
- Starting salary
- Benefits offered

TABLE 4-1 Interview between Inez and Mrs. Potts

Job Interview

MRS. POTTS:	Tell me about yourself
INEZ:	I have just completed a CNA course. I am very interested in working with the elderly. I am dependable and motivated, and I interact well with others. Though I have no former employers, I took excellent care of my mother for 2 years. She was placed in a home care hospice program, so I was able to keep her at home, where she died peacefully. The program's coordinator has written a letter of recommendation. Here is a copy.
MRS. POTTS:	Why do you want to work for us?
INEZ:	The community views your agency as delivering quality care while recognizing the value and contributions of the staff.
MRS. POTTS:	Where do you see yourself in 5 years?
INEZ:	I see myself working as a clinical care associate in the skilled unit of your facility.
MRS. POTTS:	What are your strengths and weaknesses?
INEZ:	My strengths are organization, willingness to learn, and the ability to take constructive criticism. My weakness is the need for perfection, but I have learned throughout the course that managed care requires quality with speed.
MRS. POTTS:	I will call you in several days after the interviews have been completed.
INEZ:	Thank you for your time. I will look forward to hearing from you (Figure 4-2).

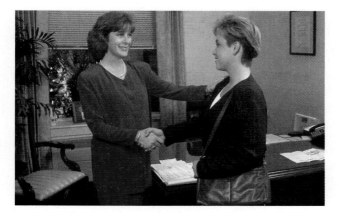

FIGURE 4-2 Always thank the interviewer before you leave the interview.

▪ Health insurance
▪ Vacation
▪ Educational opportunities

Following an interview, send a follow-up thank-you note. Express your gratitude for the opportunity to interview, and restate your interest in the position.

Job Search

Where do you start when looking for a job? Sometimes, **clinical experiences** can provide great job leads. That's why it's so important to prepare before the experience, to follow instructions, to complete assignments, to ask questions, and to demonstrate your valuable qualities. But how else can you find a position? **Networking** is another means to a job. Discussing your availability and goals with other care professionals can lead to job offers. **Job postings** in your local community hospital's personnel department can be another source of job leads.

The most extensive listing of jobs, however, is in the **classifieds**. The classified section of the newspaper, under the "Health Care" section, holds the largest list of available jobs. Let's take a look at some sample newspaper listings in Figure 4-3 to evaluate where to apply. Now, pretend that you will

CERTIFIED NURSING ASSISTANTS St. Joseph's is seeking supportive, responsible individuals F/T, P/T and W/E shifts. Send résumés to:

    Personnel Dept.
    St. Joseph's Rehab Center
    1856 Kelly Road
    East Doe, MD 08113

MENTAL RETARDATION Residential supvr. for CLA in downtown Chicago for adults with MR. Must be available to work eve. and occasional wknds. Send résumés to:

    SPED
    5621 Drummond Drive
    Chicago, IL 70021

HOME CARE CNA's needed to provide in home care to ventilator, pediatric and IV patients. Extra $$ for W/E. Call Judy at YAMA services 1-800-CAN-YAMA

FIGURE 4-3 Sample job listings in classified section of newspaper.

apply for one of these jobs, and set up an interview with your instructor. Be sure to have your résumé ready.

Some ads request responses by phone, in which case you probably will not need a cover letter. But some ads ask you to send a résumé. In this situation, you will need to type a business letter to the company. Let's look at ad 1 and type a cover letter using the format shown in Figure 4-4. Note that a cover letter has a colon (:) after the salutation, not a comma (,). In addition, note that the first name is not included in the salutation.

---

555 Knox Street
Collegeville, PA 10001

February 17, 19xx

Miss Teresa England
Director of Nurses
Sacred Heart Hospital
103 Main Street
Norristown, PA 30003

Dear Miss England:

This letter is in response to your recent advertisement in the February 14, 19xx *Philadelphia Post* for a nursing assistant.

I believe that my qualifications are a good match for your position. During my nursing assistant program at North Montco Technical Career Center in Lansdale, Pennsylvania, I have maintained a 3.6 GPA on a 4.0 scale.

I am a candidate for graduation on June 5, 19xx. Since passing my exams in January, I have worked part-time as a nursing assistant. My attendance is excellent and I am very reliable. My goal is to use my skills as a nursing assistant and to be an exemplary employee.

Enclosed is my résumé and a separate list of the skills I mastered in the nursing assistant program. I look forward to meeting you to discuss your position needs and my qualifications.

Thank you for your consideration.

Sincerely,

Paula Smith, CNA

Enc.

FIGURE 4-4 Cover letter.

Employment Opportunities for Assistive Personnel

Employment opportunities for assistive personnel are most frequently discovered in four settings: *hospitals, long-term care facilities, community mental health and mental retardation agencies,* and *home care agencies.* The opportunities for employment in each of these settings are described here, including titles, functions, and role requirements.

Hospitals

Titles and Functions

Generally, the titles of assistive personnel in hospitals include *nurse aide, nursing assistant,* and *orderly.* The nursing assistant and nurse aide perform the basic tasks listed in the above section. The multi-skilled assistant may be titled *patient care associate, care partner, clinical care associate, clinical care technician, patient care technician, clinical care assistant, nurse extender, advanced nursing assistant,* or *nursing assistant II.* There are other titles that may be used to describe the assistant who performs extended care skills. These are titles that the hospital decided to use. Assistive personnel in hospitals work under the supervision of a professional nurse (RN) who delegates tasks to the care associate.

Role Requirements

Hospitals today are hiring nursing assistants who have attended a certified nurse aide program and have passed the nurse aide competency examinations. This is important to the hospital because it ensures that the individual has met the minimum requirements for the role of a multiskilled worker. Hospitals are often willing to provide additional education and training for the expanded duty tasks, but they would prefer to employ unlicensed assistants who are already knowledgeable and competent in these expanded skills (Figure 4-5). The time and cost of training is always a consideration, and some hospitals do not have educators designated for this type of training. An applicant with expanded duty skills and knowledge will have the advantage over an applicant who does not.

It is essential for the clinical care associate to have interpersonal and communication skills, technical skills, and critical thinking skills. Hospitals want unlicensed assistants who are responsible and accountable for their actions in providing patient care. They want assistants who can troubleshoot, solve problems, and work as a team member. They need assistants who can organize their care responsibili-

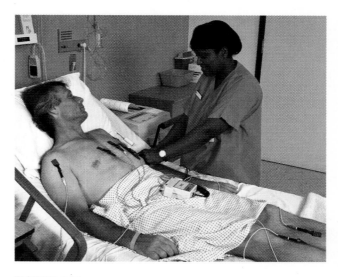

FIGURE 4-5 Clinical care assistant performing an ECG.

ties, who can communicate with team members, patients, and families, and who know the limits of their role. They do not want assistants who will jeopardize the safety of patients and perform tasks that they have not been trained for or that they are not competent to perform.

Nurses want to be assured that the care associate who works under their supervision is willing to accept delegated tasks and is accountable for job performance. They do not want someone on their team who will jeopardize their license because of irresponsible actions, lack of critical thinking, and lack of technical skills. Nurses want to delegate a task and know that the task will be performed well—that the results will be reported to them when needed. They need assistants who know normal versus abnormal results and who are not afraid to ask for help or direction when they are unsure of a procedure or the results of a task.

Nurses and care associates work together to provide patient care. Nurses will delegate some aspects of patient care to the clinical care associate. What is delegated depends on the needs of the patient, the technical skill of the associate, and the communication and critical thinking skills needed to safely perform the task. What is delegated is not determined by the associate in care; it is determined by the professional nurse. If you ever feel that you should not perform a task because of the patient's level of acuity or because of your lack of ability to perform any task safely, it is your responsibility to tell the nurse.

Long-Term Care Facilities

Titles and Functions

In long-term care (LTC) facilities, the care associate is called a *nurse aide* or *nursing assistant.* Long-term care facilities are called *nursing homes, rehabilitation centers*, or *convalescent homes*. The nursing assistant in long-term care works under the direction of a nurse to provide care for the residents. Nursing assistants in a nursing home help residents to meet their physical needs of hygiene, mobility, and nutrition as well as their psychosocial and recreational needs.

Role Requirements

In any LTC facility, the unlicensed caregiver is required to attend an educational program that is certified by the state. The graduate must pass the competency examinations of the state (Figure 4-6). The competency examinations include a written test and a skills test. In the skills test, the nursing assistant demonstrates skills selected by the examiner. Upon successful completion of the examination, the nurse aide is placed on the state's nurse aide registry. If the nursing assistant does not pass the written or practical section of the examination, the section may be retaken. The examination must be taken within two years of completing the certified nurse aide program. An LTC facility can employ a graduate for only 120 days before the assistant successfully completes the competency examinations. A certified nurse aide program must be at least 75 hours of instruction, and 37.5 hours of the program must be clinical experience in an LTC. Many certified nursing assistant programs are longer than the 75 required hours. The CNA program must include instruction in resident rights, communication skills, assisting residents with activities of daily living, nutrition, mental health needs, basic nursing assistant care skills, and death and dying. The nursing home industry is very highly regulated to protect residents' rights and to ensure

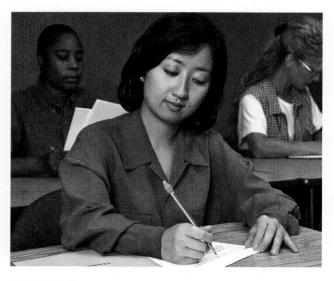

FIGURE 4-6 Nurse aide sitting for the competency exam.

adequate care. The law that regulates the LTC industry—the Omnibus Budget Reconciliation Act (OBRA)—is discussed in Chapter 2.

Community Mental Health and Mental Retardation Agencies

Titles and Functions

In community mental health and mental retardation (MH/MR) agencies, as well as hospital psychiatric and addiction units, the assistants in care are sometimes called *psychiatric technicians, mental health technicians, client care associates* or *technicians, mental health assistants, counselors, resident counselors*, and *vocational assistants*. In a hospital setting, the mental health associate works under the supervision of a professional nurse. In the community, the mental health technician may work under the supervision of a social worker, a psychologist, or a manager who has an advanced degree in psychology or a related field.

In the community, there are opportunities for employment in community living arrangements (CLAs) or community residential rehabilitation (CRR) settings. The CLA is a group home for people who have mental retardation, and the CRR is a group home for people who have a mental health or addiction diagnosis. These community homes are designed to provide residents with a home in a neighborhood that functions like any other home environment. Residents and client care counselors work together to care for the home. The resident counselor or adviser is responsible for directing and teaching the residents of the home to perform self-care skills, to travel in the community, to cook, to clean, and to manage household budgets. Resident counselors may have training as a nursing assistant and skill in counseling and teaching others. Nursing assistants may find employment in the community because they have knowledge about health and illness, possess communication skills, and may have assisted others in self-care skills or activities of daily living (ADLs).

In some states, resident counselors are educated and tested in medication administration. The required education and a successful score on the certification examination allow these assistive personnel to administer oral and topical medication to residents in a CLA. A medication record is maintained by the resident counselor who is certified to administer medications. In CRRs, resident counselors supervise the resident in the self-administration of medications. They do not administer them to residents who are capable of performing this function independently.

Some community MH/MR agencies have vocational workshops that train clients in basic vocational skills or have clients work in supportive workshops. In these workshops, clients may learn skills like the assembling or packaging of products for industries who contract with the MH/MR agency for this service. Clients are paid for their work. Assistants in this type of community work may function in the role of a teacher aide, vocational counselor, or workshop assistant. Clients may have mental retardation as well as physical disabilities. These clients will need the assistance of someone for toileting, travel to the workshop, eating, and gaining instruction in the tasks that the client will perform in the workshop. Some workshops employ people with severe mental retardation. These clients need continuous supervision and assistance in work skills and self-care skills. Nursing assistants may find employment in this type of community facility.

Some community MH/MR agencies have older adult day-care services and geriatric partial hospitalization or geriatric mental health day-care programs. This type of facility seeks nursing assistants who are listed on their state's nurse aide registry. Day hospital programs provide services to elders who have a mental health diagnosis. Older adult day-care programs provide services to elders who live with family, but who, during the daytime hours, need supervision and assistance with self-care and recreational activities. Families bring the elder to the day-care program for services while they work or when they are unavailable to supervise the elder who cannot remain safely in the home without personal supervision. In older adult partial hospitalization or mental health programs, the assistive personnel help clients with ADLs, register clients in the program, make rounds for observation, and assist in conducting recreational and supportive group activities (Figure 4-7).

Role Requirements

There are no specific educational or state requirements for working in a community group home. Generally, the MH/MR agency prefers to hire individuals who have worked in health care or in education. People who have an associate's or bachelor's degree in mental health–related fields often seek employment in community MH/MR facilities. Nursing assistants are ideal candidates for employment as resident counselors or advisers.

The agency that employs assistive personnel determines the functions and responsibilities of the position. Generally, the unlicensed assistant follows a prescribed treatment plan designed to assist the client or resident in learning self-care and vocational skills. If you work in a living arrangement, generally

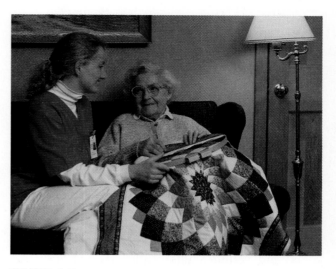

FIGURE 4-7   A mental health technician assists client working on an art project.

you will work evening and nighttime hours and assist clients in learning or completing self-care skills or household skills. The ultimate goal is to provide a home environment or work environment that enables the resident or client to perform as independently as possible. You would structure your work to promote independence and adhere to the concept of the least restrictive alternative in care. This concept is described in Unit 8. You will need to understand the principles of counseling and behavior modification, which are also described in Unit 8.

Home Care Agencies

Titles and Functions

Because the trend for home care has strengthened over the past 20 years, the need for home care aides or home health aides will rise. There are several categories of home care: insurance provider cases, Medicare cases, and private-pay cases. Medicare-driven home care proved its success in the 1970s as the number of Medicare clients increased. Medicare stipulates certain criteria that must be met before a client can receive home care services. The client must be entitled to Medicare, must be suffering from an acute illness, must be labeled "homebound," and must have a physician's order for services. In addition, the client must demonstrate a need for skilled nursing care and some rehab potential, or death must be imminent, to receive hospice services. The client receives intermittent care, generally with decreasing frequency, until discharged to self or to the care of a family member.

Since the client has an acute diagnosis and care is being delivered in the home, the home health aide must possess sharp skills and keen observation and reporting techniques because of the independent, unsupervised working environment. The primary focus of the home health aide is to deliver or to assist with personal care. In addition, the home health aide may be required to perform some of the ADL skills that the client cannot perform. Examples of this would be personal laundry, light housekeeping (bedroom, bathroom, and kitchen), grocery shopping, and meal preparation (Figure 4-8).

Insurance provider cases are steadily increasing because of the diagnostic related groups (DRGs) and the interrelated push for illness prevention. Many skilled cases once treated in an acute environment are now treated at home. Insurance cases include a wide cross section of ages. Children, adolescents, and young adults can be treated at home. Antibiotic therapy, mother-baby care post-delivery, post-surgical follow-up, and ventilator care are just a few of the problems that might require home care intervention. Once again, the clinical care associate will be called on to work with acutely ill clients in an unsupervised setting. This requires confidence, competence, critical thinking, and excellent observation and reporting techniques.

Role Requirements

Although agencies prefer certified nursing assistants, they will train individuals who can be bonded and

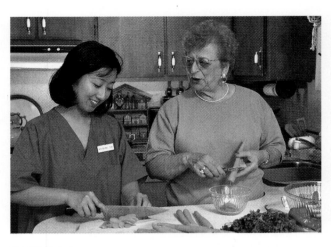

FIGURE 4-8 Home health aide assisting the client with meal preparation.

insured to perform the duties of homemaking and the nursing assistant skills used in traditional skilled nursing facility (SNF) and hospital units. Because patients are returning home more ill than in previous years, probation periods of 30 to 90 days may be implemented by the facility. Depending on the location of the agency and the community it serves, a valid driver's license and dependable transportation may be necessary.

application to practice

Use the information you learned in this chapter about the job market and the positions that you might hold upon completion of your program or course to respond to the following situations.

Learning Activities

Situation 1: Develop a résumé.

Author's Explanation: Your program instructor will review your résumé.

Situation 2: Imagine that you are going on a job interview for a home health aide (HHA) position. You have just completed a CNA course but have never held a job in health care. How will you describe your ability to fulfill the requirements of the role?

Author's Explanation: Review the description of the role of the home health aide under "Home

Care Agencies," and find the duties and tasks of the HHA. List your experience in managing a home—preparing meals, managing the house, and keeping people safe from harm—and describe your interest in caring for people in the home versus in an institution such as a nursing home.

Situation 3: Review Table 4-1. How did Inez know about the company's reputation?

Author's Explanation: Inez must have investigated the company prior to the interview. She may have talked to employees and clients of the agency.

Situation 4: Why didn't Inez state that she might go back to school in 5 years for a psychology degree?

Author's Explanation: Companies are looking for employees who are willing to make a long-term commitment.

Situation 5: Why didn't Inez mention her habit of sleeping through her alarm as one of her weaknesses?

Author's Explanation: Inez knows that successful interviewees always choose a weakness that they can present as a strength, such as having the same expectation of others as one has of oneself or wanting to do a perfect job (being a perfectionist.)

Examination Review Questions

1. Which provides the largest list of available jobs?
    a. networking
    b. job postings
    c. clinical experiences
    d. classifieds

2. Community living arrangements are group homes for
    a. drug addicts
    b. Medicaid recipients
    c. geriatric independents
    d. the mentally retarded

3. CRRs are group homes for the maximal functioning of
    a. the mentally ill
    b. ADL-compromised residents
    c. the mentally retarded
    d. geriatric residents

4. Which are the minimum state requirements for working in a group home?
    a. a bachelor's degree in mental health
    b. a nursing degree
    c. previous experience
    d. no requirements

5. A résumé includes an overview of your
    a. work history
    b. education
    c. skills
    d. all of the above

6. Employment opportunities for assistive personnel are frequent in all of the following *except*
    a. hospitals
    b. home care agencies
    c. long-term care facilities
    d. intensive care units

7. Your last action before the close of an interview should be to
    a. ask questions
    b. shake hands
    c. say "thank you"
    d. submit your résumé

8. Which of the following is the best choice for a personal reference?
    a. relative
    b. spouse
    c. in-law
    d. pastor

9. You started a new filing system at your job. The best action word for your résumé is
    a. initiated
    b. identified
    c. coordinated
    d. managed

10. Which of the following should *not* be part of your résumé?
    a. work experience
    b. personal achievements
    c. age and gender
    d. professional references

The Language of Medicine

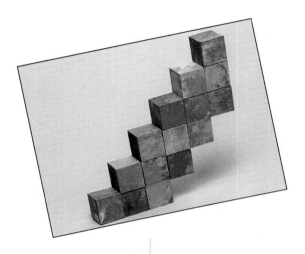

Have you ever spoken with a doctor or nurse about a health care problem? It might have seemed as though they were speaking a foreign language when they explained a problem or treatment to you. Or perhaps you could not read the doctor's prescription because there were so many symbols. You may have even thought, "This sounds like Greek to me!"

Medical terminology or the study of medical terms can also be called the *language of medicine*. It is a body of terms derived from Greek and Latin used to describe symptoms, diseases, diagnostics, and treatments. The different documents that contain medical language include post-operative reports, lab reports, nurses' notes, care plans, and medical records. To master the language of medicine, you need to be able to define, build, pronounce, and spell many terms.

Chapter 5

Medical Terms and Abbreviations

In this chapter, you will learn a simple method of building and interpreting the language of medicine. There are simple recipes to follow that will help you learn the meanings of word parts rather than memorizing whole terms. Medical abbreviations are learned best when their application to practice is understood. It is not possible to memorize every abbreviation and term, but through study and use you will become familiar with the most common. Remember, if you don't know the meaning of a term or an abbreviation, you can always find the answer in a resource manual or textbook. Relax and enjoy your study of the language of medicine.

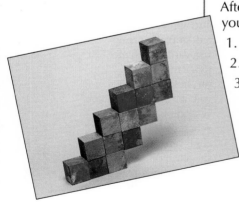

OBJECTIVES

After completing this chapter, you will be able to

1. Build medical terms
2. Pronounce medical terms
3. Define common medical abbreviations
4. Read and understand basic medical documentation
5. Define and spell all key terms correctly

k e y   t e r m s

activities of daily living (ADLs)   recipe combinations   word building
combining vowel   suffix   word root
prefix

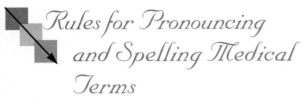

Rules for Pronouncing and Spelling Medical Terms

Let's focus on pronunciation. If you can't say a word, it's harder to spell it. Use the pronunciation key in Figure 5-1 to pronounce the words that follow.

colostomy (ko-los'-to-me)
cardiology (kar-de-ol'-o-ge)

There are four important rules to remember in addition to the pronunciation key:

The letter *c* followed by *a* or *o* has the sound of *k*.
The letter *c* followed by *i* or *e* has the sound of *s*.
The letter *g* followed by *a* or *o* has the sound of *g*.
The letter *g* followed by *i* or *e* has the sound of *j*.

Let's try saying the following words using the rules above.

Pronunciation Key

Symbol	Key Words	Symbol	Key Words
a	asp, fat, parrot	b	bed, fable, dub, ebb
ā	ape, date, play, break, fail	d	dip, beadle, had, dodder
ä	ah, car, father, cot	f	fall, after, off, phone
		g	get, haggle, dog
e	elf, ten, berry	h	he, ahead, hotel
ē	even, meet, money, flea, grieve	j	joy, agile, badge
		k	kill, tackle, bake, coat, quick
i	is, hit, mirror	l	let, yellow, ball
ī	ice, bite, high, sky	m	met, camel, trim, summer
		n	not, flannel, ton
ō	open, tone, go, boat	p	put, apple, tap
ô	all, horn, law, oar	r	red, port, dear, purr
o͞o	look, pull, moor, wolf	s	sell, castle, pass, nice
o͞o	ooze, tool, crew, rule	t	top, cattle, hat
yo͞o	use, cute, few	v	vat, hovel, have
yoo	cure, globule	w	will, always, swear, quick
oi	oil, point, toy	y	yet, onion, yard
ou	out, crowd, plow	z	zebra, dazzle, haze, rise
u	up, cut, color, flood	ch	chin, catcher, arch, nature
ur	urn, fur, deter, irk	sh	she, cushion, dash, machine
		th	thin, nothing, truth
ə	a in ago	*th*	then, father, lathe
	e in agent	zh	azure, leisure, beige
	i in sanity	ŋ	ring, anger, drink
	o in comply		[indicates that a following l
	u in focus		or n is a syllabic consonant,
ər	perhaps, murder		as in *cattle* (kat´'l), *Latin*
			(lat´'n); see full explanation
			on p. xiii]

An abbreviated form of this key appears at the bottom of every right-hand page of the vocabulary.
Source: Webster's New World Dictionary, Third College Edition ©1991, Simon & Schuster.

FIGURE 5-1 Pronunciation key.

cardiac (*c* followed by *a* has the sound of *k*)
carcinoma (*c* followed by *i* has the sound of *s*)
gastrotomy (*g* followed by *a* has the sound of *g*)
gingivitis (*g* followed by *i* has the sound of *j*)

Think of ordinary words to which each rule applies, and make a list of your own. Examples are *cardinal*, *cinema*, *gaping*, and *gin*.

Understanding Word Parts

Words are built from several components that, when examined, each have a meaning. Word components can be classified as one of the following three: *prefix*, *word root*, *or suffix*. A **prefix** is a word component that begins a word and changes the meaning of the word. A **word root** is the foundation, or major, word component. Without a word root, there is no word. Just as a prefix begins a word, a **suffix** ends a word. Prefixes and suffixes both contain *fix*. How can you remember the meaning of each? *Pre-* means "before." Therefore, a prefix begins a word. For your convenience, this chapter will mark all prefixes with a hyphen following it. Word roots will also have

a hyphen following them, but they will be in capital letters. Suffixes will begin with a hyphen.

Building and Defining Medical Terms

Building medical terms is much like a bread recipe. Certain ingredients, when mixed together in the proper order, form bread. There are many variations to bread recipes. The result is still bread even if the ingredients and the name of the bread change. There are many variations in medical term recipes, but there are "ingredient combinations" that are seen frequently. The following are the common med term **recipe combinations**.

Recipe 1—WORD ROOT + suffix (Figure 5-2)

Recipe 2—WORD ROOT + WORD ROOT + suffix (Figure 5-3)

Recipe 3—prefix + WORD ROOT + suffix (Figure 5-4)

Recipe 4—prefix + WORD ROOT + WORD ROOT + suffix (Figure 5-5)

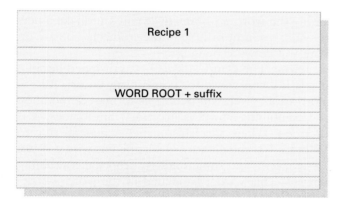

FIGURE 5-2   Recipe 1.

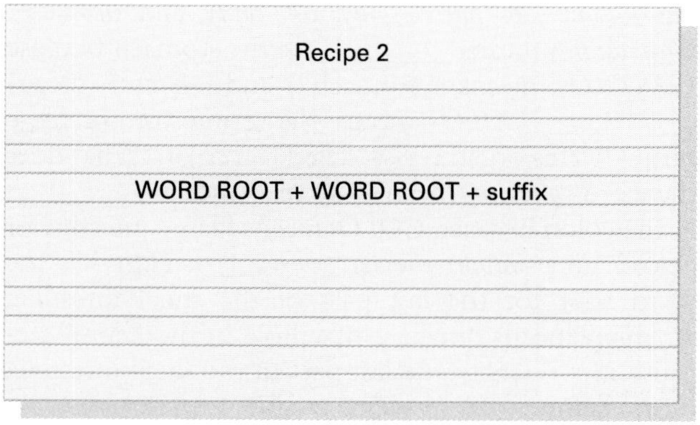

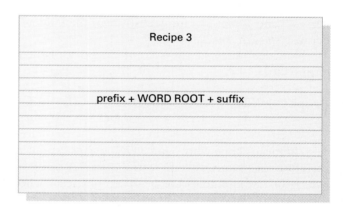

FIGURE 5-4   Recipe 3.

FIGURE 5-3   Recipe 2.

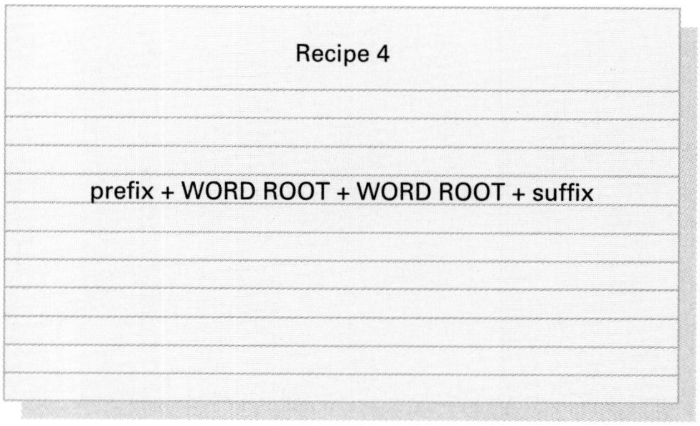

FIGURE 5-5   Recipe 4.

Recipe 5—WORD ROOT + WORD ROOT (Figure 5-6)

Let's look at the first word recipe seen in medical terminology and apply it.

Recipe 1—WORD ROOT + suffix
CARDIO- + *-logy*

The suffix *-logy* means "study of." *Cardiology* is the study of the heart because *-logy* means "study of" and *CARDIO-* means "heart." *CARDIO-* is the word root.

Let's change the word root but keep the suffix. Below is a list of word roots that refer to parts of the body. Using the first recipe, combine them with the suffix *-logy* to build other medical words.

GASTRO-   stomach
NEURO-   nerve
NEPHRO-   kidney

By combining these different word roots with the same suffix, new words can be built. This is the process called **word building**. All of the new words have a similar meaning because the suffix *-logy* is common to all the words. *Gastrology* means "study of the stomach," *neurology* means "study of the nerves," and *nephrology* means "study of the kidney" because *-logy* means "study of."

Now, let's look at the second category of med term recipes.

Recipe 2—WORD ROOT + WORD ROOT + suffix
+   *LOG-*   + *-ist*

-Ist means "one who," and *LOG-* means "study"; therefore, *-logist* means "one who studies." A *cardiologist* is one who studies the heart—a physician who specializes in the heart and heart disease.

How many other specialists can you name using the suffix *-logist*? Try to name three others. If you

said *gastrologist*, *neurologist*, and *nephrologist*, you have caught on to the concept of med term recipe building. If you did not, reread recipes 1 and 2.

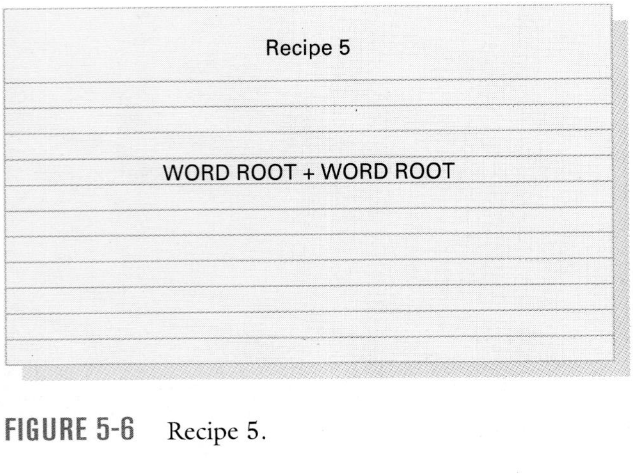

Now let's look at the *-tomy* family of suffixes and how that family applies to recipes 1 and 2. *-Tomy* means "cut into" or "incision." Therefore, *-tomy* means "cut into" or "incise."

Recipe 1—WORD ROOT + suffix
+ *-tomy*

Using the word roots *NEPHRO-* and *GASTRO-*, let's build two words with the suffix *-tomy*. *Nephrotomy* means "cut into the kidney" because *NEPHRO-* means "kidney." *Gastrotomy* means "incise the stomach" because *GASTRO-* means "stomach." Think of two other *-tomy* words you can build. Use a medical dictionary if unsure.

Recipe 2—WORD ROOT + WORD ROOT + suffix
GASTR(O)- +   *OS-*   + *-tomy*

An *OS-* is an opening, mouth, or hole. Add *OS-* to *-tomy*, and *-ostomy* means "cut a new opening." Word definition is as easy as word building. By now you should be familiar with *GASTRO-*, which means "stomach." Using recipe 2, you should be able to define the word *gastrostomy*. If you said make a new opening, mouth, or hole in the stomach, you are on your way to word defining.

Note: The *O* in *GASTRO-* was dropped because it is a hookup vowel, or **combining vowel**. All the word roots given will be in this format. Sometimes, the combining vowel is necessary. Sometimes, it is dropped. When does this occur? A general rule to follow is, "If the next word part begins with a vowel (*a, e, i, o, u*, and sometimes *y*), drop the combining vowel." That's what happened in the word *gastrostomy*. "If the word part following begins with a consonant (all the remaining letters), keep the combining vowel."

Three common surgical procedures with the ending *-ostomy* are *gastrostomy*, *colostomy*, and *ileostomy*. *Gastrostomy* means _____ in the stomach because *GASTRO-* means "stomach" and *-ostomy* means _____. *COLO-* means "large intestine or large bowel." This organ is also called the colon. What does the word *colostomy* mean? *Colostomy* means _____ in the colon because *COLO-* means "large intestine or colon" and *-ostomy* means _____. *ILEO-* is the word root for the last part of the small intestine. *Ileostomy* means "make a new hole in the ileum" because *ileo-* refers to the last part of the small intestine, or the ileum.

Let's try recipe 2 again. *ECTO-* means "out or outer" and *-tomy* means "to cut." Therefore, *-ectomy*

Recipe 5

WORD ROOT + WORD ROOT

FIGURE 5-6   Recipe 5.

CHAPTER 8

We walked next door to the shop my grandmother had owned for more than thirty years. And looking at it, it might seem as if she hadn't gotten rid of anything the entire time.

The quilt shop had a treasure hunt quality to it. While there were organized shelves with bolts of fabric lined up by color, there were just as many bolts leaning up against the wall. Fabrics of colorful flowers, cute baby animals, and Christmas prints were piled on top of one another near the cash register at the front.

To get to the rest of the shop, you had to make a semicircle around a dangerously overloaded rack of books and down an aisle that was one person deep.

If you did, you would be rewarded with a dazzling display of quilts. Eleanor had made the large, wildly colorful ones with abstract patterns that appeared to follow no rules. Nancy, on the other hand, was clearly the creator of the small, carefully constructed and elaborately quilted pieces. In the center was one of Eleanor's favorites—a small, bright log cabin quilt that Grace, the woman who taught her to quilt, had made. Each was enough to inspire even me to take up quilting.

Nancy caught me staring at the quilts. "Are you ready to make one of your own?"

"At some point," I admitted.

means "cut out, removal, excise, or excision." The word *gastrectomy* means "remove the stomach." It can also mean "excise or cut out the stomach." Almost any organ, all or in part, can be removed from the body.

Now define these *-ectomy* words: *gastrectomy, appendectomy, colectomy, nephrectomy, splenectomy.* All of them refer to the removal of something. What do the word roots mean? If you don't know, look them up in a medical dictionary.

-Itis is a suffix that means "inflammation." An inflammation is an area of the body that is red, hot, tender, and swollen. An inflammation can be caused by irritation, infection, or disease. All organs of the body can become inflamed.

Name at least five organs and their medical word roots, and combine them with the suffix *-itis*, using recipe 1. Your list might include *gastritis, appendicitis, colitis, nephritis,* and *neuritis.* If you did not name at least five, **STOP**! and reread the sections above.

-Pathy means "disease." A disease is an abnormal function of an organ or body system. It is an illness or disorder identified specifically by recognizable symptoms. Using recipe 1, build the following words using the suffix for "disease":

Disease of the heart
Disease of the nerves

Cardiopathy and *neuropathy* are the correct answers because *CARDIO-* means "heart" and *NEURO-* means "nerves." *-Pathy* means "disease."

-Osis is an ending that means "condition or state of being" as it pertains to the body. Using recipe 1, build the words that mean the same as these expressions:

Condition of the nerves
Condition of the stomach

Your answers should be *neurosis* and *gastrosis.*

Let's take a look at word recipe 3.

Recipe 3—prefix + WORD ROOT + suffix
CARD(IO)- + *-itis*

Let's take a new medical term: *carditis.* *Carditis* means "inflammation of the heart." Note that the *io* in *CARDIO-* is dropped for ease of pronunciation. Using recipe 3, add the following prefixes for variety recipes.

epi- upon or on top of
peri- around
endo- inner

Epicarditis means "inflammation on top of the heart." *Pericarditis* means "inflammation around the

heart." *Endocarditis* means "inflammation in the inner part of the heart." All three words mean "inflammation of the heart" because *carditis* means "heart inflammation."

Let's try another word-building activity using recipe 3.

Recipe 3—prefix + WORD ROOT + suffix
CYT(O)- + *-osis*

Cytosis means "a condition of cells" because *CYTO-* means "cell" and *-osis* means "condition." (Notice that when the two are joined, the combining vowel is dropped.) *-Osis* also means "increase in" when combined with prefixes that form types of blood cells. Now add the following prefixes to *cytosis*.

erythro- red
leuko- white

Add each of these prefixes to build two new words: *erythrocytosis* and *leukocytosis.*

Let's try more words with recipe 3. This time, however, you will define the words. *Hemi-* means "half." What does *hemigastrotomy* mean? If you said incision into half the stomach, you are correct. *-Ia* is a suffix that makes a word a noun. It's a polisher suffix. What does *hemicardia* mean? *Hemicardia* means "half a heart."

In recipe 4, word roots are combined with a prefix; then a suffix is added to form the word.

Recipe 4
prefix + WORD ROOT + WORD ROOT + suffix
an- + *ESTHESIO-* + *LOG-* + *-ist*

This recipe is not as common as recipes 1, 2, and 3 are. However, the principles are the same.

Some medical words are formed by combining two word roots, as in the word *cardioscope.* In recipe 5, no prefixes or suffixes are added.

Recipe 5—WORD ROOT + WORD ROOT
CARDIO- + *SCOPE-*

CARDIO- means "heart," and *SCOPE-* means "examine." A cardioscope is therefore an instrument used to examine the heart.

Let's try another.

OLFACT- smell
PHOBIA- fear

Therefore, *olfactophobia* means "fear of smell." Using the word root *PHOTO-*, meaning "light," build a word meaning "fear of light." If you said *photophobia*, you are correct.

Remember, most med terms will be formed following recipes 1, 2, and 3. Building and defining words is an ongoing process. The more you use the recipes, the easier it becomes. Remember the first time you made chocolate chip cookies? If you have made them fifty or more times since then, you probably don't need to follow the recipe any longer. The same is true when using med term recipes.

Let's return to recipe 2.

Recipe 2—WORD ROOT + WORD ROOT + suffix
CARD(IO)-   +   -itis

The word root *MYO*- means "muscle" Add this root before *carditis*, and the new word is *myocarditis*. This means "inflammation of the heart muscle."

By now, you should begin to understand the process of word building and word definition as it relates to medical terminology. Never be frightened of a large word. Try to break it down. You may not know all the parts, but in most cases, you will know part or most of the word components. Most of all, use a medical dictionary often.

Below is a list of common prefixes, word roots, and suffixes that will be used throughout the text and also in your field of study. Following the lists is a series of exercises. Complete the exercises once you have mastered the lists. Good luck!

Prefixes

a-	without
an-	without
bi-	two
tri-	three
dia-	through
homeo-	like or similar; resemblance
inter-	between
extra-	outside of; beyond
super-	above
supra-	above
quadri-	four
sub-	under

Word Roots

THROMBO-	clot
VENO-	vein
SCLERO-	hardening
ARTERIO-	artery
HEPATO-	liver
LATERO-	side
TROPHO-	development
SCOPO-	to look or examine

Suffixes

-y	the process of
-e	noun suffix; with *scopo* and *tomo* it means "the instrument to"
-ic, -al, -ary, -ous	pertaining to (adjective)

Using the lists above and the other word components you have learned, define the following terms:

1. thrombocyte
2. asepsis
3. sclerosis
4. endoscopy
5. melanoma

Analyzing Terms to Define Them

Using the lists of prefixes, word roots, and suffixes below, see if you can define the medical terms that follow.

Prefixes

Remember, prefixes come at the beginnings of words.

poly-	many; much
hypo-	less than normal
hyper-	more than normal
auto-	self
anti-	against

Word Roots

Word roots are the foundation of words. Remember, they may come at the beginning, but they are generally in the middle of a word. Some words contain more than one word root.

GLYCO-	sugar
NOCTO-	night
NEURO-	nerve
PHAGO-	eat; swallow
PATHO-	disease
RETINO-	retina
DIPSO-	thirst
URO-	urine; urination
GENO-	produce
(H)EMO-	blood (*HEMO-* is used at the beginning of a word, as in *HEMOdialysis*. The *h* is dropped when used in the middle or end of a word, as in *leukEMia*.)

Suffixes

Remember, suffixes are endings to words.

-ia condition

-y process

Analyze the following words to see if you can determine their meanings:

1. hypoglycemia
2. hyperglycemia
3. antigen
4. polyuria
5. polyphagia
6. nocturia
7. neuropathy
8. retinopathy

Answers:

1. Hypoglycemia: abnormally low blood sugar
2. Hyperglycemia: abnormally high blood sugar
3. Antigen: substance that creates a reaction in the body against itself
4. Polyuria: excessive urination
5. Polyphagia: excessive eating
6. Nocturia: night urination
7. Neuropathy: nerve disease
8. Retinopathy: retinal disease

Medical Abbreviations

Medical abbreviations provide a medical shorthand when documenting or dictating information regarding patients. Most medical abbreviations are derived from Latin. There is no easy way to learn medical abbreviations except through repeated practice. Tables 5-1 through 5-7 list medical abbreviations categorized by subject. Although they are not comprehensive, these lists have been chosen to assist you in your work as a clinical care associate.

Each session, take a list and study it with a partner. Flash cards are an excellent method for quizzing yourself or others. Post the "list for the day" on your refrigerator or bathroom mirror. Quiz yourself as you prepare dinner or perform other **activities of daily living (ADLs)**. Refer to these lists when confronted with abbreviations in future units. Many abbreviations depend on the first letter of each word, especially procedures, professions, and diagnostic studies. Others, however, require extensive study, especially bedside charting abbreviations. All the lists following are alphabetized. Your instructor may choose certain terms or require you to learn all of them. Following the lists are exercises containing medical abbreviations. Once you have mastered the lists, test your knowledge by interpreting or completing the exercises. Good luck!

TABLE 5-1   Conditions and Diseases

Abbreviation	Meaning	Abbreviation	Meaning
AIDS	Acquired immunodeficiency syndrome	DOA	Dead on arrival
ASCVD	Arteriosclerotic cardiovascular disease	DRG	Diagnostic related group
AV	Atrioventricular	DTs	Delirium tremens
BPH	Benign prostatic hypertrophy	FUO	Fever of unknown origin
CA	Cancer	Fx	Fracture
CAD	Coronary artery disease	HIV	Human immunodeficiency virus
CHD	Cardiovascular heart disease	HPV	Human papilloma virus (venereal warts)
CHF	Congestive heart failure	HTN	Hypertension
CHOL	Cholesterol	IDDM	Insulin-dependent diabetes mellitus
COPD	Chronic obstructive pulmonary disease	Mets, mets	Metastasis
CVA	Cerebrovascular accident	MI	Myocardial infarction

TABLE 5-1   Conditions and Diseases (continued)

Abbreviation	Meaning	Abbreviation	Meaning
MS	Multiple sclerosis	SLE	Systemic lupus erythromatosis
N&V	Nausea & vomiting	SOB	Shortness of breath
NIDDM	Non-insulin-dependent diabetes mellitus	Staph	Staphylococcus
OBS	Organic brain syndrome	Strep	Streptococcus
PERL	Pupils equal and reactive to light	TB	Tuberculosis
PID	Pelvic inflammatory disease	TIA	Transient ischemic attack
PKU	Phenylketonuria	TSS	Toxic shock syndrome
RA	Rheumatoid arthritis	URI	Upper respiratory infection
SIDS	Sudden infant death syndrome	UTI	Urinary tract infection

TABLE 5-2   Diagnostic Procedures and Tests

Abbreviation	Meaning	Abbreviation	Meaning
ABG	Arterial blood gas	CSF	Cerebrospinal fluid
A, B, O, AB	Blood typing groups	CXR	Chest x-ray
AFB	Acid-fast bacillus	Cysto	Cystoscopy
BE	Barium enema	D&C	Dilation (dilatation) and curettage
BP	Blood pressure	Diff	Differential
BUN	Blood urea nitrogen	DNA	Deoxyribonucleic acid
Bx	Biopsy	DPT	Diphtheria, pertussis, tetanus
CABG	Coronary artery bypass graft	ECG or EKG	Electrocardiogram
C&S	Culture and sensitivity	EEG	Electroencephalogram
CAT	Computerized axial tomography	ESR	Erthyrocyte sedimentation rate
Cath	Catheter	FBS	Fasting blood sugar
CBC	Complete blood count	GTT	Glucose tolerance test
CPR	Cardiopulmonary resuscitation	H&P	History and physical
C-section	Caesarian section	Hct	Hematocrit

TABLE 5-2   Diagnostic Procedures and Tests (continued)

Abbreviation	Meaning	Abbreviation	Meaning
HDL	High-density lipoprotein	PET	Positron emission tomography
Hgb	Hemoglobin	PFT	Pulmonary function test
Hx	History	pH	Hydrogen ion concentration (acid-base measurement)
I&D	Incision and drainage	RBC	Red blood cell
IPPB	Intermittent positive pressure breathing	Rx	Prescribe
IUD	Intrauterine device	SSE	Soap suds enema
IVP	Intravenous pyelogram	TENS	Transcutaneous electrical nerve stimulation
LASER	Light amplification by stimulated emission of radiation	TPR	Temperature, pulse, respiration
LDL	Low-density lipoprotein	TUR(P)	Transurethral resection (of the prostrate)
MMRV	Mumps, measles, rubella vaccine	Tx	Treatment
MRI	Magnetic resonance imaging	UA	Urinalysis
O&P	Ova and parasite	VS	Vital sign
OMT	Osteopathic manipulation therapy	WBC	White blood cell
PE	Physical exam	XR	X-ray

TABLE 5-3   Health Care Professionals

Abbreviation	Meaning	Abbreviation	Meaning
CCA	Clinical care associate	OT(R)	Occupational therapist (registered)
CDC	Centers for Disease Control	PA	Physician's assistant
CNA	Certified nursing assistant	PED	Pediatric
DO	Doctor of osteopathy	PT	Physical therapist
DON	Director of nursing	RD	Registered dietitian
HHA	Home health aide	RN	Registered nurse
LPN	Licensed practical nurse	RT	Respiratory therapist
MD	Doctor of medicine	ST	Speech therapist

TABLE 5-4   Pharmacology

Abbreviation	Meaning	Abbreviation	Meaning
ac	Before meals	NTG	Nitroglycerin
bid	Two times per day	pc	After meals
caps	Capsules	PDR	*Physician's Desk Reference*
cc	Cubic centimeter	q°	Every hour
D/W	Dextrose in water	qd	Every day
gr	Grain	qh	Every hour
gtt	Drops	qid	Four times per day
HS	Hour of sleep	qod	Every other day
i, ii	One, two	sl	Sublingual
IM	Intramuscular	tabs	Tablets
IV	Intravenous	tid	Three times per day
ml	Milliliter	ung	Ointment
mn	Minim	X	Ten

TABLE 5-5   Chemical Symbols

Abbreviation	Meaning	Abbreviation	Meaning
CHO	Carbohydrate	K	Potassium
CO_2	Carbon dioxide	Mg	Magnesium
Hg	Mercury	Na	Sodium
H_2O	Water	O_2	Oxygen

TABLE 5-6   Nursing Care

Abbreviation	Meaning	Abbreviation	Meaning
$\bar{a}$	Before	GB	Gallbladder
ADL	Activities of daily living	GI	Gastrointestinal
ad lib	As desired	GU	Genitourinary
adm	Admission/admitted	HOB	Head of bed
asst	Assist; assistance	hr or °	Hour
AKA	Above-the-knee amputation	HS	Hour of sleep
A.M.	Before noon	Ht	Height
AMA	Against medical advice	I&O	Intake and output
AMB	Ambulate	L	Left
approx	Approximately	LAT	Lateral
ASAP	As soon as possible	LLQ	Left lower quadrant
bilat	Bilateral	LMP	Last menstrual period
BR	Bedrest	LUQ	Left upper quadrant
BRP	Bathroom privileges	Neg	Negative
$\bar{c}$	With	NG	Nasogastric
C	Centigrade	NPO	Nothing by mouth
CBR	Complete bed rest	NS	Normal saline
c/o	Complains of	OB	Occult blood
cont	Continuous	OOB	Out of bed
dc	Discontinue	OU	Both eyes
DNR	Do not resuscitate	$\bar{p}$	After
Dr	Doctor	per	By; through
Dx	Diagnosis	P.M.	After noon
EENT	Eyes, ears, nose, throat	po	By mouth
F	Fahrenheit	post-op	Post-operative
FF	Force fluids	pre-op	Pre-operative

TABLE 5-6 Nursing Care (continued)

Abbreviation	Meaning	Abbreviation	Meaning
prn	As needed, as necessary	TPN	Total parenteral nutrition
pt	Patient	trans	Transverse
R	Right	VS	Vital sign
ROM	Range of motion	x	Times
RUQ	Right upper quadrant	yo	Year old
s̄	Without	2°	Secondary to
S&A	Sugar and acetone	⊕	Positive
sc or subq	Subcutaneously	−, neg	Negative
sed rate	Sedimentation rate	√	Check
SOB	Shortness of breath	♀ or F	Female
STAT	Immediately	♂ or M	Male
Sx	Symptoms	↑	Increase
TCDB	Turn, cough, deep-breathe	↓	Decrease
TO	Telephone order		

TABLE 5-7 Health Care Environments

Abbreviation	Meaning	Abbreviation	Meaning
AA	Alcoholics Anonymous	HMO	Health maintenance organization
AHA	American Heart Association	ICU	Intensive care unit
AMA	American Medical Association	Lab	Laboratory
ANA	American Nurses Association	MH/MR	Mental health and mental retardation
ER	Emergency room	OB	Obstetrics
GYN	Gynecology	OR	Operating room

Practice Reading Terms

Figure 5-7 shows an order sheet with multiple abbreviations. Read the following list "for understanding" of the terms. Return to the tables for any abbreviations you cannot decipher.

- Dx: CA of the Prostate with Brain Mets.
- PET scan revealed lesion R temporal lobe.
- Hx: Chronic UTI, BPH c̄ TURP, COPD.
- Admitted to ER with c/o severe head pain x 3 wks.
- PERL, neg reflexes L upper extremity.
- 75-yo white M adm c̄ SOB.
- CXR confirmed Dx TB.
- Crushing chest pain, abnormal ECG, and ↑ enzymes supported a Dx of MI.
- 1000cc .9% NS started and IV Morphine given.
- Hyperglycemia 2° IDDM.
- FBS of 410.
- 1000 D/W administered.
- I&D post-surgical abscess.
- Hgb & Hct ordered STAT.
- MRI revealed herniated disc L$_4$.
- CDC posted guidelines for AIDS and other bloodborne pathogens; blood pH 7.25.
- EEG ordered for R/O seizure disorder.
- IPPB 4 x qd ordered following PFT.
- WBCs elevated 2° infection.
- BUN elevations indicate kidney failure.
- ABGs ordered for smoke inhalation victim in ER.
- C&S of urine revealed staph and supported R/O UTI Dx.
- H&P revealed Hx of Fx.
- PE noted ↑ BP.
- ® CVA with L hemiplegia and global aphasia.
- Rx: follow-up in home with ST, OT, PT eval.
- Adm orders—amb ad lib with BRP NPO p̄ midnight.
- Dx ASCVD c̄ + 2 pedal edema bilat extremities.
- Arrived DOA in ER. CPR initiated.
- Mandatory AA after DTs.
- The AHA recommendations for ↓ risk of CHD is to ↓ chol in diet.
- The AMA is the governing body for all MDs.
- The lab reports for PKU were ⊕.
- An ↑ sed rate indicates possible autoimmune disorder such as RA, MS, or SLE.
- IVP and Cysto were neg.
- Prevention of childhood illnesses requires MMRV and DPT vaccines as part of PED exams.

- HDL and LDL levels indicate ↑ blood lipids.
- An RD was ordered for dietary counseling.
- Lorraine Lieberman was adm with FUO R/O TSS 2° strep.
- A Dx of venereal warts 2° HPV was confirmed.
- LASER therapy reduced the lesions and provided some relief of Sx.
- A TENS unit was prescribed for the intractable pain.
- The irregular periods and dysmenorrhea required a D&C.
- Mrs. Jones was in labor 24°. The baby was breech presentation and required an emergency C-section.
- A cardiac cath revealed 90% blockage of the ® coronary artery, and the patient was scheduled for a CABG.
- AFB precautions were ordered for R/O TB.
- The IUD was ineffective in preventing pregnancy.
- DNA mutations 2° illegal drug use caused congenital anomalies.
- Autopsy confirmed SIDS as cause of death.
- TIAs may lead to CVAs.
- PID can cause sterility.
- RUQ pain can be indicative of GB disease.
- Post-op orders read: TCDB q2° and prn.
- ⊕ HIV may lead to AIDS.
- NIDDM is usually late-onset.
- URIs are common in asthmatics.
- NTG sl prn chest pain.
- The PDR is a comprehensive listing of pharmaceutical agents.
- Rx ii caps bid.
- gr X ac and HS.
- Capsaicin ung apply prn to affected areas.
- ROM to ® upper extremity qid.
- HHA to asst c̄ personal care and ADL.
- CSF was cultured and found to contain blood.
- Routine adm studies include UA, H&P, ECG, CXR, and CBC c̄ diff.
- Bx revealed no malignancy.
- Dx OBS.
- GTT to R/O IDDM.
- SSE til clear prior to BE.
- XR and CAT scan confirmed Dx of hairline Fx.
- A DO is trained to perform OMT.
- TPN was initiated because of severe malnutrition 2° ulcerative colitis.
- DRGs govern type and amount of care.

ORDER SHEET

DATE	TIME	ORDERS NOTED BY NURSE	PLEASE LIST ALL DRUG ALLERGIES AND SENSITIVITIES WHEN WRITING ADMISSION ORDERS. PLEASE CHECK DRUG ALLERGIES AND SENSITIVITIES BEFORE WRITING MEDICATION ORDERS.			
			TREATMENT ORDERS	DATE	TIME	STUDY ORDERS
			POST-OPERATIVE ORDERS: OPERATIVE DAY (PAGE 1)			Tests: ☐ EKG
			1. Admit to _____			
			Preoperative diagnosis _____			
			Postoperative diagnosis _____			
			Procedure: Status Post Carotid Endarterectomy			
			Condition _____			
			Allergies _____			
			2. ☐ Vital Signs _____			
			Call HO for SBP > _____ , < _____			
			☐ Neuro✓q1h x 6hrs, then per pathway			
			☐ Arterial line to continuous heparinized saline flush			
			3. ☐ OOB to chair by evening of surgery			
			4. Diet:			
			☐ NPO except meds today			
			☐ _____ diet for breakfast in am			
			5. ☐ I&O			
			☐ Foley to straight drainage. D/C by 8 am Post-Op day 1			
			☐ JP to bulb suction. Assess drainage _____			
			6. IV ☐ 1/2 NSS + 20mEq KCl at _____ cc/hr			
			☐ D/C IV fluids when taking PO			
			7. Meds:			
			☐ Morphine Sulfate (MSO$_4$) 2-5 mg IM/sq q3-4h prn severe pain			
			☐ Acetaminophen 650mg/Codeine 30mg (Tylenol #3) 1-2 tabs			
			q4h prn moderate pain when taking orals			
			☐ Acetaminophen (Tylenol) 650mg q4h prn mild pain when			
			taking orals			
			☐ Aspirin (ASA) 325mg PO qd. Begin am POD #1.			
			☐ Other: _____			
			_____			
			MD Signature _____		Beeper # _____	
			Name (printed) _____			

FIGURE 5-7 Order sheet.

application to practice

Understanding how words are formed—joining prefixes and suffixes to word roots—and knowing the meanings of Latin and Greek words are essential to your work as a health care practitioner. Basic medical terminology should be learned and used regularly in performing patient care and other tasks assigned to you. Use the information presented in this chapter to help you resolve the problems in the situations that follow.

Learning Activities

Situation 1: You are going to attend a seminar to upgrade your skills. The topic is patient care for tracheostomy. What is a tracheostomy?

Author's Explanation: A tracheostomy is an opening made in the trachea, or windpipe. A surgical procedure is used to make the opening.

Situation 2: What is the difference between tracheotomy and tracheostomy?

Author's Explanation: A tracheotomy is an incision into the trachea. It may be performed as an emergency procedure to open the airway. A tracheostomy is a permanent opening that is made in the trachea. *OS-* means "hole," "mouth," or "opening."

Situation 3: When might a patient have a tracheostomy?

Author's Explanation: A patient might have a tracheostomy when the upper airways are permanently obstructed or when the patient requires extended care on a ventilator.

Situation 4: Today you are pulled to the urology floor. Where are you going?

Author's Explanation: You are going to the specialty area for diseases of the urinary tract. The word *urology* means "study of urine."

Situation 5: The first patient report you receive is about Mr. Harrison, who has a suprapubic cystotomy. What is this?

Author's Explanation: A suprapubic cystotomy is an incision into the bladder above the pubis.

Situation 6: The next patient had chronic nephritis and is now on hemodialysis. What is nephritis?

Author's Explanation: Nephritis is an inflammation of the kidneys. *Chronic* means "long-term." Therefore, the patient's kidney function has declined.

Situation 7: What is hemodialysis?

Author's Explanation: *Hemodialysis* literally means "breakdown of blood through." It is a procedure that removes impurities from the blood through a machine. It attempts to replace the normal function of the kidney.

Situation 8: Mr. Byrns, a longtime resident of your nursing home, was taken to the hospital for surgery of a malignant melanoma L shoulder. What is melanoma?

Author's Explanation: *Melanoma* literally means "black tumor." It is a form of skin cancer that develops from the pigmented cells, or melanocytes. It generally manifests from a wart or mole. The surgical treatment involves a wide excision of the lesion and a skin graft from the buttock or thigh over the deep wound.

Situation 9: According to hospital records, Mrs. McCartney is a 43-yo W ♀ adm c̄ severe pain RLQ, N&V, R/O appendicitis." What does this mean to you?

Author's Explanation: Mrs. McCartney is a forty-three-year-old white female admitted with severe pain in the right lower quadrant of her abdomen, nausea and vomiting. The physician is ruling out appendicitis, which means that it could be another cause, but he suspects—according to the symptoms—that her appendix is inflamed.

Situation 10: Mrs. Sandeler has just returned "p̄ a l Lobectomy for carcinoma." What is a lobectomy? What is carcinoma?

Author's Explanation: A lobectomy is the removal of one of the lobes of the lung. *Carcinoma* means "cancerous tumor."

Situation 11: Is carcinoma malignant?

Author's Explanation: Yes. *Cancer, carcinoma, malignancy,* and *neoplasm* are general synonyms.

Situation 12: You received this A.M. report from the nurse: "Mr. Lennon a 75 yo was adm last night c̄ c/o severe dyspnea, + pedal edema, and bibasilar rales. Dx R/O CHF. He is on cont O_2 @ 2 l/min. via nasal cannula. He requires pulse check at 9 A.M. Report results STAT to RN. He can be OOB ad lib c̄ BRP. HOB ↑ 45° at all times. He has a Hx of COPD." What should you do for Mr. Lennon today?

Author's Explanation: Mr. Lennon is short of breath, has fluid accumulation in his feet, and has fluid in the base of his lungs. The doctor thinks he has congestive heart failure. He is on oxygen administered through a nasal tube, and he is receiving 2 liters per minute. He requires a pulse check that must be reported immediately to the nurse. He can be out of bed as desired and has bathroom privileges. The head of his bed must be elevated at a 45° angle. He has a history of chronic obstructive pulmonary disease.

Situation 13: The nurse informs you to check the nursing chart for an update on the patient's nursing orders and ADL status. This is what you find: "NG tube to suction, NPO, c̄ sips of H_2O, IV ® arm, BR. What does this mean to you?

Author's Explanation: The patient has a nasogastric (pertaining to the nose and stomach) tube, nothing by mouth, with sips of water, intravenous in right arm, and bedrest.

Situation 14: Mr. Stark is "adm with oliguria, hematuria, and dysuria. IVP reveals pyelonephritis." What does this mean?

Author's Explanation: Mr. Stark has scanty amounts of urine formation, blood in the urine, and painful urination. The intravenous (in the vein) pyelogram record of the kidney basin shows inflammation of the kidneys and kidney basin.

Situation 15: You took a position with a MH/MR agency as a residential supervisor of three males in a halfway house. All the clients are in their fifties. One client has acromegaly, one has dyskinesia, and one is dysphasic. What can you expect from each one?

Author's Explanation: *ACRO-* means "extremities," and *-megaly* means "enlarged." This client has

enlarged extremities (hands and feet). (This condition is generally associated with tumors of the pituitary and is an endocrine dysfunction.) *Dys-* means "difficult," *KINESI-* means "movement," and *-a* is a polisher suffix. (The client's placement is probably due to a medication side effect.) *Dys-* means "difficult," *PHASO-* means "speech," and *-ic* means "pertaining to."

Situation 16: Since acromegaly enlarges the extremities, including the hands and feet, what problems might this client suffer?

Author's Explanation: He might have difficulties with fine motor skills if his fingers and toes are enlarged.

Situation 17: As a HHA, you are called by the nursing supervisor to cover four Medicare cases today. The nurse gives you a telephone order (TO) and tells you to check the care plan in each home. The first client suffers from IDDM. What disease is this?

Author's Explanation: *IDDM* stands for "insulin-dependent diabetes mellitus."

Situation 18: She requires asst c̄ transfer to shower. What are you expected to do?

Author's Explanation: Help the patient to take a shower.

Situation 19: She tells you to avoid bumping her legs because she suffers from polyneuropathy. From your understanding of medical terminology, what is this?

Author's Explanation: *Poly-* means "many," *NEURO-* means "nerve," and *-pathy* means "disease." Polyneuropathy is a disease of many nerves. (It generally involves the peripheral nerves of the extremities, which decreases sensation in the limbs. This can increase the risk of injury without the patient's knowledge.)

Situation 20: The second case is a "L CVA c̄ ® hemiplegia and aphasia. He is being seen by PT, ST, OT, RN, and HHA." What does this mean, and who is following the client at home?

Author's Explanation: This patient had a stroke (CVA) that caused right-sided paralysis (hemiplegia). In addition, the client is without speech (aphasia). He is being followed by a physical therapist, a speech therapist, an occupational therapist, a registered nurse, and a home health aide.

Situation 21: The care plan in the home states that the HHA is to assist with ROM. What does this mean?

Author's Explanation: The client is to be assisted with range-of-motion exercises by the home health aide.

Situation 22: The third case is a client "c̄ a colostomy 2° colorectal CA." What does this tell you?

Author's Explanation: The client has a new bowel opening, or a new opening was formed in the colon. The reason the colostomy was formed is because of cancer of the large intestine/rectum.

Situation 23: The fourth client is being followed by home care after an acute anterolateral myocardial infarction with subsequent necrosis. What does *anterolateral* mean? What does *myocardial* mean? What is *infarction*? What is *necrosis*?

Author's Explanation: *Anterolateral* means "pertaining to the front and the side." *Myocardial* refers to the heart muscle. *Infarction* is a part of an organ that undergoes tissue death. *Necrosis* means "condition of death."

Examination Review Questions

1. A prefix is found at the _____ of a word.
   - a. beginning
   - b. end
   - c. middle
   - d. foundation

2. A prefix that means "without" is
   - a. *an-*
   - b. *in-*
   - c. *anti-*
   - d. *hypo-*

3. The suffix *-y* means
   - a. instrument
   - b. condition
   - c. process
   - d. disease

4. The word root *PHAG* refers to
   - a. paralysis
   - b. eating
   - c. disease
   - d. speech

5. *Hypoglycemia* refers to
   - a. low blood sugar
   - b. high blood pressure
   - c. overactive pituitary
   - d. lack of sleep

6. Inflammation around the heart is
   - a. epicardium
   - b. pericarditis
   - c. endocardial
   - d. myocardosis

7. The abbreviation for "pupils are equal and reactive to light" is
   - a. PID
   - b. METS
   - c. PKU
   - d. PERL

8. The symbol for potassium is
   - a. P
   - b. pH
   - c. Ps
   - d. K

9. The common name for *CVA* is
   - a. heart attack
   - b. stroke
   - c. cardiac arrest
   - d. bypass

10. Removal of the stomach is
    - a. stomatotomy
    - b. gastrotome
    - c. gastrectomy
    - d. stomatostomy

The Body Human

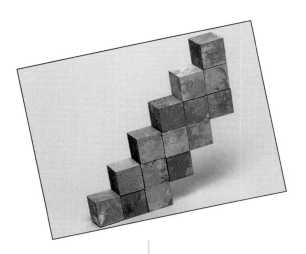

In this unit, you will be introduced to the study of the human body. The human body is a marvelously resilient and immensely capable life-form. It is more complex than the most sophisticated computer ever built, and our knowledge about the way it functions is constantly increasing. This unit will examine each system of the human body. It will provide you with information that will help you to gain an understanding of the structure and function of these systems in health and disease. Your study will help you to develop a greater awareness and appreciation of your patients' conditions, the significance of your observations, and the purpose and principles underlying your actions in providing care.

Chapter 6

The Body as a Whole

There are two sciences involved in the study of all living organisms: *anatomy* and *physiology*. **Anatomy** is the study of the structure of an organism. **Physiology** is the study of the function of an organism. An **organism** is a life-form, a living being that is made of many structures that are dependent on one another. You are an organism. All of the structures in your body relate to one another, and they work together to function as a whole human being.

Take, for example, a car. A car has many parts, or components, within it. Each part has a name, and each part belongs to the car's reference system—the electrical system, the exhaust system, and the fuel system. Each part is made of some kind of material specific to the structure and function of that part. Each system of the car, along with the parts that make up that system, provides a valuable and unique function. Each system must function properly for the car to run.

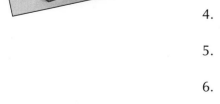

OBJECTIVES

After completing this chapter, you will be able to

1. Distinguish between the sciences of anatomy and physiology
2. Describe the structural units approach of the body
3. Discuss the structures and functions of the main parts of the cell
4. List the four types of tissues found in the body
5. List the systems of the human body
6. List the organs of each body system
7. Describe the function of each body system
8. Define the anatomical directions
9. Locate the cavities of the body
10. Name the organs in each body cavity
11. Name the quadrants
12. Define and spell all key terms correctly

k e y   t e r m s

anatomy	genes	organelles
anterior (ventral)	genetic code	organism
cell	genetic material	organs
cell membrane	hormones	physiology
chromosomes	inferior	posterior (dorsal)
connective	lateral	quadrants
cytoplasm	medial	superior
DNA	mitosis	system
endocrine glands	muscular	tissue
epithelial	nervous	
flagella	nucleus	

Structural Units

In the study of human anatomy, the most useful method for identifying structures is based on the *structural units approach*. The structural units approach is based on four levels of detail: *cell, tissue, organ,* and *system* (Figure 6-1).

Cells

The body is composed of millions of microscopic units called cells. The **cell** is the basic building block of all organisms. (The word *cell* is derived from the word root *cell/o,* meaning "hidden chamber.") Until the nineteenth century when the microscope was

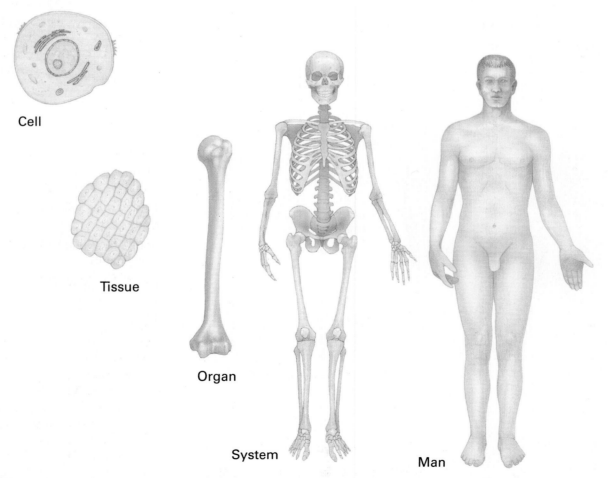

Cell

Tissue

Organ

System

Man

FIGURE 6-1   The four structural units on which all living organisms are based: cell, tissue, organ, and system.

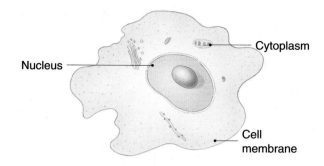

FIGURE 6-2 Cell structure.

developed, the cell was hidden from scientists. The cell was nature's little secret. Each animal cell is composed of three main structures: the *cell membrane*, the *nucleus*, and the *cytoplasm* (Figure 6-2).

Cell Membrane

The **cell membrane** acts as a *boundary* between the contents of the cell and the environment outside. The cell membrane allows substances like glucose (sugar), oxygen, and water to enter the interior of the cell, and it permits waste products like carbon dioxide to leave the cell. The membrane is the cell's interface with the world around it; all interactions with the environment inside and outside of the cell involve some part of the membrane. The cell membrane is *selective* in the substances it permits to enter and to leave the cell. For example, brain cells allow substances that are *fat-soluble* to enter, and they do not allow water-soluble substances to enter. This means that medications that enter brain cells must be able "to mix" and "to dissolve" in a fatty environment. Think of what results when you pour a teaspoon of oil in a glass of water. The oil beads up on the top surface of the water; it does not dissolve. On the other hand, sugar, salt, and other substances would eventually dissolve or mix evenly throughout the glass of water.

Nucleus

The **nucleus** is often called the *brain* of the cell because it directs all of the cellular activities. You can also imagine the nucleus as a "reference library" because of all of the information that it stores. Inside the nucleus is a "file" of information that contains the **genetic material** for that particular cell. This genetic material is called **DNA**. The DNA molecule is shaped like a *twisted ladder*. The matching pieces on each step of the ladder are amino acids that form a **genetic code**, much like a credit card code or a personal identification number. DNA serves as a blueprint for the cell, enabling it to duplicate itself and produce an exact replica. DNA also provides the information the cell

needs to carry out its life functions. DNA is the material of which **genes** are composed. Genes contain the heritage of each organism passed on to individuals by their ancestors. Genes are our anatomical and physiological inheritance.

If you have blue eyes, you inherited these blue eyes because during your conception, you received the blue eye gene from your mother and your father. Every aspect of your appearance is the result of the genetic information given to you by your parents. Unless you are an identical twin, there is no one in the world with the same genetic code as you. Even your brothers and sisters do not have the exact genetic code that you have. While you and your siblings may look and act alike and even have the same diseases or conditions, you are the result of a unique alignment (matching) of your parent's genetic information.

Genes align themselves along structures called **chromosomes**. In every cell of the body, there are twenty-three pairs of chromosomes. When cells reproduce themselves, they pass on the full complement of twenty-three chromosome pairs. This process is called **mitosis**. However, sex cells (eggs and sperm) contain only half of the genetic information. The egg from the female carries twenty-three chromosomes, and the sperm from the male carries twenty-three chromosomes. When these two cells unite and the egg is fertilized, the result is an offspring with twenty-three chromosomes from each parent, or twenty-three pairs of chromosomes. Figure 6-3 illustrates DNA and chromosome pairs.

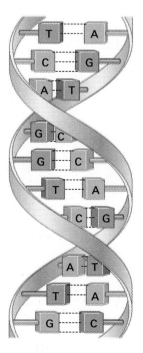

FIGURE 6-3 DNA and chromosome pairs.

Cytoplasm

The **cytoplasm** of the cell is a jellylike substance outside of the nucleus and within the cell's membrane. The cytoplasm contains water, minerals, and little organs called **organelles**. The organelles are the structures that carry out digestive, respiratory, and circulatory functions. Organelles also carry out metabolic functions; that is, they build up and break down molecules of fat, protein, and carbohydrates to produce or release energy for the cell, to manufacture new substances, and to construct daughter cells.

The cell is the fundamental unit of life. Nothing smaller than a cell is truly living—that is, capable of independent existence within its environment and of self-replication. Cells are highly specialized in their structure and functions. In the human body, there are more than two hundred different types of cells. They can be categorized into *three* main groups, according to their pattern of reproducing (Figure 6-4).

The cells in the first group, including muscle and nerve cells, usually do not reproduce, although they are able to repair themselves if their genetic informa-tion is not damaged. The cells in the second group have a moderate ability to divide if damaged through disease or injury. Hepatocytes (cells of the liver) are in this group. The third group contains cells that actively replicate because they are continually lost or have a naturally short life span. Blood cells and skin cells are included in this third group. Red blood cells live approximately 120 days, and skin cells are shed constantly from the surface of the skin. To keep up with the process, new cells are reproduced continually.

In the human body, cells are classified by their appearance and function. In fact, the structure of a cell, tissue, or organ can determine its function, and vice versa. For example, red blood cells (RBCs) are concave in shape; that is, they have a depressed (sunken in) surface designed to carry oxygen and carbon dioxide throughout the body. Sperm cells have long, whiplike "tails" called **flagella** that help them to move (swim) through fluid to get to their destination. They must leave the male body and move through the female body into the pelvic cavity to fertilize the egg in order to reproduce.

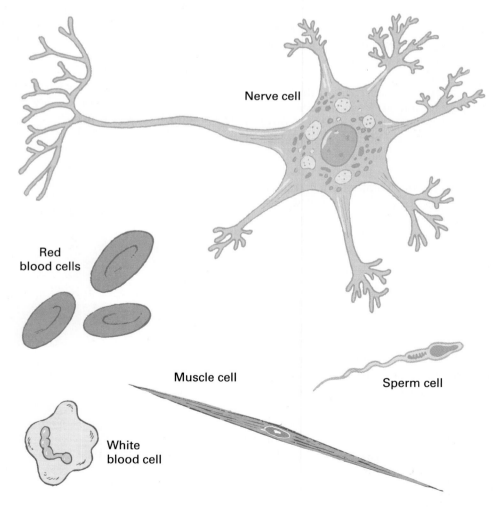

FIGURE 6-4 Cells grouped by their reproductive nature.

Tissues

Cells of similar function unite to form tissues. A **tissue** is a combination of cells that carries out a specific function. The structure and function of tissues are closely related.

Types of Tissues

Tissues are distinguished from one another on the basis of differing textures, composition and arrangement, and properties. There are four principle types of tissues: *epithelial, connective, muscular,* and *nervous.* An example of each type is shown in Figure 6-5.

- **Epithelial** tissue is found in the skin, in the lining of the digestive tract, and in glands. Epithelial tissue is designed to secrete and to absorb substances. What does the skin secrete? The skin secretes sweat and oil. Many substances are absorbed by cells that line the digestive organs: water, salts, nutrients, and vitamins, for example. This lining secretes digestive juices, such as hydrochloric acid and various enzymes, which are needed to break down food. For the cell membrane to absorb nutrients and for the organelles to use these nutrients for cellular activity, they must be broken down into very small substances called *molecules.*

- **Connective** tissue includes the fibrous tissue that holds the body together. Cartilage, tendons, and bones are made of connective tissue. The fat found in the body is made of a type of connective tissue called *adipose tissue.* Adipose tissue supports and protects organs like the kidneys, which are surrounded by a capsule of this fatty tissue. Connective tissue is found in many body structures because it holds other tissues together or because it connects different types of tissues that make up the organs of the body.

- **Muscular** tissue is composed of special cells that are designed to contract or to pull together to produce movement. In fact, muscular tissue is responsible for all of the movements of the body. It is found in the blood vessels, digestive organs, and heart and on the skeleton. Muscular tissue is classified by its appearance, location, and function.

- **Nervous** tissue, the fourth type of tissue, is composed of nerve cells called *neurons.* This highly specialized type of tissue is designed to receive messages from the environment, to send messages to the brain, and to direct and control the reactions of the body. Nerve cells have structures that extend from the body of the nerve cell to receive and deliver messages throughout every surface of the body. All voluntary and involuntary actions of the body and all perceptions (the senses of hearing, touch, taste, smell, and vision) are under the control of nervous tissue.

Organs

Tissues are joined together to form organs. Most **organs** are made of several types of tissues. For example, the stomach is composed of muscle tissue, connective tissue, and epithelial tissue; and it is controlled by nervous tissue. Tissues are arranged to form a particular structure and to produce a particular function. Every organ in the body has a unique structure or appearance. The structure is related to the specific function or to the many functions that the organ is capable of producing.

The skin, which is both an organ and a system of the body, is designed to release heat through the secretion of sweat and to absorb and hold heat in the body. Which type of tissue is responsible for this function of the skin? You are correct if you remembered that it is epithelial tissue. The skin also has muscle fibers that help it in the function of regulating body temperature. What happens to your skin when you are cold? You get goose bumps because the muscle fibers contract to pull the tissues closer together to keep the heat in your body. The skin is very elastic. It stretches around the skeletal muscles of the body, and it stretches as our bodies grow in length and width. Sometimes, the skin is left with scars from stretching beyond the capacity of its elasticity, and then stretch marks are present. The skin is also an organ of perception. It is a sense organ that makes you aware of touch, temperature, texture, and pressure. What type of tissue has this function? Nerve fibers present throughout the surface of the body allow us to feel through the nervous tissue in the skin. Connective tissue unites the tissues of the skin, and adipose tissue cushions the skin.

Systems

The highest-level structural unit that is used for reference is a system. A body **system** is made of various organs that act together to produce specific functions of the body. The organs of a body system may be located close to one another or scattered throughout the body.

The organs of the digestive system are connected and form a long tube called the *alimentary canal.* These organs, which digest food, begin at the mouth and end at the anus. This long tube is composed of smooth muscle and is lined with a mucous membrane capable of absorbing and secreting substances in the process of digestion. Other organs outside of the alimentary canal assist in the digestion of food. These are called *accessory organs,* and they include the liver, gallbladder, and pancreas.

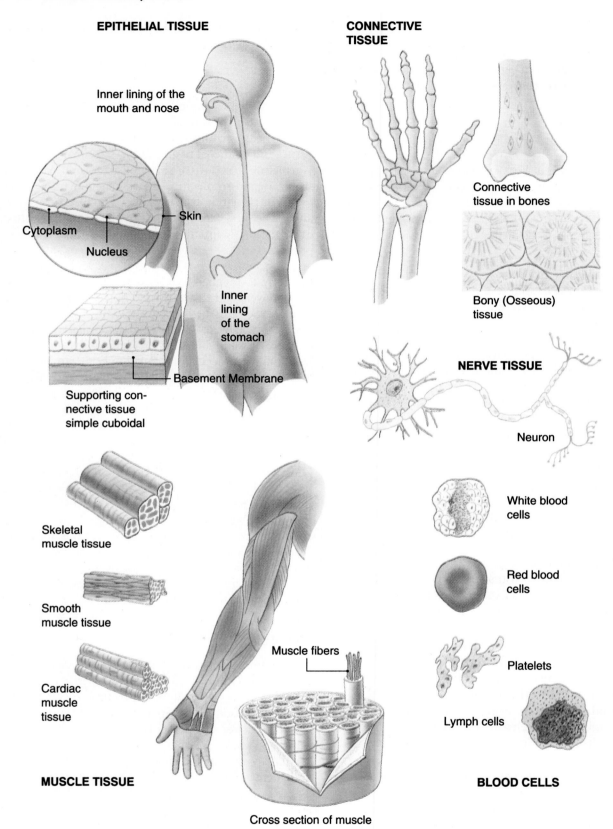

EPITHELIAL TISSUE

Inner lining of the mouth and nose

Cytoplasm

Nucleus

Skin

Inner lining of the stomach

Basement Membrane

Supporting connective tissue simple cuboidal

CONNECTIVE TISSUE

Connective tissue in bones

Bony (Osseous) tissue

NERVE TISSUE

Neuron

White blood cells

Red blood cells

Platelets

Lymph cells

BLOOD CELLS

Skeletal muscle tissue

Smooth muscle tissue

Cardiac muscle tissue

Muscle fibers

MUSCLE TISSUE

Cross section of muscle

FIGURE 6-5   Four types of tissues.

The nervous system is scattered throughout the body and extends to every part of the body. The main organs of this system are the brain and spinal cord, which are connected, but divisions of this system send nervous messages to every organ.

The endocrine system is composed of organs called **endocrine glands**, which are located in the brain, abdomen, pelvis, neck, and chest. (*Endo-* is a prefix meaning "within" or "inside.") Endocrine glands secrete chemicals called **hormones** directly into the bloodstream. These glands are different from exocrine glands (*exo-* means "outside" or "outer"), which secrete substances outside of the bloodstream. Saliva is produced in the exocrine glands called *salivary glands.* It is secreted from the salivary glands into the mouth. The endocrine system is responsible for many functions in the body. Even though these organs are spread throughout the body, they work together and relate to one another by their chemical messengers, **hormones**.

Table 6-1 lists the systems of the body human, identifies the organ or organs that make up each system, and describes the function or functions of each system.

Anatomical Systems of Reference

Anatomists use special terms to refer to the location, direction, and position of body structures. The human body is so complex that we need systems of reference to aid us in rapidly and accurately identifying and locating the part of the body or organ being described. Figure 6-6 identifies anatomical directions used in referring to the body.

TABLE 6-1   Systems of the Body Human

System	Organ	Function
Integumentary	Skin	Regulation of body temperature, organ of sensation
Skeletal	Bones	Protection of internal organs, movement, framework of body, production of blood cells, support
Muscular	Skeletal muscles	Movement, posture, production of heat
Nervous	Brain, spinal cord, nerves	Coordination, control of body functions, perception and sensation
Cardiovascular	Heart, blood vessels, blood, lymph nodes and vessels	Circulation
Respiratory	Lungs, larynx, bronchi, trachea, nose, pharynx	Respiration
Digestive (gastrointestinal)	Stomach, mouth, colon, small intestine, liver, gallbladder, pancreas, esophagus	Absorption of nutrients, excretion of waste
Urinary	Kidney, bladder, ureters, urethra	Excretion of waste, production of urine
Reproductive	Testes, penis, ovaries, uterus, fallopian tubes, breasts, vagina, seminal glands	Reproduction of the species
Endocrine	Pituitary, adrenal, thymus, thyroid, parathyroid glands; pancreas, testes, ovaries	Production of hormones

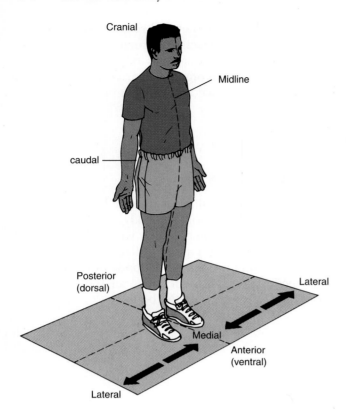

FIGURE 6-6 Anatomical directions.

Anatomical Directions

Directional terms describe anatomical direction and identify whether some body part is above, below, on the side, or in the middle. **Superior** means "above" or refers to the upper portion of the body or of an organ. What is the most superior structure of the human body? The head is the most superior part of the body. The neck is superior to the shoulders. **Inferior** means "below" or refers to the lowermost portion. The neck is inferior to the head, and the ankle is inferior to the knee.

Anterior and **ventral** refer to the front side of the body or structure. Ventral refers specifically to the belly side of an animal. The breasts and the belly are on the anterior surface of the human body. How would you locate a dog's anterior, or ventral, surface? The anterior surface of four-legged animals faces the ground when they stand on all four legs.

Posterior and **dorsal** refer to the back side of the body or structure. The buttocks and spine are on the posterior surface of the body. When you pet a dog by stroking its back, what surface are you touching? You can feel the dog's spine, so it is the posterior surface.

The term **medial** refers to the middle or midline. The term **lateral** refers to the side. These directional terms are described when the body is in

anatomical position, standing erect with the palms up (see Figure 6-6).

You will hear these terms used in describing diagnostic and surgical procedures. When an x-ray technician takes a chest x-ray, the pictures are taken from posterior to anterior and lateral surfaces of the thorax (chest cavity). The doctor's order would be written, "Chest X-ray PA & Lateral."

Reference Cavities

The second set of reference terms describes the cavities (spaces) of the body. Think of a hatchback car. The ventral cavity houses the motor, and the dorsal cavity is the trunk. Figure 6-7 shows the position of the ventral and dorsal cavities of the human body and identifies the smaller cavities within each.

Ventral Cavity

The ventral cavity is divided into three smaller cavities: thoracic, abdominal, and pelvic. The chest is called the *thoracic cavity*, or the *thorax*. The lungs, esophagus, and heart are located in the thoracic

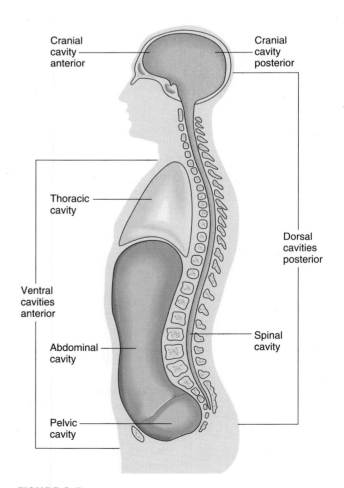

FIGURE 6-7 Body cavities.

cavity. The diaphragm, the large muscle that aids the lungs in the mechanics of breathing, separates this cavity from the abdomen. The *abdominal cavity* contains the organs of the digestive system and the kidneys. The *pelvic cavity* houses the bladder, the reproductive organs, and parts of the intestine. There is no physical boundary between the abdominal and pelvic cavities. Sometimes, the two together are called the *abdominopelvic cavity*.

Dorsal Cavity

This posterior cavity is divided into two cavities: cranial and spinal. The *cranial cavity*, or the *cranium*, contains the brain. The *spinal cavity* contains the spinal cord.

Quadrants

Imaginary lines can be drawn horizontally and vertically to separate the abdomen into four areas called **quadrants**. These quadrants can be used to designate organ location, pain, or lesions across the abdomen. The axes (the horizontal and vertical lines) pass through the umbilicus (navel or belly button). Figure 6-8 illustrates the quadrants of the abdominal cavity.

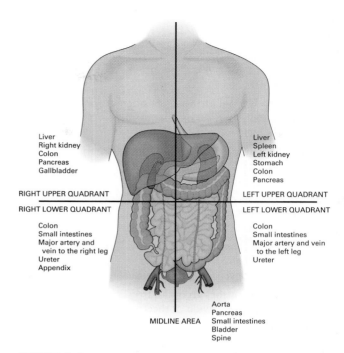

FIGURE 6-8   Quadrants of the abdominal cavity.

---

application to practice

Learning Activities

Situation 1: Your patient has right upper quadrant pain. Exactly where is his pain?

Author's Explanation: Draw an imaginary line vertically and horizontally over the abdomen through the umbilicus to create 4 equal areas. These areas are called quadrants. Therefore, the top right area is the right upper quadrant. There are several major organs located in this quadrant including the liver and gallbladder.

Situation 2: The physician's order reads for a posterior/lateral x-ray of the thorax. What body part will be x-rayed?

Author's Explanation: The thorax is the chest. Posterior means back and lateral means side. Therefore, the chest will be X-rayed from the back and side.

Situation 3: The lateral bone of the forearm is fractured at the distal end of the bone. Exactly where has this fracture occurred?

Author's Explanation: When the body is in anatomic position, the palms are facing up. The radius runs along the thumb side of the hand. Therefore, the radius is the lateral bone. The distal end is the point furthest away from the point of origin. The point of origin is the shoulder. Therefore, the radius bone is broken closest to the wrist.

Situation 4: A patient is told that a mass was found in the pelvic cavity. Where is this mass?

Author's Explanation: The pelvic cavity is inferior or below the abdominal cavity and lies behind the pubic bone. It houses the reproductive and urinary organs. The mass is somewhere behind the pubic bones between the hips.

Situation 5: You are instructed to swab a patient's wound for cytology studies. What laboratory will receive this specimen?

Author's Explanation: You will send the specimen to the lab department that studies and analyzes cells.

Examination Review Questions

1. Which organ is housed in the thoracic cavity?
   a. intestines   c. brain
   b. spinal cord   d. heart

2. Which of the following is considered a dorsal cavity?
   a. cranial   c. abdominal
   b. thoracic   d. pelvic

3. The appendix is located in which quadrant?
   a. RUQ   c. LUQ
   b. RLQ   d. LLQ

4. The ____ is considered to be the "brain" of the cell.
   a. membrane   c. DNA
   b. nucleus   d. cytoplasm

5. The tissue found in the glands is
   a. epithelial   c. muscle
   b. connective   d. nervous

6. What distinguishes an organ from a tissue?
   a. An organ is made of the same tissue.
   b. A tissue is made of different cells.
   c. An organ is made of different tissue.
   d. A tissue is structurally more complex.

7. Which body system produces hormones?
   a. respiratory   c. endocrine
   b. nervous   d. circulatory

8. The neck is anatomically _____ to the shoulders.
   a. inferior   c. dorsal
   b. superior   d. ventral

9. Genes are composed of
   a. chromosomes   c. mitosis
   b. DNA   d. cytoplasm

10. The nervous system is responsible for
    a. excretion   c. respiration
    b. reproduction   d. coordination

C h a p t e r   7

The Skin

The skin is considered to be both an organ and a system. The system is referred to as the **integumentary system**. The skin is the largest organ of the body. It covers approximately 1.6 to 1.9 square meters of surface in the average-size adult. The weight of this amount of skin is about 20 pounds, and this makes it the heaviest organ of the body. Numerous structures interact in each square inch of skin. The skin is a marvel in its design. For example, consider your little finger, which is composed of thousands of cells. Fitting into this tiny structure are sweat glands, nerve endings, blood vessels, oil glands, and hair follicles.

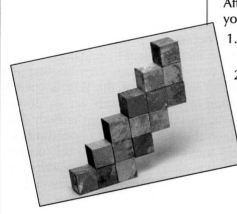

OBJECTIVES

After completing this chapter, you will be able to

1. Name the structures of the integumentary system
2. Describe the functions of the integumentary system
3. Describe the common conditions and diseases of the integumentary system
4. List the observations about the skin that you should report to the nurse
5. Apply your knowledge of the skin to problem-solving strategies in care delivery
6. Define and spell all key terms correctly

	key terms	
acne	duoderm	melanin
arrectores pilorum	epidermis	psoriasis
cyanosis	first-degree burns	second-degree burns
decubitus ulcers	hives	third-degree burns
dermis	integumentary system	

Structures of the Skin

The skin is composed of two distinct kinds of tissues. The outer surface, or *epidermis,* is made up of several layers of epithelial tissue. (The prefix *epi-* means "upon," and the word root *derm-* means "skin.") The second layer of skin is called the *dermis.* The dermis is made of connective tissue.

Epidermis

The **epidermis** is composed of cells that reproduce continually because they are shed continually each day. As you learned in Chapter 6, the third type of cells that reproduce continually is the skin cell. Epidermal cells are also the cells that generate the color of the skin. A chemical called **melanin** determines the color of a person's skin. The more melanin your skin cells produce, the darker the color of your skin. Melanin production is stimulated by a hormone called the *melanocyte-stimulating hormone,* which is produced in the pituitary gland. This hormone is released in relation to one's exposure to sunlight. And genetically, by your DNA history, it predetermines your skin color. If you are Caucasian, you will notice the burn or tan of your skin when it is exposed to ultraviolet (UV) sun rays. People who have more melanin may not appear to change color so easily, but their skin generates more melanin, and dark-skinned people sunburn, too. What should everyone use when he or she is going to be in the direct UV rays of the sun? Sunscreens help to protect the skin from these damaging rays. Also, certain medications will make one more vulnerable to the ultraviolet rays of the sun and will create severe sunburn when the skin is exposed to the sun for even short periods of time.

Dermis

The **dermis** is composed of connective tissue. In the dermis, cells are scattered about, with many elastic fibers between them. Some of the skin cells of the dermis store fat. Dermal fat cells and elastic fibers usually decrease with age, and this causes wrinkles in the skin. The dermis is rich in tiny blood vessels called "capillaries." The dermis also contains hair follicles, sweat glands, nerves, and oil (sebaceous) glands. Small involuntary muscle fibers are also present in the dermis.

Oil glands help to moisturize the hair follicles and the epidermis. Sweat glands help to cool the skin surface by releasing sweat (water and salts). The palms, the soles of the feet, the scalp, and the armpits contain at least three thousand sweat glands per square inch. Muscle fibers help to keep the heat in the body. These fibers are called **arrectores pilorum**, which is Latin for "erectors of hair." Think of your skin's reaction to cold and to some emotions, especially fear and anger. Have you ever been so angry that your hair stood on end? Nerve cells help to keep us aware of many sensations in the environment.

Figure 7-1 shows a cross section of the skin.

Functions of the Skin

The skin is often called the "body's first line of defense." This is because it protects us in so many ways. Skin that is intact (uncut or undamaged) protects us against pathogens, those microbes that produce infection. The surface of the skin is covered with many microorganisms, which act to destroy these pathogens, thereby protecting the body from infections. When the skin is cut, an opportunity exists for helpful microbes and harmful microorganisms to enter and produce infections. The skin helps also to prevent the entrance of harmful chemicals.

The skin helps to control body temperature through the evaporation of sweat, which decreases body temperature; and the contraction of tiny muscle fibers in the skin helps to contain heat in the body. Also, fluid volume is controlled partially by sweating because sweat contains water and salt. Changes in the volume of blood flow to the skin help to maintain body temperature and blood pressure. The nerve cells of the skin alert the body of dangers and pleasures in the environment. The melanin in the skin protects us by preventing the harmful rays of the sun from entering the interior of the body. However, exposure to the sun is damaging because of these UV rays.

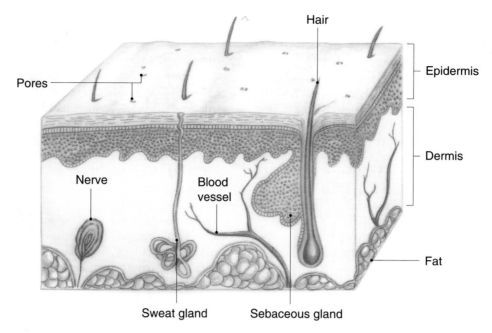

FIGURE 7-1   A cross section of the skin.

Common Conditions and Diseases of the Skin

Acne is an inflammatory disease of the sebaceous glands. Acne is commonly referred to as pimples. Acne generally appears in the areas with the richest oily secretions, such as the face, neck, upper chest, back, and shoulders. It usually develops in puberty and adolescence but can continue in adulthood.

Hives is a skin condition that usually develops as the result of an allergic reaction to foods, medications, and products applied to the skin. Hives appear as raised patches that are white in the center and raised at the edges of the wheal. Hives create severe itching. They may be the first sign of an allergy and indicate that the food, medication, or product must be avoided to prevent a more severe allergic reaction.

Psoriasis is a chronic inflammatory disease that is not infectious or contagious. The cause is unknown. The inflammatory response produces redness and dries with white or silver patches of scaly or flaky skin.

Burns are described in degrees of injury to the layers of the skin (Figure 7-2). Superficial burns (**first-degree burns**) involve injury to the epidermis only. Sunburn, which appears as redness at the surface, is an example of a first-degree burn. Partial-thickness burns (**second-degree burns**) involve injury to the dermis and are characterized by blisters on the surface. Full-thickness burns (**third-degree burns**) involve injury of the epidermis, dermis, and underlying tissues, with complete destruction of all layers of the skin.

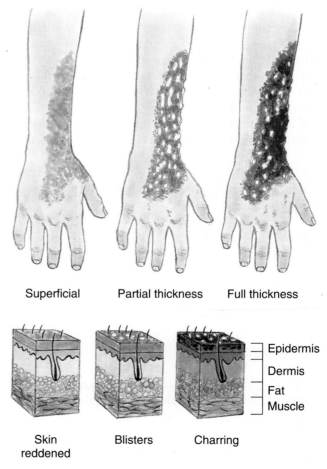

FIGURE 7-2   Severity of burns.

application to practice

The clinical care associate is the person who most often has the opportunity to prevent trauma to the skin by efficient care. The clinical care associate is also the person who has the greatest opportunity to observe the skin and report any findings. The nurse counts on the clinical care associate to care for the patient's skin and to report any observations that indicate a change in the patient's condition. What you see and feel are essential to the care of the skin. You are the first line of defense in the protection of the patient's skin.

Consider the following situations, using the information that you learned about the structure and function of the skin.

Learning Activities

Situation 1: What will you need to know about your clients/residents when you plan to take them on a picnic? Think of the resident of a long-term care (LTC) facility who is fair and bald. How will you protect his skin?

Author's Explanation: Be sure to apply sunscreen to the skin, and encourage the resident to wear a hat. Sunglasses should also be worn when a person will be outside in bright sunlight. Even with these protective measures, your clients should not be exposed to the sun and heat for any extended period of time. Even on cloudy days, the harmful rays of the sun can cause damage to the skin. Patients with dark skin should also wear sun protection.

Situation 2: Would you need to know if any residents are particularly sensitive to the sun (photosensitive)?

Author's Explanation: Yes. Some medications make the skin especially sensitive to the sun, and a person may get a sunburn in a very short period of time. You will need to ask the nurse about residents who should avoid any exposure to the sun. Medications like birth control pills, sulfa drugs, antidepressants, and antipsychotics cause the side effect of photosensitivity.

Situation 3: If you were to take residents in your LTC facility to a picnic on a hot summer day, you would need to consider another potential risk. This risk is not related to the UV rays of the sun, but the effects of heat. What would you observe about the skin in relation to being outdoors on a summer day?

Author's Explanation: You would notice redness or increased skin color and sweating. The skin would also feel warm. However, if the person has been sweating profusely, you would find that the skin is clammy, maybe even cool as the sweat evaporates. Always ask the nurse about any special precautions or instructions when you take clients to outdoor activities, especially in the heat. Excess loss of water and salts from the body can affect the heart, blood pressure, the kidneys, and even the brain.

The loss of salt and water from the body can cause dehydration. Dehydration can affect the conduction system of the heart and lead to abnormal beats in the rhythm of the heart. Loss of water and salts from the body can lead to abnormal nervous activity in the brain. Careful observation of the skin may help you to see the signs of potential dehydration. Watch for excessive sweating, and do not fail to replace this fluid loss. Fluids can be replaced with water or juice. Talk with the dietitian or nutritionist at your facility about proper fluid replacement. Alcohol-containing beverages and caffeinated drinks, such as coffee, tea, and soda, are not good choices for fluid replacement since alcohol and caffeine increase the loss of water from the kidneys.

Situation 4: As you rub a client's dark skin with a white washcloth, the washcloth becomes darker. What do you think about this effect? This is more apparent when the client's skin is very dark. Why?

Author's Explanation: This is not an abnormal event. Epidermal cells are exfoliated (shed) when you rub the surface of the skin. This is not noticeable in fair-skinned people. However, skin cells are continually rubbed away in all people, and they continually reproduce new cells.

Situation 5: In your work, you should always notice the patient's skin color and any changes in it. What would you do if you noticed that a patient's skin color was flushed, or if the skin tone changed to a gray or bluish color?

Author's Explanation: Any change in skin color should be reported to the nurse. Red or flushed color indicates that there is increased blood flow to the skin and increased oxygen content in the blood. Flushed or red skin could be an indication of increased body temperature or fever. In this instance, the skin would also feel warm. This increased oxygen may not be a positive sign

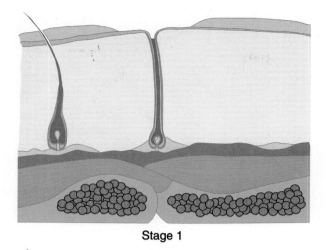
Stage 1

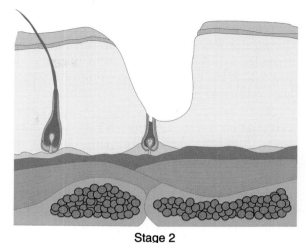
Stage 2

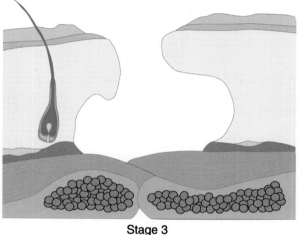
Stage 3

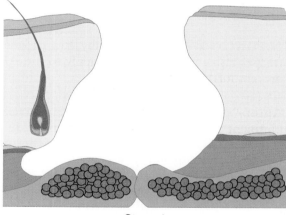
Stage 4

FIGURE 7-3 Stages of skin breakdown.

in patients who suffer from chronic lung disease. This is especially true if a patient with Chronic Obstructive Pulmonary Disease (COPD) is receiving oxygen therapy. The oxygen flow meter may be set too high, and this can be very dangerous. Immediately call the nurse for a suddenly flushed (pink to red) skin color in a patient receiving oxygen. A gray or bluish tint to the skin, called **cyanosis** (*cyano*-means "blue"), indicates that the person is not getting enough oxygen. In either case, a change in skin color should be promptly reported to the nurse. Skin color also changes with pressure to the skin. If you sit with your knees crossed, you may see that the epidermis is reddened in the areas that had the greatest pressure.

Situation 6: Imagine a patient who is immobile and remains in one position until you change the position. If left in a supine position for two or more hours, what will you note about the areas of the skin where the pressure of body weight rests?

Author's Explanation: The skin that lies over protruding bones will be reddened when you change the position. For some people, the skin will be affected in an hour or less.

Patients who are immobile are at great risk for skin breakdown. You should consider the patient's nutritional status, age, ability to control bowel and bladder functions and sensory awareness in the care of the skin. A combination of pressure, heat, moisture and darkness create an environment that is ripe for the growth of harmful microbes and skin breakdown.

The result of these hazards to the skin is the development of **decubitus ulcers** (pressure sores). The stages of skin breakdown are described in Figure 7-3.

Situation 7: Consider the factors that lead to skin breakdown and pressure sores. What actions can you take as a clinical care associate to prevent the development of decubitus ulcers?

Author's Explanation: Skin should be kept clean and dry. Patients who are incontinent should be washed and dried well whenever they are incontinent of urine or feces. Washing and drying the area will prevent the harmful acids and enzymes in urine and stool from breaking down the cells of the epidermis. Reposition the patient at least every two hours.

Situation 8: Consider a baby who is left in soiled diapers for even a short period of time. What will the results be?

Author's Explanation: Diaper rash will develop, and red, tender skin will result. Diaper rash is painful, and even water can cause the skin to sting. Adults who are not able to control their excretions, or who are unable to toilet themselves, also develop excoriation of the skin.

Situation 9: If your baby had excoriation (diaper rash), what would you apply to the skin to prevent further breakdown?

Author's Explanation: You would choose an ointment that soothes and protects the skin and acts as a skin barrier, such as a petroleum-based ointment. You would also change the baby frequently and keep the area clean and dry.

Adults need the same treatment. Your agency will have products called *incontinence products* that create a barrier for the skin. These skin barriers add a protective film over the skin to prevent the harmful contents of urine and feces from penetrating the skin. If you have a spray skin barrier, spray some on your hand and notice that when you apply water to this area the water beads up and rolls away. This barrier may sting when it is applied to excoriated skin. Tell the patient to expect some stinging. In addition, the skin needs to be nourished by eating the proper balance of protein, carbohydrates, and fats if it is to remain healthy.

Situation 10: Based on your current knowledge of nutrition, what should you encourage patients to eat to heal damaged skin? To maintain healthy skin? If you are unsure, what member of the health care team can provide the answers?

Author's Explanation: Healing requires a diet that is adequate in its protein content and that provides all essential nutrients, including a balance of vitamins and minerals. When healing is needed, carbohydrates and fats must also be present in the diet to spare the proteins that are necessary to build new tissue. If you were unsure of this answer, you could have consulted a nutritionist or dietitian.

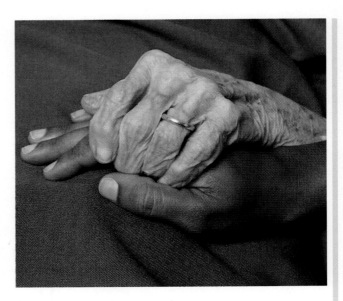

FIGURE 7-4 Elderly skin.

Situation 11: If you are caring for a patient who is eighty years old and is unable to move independently, what should you consider?

Author's Explanation: Remember that skin breakdown can occur with immobility because of the pressure of body weight on bony prominences as they press against the skin. Patients of all ages will be affected by this immobility factor. Because this patient is older, the skin is less elastic, thinner, drier, and more fragile than that of younger patients. This is a normal aspect of physical aging. Sometimes you will notice that the elder client's skin is so thin that it easily tears with any rubbing or pressure. The term *onion skin* is frequently used to describe thin, transparent, and fragile skin in elders. Notice the skin of an onion. The outer layer of the skin is dry and easily tears away when you handle it. Figure 7-4 is an example of elderly ("onion") skin.

Situation 12: What important care measures should you employ as a clinical care associate when caring for older clients? (Remember that the skin of elders is thinner and drier than younger adult skin.)

Author's Explanation: Generally, an elder's skin does not need to be washed with soap every day. Only areas of the skin that are affected by sweat and other body fluids (such as urine or stool if the person is incontinent) should be washed with soap and water daily. Lotions should be applied to enrich the epidermis with lubrication. When you dry thin or fragile skin, be careful not to rub the skin; pat the skin dry. "Onion skin" will tear easily, allowing infection to occur. Observe the elder's skin for any discoloration or changes

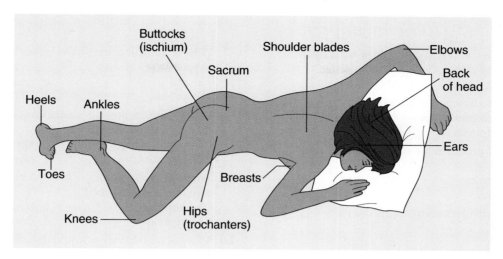

FIGURE 7-5   Bony prominences.

in pigmentation. Report these observations to the nurse.

Situation 13: The force of body weight against bony prominences puts excessive pressure on the skin over the bones. (Figure 7-5 illustrates the bony prominences.) Which areas of the body have bony prominences (places where the bones protrude)?

Author's Explanation: The hips, heels, ankles, knees, lower back area of the skull, the shoulders, and the buttocks are especially vulnerable to pressure sores.

Situation 14: What can you do to prevent prolonged pressure in these areas?

Author's Explanation: Be certain to turn your clients at least every 2 hours. Some patients will need to be turned more frequently to prevent pressure sores. In this case, a "turning schedule" is often posted at the bedside to ensure that patients are turned regularly. Areas of the skin that press against each other should be cushioned with pillows or protective cushions. Place pillows between the knees when patients are lying on the right or left sides, and use heel cushions. Always turn the patient as frequently as possible to prevent the development of pressure sores. In addition, eggcrate mattresses, water or air mattresses, and heel and elbow protectors can be ordered by the nurse or doctor.

When pressure sores are in the early stages, treatments such as the application of duoderm dressings can prevent further breakdown of the skin. **Duoderm** acts like a second skin. (*Duo-* means "two" and *derma* means "skin.") The pro-

cedure for applying a duoderm will be discussed in the skills unit.

If you apply hot or cold packs to the skin, be certain to check the skin at least every 10 minutes. Observe for changes in skin color: red, blanched (white), or gray-blue discoloration. If a patient has decreased blood flow to the area or has nerve damage, there will be no sensation of the damage and pain created by heat or cold. When you apply hot or cold packs to the skin to decrease swelling or to promote comfort, position these applications slightly above or below the site of injury. Place a towel between the skin and the hot or cold application. This will help to decrease the direct pressure of the hot or cold pack on the site of injury.

Always measure the temperature of the water before placing a patient in a tub bath. Measuring the temperature will help to avoid burns and discomfort to the patient. Bathwater should not be hotter than 110°F.

Situation 15: You apply a cold pack to a patient's arm to reduce the swelling from a wrist sprain. What will you observe if the cold pack is too cold and is obstructing blood flow to the area?

Author's Explanation: The skin will blanch (turn white) or become pale. It will surely feel cold. If you see this, remove the cold pack, and tell the nurse what you observed as soon as possible. Do not be afraid that you will be accused of neglect or improper patient care. Failing to report any observation could place the patient in danger. Do not fear accusation; think about the patient's well-being and your ethical duty to do what is best for the patient.

Examination Review Questions

1. The dermis is composed primarily of what tissue?
   a. epithelial
   b. muscular
   c. connective
   d. nervous

2. Which is *not* a function of the skin?
   a. pathogen protection
   b. fluid elimination
   c. temperature control
   d. allergy prevention

3. Which gland produces the oil that moisturizes hair follicles?
   a. sudoriferous
   b. sebaceous
   c. sweat
   d. salivary

4. A burn that involves injury to the dermis is a ____- degree burn.
   a. second
   b. superficial
   c. partial
   d. third

5. A chronic inflammatory skin disease of unknown etiology is
   a. hives
   b. psoriasis
   c. acne
   d. wheal

6. Which of the following is not a precaution for elderly skin and the sun?
   a. Replace fluids.
   b. Provide head covering
   c. Apply sunscreen.
   d. Avoid the sun.

7. What is the skin color that indicates lack of oxygenation?
   a. red
   b. yellow
   c. gray
   d. white

8. Which of the following is *not* a consideration for potential skin breakdown?
   a. immobility
   b. incontinence
   c. age
   d. race

9. Which of the following is *not* a primary health measure for pressure ulcers?
   a. nutrition
   b. eggcrate
   c. positioning
   d. duoderm

10. What skin observation would denote that a cold pack was obstructing blood flow?
    a. blanching
    b. erythema
    c. cyanosis
    d. flushing

The Skeletal System

Imagine that the framework of your body is a solid piece of steel. Can you see yourself crossing your legs or running for the bus? I don't think so! Your knees wouldn't bend, and your hips would be rigid. Unlike steel, the bones of the skeleton are living structures that perform many vital functions for your body. Bones are like the branches of a living tree. The outer surface of a tree branch is hard, and the spongy inner core nourishes the tree. In most winds, a strong, healthy tree branch will only bend, but if bent forcefully, it will snap and break.

Like branches, the outer surface of a bone is hard, and the spongy, inner core nourishes the body. Together, the bones form the human skeleton. In this unit, you will learn the structures and functions of the skeletal system.

OBJECTIVES

After completing this chapter, you will be able to

1. Differentiate between long, short, flat, and irregularly shaped bones
2. Identify the bones of the arms, legs, chest, vertebrae, hands, feet, skull, and hips
3. Describe at least three functions of the skeletal system
4. Describe the changes that occur in bones and joints in the aging process
5. Describe common conditions and diseases of the skeletal system
6. List the observations about the skeletal system that you should report to the nurse
7. Apply your knowledge of the skeletal system to problem-solving strategies in care delivery
8. Define and spell all key terms correctly

appendicular
articulation
axial
bone spurs
calcium
cancellous
cartilage
compact
compound fracture
concave

convex
diaphysis
epiphysis
etiology
fractures
gout
herniated intervertebral disc
intervertebral disc
joints
kyphosis

ligament
lordosis
nucleus pulposus
osteoarthritis
osteoporosis
rheumatoid arthritis
scoliosis
simple fracture

Structures of the Skeletal System

The bones of the skeleton are classified as *long, short, flat,* or *irregularly shaped.* Long bones are found in the arms and legs. Short bones are found in the fingers and toes. Flat bones include the sternum (breastbone) and ribs. And irregularly shaped bones are found in the wrist, ankles, spine, face, and cranium.

Appearance and Structures of Long Bones

An examination of a typical long bone (such as the femur, or thighbone) reveals two distinct types of bone tissue: *compact* and *cancellous.* **Compact** bone tissue is dense and strong. **Cancellous** bone tissue is spongy and porous.

In long bones, the central shaft of the bone is called the **diaphysis**, and each end of the long bone is called the **epiphysis**. Compact tissue is found in the interior portion of the diaphysis. This provides mechanical strength for the portion of the bone that bears the greatest strain. In the epiphyses of long bones, the cancellous tissue contains the red bone marrow, which produces the blood cells.

Divisions of the Skeletal System

The two subdivisions of the skeletal system are known as the *axial* skeleton and the *appendicular* skeleton. The **axial** skeleton includes the bones of the cranium, face, spinal column, and chest. The axial skeleton is the axis to which the extremities, or appendages, attach. The **appendicular** skeleton includes the shoulder girdle, arms, hands, hips, legs, and feet. The appendages of the body are the extremities. Figure 8-1 provides anterior, lateral, and posterior views of the bones of the skeletal system.

(Note: Your instructor will determine the bones that you must learn for this course.)

The Vertebral Column

After birth, the normal curves of the spine are formed to accommodate the natural movements of the human body. When a baby begins raising the head, this creates the S curve of the cervical vertebrae (the neck bones). Walking and standing erect create the inward curve of the lumbar region (the waist area). The vertebrae begin as small bones in the neck and progressively become larger through the thoracic vertebrae (posterior chest area). The largest vertebrae are found in the lumbar area. The structure of the vertebral column is determined by function. The largest bones of the spine are found in the area of the body that bears the greatest weight and pressure of movement. The spine has *four normal curves.* The cervical area is **concave** (curved inward), the thoracic area is **convex** (curved outward), the lumbar area is concave, and the sacral and coccygeal (buttocks area) are convex. Figure 8-1 illustrates the normal curvature of the spine.

Abnormal Curves of the Vertebral Column

The normal curves of the spine can become exaggerated as a result of injury, poor posture, or disease. The terms used to describe these abnormal curves are derived from the Greek language. The abnormal curve of the thoracic vertebrae is **kyphosis**; it is commonly called *hunchback* because *kyphos* means "hump." People with chronic lung diseases often develop this abnormal curve, as do people who posture the chest region in a forward hunch. An exaggerated concave or anterior curve of the lumbar area is called **lordosis**. In Greek, this means "curving forward." People often refer to this as *swayback.* This poor posture often develops in women who wear high heels for their everyday work and leisure shoes. High heels thrust the weight of the body forward, and in addition to an exaggerated lumbar curve, the heel bears most of the

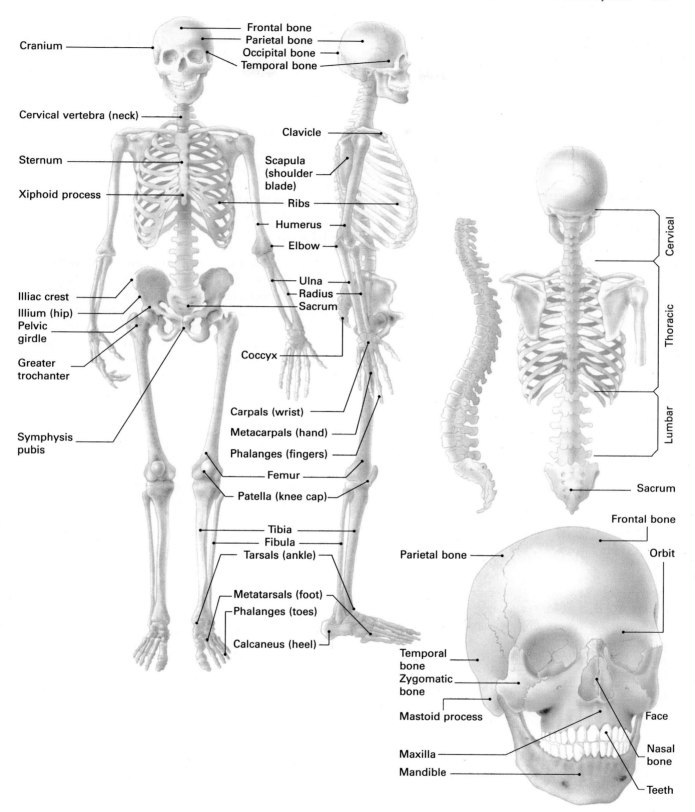

FIGURE 8-1   Anterior, lateral, and posterior views of the skeletal bones.

body weight. The word used to describe a sideways curve of any section of the vertebrae is **scoliosis**, which comes from *skolios*, the Greek term for "crooked." Fast, uneven growth of the back muscles is often the cause of this abnormal curvature of the spine.

Intervertebral Discs

Between each vertebra is a cushion that helps to absorb shock and prevent friction. This cushion, called an ***intervertebral disc***, is made of a pulpy, gelatin-like substance called the **nucleus pulposus**. Exaggerated motions and extremes in body movement can cause harm to these discs. If you bend and twist at the waist, you force the lumbar region vertebrae to move in a manner that they are not designed for. As a result, you may cause a herniation of the intervertebral disc. An example of disc herniation is shown in Figure 8-2.

When disc herniation occurs, it creates an abnormal protrusion or herniation of the nucleus pulposus. This puts pressure on the spinal nerves in the area of herniation, creating a great deal of pain and perhaps requiring surgical repair. Surgery is indicated when the herniation cannot resolve itself within a designated period of time and when the pressure on the nerve is creating a loss of function in the body part that the involved nerve controls.

Articulations

The **joints** of the body are called *articulations*. An **articulation** is the union of two or more bones. Every bone of the human body except one articulates (relates to) at least one other bone. The hyoid bone is the exception. The hyoid bone is found at the base of the tongue and supports it. This bone does not articulate any other bone.

There are three types of joints. *Fixed joints*, like the bones of the cranium, do not allow for any movement. *Slightly movable joints* are found at the wrists

and the ankles. This type of joint allows for some movement. The vast majority of bones in the body form *freely movable joints*. This type of joint allows for movement in one or more directions. Freely movable joints allow for hinge-type action, pivoting action, gliding action, or circular action. Freely movable joints are protected by a capsule that contains fluid and that lubricates the movements of these articulations.

The ends of bones, known as the ***articular surfaces***, are covered with a tough connective tissue called **cartilage**. Cartilage acts like a rubber cushion, softening the shock of movement.

Ligaments

A **ligament** is a tough, fibrous band of connective tissue that connects one bone to another. Ligaments are durable structures. However, they are capable of damage and can tear as a result of injuries and trauma. Torn ligaments are most common in the knees, especially in sports injuries that result from excessive weight and force at the site of the ligament connection.

Functions of the Skeletal System

The skeletal system, the 206 bones of the body human, has several functions. First, it serves as a *framework* for the body. The skeleton is a supporting structure, and in this way, it is like the wooden frame of a building. Imagine your body without this framework. You would collapse into a heap of muscles and organs!

The second function of the skeletal system is *protection*. The hard bony structures of the skeleton protect delicate internal organs. The cranium (skull) protects the very delicate organ of the brain, and the rib cage and sternum protect the heart and lungs.

Another function of the skeletal system is the *production of blood cells*. Bone marrow, found within certain bones, is the site for blood cell production. When you cook soup, you might use beef or chicken bones to make the stock. The marrow is the portion of the bones that makes the stock rich in flavor. The bone marrow is most active at the ends of long bones, like the thighbone. As we age, the bone marrow becomes less active, and although our bones continue to produce blood cells, the production is slower. In babies and children, red marrow is found in the epiphyses of the humerus (upper arm) and the femur. (This gradually decreases throughout the developmental years.) In adults, the ribs, vertebrae, sternum, and hips contain the red marrow.

Bones provide a place of attachment for the skeletal muscles. Therefore, the fourth function of

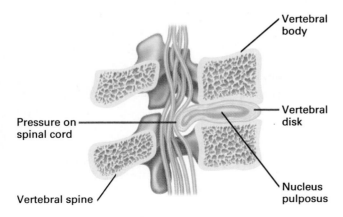

FIGURE 8-2 Disc herniation.

Vertebral body

Vertebral disk

Nucleus pulposus

Vertebral spine

Pressure on spinal cord

bones is to act as an *anchor* for the muscles. Together, the bones and skeletal muscles make movement possible.

The last function of the skeleton is the *storage of minerals*. Most important, the bones store **calcium**. Calcium is deposited in bones, and approximately 98 percent of it is stored in the form of a salt. The calcium that is stored in bones serves to give them strength and stability of shape. The calcium that remains in blood and body fluids is used in vital chemical reactions. Calcium is released from the bones in response to the needs of the body and the availability of calcium in the blood. Hormones regulate the deposit of calcium into the bones and the removal of calcium from the bones.

When your blood lacks calcium, this mineral will be removed from your bones. Calcium is needed to carry out the functions of the muscles, the nerves, and the heart. Depletion of calcium from the bones causes brittle bones. It is important that your body has the required amount of calcium to carry out essential functions. When women are pregnant, they need more calcium for the development of the fetus. If the mother does not receive the required calcium from her diet and from vitamins, the calcium from her bones will be released so that the baby can grow.

Conditions and Diseases of the Skeletal System

Osteoarthritis is the form of arthritis that often occurs as a result of the aging process. Approximately thirty million Americans over the age of sixty-five experience the pain of this condition. It is the most common chronic condition of elders. Osteoarthritis is the degeneration (decline and destruction of the structure and function) of the cartilage that covers the surface of the bones that form joints. In this condition, excess bone grows along the joint edges of the bones. These growths are called **bone spurs**. Degeneration of the articular cartilage results in the loss of the protective covering, which causes the inflammation of the joints. Weight-bearing joints are most affected. People with osteoarthritis have decreased agility and mobility, and they often experience pain. Movement should be slower, but exercise of these joints is necessary to prevent further loss of function. Anti-inflammatory medications, like aspirin, are prescribed to decrease the inflammation and pain.

Rheumatoid arthritis is a systemic disease (affecting more than one body system) with widespread involvement of the connective tissues. Remember that connective tissue is found in many body organs.

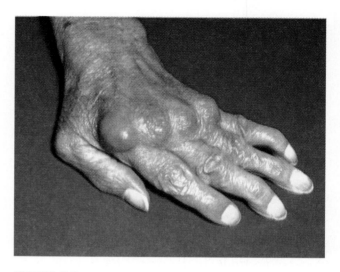

FIGURE 8-3 Arthritic joints. James Stevenson, Science Photo Library, Photo Researchers, Inc.

This condition is familial. The **etiology** (cause) of this condition is unknown, but it is thought to be related to an antigen-antibody reaction. Rheumatoid arthritis causes inflammation of the joints and the membranes that surround them (Figure 8-3). Swelling and the loss of mobility result. Other connective tissues are also affected. This disease process begins earlier in life than osteoarthritis. Anti-inflammatory medications are prescribed to decrease the pain and inflammation.

Gout, or gouty arthritis, is a form of arthritis that is caused by the deposit of uric acid crystals in and around the joint tissues. This results in inflammation, pain, and swelling of the joints. The large toe is most often the affected joint. Those who suffer from gout should avoid foods that are rich in uric acid. The nutritionist or the physician should give the patient a list of these foods. Medications to control uric acid levels in the blood might also be prescribed.

A **herniated intervertebral disc** results from the protrusion of the nucleus pulposus (the pulpy, elastic substance that is found in the center of the discs). This can be caused by sudden exertion, compression, or insult to the disc. The herniation of this substance in any area of the spinal column causes pressure on the spinal nerves in that particular area. This is very painful, and it can cause temporary or permanent loss of function to the affected body part. The area most prone to disc herniation is the lumbar region of the spine. The nerve usually affected is the sciatic nerve. Pain radiates down the leg and into the foot. Herniation sometimes requires surgical repair. The discs lose their resiliency with the aging process.

Osteoporosis is a condition that results from the loss of calcium from the bones. This makes the bones porous and brittle, and they can be easily broken. Lack of calcium in the diet, lack of exercise (weight bearing is important for the deposit of calcium into bones, especially the long bones), and the lack of the hormone estrogen in postmenopausal women are believed to be the causes. Postmenopausal Caucasian women have the highest incidence of osteoporosis. Women of other races also have a higher incidence of this condition than males of any race.

Fractures are broken bones (Figure 8-4). A broken bone is called a **compound fracture** when the bone protrudes through the skin. Compound fractures are dangerous because of the risk of infection, and surgery is required to correct the damaged bone and skin. With a **simple fracture**, the bone does not protrude. In this type of fracture, the bone is immobilized usually with a plaster of paris cast. Bones heal best when the fracture ends are repositioned accurately and tightly. Plaster casts must not be allowed to get wet because water deteriorates the cast. Plastic is another substance that is used to make casts.

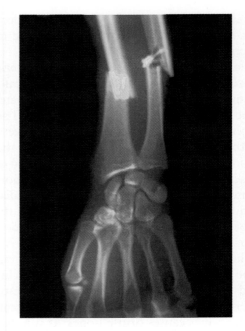

FIGURE 8-4   Enhanced color x-ray of bone fractures. Scott Camazine, Photo Researchers, Inc.

application to practice

As a clinical care associate, you will be responsible for walking patients and assisting them with daily living activities. You will also be responsible for preventing injury to the patient's skeleton and for assisting patients in maintaining healthy bones. Consider the information that you have learned about the human skeletal system in this chapter, and apply it to the following situations.

Learning Activities

Situation 1: Consider the functions of the skeletal system. Which functions can you observe? Also list the functions for which you can provide care as prescribed by the doctor and nurse.

Author's Explanation: Some of the functions that you will observe and for which you will provide care are

- Insult or injury to the supportive and protective functions
- Potential for injury to the bones (steady/unsteady on feet)
- Decrease, change, or lack of movement of a limb or section of the skeleton
- Signs of infection, bleeding, or anemia due to decreased bone marrow functions (these will be discussed in Chapter 11, The Circulatory System.)

- Signs and symptoms of fractures of the bones
- Pain and swelling of joints
- Pain associated with specific movements
- Dietary intake of nutrients that contain sources of calcium
- Crystal-like substances in the urine
- Changes in posture or shape in any bone or part of the skeleton

Situation 2: You are assigned to assist a patient with ambulation (walking), and you noticed that he is limping. He seems to be protecting the right leg, bearing more weight on the left side. What should you do?

Author's Explanation: Assist the patient back to his room, and ensure his safety in a chair or in bed. Report your findings to the nurse. Ask the patient whether he is experiencing any pain. Ask about assistive devices that he uses for walking (cane, crutches, walker) at home. Do not allow the patient to go without assistance until the nurse, doctor, or physical therapist has made an evaluation.

Situation 3: You are assigned to assist a patient with ambulation, and she uses a cane. What is the correct procedure for assisting this patient?

Author's Explanation: The patient should hold the cane in her hand on the unaffected side of the body. (If the patient has right-sided weakness, the cane should be held in the left hand.) The affected leg should move forward along with the cane before the patient moves the unaffected leg forward. While you are assisting the patient, you should walk beside her on the affected side. Look for any obstructions or hazards in the environment, and remove them.

Situation 4: You are assigned to Mr. Abdul, who is unable to move or stand without assistance because he has had a stroke. The stroke affected his left leg, causing severe weakness. He spends much of his day immobile, remaining in bed or in a lounge chair. What can you do to provide weight bearing activity for Mr. Abdul?

Author's Explanation: Periodically, you should provide Mr. Abdul with the opportunity to stand and hold onto a secure surface so that his legs can bear the weight of his body. Once Physical Therapy has prescribed a walking regimen, you should walk him as frequently as possible to prevent calcium loss from the bones.

Situation 5: Mrs. Cammarota has had a stroke, which affected the left side of her body. She

has been admitted to your long-term care facility for rehabilitation. She has weakness of the left arm and leg and needs assistance with activities of daily living (ADLs). She is left-handed. With which ADLs will Mrs. Cammarota require your assistance?

Author's Explanation: You should check with the nurse to find out what her assessment of the resident revealed so that you can assist Mrs. Cammarota with necessary ADLs. You will most likely assist her with eating, dressing, mouth care, changing positions while in bed, and walking.

Situation 6: What information do you need to know before you get Mrs. Cammorata out of bed to walk her?

Author's Explanation: You need to know if she uses a cane or walker and how far you should walk her. You also need to know if Physical Therapy wants to observe her ambulation and whether she has been evaluated yet. You need to know how much assistance she needs to get out of bed (OOB) and whether she has had any dizziness upon getting OOB. It would also be useful to know how Mrs. Cammorata is accepting her physical limitations and her rehabilitation.

Examination Review Questions

1. Which bone is considered a long bone?
   a. leg
   b. wrist
   c. ankle
   d. cranium

2. The abnormal curvature of the spinal column known as *hunchback* is
   a. lordosis
   b. kyphosis
   c. scoliosis
   d. psoriasis

3. The conective tissue that binds bone to bone is
   a. tendon
   b. ligament
   c. cartilage
   d. disc

4. Which joint is considered freely movable?
   a. hip
   b. wrist
   c. elbow
   d. knee

5. Which of the following is *not* a function of the skeletal system?
   a. framework
   b. support
   c. protection
   d. movement

6. The production of red blood cells would occur in which bone?
   a. femur
   b. cranium
   c. sternum
   d. patella

7. Which skeletal disease is a direct result of normal aging and the associated wear and tear on bones?
   a. osteoporosis
   b. osteoarthritis
   c. rheumatoid arthritis
   d. gout

8. What is caused by uric acid deposits in and around the joint?
   a. rheumatoid arthritis
   b. osteoarthritis
   c. osteoporosis
   d. gout

9. The risk of infection is greatest with which kind of fracture?
   a. simple
   b. compound
   c. greenstick
   d. hairline

10. Which bone belongs to the axial skeleton?
    a. tibia
    b. humerus
    c. radius
    d. scapula

Chapter 9

The Muscular System

Every body movement is the result of the contraction and relaxation of muscles. Muscles make actions possible. Muscular activities are both external and internal. The external actions involve movement of the bones. The internal actions move food and waste products through the digestive tract and move blood through the vessels and the heart. The act of breathing is accomplished with the aid of the respiratory muscles. Muscles are described by their appearance, their location, and the action they generate. There are three types of muscle: *skeletal,* *smooth,* and *cardiac.* Each type will be examined in terms of its unique structure and function.

OBJECTIVES

After completing this chapter, you will be able to

1. Name the structures of the muscular system
2. Describe the functions of the muscular system
3. List the location of each major skeletal muscle
4. Compare and contrast the types of muscles
5. Describe the conditions and diseases of the muscular system
6. List the observations about the muscular system that you should report to the nurse
7. Apply your knowledge of the muscular system to problem-solving strategies in care delivery
8. Define and spell all key terms correctly

key terms

abduction	involuntary	paraplegia
adduction	isometric	quadriplegia
atrophy	isotonic	skeletal
contractures	muscle tone	smooth visceral
extension	myasthenia gravis	striated
flexion	myocardium	striated branching
hemiplegia	origin	tendons
hypertrophy	paralysis	voluntary
insertion		

Skeletal Muscle: Structure and Function

Skeletal muscle is made of fibers that have a striped appearance; this type of muscle tissue is called **striated** muscle tissue. It is called **skeletal** muscle because these are the muscles that are attached to bones and move the bones of the body. It is also called **voluntary** muscle tissue because the individual controls the movement of the skeleton. You make the decision to move a body part, and nerves stimulate the muscle to move. You voluntarily walk, smile, raise your hand, and so on. The fibers of skeletal muscle are thin and sometimes very long. They can be one thousand times longer than their width. The muscles in front of the thigh are an example of this. These muscle fibers stretch the length of the longest bone in the body, the femur.

Muscle cells produce heat in the process of breaking down nutrients. Because muscle cells are highly active and numerous, they are a major source of the body's heat. Skeletal muscles are a main source of maintaining a constant body temperature. They are named by their *location* (for example, the anterior tibialis), *action* (abductor), *shape* (trapezius), *origin* and *insertion* (sternocleidomastoid), *divisions* (triceps, biceps), or the *direction* of the fibers (oblique). Posterior and anterior muscle groups are depicted in Figures 9-1 and 9-2.

Movement of Skeletal Muscles

Skeletal muscles are attached usually to two bones, spanning across the joint between the bones. As the muscle fibers contract, movement is created at the joint. The bone that *remains stationary* (does not move) has the muscular attachment called the **origin**. The bone that *moves* as a result of the contraction of the muscle has the end of the muscle called the **insertion**. Muscles are attached to bones by **tendons**, which are nonelastic cords that act as anchors

for the muscle. Generally, more than one muscle produces a single movement. Groups of muscles work together to move and stabilize the bone or bones they control. Remember two concepts when learning muscle groups. First, for every action, there is an opposite action. For example, the biceps flex. Opposite the biceps, the triceps extend. Second, muscle groups superior to (above) the joint move that joint. An example is the bicep-tricep group. They are superior to the elbow, and they move the elbow joint. The muscles of the forearm move the wrist, and so on.

Types of Skeletal Muscle Movements

It is important to understand the directions in which muscles are designed to move. When you learn to perform range-of-motion (ROM) exercises, you need to know the terms for these motions and especially the directions in which you should move the patient's muscles. You do not want to put muscles through a range of motion that they are not designed to perform naturally.

The following terms and illustrations describe the normal range of motion of joints and muscles. **Flexion** is an action that reduces the angle of a joint. Imagine bending your lower arm upward and bulging your biceps muscle. This is flexion. **Extension** is the opposite of flexion; extension makes the angle of a joint larger. When you straighten your lower arm, this is extension.

Abduction means moving a part away from the midline of the body. When you move your arm or leg away from the center of your body, this is abduction. Look at Figure 9-3 to see the muscles whose main function is abduction. **Adduction** means moving a part toward the midline. Move your arm or leg in toward the center of your body. This is adduction. Remember that *ab-* means "away from," and *ad-* means "toward." This will help you to distinguish abduction from adduction. Think of *ad-* as *add*ing to the body!

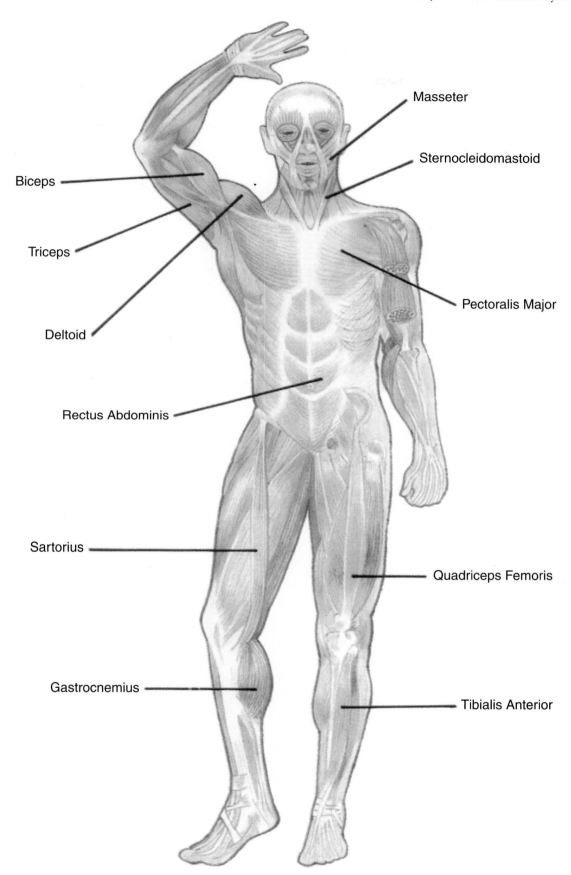

Masseter

Sternocleidomastoid

Biceps

Triceps

Pectoralis Major

Deltoid

Rectus Abdominis

Sartorius

Quadriceps Femoris

Gastrocnemius

Tibialis Anterior

FIGURE 9-1   Anterior muscle groups.

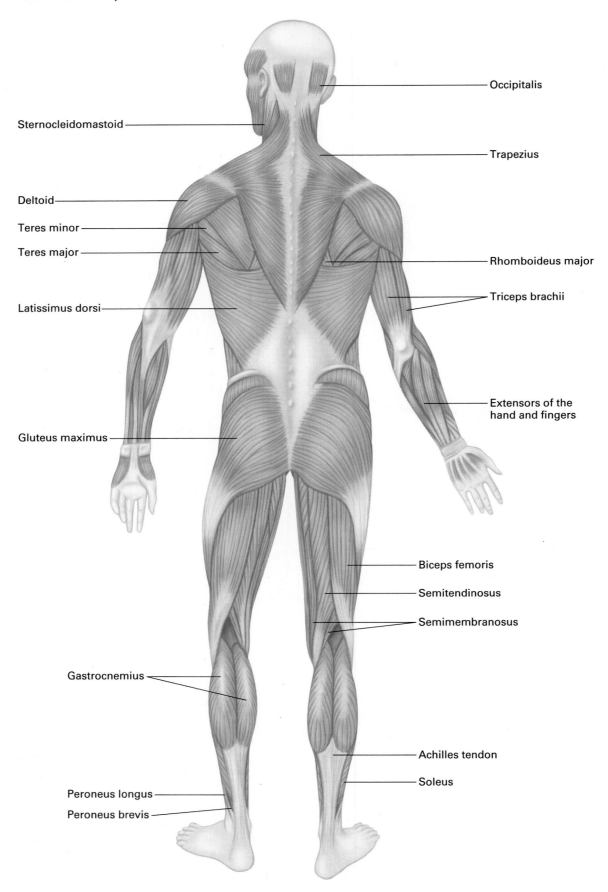

Occipitalis

Sternocleidomastoid

Trapezius

Deltoid

Teres minor

Teres major

Rhomboideus major

Triceps brachii

Latissimus dorsi

Extensors of the
hand and fingers

Gluteus maximus

Biceps femoris

Semitendinosus

Semimembranosus

Gastrocnemius

Achilles tendon

Soleus

Peroneus longus

Peroneus brevis

FIGURE 9-2   Posterior muscle groups.

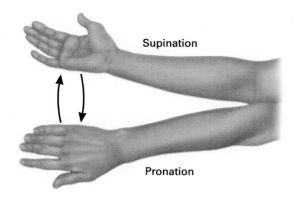

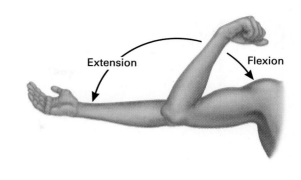

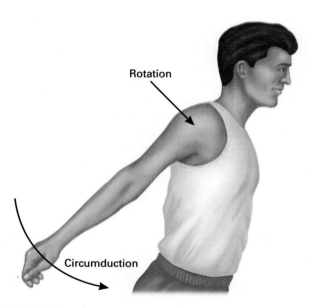

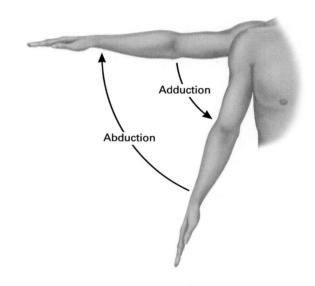

FIGURE 9-3   Movements produced by muscles.

Skeletal Muscles Used for Intramuscular Injections

Medications are sometimes given directly into a muscle. The most commonly used muscles for intramuscular (IM) injections are the deltoid, gluteus medius, and, in small children, the vastus lateralis (part of the quadriceps group). The nurse, physician, or medical assistant must know the procedure and the structure of these muscles to inject intramuscular medications safely.

Smooth Muscle: Structure and Function

Smooth muscle tissue works involuntarily. It is the type of muscle tissue found in the digestive organs, the blood vessels, the skin, and some of the organs of the urinary system. It is called **smooth visceral** muscle—"smooth" because of its nonstriated appearance, and "visceral" because it is found in the viscera (internal organs).

Cardiac Muscle: Structure and Function

The type of muscle tissue found in the heart is called **striated branching** muscle tissue—"striated" because it has the striped appearance of skeletal muscle, and "branching" because the muscle fibers overlap and branch around one another, making the muscle tissue more durable and strong. This muscle tissue contracts and relaxes every second of your life, and its function determines its structure. On the average, this muscle will produce movement seventy-five times per minute. Cardiac (heart) muscle, or the

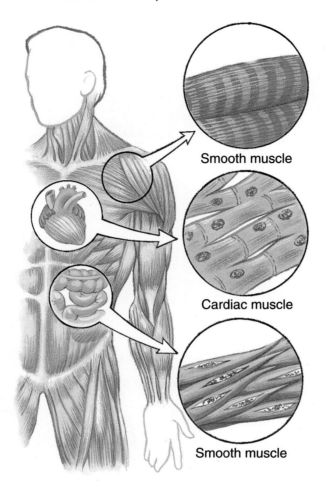

Smooth muscle

Cardiac muscle

Smooth muscle

FIGURE 9-4   Characteristics of muscle tissue.

myocardium, is not voluntarily controlled; it is **involuntary** muscle tissue. You do not have to think about and decide to move this muscle. Cardiac muscle is controlled by a center in your brain that automatically stimulates the myocardium.

Figure 9-4 illustrates the characteristics of different types of muscles.

Muscle Tone

Muscle tone refers to the state of tension of the muscles. Muscle tone is the muscles' constant state of contraction. A contraction that does not produce movement is called **isometric**; this type of contraction helps to tone the muscles. Unconsciously, muscles are stimulated by the brain and spinal cord. The muscular system is in a constant state of readiness. The increase or decrease in stimulation depends on the level of activity of the nervous system. In restful states, the tone decreases. In times of excitement, it increases. Muscle tone helps to maintain posture. When tone decreases, posture deteriorates. Good

muscle tone helps us not only to look good, but to feel good and to recover more quickly from disease and injury.

Exercise and Its Benefits

Regular exercise helps to maintain good skeletal muscle tone. Other benefits include its effects on smooth and cardiac muscle. **Isotonic** muscular contraction is the form of exercise that generates movement of the muscles. Isometric contractions do not generate movement but do improve muscle tone. To distinguish these two forms of contraction, think of isotonic as aerobic exercise. When you press your hands tightly together, you contract the bicep muscles, but you do not move the arm bones. Improved heart activity, blood pressure, and digestive functions are some of the benefits of aerobic exercise. When patients are bed-bound, their muscle tissues can easily lose tone and work less efficiently. Routine exercise is essential to their recovery. Bed-bound patients can do isometric or isotonic exercises to prevent the loss of muscle tone. Simple ROM exercises and isometric contractions can help to prevent the loss of strength and tone of the muscles.

Conditions and Diseases of the Muscular System

The major problems of the muscular system involve disorders such as paralysis, weakness, pain, atrophy, and cramps.

Contractures result from the shortening of the muscle fibers when they are in a resting state. They occur when individuals are immobilized for periods of time and when their limbs are not positioned in proper alignment. The muscles readjust to the position of the resting state of a flexed arm or leg. Contractures must be rehabilitated by the progressive lengthening of the muscles through exercise. They can be prevented by proper positioning and active (performed by the patient) or passive (performed by someone else) range-of-motion exercises. Figure 9-5 shows an example of a contracture.

Paralysis results from trauma, infection, or injury to the brain or spinal cord. When all four limbs are paralyzed, this is called **quadriplegia**. **Paraplegia** means paralysis from the waist down to the toes. **Hemiplegia** is usually due to a stroke and results in paralysis on either the right or left side of the body.

Atrophy is the shrinking or deterioration of muscles. The affected muscles are weak and smaller than normal. Atrophy results from lack of movement of the muscle due to paralysis, nerve damage, immobilization,

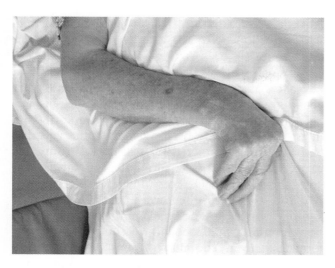

FIGURE 9-5   Contracture of the arm.

or prolonged bed rest. If you ever had a cast on an arm or leg, you saw the atrophied muscles when the cast was removed. The opposite of atrophy is **hypertrophy**. Hypertrophy is the overdevelopment of muscles. This results from overexercising. Imagine a body builder who lifts weights extensively, and you will see hypertrophy. This is not necessarily a healthy state, especially if the body builder used steroids to enlarge muscle tissue growth. Hypertrophy of the myocardium is not a healthy muscular state.

Myasthenia gravis is a disease that causes severe muscular weakness (*myo-* means "muscle," *asthenia* means "weakness," and *gravis* means "severe"). This disorder is characterized by easy fatigue of muscles and general muscular weakness. It involves the impairment of signal conduction between the muscles and the nerves that innervate them.

application to practice

As a clinical care associate, your tasks in patient care will involve assisting patients in exercise and ambulation. You will also observe, record, and report your observations and assigned interventions that affect all types of muscular tissues, including cardiac and smooth muscles. Use the information that you learned about the muscular system in this chapter, and apply it to the following situations.

Learning Activities

Situation 1: What observations can you make about the condition or state of health of the muscular system? Consider each type of muscle tissue in your response.

Author's Explanation: Observations of the *skeletal* muscles include the individual's ability to perform activities of daily living. You can observe the patient's ability to walk, talk, chew, swallow, make facial expressions, write, eat, and perform personal hygiene. If a patient complains of pain with a specific movement, you should note this and report it. If a patient has difficulty walking, bending, lifting, or performing certain movements, you should observe the limitation in movement and report it to the nurse. If a patient complains of weakness or of being easily fatigued with activity, be sure to report this as well. Note the tone of the skeletal muscles, and compare the strength and size of muscles on both sides of the body. Observe and report any contractures or atrophy of muscles. If you assist

the patient with ROM exercises, position transfers, or ambulation, always report the patient's response, your observations, and any complaints or abnormalities noted. Complaints of muscle cramps should also be reported.

Observation of the *smooth* muscles are a less obvious process because you cannot see these muscles. Smooth muscles of the digestive system may lack tone. This can result in difficulties with the digestion of foods and the elimination of wastes. Patients who have been dependent on laxatives often suffer from constipation. However, there are other causes of constipation. Indirectly, you note the condition of smooth muscle in the blood vessels when you measure blood pressure. Once again, there are many other factors that affect the condition of blood vessels and blood pressure. The urinary bladder and its ability to store and release urine is a measure of the muscle tone of the bladder. Numerous factors impact the control of the bladder and the bowels; nonetheless, the condition of these smooth muscles affects the healthy functioning of these organs.

Cardiac muscle must be observed indirectly, also. The state of the myocardium is assessed by the force and strength of its contractions. When you measure pulse, you should always note the rhythm of the heartbeat and feel the force of each beat. Note if it is weak, thready, bounding, or forceful, and report any changes in the rhythm and strength. (In Chapter 11, "The Cardiovascular System," you will learn more about the measurement of pulse.) Measuring blood pressure also reveals information about the state of health of the myocardium. Any complaints of chest pain should be reported immediately to the nurse. This could be a sign of a myocardial infarction (MI), or a heart attack. An MI means that the muscle of the heart is in danger due to a lack of blood flow to this muscle.

Situation 2:
Mrs. Grace has suffered a stroke. You are assigned to provide physical care for her. She was admitted to the hospital two days ago, and the stroke has affected her right side. As you begin to assist her with her bed bath, you see that her right hand is bent back and is fixed in this position. What do you do?

Author's Explanation: You should inform the nurse immediately of this finding because she did not tell you about this contracture of the right hand. Mrs. Grace will need a Physical Therapy (PT) evaluation and a rehabilitation treatment plan. Be sure to position her body in correct alignment and to position the arms and legs in the position of function. Mrs. Grace will need range-of-motion exercises (these will be reviewed in Chapter 25). Once PT has evaluated Mrs. Grace, you will assist her with these exercises. Be sure to keep her feet in the position of function to prevent foot drop. Sneakers can be worn even in bed to keep the feet in good position. A small ball or other device should be kept in her right hand to keep the fingers in proper position. Physical Therapy may recommend a splint for the right hand to correct the contracture and to prevent further deformity to the hand. Nursing care is essential to the recovery of a patient who has had a stroke. Rehabilitative exercise, immediate care, and prevention of further injury to the musculoskeletal systems are imperative in the patient's recovery.

Situation 3:
Mr. Sherone is a forty-year-old man who was in a car accident and has had injury to his spinal cord at L4 (lumbar vertebra 4). As a result of this injury, he has paraplegia. He was admitted to your rehabilitation unit yesterday. The first goal he has set with his physical therapist is to learn to transfer himself from bed to wheelchair. Mr. Sherone was in the spinal cord unit at the university hospital for three weeks. Today, he will begin to learn this transfer technique. The nurse tells you that Mr. Sherone will need assistance with his activities of daily living (ADLs). She wants you to encourage him to perform active ROM exercises of the upper extremities and passive ROM to the lower extremities. He is also on a bowel-retraining program. How will you plan to proceed with your A.M. care? What do the nurse's instructions mean to you?

Author's Explanation: After introducing yourself, you will need to ask Mr. Sherone how you can assist him with care. Ask him how he was assisted in the hospital with his grooming needs. Also ask him how he has been able to turn in bed and what grooming items he wants you to prepare for his use. Since Mr. Sherone has an L4 injury, you know that he is unable to move his lower extremities and that he has a urinary catheter. He will be able to use his upper body to assist or to turn independently so that you can wash his back. You know that the nurse has told you to perform the lower-body ROM exercises and that you are to encourage him to do the upper-body exercises independently. Request detailed information from the nurse about Mr. Sherone's bowel-retraining program and how the nurse will proceed with this program.

Observe Mr. Sherone doing the upper-body exercises to see that he performs them properly, and observe how much upper-body strength he appears to have. While you provide for his privacy in bathing, you should keep his call bell in reach so that he can call you when he has finished his part in the A.M. care. Keep his side rails up so that he will be safe and so that he can use the top rails to help with moving in bed. You should observe the skin condition and the state of his muscle tone. Observe his feet for foot drop and his heels for pressure ulcers. Keep pressure off his heels, and assist or remind him to turn from side to side as much as possible. This will help to keep his back free from pressure sores. Observe all bony prominences for any signs of skin breakdown. ROM exercises should be performed according to the orders. Observe his urinary drainage bag for the quantity and color of urine and for any sediment (these observations will be discussed in Chapter 14, The Urinary System). Note and report if he has a bowel movement and the results of his bowel-retraining regime.

Situation 4:
Mr. Sherone has been your patient for three days, and you notice that the pressure ulcer on his coccyx has progressed from stage 1 to stage 2. Ever since the physical therapist has taught him to transfer from bed to chair, he has remained out of bed (OOB) for at least four hours at a time. You know that he should not remain in one position for more than two hours, but he seems so much happier when he is OOB in his wheelchair and roaming about the rehab unit. You want to promote this independence, and you want to see him happy. In addition, Mr. Sherone has not worn anything on his feet except his soft slippers since he arrived on your unit. He says, "My feet don't work, and I feel stupid wearing shoes." What will you do?

Author's Explanation: First, report to the nurse your finding about the change in the stage of the pressure sore, and explain about the slippers. After the nurse has assessed Mr. Sherone's coccyx, follow the nurse's directions for care of the site. You and the nurse should talk to Mr. Sherone about the need to wear supportive shoes so that he will keep his feet in proper alignment and prevent foot drop. Ask him if he is willing to return to bed every two hours for short periods of time to decrease the prolonged pressure on his coccyx. Encourage his desire to move independently about the unit, and emphasize the need to prevent an advanced-stage pressure ulcer on his lower spine.

Situation 5: You are assigned to Mrs. Polaski, who has myasthenia gravis, is very weak, and tires easily. The nurse instructs you to perform passive ROM exercises to all extremities. One day, while you are performing an exercise that moves the arms away from the midline of the body, she screams in pain when you abduct the left arm. What do you do?

Author's Explanation: Stop this exercise. Continue with the other ROM exercises, and report to the nurse immediately the pain that you observed on abduction of the left arm.

Examination Review Questions

1. What is another name for involuntary muscle tissue?
   a. striated
   b. visceral
   c. nonstriated
   d. branching

2. How is skeletal tissue attached to bone?
   a. ligament
   b. cartilage
   c. tendon
   d. bursa

3. Moving away from the midline is called
   a. extension
   b. adduction
   c. flexion
   d. abduction

4. Which is capable of full ROM?
   a. knee
   b. wrist
   c. neck
   d. hip

5. Smooth muscle is also termed
   a. striated
   b. visceral
   c. voluntary
   d. skeletal

6. When muscular exercise does not produce movement, it is
   a. aerobic
   b. isometric
   c. isotonic
   d. anaerobic

7. A shortening and tightening of skeletal muscle is called
   a. atrophy
   b. contracture
   c. paralysis
   d. anomaly

8. Paralysis of one side of the body is
   a. biplegia
   b. paraplegia
   c. quadriplegia
   d. hemiplegia

9. The chest muscles are also called the
   a. triceps
   b. latissimus
   c. pectoralis
   d. biceps

10. The muscle commonly used for IM injections in children is the
    a. deltoid
    b. quadriceps
    c. gluteus medius
    d. vastus lateralis

Chapter 10

The Nervous System

To comprehend and appreciate the most majestic, sensational information-processing machine known, the human nervous system, you must use this multifunctional system. The nervous system is the system that makes us realize our aliveness. It works with lightning speed to relay messages and to react to these messages. It is so miraculous that it responds to messages that we are unaware of receiving. Although the human nervous system is designed exactly the same in each human being, it is precisely this system that makes your thoughts, your feelings, and your behavior uniquely *you*. Many students fear the study of this system because of its complexity and elusiveness. However, it will be presented in a manner that will highlight the most essential facts that you can apply to practice. Enjoy the learning.

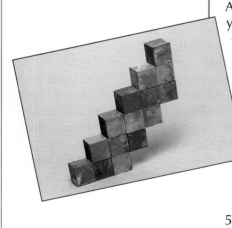

OBJECTIVES

After completing this chapter, you will be able to

1. Name the organs of the central nervous system
2. Describe the overall functions of the nervous system
3. List and describe parts of a neuron
4. List the structures and functions of the peripheral nervous system
5. Describe the conditions and diseases of the nervous system
6. List the observations about the nervous system that you should report to the nurse
7. Apply your knowledge of the nervous system to problem-solving strategies in care delivery
8. Define and spell all key terms correctly

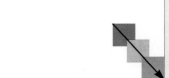

acoustic nerve	frontal lobes	parietal lobes
adrenaline	glioma	Parkinson's disease
autonomic nervous system (ANS)	grand mal	peripheral nervous system (PNS)
axon	hydrocephalus	petit mal
benign	hypothalamus	pinna
brain stem	incus	pons
cell body	inner ear	presbyopia
central nervous system (CNS)	interneurons	pupil
cerebellum	iris	remission
cerebral vascular accident (CVA)	malignant	retina
cerebrum	malleus	rods
choroid	medulla oblongata	sclera
concussion	meninges	sensory
cones	meningitis	spinal nerves
constrict	metastasis	stapes
corpus callosum	midbrain	status epilepticus
cranial nerves	middle ear	stroke
dendrites	motor	sympathetic
dilate	multiple sclerosis	synapse
embolus	neurochemical	temporal lobes
epilepsy	neuron	thalamus
epinephrine	occipital lobes	thrombus
exacerbation	olfactory bulb	transient ischemic attack (TIA)
external ear	parasympathetic	tympanic membrane

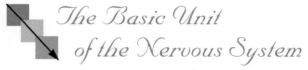

The Basic Unit of the Nervous System

The basic structure or unit of the nervous system is the **neuron**, or nerve cell (Figure 10-1). The body human has billions of neurons. They can be as small as 4/1,000 of a millimeter thick—many times thinner than a hair. The structure of a neuron is like no other cell. Most neurons look like a miniature replica of a tall, bushy-topped tree, like a beech or oak tree. There are three main parts to a neuron: the *axon*, the *dendrites*, and the *cell body*.

The **axon** is the long fiber that extends from the cell body. Axons may be as short as 1/100 of an inch or as long as three feet. Axons conduct messages away from the cell body. They are coated with a whitish insulation called a *myelin sheath*. Myelin is much like the protective covering of an electric or telephone wire. When one of these wires is frayed or damaged, it does not conduct electricity or telephone messages efficiently. When myelin is damaged or inflamed, the axon is unable to conduct the messages away from the cell body effectively.

The **dendrites** are short projections that protrude to form a treelike mass of short branches extending from the cell body. Thousands of dendrites may extend from one neuron. The dendrites are the spiky branches. Dendrites conduct messages to the cell body. They send information to be processed much like transformers. Axons and dendrites are extensions of the cell body, and they contain the cytoplasm of the nerve cell.

The **cell body** contains the nucleus of the neuron. Because it contains the nucleus, the cell body is the "brain" of the nerve cell. It functions to change the nature and direction of the signals that pass through it. Like a telephone switchboard, the cell body processes the incoming message (from dendrites) and determines which direction to send the outgoing message (to the axon).

Types of Neurons

There are three types of neurons: *sensory* neurons, *motor* neurons, and *interneurons*.

- **Sensory** neurons bring messages to the brain and the spinal cord. They relay information from the body and the environment to the brain for interpretation. If the chair on which you are sitting is hard, you will feel this because the sensory nerves in your buttocks are sending signals about this sensation to the touch and pressure center of your brain. If you are staring out the window at the

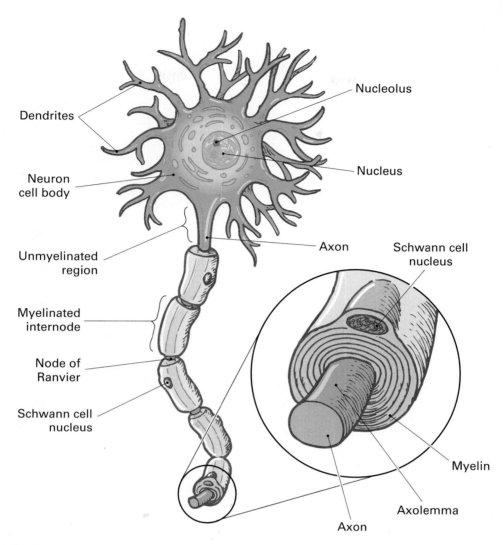

Dendrites

Nucleolus

Neuron
cell body

Nucleus

Unmyelinated
region

Axon

Schwann cell
nucleus

Myelinated
internode

Node of
Ranvier

Schwann cell
nucleus

Myelin

Axolemma

Axon

FIGURE 10-1   A neuron.

scenery, the sensory nerve (optic nerve) in your eyes is sending this message to your brain. Your perception of the beauty or horror of the scene is interpreted in the visual center of your brain.

Motor neurons carry messages away from the brain and the spinal cord. If your brain interprets the sensation that your buttocks are uncomfortable, you will most likely start to shift your position. This is a motor response. Motor responses involve conscious and unconscious (voluntary and involuntary) responses or reactions. If the scenery outside the classroom window imposes a threat—you see the funnel of a tornado, for example—your body will prepare to fight or flee the situation. The reactions of your heart, muscles, and other body organs are also motor responses.

Interneurons carry messages between sensory and motor neurons. Interneurons are found only in the brain and spinal cord. They form a net-

work for interconnection between sensory and motor nerves. They make it possible to coordinate complex reactions. For example, when you see what looks like a tornado coming your way, the brain does not have time to interpret all of the possible results. Your "switchboard operator" relies on advanced "telecommunication" fibers to connect input messages to output responses automatically. The interneuron makes the automatic connection without the intervention of the operator to direct the messages.

Each sensory neuron receives only one type of sensation or perception, and each motor neuron generates only one type of reaction or behavior. Therefore, the nerve in your little finger that will receive the message that something is burning your skin will not receive the message that a pin is piercing your skin. Each neuron is specialized to receive and send a specific message.

Transmission of Signals

When the ends of a dendrite are stimulated, sodium and potassium salts rapidly exchange positions from inside and outside the cell membrane. Sodium moves in, and potassium moves out. This creates a wave of electrical stimulation along the length of the entire nerve cell. These messages are sent as fast as 100 meters per second. As the sodium and potassium change places, a resting neuron becomes an excited neuron.

To transmit a message from one nerve to another, the neurons must meet at a juncture (meeting space) between the two neurons called a **synapse**. This is the place where a signal is passed on from one neuron to the next. When a sensory signal reaches the end of an axon fiber, a neurochemical is released. (A **neurochemical** is a protein substance that sends a message.) This **neurochemical** is necessary to pass the message on to the dendrites of the next neuron. Some neurochemicals are hormones, like **adrenaline**, which is also called **epinephrine**. This neurochemical stimulates or accelerates reactions. Other neurochemicals slow reactions or simply relay the signal onto the next neuron. An excess or a lack of any neurochemical changes the body's receiving or relaying of messages.

Today, scientists are discovering more information about neurochemicals and the body-mind responses to an excess or lack of certain neurochemicals. Actions and new functions that some neurochemicals suppress and stimulate are continually being revealed in the physiology of all animals. A new generation of antidepressant medications, which block serotonin (a neurochemical) uptake, are being used to treat depression because of the newfound correlation between an increase in serotonin and clinical depression.

Divisions of the Nervous System

The nervous system is divided into two main divisions: the *central nervous system (CNS)* and the *peripheral nervous system (PNS)*. The peripheral nervous system can be subdivided further into the *cranial nerves* and *spinal nerves* and the *autonomic nervous system (ANS)*. The divisions of the nervous system are shown in Figure 10-2.

The Central Nervous System: Structures and Functions

The **central nervous system (CNS)** is composed of the brain and the spinal cord. It is called the CNS because it is located in the center of the body and because it is the center for processing all nervous ac-

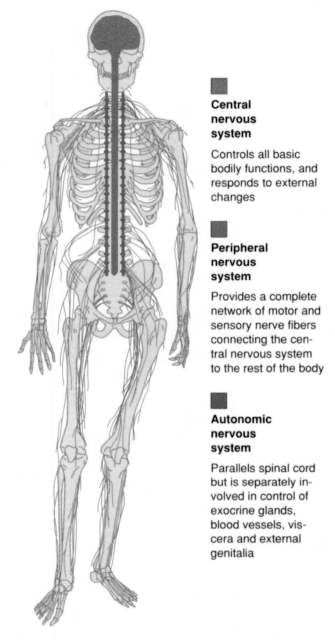

Central nervous system

Controls all basic bodily functions, and responds to external changes

Peripheral nervous system

Provides a complete network of motor and sensory nerve fibers connecting the central nervous system to the rest of the body

Autonomic nervous system

Parallels spinal cord but is separately involved in control of exocrine glands, blood vessels, viscera and external genitalia

FIGURE 10-2   Divisions of the nervous system.

tivity. A description of the structures of the CNS and their functions follows.

The Brain

The brain is composed of the *cerebrum, brain stem, interbrain,* and *cerebellum*. Each of these sections of the brain has several parts or sections that control various functions of the body. The brain is an enormously complex organ. It is housed in the protective bones that compose the cranium (skull).

Cerebrum   The largest section of the human brain is the **cerebrum**. The cerebrum of humans is larger than in any other animal. This is the part of the brain that makes us uniquely human. The cerebrum is what makes us think, reason, imagine, create, see, hear, feel, smell, and taste. The cerebrum is divided into two hemispheres, or halves: the *right hemisphere* and the *left hemisphere*. They are connected by a small bridge of tissue, the **corpus callosum**. The right and the left cerebral areas each have matching sections or lobes. Each cerebral hemisphere is composed of four lobes. Figure 10-3 identifies the two hemispheres and the four lobes of the brain.

The lobes of the cerebrum are named by the bones that encase them. They are the *frontal, temporal, parietal,* and *occipital lobes.*

- The **frontal lobes** are located in the front of the cerebrum, beneath the frontal bones. They are responsible for conscious and voluntary motor activities. Such activities include walking, writing, and playing ball. Verbal and written speech centers control the muscles of the tongue, the voice box, and the hand and arm.

- The **temporal lobes** are located at the lower sides of the cerebrum, around the area of the ears. The temporal lobes are responsible for hearing and the interpretation of sound and spoken language.

- The **parietal lobes** are located on the top sides of the cranium. These lobes are responsible for the sense of touch, including the perception and sensation of pain, pressure, and temperature. The parietal lobes help us to judge distance, size, and shape.

- The **occipital lobes** are located at the posterior base of the cerebrum. The occipital lobes are responsible for sight and the interpretation of vision. The interpretation of written language also occurs in the occipital lobes.

The sense of smell is accomplished at the core of the cerebrum in the **olfactory bulb**. Nerve fibers in the nose send messages to this site for interpretation.

Each lobe is known to be responsible for distinct functions. Nerves travel up the spinal cord to the brain and the cerebrum. These nerves cross over into the brain stem to the opposite side. Therefore, the left side of the cerebrum controls the right side of the body. When a person has a stroke in the left side of the brain, it is the right side of the body that is affected. Figure 10-4 provides a sagittal view (left plane and right plane) of the brain.

Brain Stem   The **brain stem** is the portion of the brain that connects to the spinal cord. It consists of three sections: *medulla oblongata, pons,* and *midbrain.*

- The **medulla oblongata** is a bulb-shaped protrusion that sits just inside the cranium above the spinal cord. The medulla contains reflex centers that control three vital functions: respiration, heart rate, and blood pressure. Obviously, this is a vital structure because of these basic life functions: control of the muscles of respiration, the heart rate, and the constriction of blood vessels to maintain blood pressure. Vomiting, coughing, and hiccuping are also controlled in the medulla.

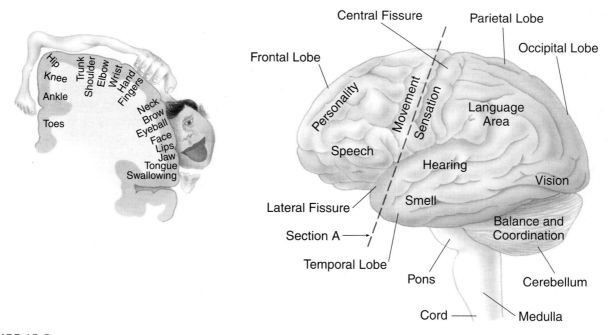

FIGURE 10-3   Lateral view of the brain.

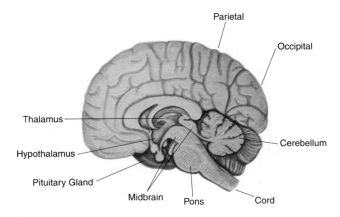

FIGURE 10-4 Sagittal view of the brain.

- The **pons** is located directly above the medulla. It serves as a relay station by sending messages from the medulla to higher centers of the brain. It also contains reflex centers for some of the cranial nerves.
- The **midbrain** rests on top of the pons. It is a reflex center for hearing and eye movements. It is also involved in motor coordination.

Interbrain   Located anterior to the midbrain are two structures in the interbrain. These are called the **thalamus** and the **hypothalamus**.

- The **thalamus** acts as a relay center for sensory information that is being sent to the brain. Sensory impulses that are sent from anywhere in the body pass through the thalamus to direct the message to the appropriate center of the brain.
- The highest level of unconscious and autonomic control is accomplished by the **hypothalamus**. Body temperature, hunger, and thirst are regulated here. This structure also controls many functions of the pituitary gland.

Cerebellum   The **cerebellum** is sometimes called the *little brain* because of its appearance. It is located under the occipital lobe. This structure is involved in the production of normal body movements. The cerebellum helps to produce smooth, coordinated body movements and to maintain equilibrium and normal posture. The gait (the way in which someone walks) is coordinated by this structure.

Meninges

The **meninges** are the protective coverings, or membranes, that protect the spinal cord and brain. The meninges are comprised of three layers: the *dura mater*, the *arachnoid*, and the *pia mater*. The outermost layer is the dura mater, which literally means "tough mother." The middle layer is the arachnoid, and this means "spider-like." The innermost layer that lies directly on the brain and spinal cord is the pia mater, which means "delicate mother." In the arachnoid layer, *cerebrospinal fluid (CSF)* flows to bathe and protect the brain and spinal cord. The CSF is made in the ventricles of the brain by a network of capillaries that filter blood.

To imagine the structure of the meninges, think about the layers of an orange. On the outside is the tough, outer orange skin; this is like the dura mater. Just inside the tough orange skin is a weblike mesh of white rutin. The rutin is like the middle layer of meninges, the arachnoid membrane. Closest to the orange pulp is a thin membrane that can be removed delicately from each orange section. This almost transparent membrane is like the pia mater. Most people have heard of the disease called *meningitis*. When the meninges become invaded by a virus or a bacteria, they become inflamed. The spinal cord and brain may be affected. These membranes protect the brain and spinal cord.

The Peripheral Nervous System: Structures and Functions

As noted earlier, the **peripheral nervous system (PNS)** is made up of the cranial and spinal nerves and the autonomic nervous system. Explanation of each of these components follows.

Cranial Nerves

There are twelve pairs of **cranial nerves**. These nerves originate in the brain, and they are referred to by both a name and a number. Basically, these nerves send sensory messages to the brain, or they send motor messages away from the brain. Except for the vagus nerve (X), cranial nerves control sensations and motor responses from the shoulders, neck, and face. These are the nerves that send sensory information to the brain centers for interpretation of sight, hearing, taste, smell, and feel—everything that touches our face, throat, and eyes. They also control eye movements, swallowing, tongue movements, shoulder movements, and throat movements. They allow us to swallow, speak, smile, frown, shrug our shoulders, turn our head, constrict and dilate our eye pupils, and stick out our tongue. The vagus nerve is involved in controlling the internal organs of the heart, lungs, and digestive tract.

Spinal Nerves

The thirty-one pairs of **spinal nerves** enter and exit all along the spinal cord. The connection of the nerves with the spinal cord is illustrated in Figure 10-5. The spinal nerves are involved in sensation and movement of the arms and legs. They connect with nerves of the central nervous system and the autonomic nervous system.

The Autonomic Nervous System: Structures and Functions

The **autonomic nervous system (ANS)** is a subsystem of the nervous system that is involved with involuntary and automatic control of the glands and organs of the entire body. These motor nerves affect the responses of the glands and the internal organs that control all body functions under stress and normal conditions of living.

There are two subdivisions of this system. Simply put, the **sympathetic** division is referred to as the *fight-or-flight* division because it readies the internal organs and muscles for stressful situations. Consider a situation that is stressful for you, and think about the physiological response of your body. Your heart starts to beat faster and stronger, your breathing is deeper and faster, your mouth is dry, your pupils are dilated, your skin is flushed, and you feel nervous, but energized. You are ready to fight or run from whatever is threatening you.

The second division of the ANS is the **parasympathetic** division. Nerves that control parasympathetic responses essentially stimulate the body during normal conditions of life. Your heart beats at a regular rate, and your respirations are within normal limits. Your blood pressure is stable, your digestive functions are not disrupted, and your muscles and skin have a normal supply of blood. The ANS receives and sends information to and from the CNS. You can only become aware of stressful and nonstressful events if the CNS is intact and in harmony with the ANS and the PNS.

While the divisions of the nervous system have specific functions and structures, they do not work as separate or isolated systems. The entire nervous system works as a unified system to receive sensations and perceptions and to control motor responses and reactions of the internal and external environment. For example, your nerves in sensory organs (PNS) receive messages from the environment. These messages are directed to the spinal cord and brain (CNS). In the CNS, these messages are processed, and a response is determined. If the message is stressful or alarming, nerves of the sympathetic division of the ANS prepare the organs of the body to respond. If the messages are nonstressful, the parasympathetic nerves and other peripheral nerves continue to steadily regulate the body's routine functions.

Special Sense Organs: Structures and Functions

Two of the special sense organs of the human body are the *eye* and the *ear*. Detailed descriptions of the structures and functions of each of these organs follow.

The Eye

When you look at a person's eye, you see only a portion of the entire structure. See Figure 10-6 for an illustration of the eye. There are three coats, or layers, that compose the eye: the *sclera*, the *choroid*, and the *retina*.

Sclera

The **sclera**, a layer of tough connective tissue, is commonly called the *white of the eye*. This is only the anterior portion, and the sclera is continuous to the posterior part of the eyeball. There is a thin transparent membrane lying over the sclera that is called the *cornea*. On top of the cornea is another protective membrane known as the *conjunctiva*. This is a mucous membrane that helps to keep dirt and dust particles from irritating the cornea. The conjunctiva also lines the upper and lower eyelids.

Choroid

The **choroid** is the second continuous layer of the eyeball. In the frontal portion of the choroid are two special involuntary muscles: the *iris* and the *pupil*. The **iris** is a doughnut-shaped muscle that is the colored part of the eye. In the center of the iris is an open area called the **pupil**. The iris has muscle fibers

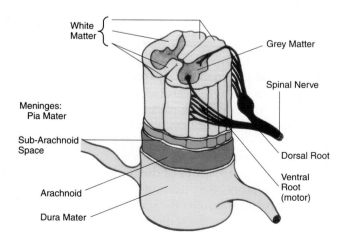

FIGURE 10-5 Segment of the spinal cord with spinal nerve.

White Matter

Grey Matter

Spinal Nerve

Meninges: Pia Mater

Sub-Arachnoid Space

Dorsal Root

Ventral Root (motor)

Arachnoid

Dura Mater

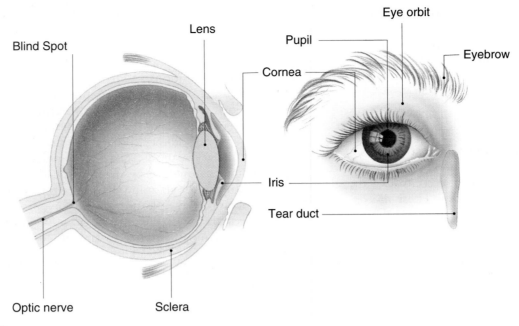

FIGURE 10-6   The eye.

that are arranged like the spokes of a wheel. These control the opening and closing of the pupil. When the pupil **dilates** (gets larger), it allows more light to enter. Under normal circumstances, the pupil dilates in dim light or darkness. And when the pupil **constricts** (gets smaller), this restricts the amount of light that enters. Normally, the pupil constricts in the presence of bright light.

Behind the iris and pupil lie the ciliary muscle and the lens. The lens is held in place by a ligament that attaches it to the ciliary muscle. When you look at a distant object, the ciliary muscle relaxes and flattens the curve of the lens. When you read or look at something close, the ciliary muscle contracts and bulges the curvature of the lens. Changes in the ciliary muscle are designed to allow more light to enter and focus on the interior of the eye. As we age, the lens loses its elasticity and can no longer accommodate enough to bring near objects into focus. This is called **presbyopia** (literally, "old vision").

Retina

The innermost layer of the eye is the **retina**. This layer of the eyeball is very vascular. Changes in the blood vessels are seen with retinal deterioration associated with certain diseases like *diabetes mellitus*. There are two specialized types of microscopic receptors that respond to light rays that enter the retina: *rods* and *cones*. **Rods** are sensitive to dim light and are needed for good night vision. **Cones** are sensitive to bright light and are important for good

vision in daylight and for color vision. The cranial and optic nerves transmit messages from the retina to the visual center of the cerebrum. When the eye is examined with an ophthalmoscope, the condition of the retina is being examined. Fluid fills the hollow portion of the eyeball. This fluid helps to maintain the shape of the eyeball and to bend light rays to focus on the retina.

The Ear

The ear has three main sections: *external, middle,* and *inner.* See Figure 10-7 for an illustration of the ear. The **external ear** is what you can see protruding at the side of the head. The flap of the ear, the **pinna,** acts to collect sound waves, which move along the external ear canal to the eardrum. The **middle ear** is a tiny hollow structure in the temporal bone. The **tympanic membrane** (eardrum), is the separation between the external ear and the middle ear. When sound waves strike the eardrum, a mechanical chain of events is created that causes movement of three tiny bones. The **malleus, incus,** and **stapes**—the three bones of the middle ear—strike each other in sequence, allowing sound waves to enter the inner ear. Within the structures of the **inner ear** are microscopic receptors for hearing and balance. The **acoustic nerve** transmits the impulses received in the hearing receptors to the temporal lobe for interpretation of the sounds heard. When there is an infection or inflammation in the inner ear, hearing and equilibrium (balance) can be affected.

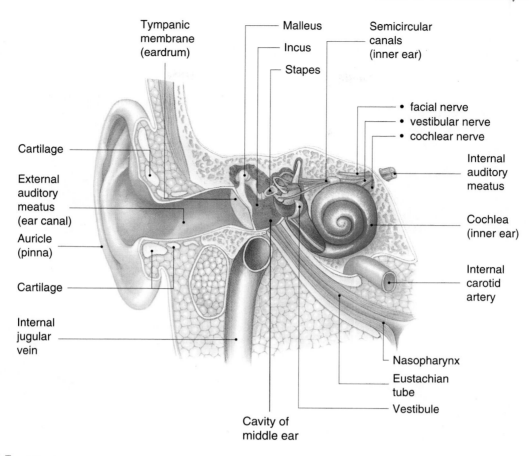

FIGURE 10-7   The ear.

Conditions and Diseases of the Nervous System

Multiple sclerosis is a disease of the CNS that results from inflammation or loss of the myelin coating on multiple nerve fibers throughout the CNS. Many theories exist about the cause of this disease, but the actual cause is not known. Symptoms vary in nature and severity. Disturbances of gait, vision, and motor coordination are often seen. There may also be paralysis. This disease is characterized by **exacerbation** (flare-up of symptoms) and **remission** (disappearance of symptoms). The symptoms can disappear for months or years and return without warning. Treatment varies and depends on the presenting symptoms.

Meningitis is an inflammation of the meninges. The inflammation of these membranes is caused by an infection that often begins with signs of a respiratory infection. Babies are most vulnerable to infection of the meninges. Symptoms include stiffness of the neck, pain, fever, chills, body rash, and headache. A spinal tap or lumbar puncture is performed to diagnose meningitis. The cerebrospinal fluid will show evidence of the infectious agent. The CSF is normally clear, but when the meningococcus is infecting the meninges, it will be a milky color.

A **cerebral vascular accident (CVA)** is commonly called a **stroke**. Strokes are caused by

- Hemorrhage
- **Thrombus**—a blood clot that forms in a blood vessel in the brain
- **Embolus**—a blood clot that travels to the brain

Figure 10-8 illustrates these three causes of stroke. The symptoms that result are determined by the severity and location of the vascular accident. The symptoms usually appear abruptly and may be subtle at first, and then within minutes or hours they can become severe. What seems like blurred vision, a headache, and slurred speech can progress to loss of vision and aphasia (speech disturbances). Consciousness may be lost, and coma may result. Paralysis of one side of the body is common, and this is called *hemiplegia*. The paralysis will be on the opposite side of the body from where the hemorrhage or clot occurred in the brain. Sometimes people suffer "ministrokes" or TIAs. A **transient ischemic attack (TIA)** occurs when blood flow is hampered for brief periods of time, and mild strokelike symptoms are noted.

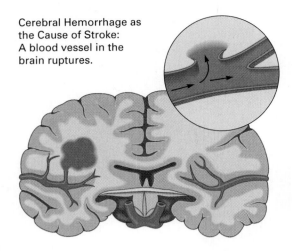

Cerebral Hemorrhage as the Cause of Stroke: A blood vessel in the brain ruptures.

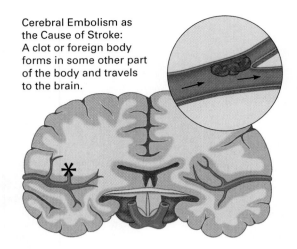

Cerebral Embolism as the Cause of Stroke: A clot or foreign body forms in some other part of the body and travels to the brain.

STROKE

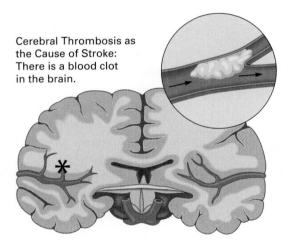

Cerebral Thrombosis as the Cause of Stroke: There is a blood clot in the brain.

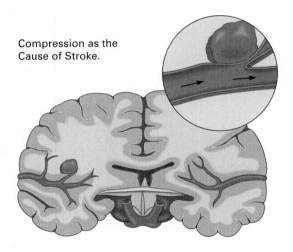

Compression as the Cause of Stroke.

FIGURE 10-8   Causes of stroke.

When blood flow and oxygen return to the portion of the brain that is affected, the symptoms abate (go away). These should not be ignored because they are often a warning sign of what could become a CVA if the underlying problem is not corrected. High blood pressure is an underlying cause of many strokes.

Parkinson's disease is characterized by motor disturbances. Most often there is a tremor, especially when the person is at rest, and it is most apparent in the hands. Shaking of the head is sometimes seen. There is rigidity of muscles. The facial expression is often fixed and does not show emotion. Speech may be garbled and soft, and frequently the person has what is known as forward propulsion. This is seen when a person with Parkinson's tries to stop walking at a given spot but continues to move forward as though being pushed. Medications are used to decrease the stiffness and rigidity. A neurochemical, *dopamine*, which is lacking in this patient, is given in the form of a medication called *L-Dopa*.

Spinal cord injuries are the result of trauma to any part of the spinal cord. The symptoms that result are directly related to the severity and location of the injury. When injuries are high in the spinal cord (cervical area), the results can mean quadriplegia, inability to control the muscles of respiration, and sometimes even death. A ventilator may be required to breathe mechanically for this person. When spinal cord injuries occur, there is a loss of function from that area of the spinal cord down the body. If the lumbar spine is traumatized, this could result in paralysis of the lower extremities (paraplegia).

Epilepsy (seizure disorder) may be caused by trauma or infections of the brain or by an unknown cause. Sometimes, seizure disorders begin when there has been no insult to the brain but there is a family history of epilepsy. Epilepsy is not a mental illness. The person with epilepsy suffers from seizures or convulsions. There are many types of seizures, and they take very different forms. Some seizures may be almost unnoticeable. The person may "blank out" or stare for several seconds. This is called a **petit mal** seizure. The most dramatic form of seizure is a **grand mal** seizure, or generalized seizure. This appears with a sudden loss of consciousness, falling to the ground, and muscle contractions, followed by relaxation of the muscles. Sometimes, the person may become incontinent of bowels and bladder. The airway may be obstructed by the tongue, and frothing of saliva and biting of the tongue may result when the jaw is clenched. These seizures may last from 1 to 5 minutes. If they last longer, they can be life-threatening. If a seizure stops and begins again suddenly, the situation is life-threatening and must be treated immediately. This condition of continuous seizure activity is called **status epilepticus**.

Following a grand mal seizure, the person may have a headache, forget what happened, and feel exhausted. Medications are used to treat and control seizures. An electroencephalogram (EEG) is done to definitively diagnose the type of seizure that occurred. Abnormal and rapidly discharged impulses are detected in specific sections of the brain. This identifies the location of the disturbance and the type of seizure.

Hydrocephalus literally means "water in the head." This condition occurs when there is obstruction of the circulation of the CSF. This condition is usually evident at birth and is characterized by enlargement of the head and prominent veins in the head. Hydrocephalus can be corrected surgically with the placement of a shunt that diverts the CSF into the venous circulation. If treated soon after birth, disabilities can be prevented.

Tumors can develop in the brain at any time of life, and these may be the primary site of cancer. Some tumors are **benign** (noncancerous), and others are **malignant** (cancerous). The malignant tumor may be the result of the spread of cancer **(metastasis)** from another site in the body. The tumor may be operable, meaning that it can be removed surgically. It may be inoperable due to the location and type of the tumor growth. Inoperable tumors are treated with chemotherapy and radiation therapy to shrink the size of the tumor and to halt its spread and growth. The symptoms that result from brain tumors vary and depend on the location of the tumor.

Concussion is defined as a temporary loss of consciousness as the result of a blow to the head. Even if consciousness is not lost, a concussed person may experience dizziness, headache, fatigue, nausea, vomiting, and changes in sleep and mood. The concussion may be the result of a skull fracture that may cause a blood clot, hemorrhage, or lesions of brain tissue. The symptoms of the trauma may be more severe than concussion and may result in seizures, coma, paralysis, and even death. Sometimes, the symptoms from a blow to the head may not appear for days or weeks.

application to practice

The clinical care associate is often involved in the care of patients with spinal cord injuries or other conditions of the nervous system. Your observations and clinical findings can assist the nurse and the team in the care and treatment of patients with nervous system disorders. Consider the information about the nervous system that you just learned, and relate this knowledge to the following patient care situations.

Learning Activities

Situation 1: Miss Jones is seventeen years old. She was admitted to your pediatric unit last night following a car accident. She suffered a skull fracture that did not lacerate the brain. You are assigned to care for her, and the nurse's report reveals the following information. She is complaining of a headache, dizziness, and nausea. She is able to speak and to voluntarily move her limbs, and she has not lost consciousness. She is NPO (nothing by mouth) until 12 noon and on bedrest. You are to observe her for signs of neurological changes and to assist her with a.m. care. Upon entering her room, you see that she is getting out of bed. She tells you that she has to go to the bathroom to use the toilet and to get a drink of water. Describe how you will proceed.

Author's Explanation: You should tell Miss Jones that she has to return to bed, and assist her so that she does not fall. Explain why she is to stay in bed and that she will need to use the bedpan until her doctor says that she can be out of bed (OOB). Remind her that she cannot eat or drink anything until noon. Ask her about her head pain and the dizziness and nausea. Observe her speech and movements, and assure her that you will be available to assist her. Consider her age and the embarrassment of using a bedpan and the impact of restricting her freedom to get out of bed and to eat. Report any changes that you notice about her speech, movements, and level of consciousness and any complaints. Also inform the nurse of her desires, including getting OOB and drinking fluids.

Situation 2: Mr. Weatherby is a sixty-eight-year-old man who was admitted to the emergency room (ER) two hours ago. When you arrive, you get a report about Mr. Weatherby. The nurse tells you that he had a CVA. A computerized axial tomography (CAT) scan revealed a blood clot in the left frontal lobe. What impairments do you expect he will have?

Author's Explanation: Since the stroke resulted from a clot on the left side of the cerebrum, you expect to see the impairments on the right side of the body. Because it was the frontal lobe, you will probably see weakness or paralysis of the right arm, leg, and facial muscles. He may be unable to speak or swallow, and he may be unconscious.

Situation 3: Mrs. Gabet is a forty-two-year-old woman who has a **glioma** (tumor of the glial cells of the brain) in the right occipital lobe. She is being admitted to your oncology unit for chemotherapy and radiation. You are to orient her to her room, take her vital signs, chart her height and weight, and complete an inventory of her belongings. What symptoms do you expect Mrs. Gabet to have, and what assistance do you think you will need to provide for her care?

Author's Explanation: Since the tumor is in the right occipital lobe, she will probably have impaired vision or blindness in the left eye or both eyes. She is probably depressed and fearful of her condition and upcoming treatments. When you orient her to her room, you should walk around the room by her side. Depending on the severity of her visual impairment, describe in words the location of the items and furniture in the room. If she is unable to see in one eye, you should stand or sit on her opposite side to make it easier for her to see you. When her lunch tray arrives, help her to arrange the food on her tray in a clockwise direction so that she can determine how she will eat her food. Always announce yourself by name when you enter her room so that she knows who is present. Describe the usual order of daily events on this unit. Put her call bell and any items that she needs and wants within easy reach. If her visual impairments are severe and she is unable to navigate around in her room, tell her to ring the call bell whenever she needs assistance to move about. Inform the nurse of the patient's height, weight, and vital signs and the observations that you made about her physical and emotional condition and her safety.

Situation 4: Bobby Esposito is a six-year-old boy who fell last week while riding his bike. His mother has brought him to the doctor's office for a checkup because of complaints of a headache and excessive sleeping. Yesterday, he came home from school with a bruise over his left eye, and he does not remember how he got the bruise. As you enter the examination room to take his vital signs, you hear him cry out. He falls to the ground and begins to have jerking movements of his limbs. He arches his back, and you see frothy saliva coming from his mouth. What do you do?

Author's Explanation: Call for the doctor or nurse, and remain with Bobby. Protect his head from injury, and loosen any tight clothing. Move furniture out of the way so that he will not injure himself by striking anything with his arms or legs. If possible, turn his body or his head to the side so that he will not choke on his saliva. Observe the time the event began, and monitor his breathing. Do not try to open his mouth to prevent tongue biting because of potential injuries to yourself or to him. Do not restrict his limbs or restrain his movements. This also can cause injury. Note the time the seizure stops. When the seizure stops, tell Bobby where he is, and allow him to rest in a safe place. Check for any injuries, including his tongue. See if he has been incontinent of urine or stool. Take his vital signs, reassure him of his safety, and do not leave him alone. Describe exactly what you saw and heard to the doctor and the nurse.

Examination Review Questions

1. The nerve cell component that conducts messages away from the neuron is the
   - a. neuron
   - b. cell body
   - c. axon
   - d. dendrite

2. The nerve cell component that contains the nucleus is the
   - a. dendrite
   - b. cell body
   - c. axon
   - d. neuron

3. Which nerve cell transmits messages to the brain?
   - a. sensory
   - b. motor
   - c. neuron
   - d. interneuron

4. Nerve impulses must fire across a junction between neurons called the
   - a. neurochemical
   - b. epinephrine
   - c. adrenaline
   - d. synapse

5. Which nervous system division is composed of the brain and spinal cord?
- a. sympathetic
- b. central
- c. peripheral
- d. autonomic

6. The part of the brain responsible for higher-level functions such as thinking is the
- a. cerebellum
- b. midbrain
- c. cerebrum
- d. interbrain

7. The _____ base of the cerebrum is responsible for sight.
- a. frontal
- b. temporal
- c. parietal
- d. occipital

8. The brain structure that regulates body temperature is the
- a. thalamus
- b. hypothalamus
- c. pons
- d. medulla

9. An inflammation of the membrane that covers the spinal cord causes
- a. muscular dystrophy
- b. encephalitis
- c. multiple sclerosis
- d. meningitis

10. A right CVA causes
- a. left hemiplegia
- b. rigid movement
- c. right hemiplegia
- d. flaccid movement

Chapter 11

The Circulatory System

Circulation is the continuous movement of blood and lymph fluid throughout the body. All of the systems and organs depend on the circulatory system. Arteries carry blood with oxygen and nutrients to each cell, and veins carry away the cell's waste products. If the circulation is not adequate, cells die. When the cells die, tissues begin to die, and the organs stop working properly. This may cause an entire system to stop functioning.

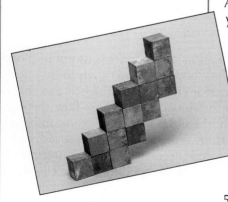

OBJECTIVES

After completing this chapter, you will be able to

1. Name the organs of the circulatory system
2. Describe the functions of the circulatory system
3. Describe the location and function of each organ
4. List the functions of the heart and blood vessels
5. Describe the conditions and diseases of the circulatory system
6. List the observations about the circulatory system that you should report to the nurse
7. Apply your knowledge of the circulatory system to problem-solving strategies in care delivery
8. Define and spell all key terms correctly

key terms

albumin
anemia
aneurysms
angina
angina pectoris
antibodies
antigens
aorta
arrhythmias
arterioles
artery
atrioventricular (AV) node
bicuspid
blood pressure
bradycardia
capillaries
cardiac catheterization
cardiomegaly
cardiovascular (CV)
central venous pressure
centrifuge
congestive heart failure
Cooley's anemia
coronary arteries
coronary artery disease (CAD)
dysrhythmias

endocardium
erythrocytes
force
globulins
hemoglobin
hemophilia
hypertension
hypotension
leukemia
leukocytes
leukopenia
lymph
lymph nodes
lymph vessels
lymphatic system
mitral
mitral valve prolapse
myocardial infarction (MI)
myocardium
neutropenia
occlusion
pain scale
pericardium
phagocytes
phlebitis
plasma

platelets
pulse
pulse points
radial artery
rate
Rh factor
rhythm
septum
shock
sickle-cell anemia
sinoatrial (SA) node
sphygmomanometer
spleen
tachycardia
telemetry
thrombocytes
thrombocytopenia
thrombophlebitis
thymus gland
tonsils
tricuspid valve
valvular diseases
vein
venules

The Circulatory System: Structures and Functions

The circulatory system includes the **cardiovascular (CV) system** and the lymphatic system. The term *cardio-* means "heart," and *vascular* refers to blood vessels. The function of the cardiovascular system is to circulate blood. Blood transports nutrients, oxygen, carbon dioxide, waste products, and chemical substances to and away from the cells of the body. The organs of this system include the heart, arteries, veins, capillaries, and blood. Blood is a special type of tissue. The lymphatic system includes the lymph ducts, lymph fluid, lymph nodes, and lymphatic vessels, and the accessory organs to the immune system.

The primary functions of the circulatory system are

1. Transportation or circulation of oxygen and carbon dioxide
2. Transportation of hormones
3. Transportation of nutrients and waste products
4. Protection against infection
5. Prevention of hemorrhage

The Heart

The primary function of the heart is to pump blood throughout the body. Blood constantly flows through the interior chambers of the heart so that it can be sent to the lungs. Blood must flow through the capillaries of the lungs so that oxygen can be absorbed and carbon dioxide can be removed. After blood is oxygenated ("refueled") in the lungs, it returns to the heart to be pumped to all the cells of the body. An illustration of the heart is provided in Figure 11-1.

The heart is located on the left side of the thoracic cavity between the lungs. It is protected by the sternum (breastbone) and the ribs. The heart is a three-layer muscular organ that is surrounded by a double-layer protective membrane called the **pericardium**. The muscular layer of tissue is called the **myocardium**, and the inner lining of the heart is called the **endocardium**. The heart is divided into right and left sides by a wall of tissue called the **septum**. The septum separates the blood that flows through the interior of the heart. The blood on the

The Heart

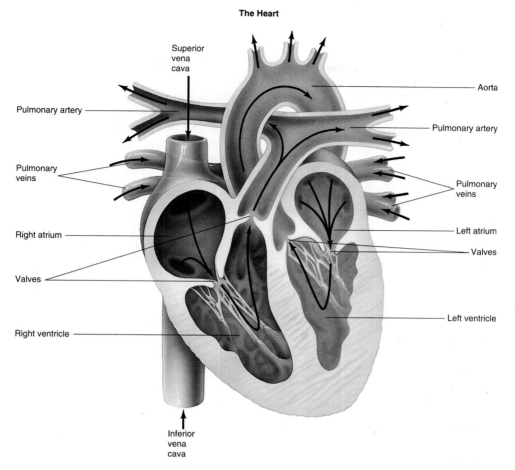

Superior
vena
cava

Pulmonary artery

Pulmonary
veins

Right atrium

Valves

Right ventricle

Inferior
vena
cava

Aorta

Pulmonary artery

Pulmonary
veins

Left atrium

Valves

Left ventricle

FIGURE 11-1 The heart.

right side of the heart is returning to the heart from all over the body. This blood is rich in *carbon dioxide* and poor in *oxygen* (deoxygenated blood). Blood from the right side is pumped to the tiny blood vessels (capillaries) in the lungs that surround microscopic air sacs (Figure 11-2). When blood reaches these capillaries, the carbon dioxide (CO_2) escapes to the air sacs. The oxygen (O_2) from the air sacs then enters the blood in the capillaries. This newly oxygenated blood (rich in oxygen) returns to the left side of the heart to be pumped throughout the body. The exchange of O_2 and CO_2 is the most vital homeostatic (referring to a steady or balanced state) mechanism of the body because the most essential element of life is oxygen.

The right and left sides of the heart are further divided into upper and lower sections called *chambers*. The upper chambers are called the *atria*. The lower chambers are called the *ventricles*. Between the right atrium and the right ventricle is a valve called the **tricuspid valve**. The purpose of any valve is to prevent the backflow of blood. When the tricuspid valve opens, it allows blood to flow into the right ventricle, and then it closes to prevent backflow. This blood then travels through a large blood vessel called the

pulmonary artery to the lungs. Between the left atrium and the left ventricle is another valve called the *bicuspid valve* or *mitral valve*.

With each heartbeat, the valves open and close. The opening and closing of the heart valves create the "lubb-dupp" sounds that can be heard through a

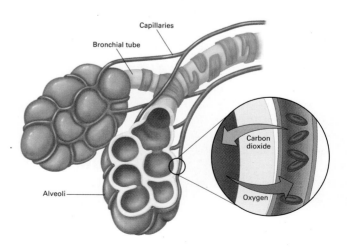

Capillaries

Bronchial tube

Carbon
dioxide

Oxygen

Alveoli

FIGURE 11-2 Carbon dioxide escapes from the blood to the air sacs, and oxygen enters the blood from the air sacs.

stethoscope. Heart sounds indicate the state of health of the heart valves. Figure 11-3 shows the flow of blood through the heart valves.

When these valves are weakened, what happens to the flow of blood? It backs up! This creates congestion. Congestion of the blood flowing to and from the heart is known as *congestive heart failure* (CHF). There are numerous causes of this condition, but one is valve failure. To help you more fully understand this condition, consider the following analogy.

Imagine that you are traveling on a highway and there is a steady flow of traffic going south. Suddenly, the right lane is blocked by a truck that has broken down. The southbound traffic begins to back up, creating a traffic jam. The highway becomes congested by this backup of traffic. Just as highways are a means of transportation for motor vehicles, blood vessels are a means of transportation for blood. When traffic can't move because of an obstruction, motor vehicles are congested in that area.

When valves, heart muscle, or blood vessels are obstructed, damaged or weakened blood becomes congested in the area due to the backflow of blood.

There are two other valves in the heart, and they are shaped like a half-moon. These *semilunar valves* (*semi-* means "half," and *lunar* refers to the moon) prevent the backflow of blood that is going to the lungs and blood that is returning to the heart from the lungs. These valves lie between the heart and the blood vessels that serve as the routes out of the ventricles. They are like the north- and southbound lanes of a highway.

Imagine the lungs as the city of Los Angeles. The pulmonary artery is a one-way freeway leading to the city (the route to the lungs), and the pulmonary veins are a one-way freeway leaving the city (the route from the lungs). The exit ramp into LA is the pulmonary semilunar valve. Like a vehicle, blood travels on the highway of the pulmonary artery, the main highway into the lungs. The business that must take place

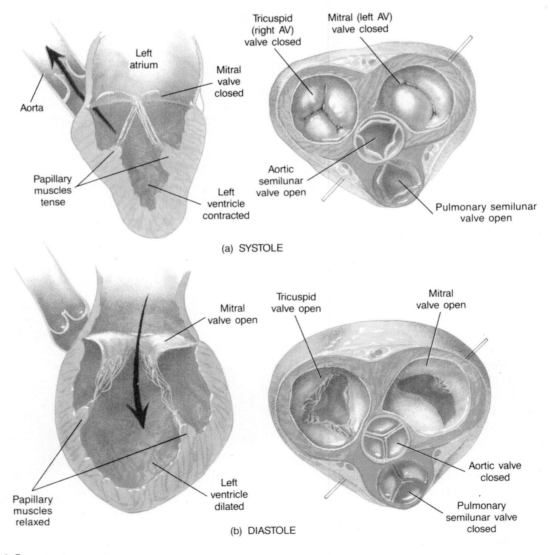

(a) SYSTOLE

(b) DIASTOLE

FIGURE 11-3   The heart valves.

there is to drop off one passenger (carbon dioxide) and to pick up a different passenger (oxygen). After the business is completed, the blood exits the lungs via the pulmonary veins. The new destination is the left ventricle, which pumps blood to another highway, the aorta, the largest artery in the body. The next exit ramp is the aortic semilunar valve, as blood exits en route to the aorta. The trip is complete, and the vehicle (blood) now passes through all the suburbs (organs of the body) to drop off and pick up more passengers (oxygen and carbon dioxide). Every minute, this trip is completed at least sixty times.

The heart beats approximately sixty to one hundred times per minute in the adult body. Newborn babies and small children have faster heart rates. When the heart beats above the normal rate, this condition is called **tachycardia** (*tachy-* means "fast"). When the heart beats below the normal range, the term used is **bradycardia** (*brady-* means "slow").

The heart is often said to be the size of one's fist. When the heart muscle is unhealthy due to disease or congestion, it is enlarged, and the muscle is stretched and weak. This is called **cardiomegaly** (*megaly* means "enlargement" or "large"). As the heart ages, it may enlarge. As a result of this enlargement, it beats faster to compensate (make up) for the lack of muscle strength in the act of pumping blood.

The heart, like any other organ, needs its own blood supply. The blood vessels that supply the nutrients and oxygen to the heart are called the **coronary arteries**. When these blood vessels become clogged due to fatty deposits, coronary artery disease (CAD) exists. As a result of the plaque (buildup of fat) on the walls of these blood vessels, blood flow is obstructed. The vessels become narrow and hardened. When a muscle does not receive oxygen and nutrients, it suffers spasms and pain. When the heart muscle does not receive enough oxygen, the tissue may die. Then a heart attack results. A heart attack is often referred to as a *myocardial infarction* (MI). Scar tissue forms in the area of the heart that did not receive the oxygen. This is the infarction. The coronary arteries can become diseased due to substances in the blood that clog these vessels. Fat and nicotine are two substances that cause the obstruction and hardening of the coronary arteries. Some people have momentary periods of heart pain due to lack of blood flow and oxygen. This is called **angina**.

The Electrical Stimulating System of the Heart

Throughout the myocardium is nervous tissue that stimulates the heart cycle (Figure 11-4). A chain of events sets the rate and rhythm of the heartbeat. The heart has a "pacemaker" called the **sinoatrial (SA) node**. This cluster of specialized nervous tissue sets the chain of events into action. Just as the leader of a

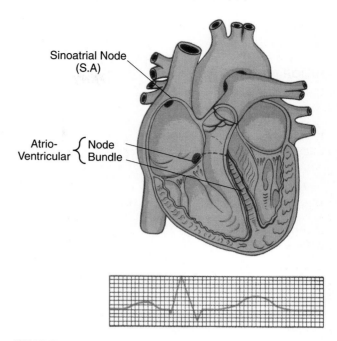

FIGURE 11-4   Nervous tissue stimulates the heart, regulating the rate and rhythm of the heartbeat.

marching band sets the timing for the march, the SA node sets the pace for the rate of the heart. Neurochemical messages pass from the SA node to the **atrioventricular (AV) node** to the *bundle of His* to the *Purkinje fibers*. This cycle is repeated at least 60 times a minute throughout one's lifetime. When an electrocardiogram (ECG) is performed, it generates a picture of the electrical activity of the heart. An ECG will provide information about the regularity of the heart's rate and rhythm. This diagnostic test will be discussed in Chapter 26.

Blood Vessels

Arteries, veins, and capillaries are all blood vessels. These are the highways through which blood travels. Just as highways are routes to streets that extend through towns, so arteries and veins are the major highways that exit to main streets that lead to and from the organs of the body. These main streets have turnoffs to small streets that travel within the tissues of the body. And these small streets are routes to even smaller streets that take us to houses or buildings like the cells.

To get to school or work each day, you might take a freeway. Perhaps you exit the freeway to Main Street and turn right onto Market Street, where your school or hospital is located. Large arteries and veins have to transport blood to microscopic cells within large organs. To accomplish this, blood vessels must have smaller and smaller routes. Figure 11-5 depicts the arteries and veins of the human body through which blood flows.

MAJOR ARTERIES

MAJOR VEINS

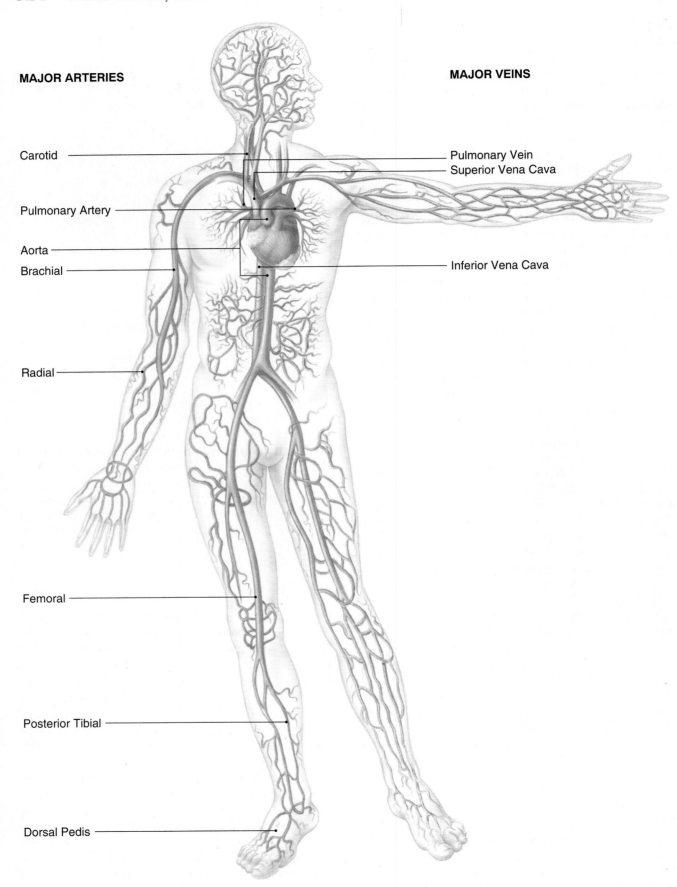

Carotid

Pulmonary Artery

Aorta

Brachial

Radial

Femoral

Posterior Tibial

Dorsal Pedis

Pulmonary Vein
Superior Vena Cava

Inferior Vena Cava

FIGURE 11-5   Arteries and veins of the human body.

Arteries

An **artery** carries blood that is pumped from the heart to all parts of the body. Pulse and blood pressure can be measured in the arteries. The force of the heart's contraction can be felt or heard as blood is pumped through the arteries.

Arteries carry blood that is oxygenated. The only artery in the body that does not carry blood that is rich in oxygen is the pulmonary artery. Where is this artery located? Why is it called an artery if it does not carry oxygenated blood? You can find this answer if you reread the section above on the route blood takes to and from the lungs.

The largest artery in the body human is the aorta. The **aorta** is the artery that receives blood pumped by the left ventricle.

Arteries are made of three layers of tissues, and so are veins. Structurally, they are alike, except that veins have valves and arteries do not. Why? The next section on veins will give you the answer. The smallest arteries are called **arterioles**. These carry blood from the arterial ends of the capillaries.

Veins

A **vein** is a blood vessel that carries blood to the heart. The largest veins of the body are the *superior vena cava* and the *inferior vena cava*. Veins converge from the upper and lower extremities to carry blood into the right atrium. This venous blood is deoxygenated (poor in oxygen). It is sent to the capillaries of the lungs to exchange carbon dioxide and oxygen in the air sacs. Veins have valves because, unlike arteries, they do not have the pumping action of the heart to push the blood. (Remember that the function of a valve is to prevent the backflow of blood.) Blood that leaves the lower extremities has to be pushed uphill against gravity to return to the heart. Without the valves, the venous blood of the feet would be congested by the backflow of blood. Varicose veins are the result of weakening of the valves in the veins. The smallest veins are called **venules**. These lead to the venous end of capillaries.

Capillaries

Capillaries are microscopic vessels that have only one layer of epithelial cells. There are millions of capillaries in the body. If all of the capillaries of the body were extended end to end, they would cover an area over 60,000 miles long. Capillaries are just wide enough to allow blood cells to travel through in single file. Each capillary has a venous end and an arterial end (Figure 11-6). Capillaries are the secret to the cellular exchange of nutrients, waste products, and the blood gases (oxygen and carbon dioxide). Remember that each cell has a life of its own and re-

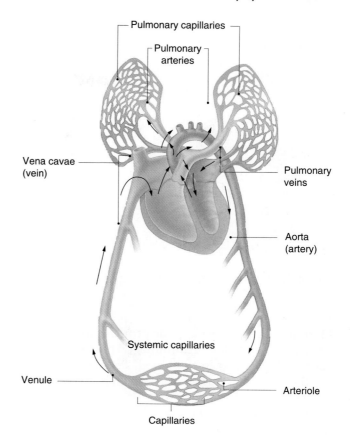

FIGURE 11-6   Venous and arterial ends of a capillary.

quires all of the same substances as the entire body does to maintain life. Since capillaries are made of epithelial cells, they can absorb and secrete substances into and out of cells.

Blood

The foremost function of blood is to transport O_2, cellular nutrients, and waste products. Oxygen and nutrient molecules are transported to the cells of the body. The lungs are the site for the absorption of oxygen from the environment into blood. Carbon dioxide is a cellular waste product, and it is transported in blood to the lungs to be exhaled into the environment. The kidneys are the site for removing other cellular waste products from the blood. Hormones are also transported via the blood.

Contained within blood are a number of components (Figure 11-7). When blood is drawn for examination, it can be separated into several components so that each component can be studied individually. Spinning a tube of blood at great speed in a machine called a **centrifuge** separates the whole blood into its components: plasma and formed elements. Formed elements are the blood cells. There are three types of blood cells: *red blood cells*, *white blood cells*, and *platelets*.

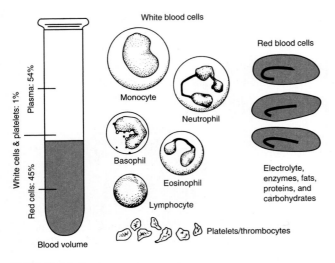

FIGURE 11-7   The blood and its components.

Plasma

Plasma contains water and the protein substances albumin and globulins. **Albumin**, or plasma protein, helps to hold water in the blood. Plasma albumin is like the white of a chicken egg, which is called the albumen. **Globulins** are proteins that help to provide the body's immunity because they contain antibodies. **Antibodies** help us to fight infections caused by bacteria and viruses. Bacteria, viruses, and chemicals are foreign substances called **antigens**. Antibodies are formed in response to the presence of an antigen. Antibodies are built in the blood by natural and acquired immunization. If you had German measles (rubella) as a child, you developed a natural immunity: You developed antibodies to prevent you from getting rubella again. If you were given the rubella vaccine, you developed an acquired immunity: You built the antibodies because you were injected with the German measles vaccine. The level of a specific antibody can be measured in the blood to determine if one has immunity to certain diseases.

Red Blood Cells

Red blood cells (RBCs) are also called **erythrocytes** (Figure 11-8). (*Erythro-* means "red"; *cyte* means "cell"). The function of red blood cells is to carry oxygen and carbon dioxide in the blood. A molecule called **hemoglobin** carries these gases on the RBC. In every cubic millimeter of blood, there are 4.2 to 6.2 million erythrocytes. A lack of red blood cells or hemoglobin creates a condition known as *anemia*. (*Hemo-*, *hemato-*, and *-emia* are medical terms for "blood.")

White Blood Cells

White blood cells (WBCs) are also called **leukocytes** (*leuko-* means "white"). The major types of WBCs are *lymphocytes*, *monocytes*, and *neutrophils*. The normal range of leukocytes per cubic millimeter of blood is 5 to 10 thousand. When infection is present, the number of WBCs increases to help the body fight the infection. Some white blood cells devour microorganisms. They are called **phagocytes** (*phago-* means "eat"). White blood cells fight infection in another way. Some WBCs produce antibodies in response to the foreign organism or antigen. The antibodies either kill or alter the antigen and make it harmless. A lack of leukocytes is called **leukopenia** (*-penia* means "deficiency"). When the blood lacks neutrophils, the condition is **neutropenia**. A type of protective isolation called *neutropenic precautions* will be discussed later in this chapter under "Application to Practice."

Platelets

Platelets are blood cells called **thrombocytes** (the root *thrombo-* means "clot"). Platelets help the blood to clot when there is an injury causing bleeding. The normal range of platelets is 130,000 to 400,000 per cubic millimeter of blood. **Thrombocytopenia** is a lack of clotting cells. This condition causes bruising and bleeding. Platelets rush to the site of injury in a blood vessel, and they plug the site to prevent excessive bleeding. As blood flows to this site, the platelets release certain factors that start a chain reaction to produce a blood clot. When platelet factors are not present, the clot formation is halted, and hemorrhage can occur. Inherited conditions like **hemophilia** are the result of a missing gene on the X chromosome. This is the gene that directs platelets to produce factor #8. People with hemophilia have a bleeding disorder, and when injured or through spontaneous bleeding into the joints, they can hemorrhage. This platelet factor can be given to the hemophiliac through an intravenous infusion.

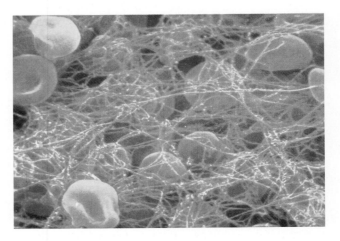

FIGURE 11-8   Red blood cell. Science Photo Library, Photo Researchers, Inc.

Blood Types

Blood types are inherited through the gene for blood group or type. There are four blood types: *A, B, O,* and *AB.* Another identifying characteristic of blood types is the **Rh factor**. This is also inherited. If you have this factor, you are Rh-positive. If you do not have this factor, you are Rh-negative. Type O+ is the most common blood type, and AB– is the least common. A blood test can determine both the blood type and the Rh factor. Blood type is determined by the presence of a specific antigen. The presence of antigen A results in type A blood. The presence of antigen B results in type B blood. If antigens A and B are present, the result is AB blood type. If neither antigen is present, the person is typed as having O blood. Remember, the presence of an antigen results in the production of antibodies to fight against the antigen. This is why it is so important to give the correct blood type when patients need a blood transfusion. Before a blood transfusion is given, a blood test is performed called a *Type and Screen* or *Type and Cross Match.* If the incorrect blood type is given, the person will have a severe reaction that could be fatal. This happens when the patient's blood antibodies reject the presence of the foreign antigen in the blood being transfused and destroy the blood. In an emergency, only type O– blood can be administered. Why? Because type O– has no antigens and no Rh factor to create the antigen-antibody reaction.

Pulse

Pulse is measured by placing the fingertips over an artery that lies close to the surface of the body. There are several major **pulse points**: temporal, carotid, brachial, radial, femoral, popliteal, and dorsalis pedis. The artery usually used to measure pulse is the **radial artery**. Several characteristics are used to describe the pulse: **rate** (fast or slow), **force** (weak or strong), and **rhythm** (regular or irregular). Each beat felt is the result of one contraction of the left ventricle. The rate is measured by counting each pulsation felt by the fingertips. The force and rhythm of each beat indicate the strength and the regularity of the rhythm of the heart's contraction. All of these characteristics should be noted when measuring pulse. The procedure for measuring pulse will be discussed in Chapter 25.

Blood Pressure

Blood pressure is the measurement of the pressure exerted in blood vessels as blood is forced through the circulatory system. Blood pressure is routinely measured in an artery; however, pressure is present in capillaries, and it can be measured in veins. Venous pressure is measured by inserting a catheter into the large veins near the heart; the **central venous pressure** is measured in this way.

Arterial blood pressure is measured by placing an inflatable cuff over an artery and increasing the pressure against the artery to obstruct the flow of blood in that location. When the cuff is deflated, the blood begins again to flow through the artery. With the use of a stethoscope, you can hear the pounding of the blood as it flows. The brachial artery is generally used to measure blood pressure. A device called a **sphygmomanometer** is used to measure the arterial blood pressure in terms of millimeters (mm) of mercury. The sounds that are heard when listening for blood pressure indicate the pressure in the artery when the heart is contracting and relaxing. The average blood pressure for an adult is 120/80 mm of mercury. The normal range for blood pressure is 140/90 to 90/60 mm of mercury. Blood pressure higher than 140/90 is a condition known as **hypertension** (high blood pressure). When blood pressure is low, it is called **hypotension**. The procedure for measuring blood pressure will be discussed in Chapter 25.

Many factors influence blood pressure, including these:

1. The vasomotor center in the medulla constricts and dilates blood vessels, making them wider or narrower and increasing or decreasing the force of blood flow.

2. The cardiac center of the medulla influences the rate and strength of the heart's contractions.

3. The vasomotor center is sensitive to chemical substances in the blood, such as O_2 and CO_2, and the acid content in the blood.

4. The condition of the inner walls of the arteries affects their elasticity (their ability to dilate and constrict). Arteriosclerosis reduces their elasticity.

5. The volume of blood or fluid in the blood affects blood pressure. When blood volume is decreased due to hemorrhage, blood pressure decreases. When volume is excessive, it raises blood pressure.

6. The condition of the myocardium and its ability to contract influences blood pressure.

7. Emotions stimulate the nervous system's response to stressful and nonstressful life events, affecting blood pressure.

8. Lifestyle—including eating, drinking, and smoking habits—influences the condition of the heart and blood vessels and consequently influences pulse and blood pressure.

9. Genetics predispose some individuals to heart disease and hypertension.

Pulse and blood pressure are essential measurements of the cardiovascular system. They provide valuable information about a person's state of health.

The Lymphatic System

The **lymphatic system** is made of lymph capillaries, which lead to larger lymph vessels directed to the thoracic cavity, as shown in Figure 11-9. Lymph vessels drain and filter tissue fluid and return vital substances like blood protein to the venous system. The fluid in these vessels is called **lymph**. Throughout lymphatic vessels are valves that allow lymph to flow in only one direction. Also present throughout these vessels are **lymph nodes**, which filter the lymph fluid before it returns to the venous blood. The lymph nodes produce antibodies, globulins, and lymphocytes. An important function of lymph nodes is to filter bacteria and inflammatory products before lymph returns to the blood. At times, the lymph nodes in the neck, armpits, or groin become enlarged because of the accumulation of filtered infectious and inflammatory substances. If you've ever had a respiratory infection, you may have felt the enlarged or swollen lymph nodes in your neck. **Lymph vessels** surround the intestines and absorb globules of fat from digested foods and deposit this fat in tissues of the body.

Accessory Organs for Immunity

Three organs work with the lymphatic system to produce immunity to disease and to help to fight infections. These are called accessory organs. They are the *tonsils, thymus gland,* and *spleen.* Figure 11-10 provides an illustration of each of these organs.

The **tonsils** are located on the right and left sides of the back of the mouth above the entrance to the throat. The function of the tonsils is to guard the entrance to the digestive and respiratory organs. The tonsils trap bacteria to localize the infection. When they become inflamed, they are red and swollen and may have pus around them.

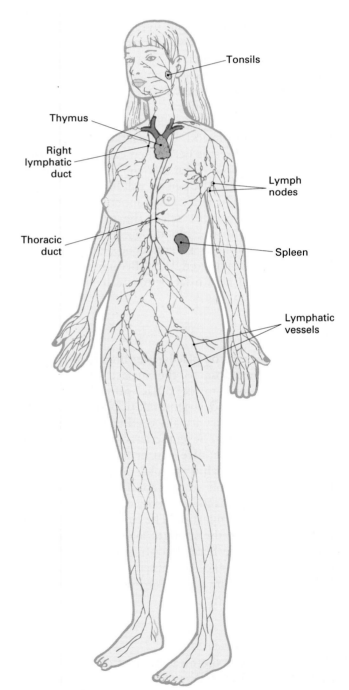

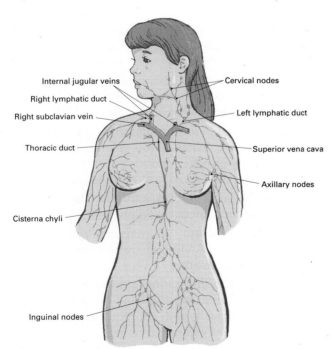

FIGURE 11-9   The lymphatic system.

FIGURE 11-10   Tonsils, thymus gland, and spleen.

The **thymus gland** is located under the sternum in the center of the thoracic cavity. The thymus gland gradually shrinks in size as the body matures. Early in life, it releases a substance that helps to prepare the lymphatic system to develop the immune response. The thymus also produces lymphocytes.

The **spleen** is an organ that lies in the upper left abdomen beneath the diaphragm and under the lower ribs. It is very vascular, which means that it has many blood vessels running through it. The spleen's functions include destroying old red blood cells, filtering microorganisms, storing blood, producing antibodies, and stimulating bone marrow to produce blood cells.

Conditions and Diseases of the Circulatory System

Coronary artery disease (CAD) is the obstruction and narrowing of blood vessels that supply blood to the heart. Plaque builds up on the inner walls of these arteries and obstructs the flow of blood. The disease of these arteries can lead to angina and to myocardial infarction. Lifestyle change, medication, and diets low in salt and fat are treatments for CAD. Sometimes, surgery is required to repair the coronary arteries. **Cardiac catheterization** is a diagnostic procedure for the definitive diagnosis of CAD. Cardiac catheterization indicates which coronary arteries are diseased and how much **occlusion** (blockage) is present. The catheter that is passed through the femoral artery is threaded up to the heart and into the coronary arteries. A dye is injected so that the catheter and the blood vessels can be seen on a screen like an x-ray monitor. After the procedure, a sandbag is placed over the femoral artery to prevent hemorrhage from the artery. The pulses in the feet must be checked by palpation (feeling). This is done to be sure blood is flowing adequately to the feet. The patient must lie flat and must not move or bend the leg that was used for catheterization. Following cardiac catheterization, the patient's pulse, blood pressure, and ECG are monitored closely by nursing staff. Atherosclerosis and arteriosclerosis are the major causes of CAD. Figure 11-11 depicts the conditions of a normal artery and an artery with atherosclerosis. Figure 11-12 shows a procedure for CAD called *balloon angioplasty.* This treatment is done during a cardiac catheterization.

Angina pectoris is a condition that is characterized by tightness and pain in the chest. It is caused by an inadequate supply of oxygen to the myocardium. Anginal attacks are usually brought on by exertion and emotional stress. They are usually brief

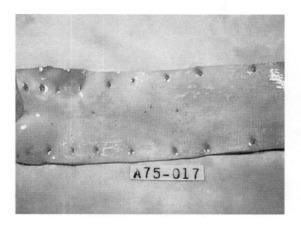

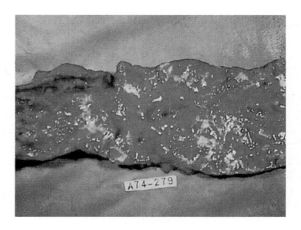

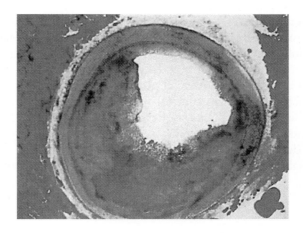

FIGURE 11-11   A normal artery and an artery with atherosclerosis.

and relieved by rest and nitroglycerin, a powerful medication that dilates blood vessels.

Myocardial infarction (MI) is a heart attack (Figure 11-13). Lack of O_2 secondary to CAD causes necrosis (death) of some portion of heart muscle, and this causes scarring of the myocardium. The warning signs of an MI are crushing chest pain, pain radiating to the neck and left arm, pain between the shoulder blades, or jaw pain, sweating, and

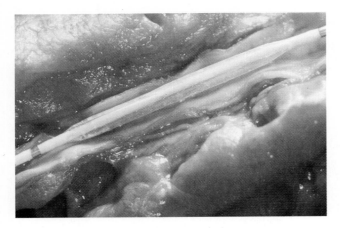

FIGURE 11-12   Balloon angioplasty. Southern Illinois University, Photo Researchers, Inc.

shortness of breath. Myocardial infarction can have less pronounced warning signs, such as feelings of indigestion. In this case, the individual may ignore or misread the signs. Changes in an ECG are seen following an MI. Blood levels of certain enzymes are elevated following an MI. The heart rhythm and rate are abnormal and irregular during and immediately following a heart attack.

Aneurysms are abnormal dilatations (swellings or enlargements) of an arterial vessel resulting from a congenital (present at birth) malformation or weakness of the vessel wall. The most common sites are cerebral arteries and the aorta. The weakened wall creates a "bubble" that is further weakened with each pulsation of the artery. Eventually, this weakened area gives way, and the blood leaks into surrounding tissue. If the break is small or the aneurysm is detected before it breaks, surgical resection is performed. If the weakened area bursts, gross hemorrhage will ensue. Abdominal aortic aneurysms are seen in older adults. Cerebral aneurysms are found mostly in young adults. Prognosis is good if detected and treated before gross hemorrhage occurs. Cerebral resection may result in residual symptoms, depending on the artery involved because nerve cells may be damaged. Nerve cells do not regenerate.

Leukemia (literally, "white blood") is a disease known as *white blood cell cancer*. It is characterized by an abnormally high leukocyte (WBC) count. The enormous white blood cell count consists of hundreds of thousands of immature WBCs that essentially render the individual helpless to fight infections. Leukemia can be acute or chronic in nature. This form of "blood cancer" is treated with chemotherapy agents. Bone marrow transplants are sometimes successful in treating acute forms of leukemia. Acute forms can be fatal because of the complications of infection or the treatments for the various forms of leukemia.

Valvular diseases are diseases of a heart valve. The valve most frequently affected by diseases is the **mitral** (or **bicuspid**) valve, which lies between the left atrium and the left ventricle. Severe cases of mitral valve disease are treated surgically. The valve can be replaced with a plastic device that performs in a similar fashion. Rheumatic heart disease was once the chief cause of stenosis (narrowing) of this valve. Today, subacute infections are caused by the streptococcus bacterium, a harmful pathogen that causes "vegetation" (bacterial growth) around the cusps of this valve. This is why it is important to evaluate all sore throats and take action to treat strep throat immediately.

Some people are born with a congenital weakness of the mitral valve called **mitral valve prolapse**. In this condition, the cusps of the valve are weak and unable to close perfectly. Some people experience symptoms, and others may live many years with no awareness of any symptoms. Treatment is indicated by the nature of the symptoms that are present. When the mitral valve fails, blood accumulates and causes congestion in the left atrium and the lungs. The resulting condition is known as *left-sided heart failure with pulmonary edema*.

The aortic semilunar valve is another heart valve that may fail to perform efficiently. Aortic insufficiency may result in aortic stenosis. The opening of this semilunar valve is narrowed, causing obstruction of blood flow between the left ventricle and the aorta.

When the heart valves are diseased, the heart compensates by beating faster or irregularly, and the force of the contractions are eventually weakened. This leaves the heart with less durability and efficiency. The rate and character of the heart rate and rhythm become irregular, the blood pressure varies, the myocardium swells, the blood redistributes itself, and congestion results in various areas of the body.

Congestive heart failure is a syndrome. This means that the signs and symptoms of congestive

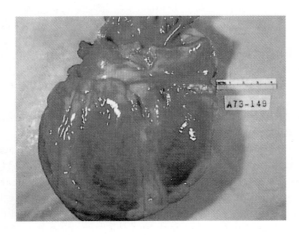

FIGURE 11-13   Myocardial infarction.

heart failure "run along together" and present a clinical picture that may be the result of any number of conditions. The severity of symptoms varies considerably between individuals. The underlying causes also vary. Some underlying causes include weakening of the heart muscle or valves, increased and excessive overload of fluid in the circulation, dysrhythmia of the heart, and pulmonary congestion.

Cardiac **arrhythmias** (or **dysrhythmias**) consist of a variety of irregular rates or rhythms of the heartbeat. (The terms *arrhythmia* and *dysrhythmia* are used interchangeably). The underlying causes range from disruption of the nervous system, the nervous system's control of the rate and rhythm of the heart, damage to the muscle of the heart, imbalance of electrolytes or salts in the circulation, and the effects of medications on the heart. Either the atria or the ventricles may be out of rhythm or beat too fast or too slow. The pacemaker of the heart, the SA node, may be diseased and fail to stimulate regular rate and rhythm. The dysrhythmia is usually detected by an ECG, or the patient may complain of symptoms of irregular sensations or palpitations that are not seen when the ECG is performed. In this case, the physician may order a twenty-four-hour monitoring of the heart rate and rhythm with the use of a Holter monitor. If the patient is admitted to the hospital and cardiac problems are detected or suspected, the patient may be put on **telemetry**. Telemetry is a process of measuring (*-metry*) by distance (*tele-*). In this case, the electrical activity of the patient's heart is monitored constantly for dysrhythmia.

Shock can result from a number of underlying causes, including cardiac failure, neurological trauma, fluid loss, and hemorrhage. Most commonly, shock is associated with hypovolemia, a decrease in the volume of blood. Symptoms of shock include rapid, thready pulse; rapid respirations; decreased blood pressure; cold, clammy skin; and unconsciousness. The blood pressure may not be audible with a stethoscope. It may be necessary to obtain pressure by palpation of the systolic pressure. Immediate treatment is necessary. Blood volume must be increased by intravenous fluids and blood transfusions. Whatever caused the shock must be treated promptly to prevent death.

Phlebitis is the inflammation of a vein. Phlebitis is most common in leg veins and results from ineffective venous return to the heart. The inflamed area can lead to the formation of a thrombus (clot), and **thrombophlebitis** results. Medications to prevent clotting, called *anticoagulants*, are given. The leg is rested so the clot will not dislodge and travel to another vein. When this happens, an embolus results. Phlebitis can result from irritation of a vein caused by intravenous medications. The skin around the vein is warm and reddened and painful. If IV medications are required, the intravenous catheter is removed, and another vein is chosen for the catheter insertion.

Anemia (literally, "without blood") can be caused by blood loss, a lack of erythrocytes, a lack of iron, malabsorption syndromes of the small intestine, a low hemoglobin level, cancer, and genetic conditions. **Sickle-cell anemia** and **Cooley's anemia** are two forms of genetically caused anemia. Sickle-cell anemia is found predominately in African Americans, and Cooley's anemia in people from Mediterranean countries, such as Italy and Greece. Treatment depends on the cause of the anemia.

application to practice

The clinical care associate is often involved in monitoring patients with circulatory system conditions and diseases. Your observations and clinical findings can assist the nurse and the team in the care and treatment of patients' cardiovascular functions and health. Apply the information that you have learned in this chapter to the following situations.

Learning Activities

Situation 1: Mrs. O'Maley is a forty-two-year-old woman who was admitted to the critical care unit (CCU) yesterday. She arrived in the emergency room (ER) with complaints of dizziness, palpitations, and sweating that occurred when she was doing her morning exercises. She was found to have an irregular ECG with multiple premature ventricular contractions (PVCs) and ventricular tachycardia. What is your understanding of ventricular tachycardia? What test was used to detect this condition? How will her heart status be monitored in the CCU?

Author's Explanation: Mrs. O'Maley has an abnormal heart rate. Her ventricles are beating too fast, and at times, her ventricles beat before her atria. This means that the lower chambers of the heart beat before the upper chambers. An ECG was done in the ER to detect this, and she was admitted to the CCU to have continuous telemetry monitoring of her heart rate and rhythm. Her condition could be life-threatening, and she will be given medications to regulate her heart rate and rhythm.

Situation 2: Mr. Vegas is a seventy-six-year-old man and a resident in your long-term care facility. You have known him for a year. His diagnosis is CHF. He is sometimes short of breath, and you know he takes a medication for his heart. The nurse always reminds you to take his pulse before the 8:00 A.M. medication is given. When you enter his room at 7:30 A.M., he is sitting in a chair, and his breathing is labored. When you look at his feet, you see that they are puffy and his slippers are too tight for his feet. You take his vital signs, and these are your findings: pulse 106, respirations 34, blood pressure 168/102, temperature 98.4°F. What will you report to the nurse, and when will you report these findings?

Author's Explanation: Go immediately to the nurse and inform her of Mr. Vegas' struggle with breathing. Tell the nurse about his swollen feet, and report his vital signs.

Situation 3: Which of Mr. Vegas' vital signs are abnormal, or out of normal range?

Author's Explanation: His pulse is higher than the normal range for an adult (100 per minute). His respirations are rapid because 12 to 20 is average. His blood pressure is above the average of 120/80, and anything above 140/90 is considered to be high blood pressure.

Situation 4: Why do you think Mr. Vegas' feet are swollen? Why is his breathing loud and labored?

Author's Explanation: He has congestive heart failure. His heart is stressed and unable to handle the pumping of blood to and from the right side of the heart. As a result, blood becomes congested, and tissue fluid is leaking into the extracellular space of soft tissue in the lower extremities. His lungs are also full of fluid because the left side of the heart is unable to receive or pump out the returning blood from the lungs.

Situation 5: Mr. Smythe is a twenty-two-year-old with a diagnosis of acute leukemia. He is admitted to your oncology unit for chemotherapy. He is placed on neutropenic precautions. Why?

Author's Explanation: Remember that neutrophils are a type of white blood cell and that white blood cells protect the body from infections. Since Mr. Smythe has leukemia, he is manufacturing an excessive number of immature white blood cells, which are unable to help defend against possible infection.

Situation 6: The sign on Mr. Smythe's door reads "NEUTROPENIC PRECAUTIONS: Anyone who enters must wear a mask. Do not bring fresh fruit or flowers into the room." Why does the sign have these warnings?

Author's Explanation: This patient is at risk for infection because his white blood cells are malfunctioning. *Anyone* who enters his room could breathe out microbes. Fresh fruit and flowers have microbes present on them, and these could cause infection for this patient.

Situation 7: Sue Le is 10 years old. She was in an auto accident and was admitted to the trauma unit at your university hospital. She is receiving blood transfusions because she had multiple injuries that resulted in hemorrhage. You heard the physician say that she had a lacerated spleen. Does the injury to her spleen have anything to do with the hemorrhage? One of your duties is to pick up blood products from the blood bank. The first time you are sent, you pick up a pint of whole blood identified as B+. A few hours later, you are asked to get a unit of packed cells. What does the B+ blood indicate to you about Sue's blood type? What is the difference between the unit of whole blood and the unit of packed cells?

Author's Explanation: Remember that the spleen stores blood and that it is a very vascular organ. The spleen also stimulates bone marrow to produce blood cells. Laceration of the spleen is definitely one of the causes of her hemorrhage. The whole blood marked B+ means that Sue has B+ blood. The nurse must carefully check the unit of blood with another professional nurse before she begins the transfusion. Giving the wrong blood type could result in a blood transfusion reaction. This is very serious and could be fatal. The unit of packed cells contains only blood cells and no other blood components.

Situation 8: At 9:00 P.M., you are asked to take Sue's vital signs before the nurse hangs the blood and to check them again 5 minutes and 15 minutes after the transfusion is started. The nurse hangs the blood at 9:10 P.M. These are your results at 9:00 P.M.: temperature 98°F, pulse 120, respirations 28, blood pressure 68/40. Why are her pulse and respirations so rapid and her blood pressure so low?

Author's Explanation: The patient is exhibiting shock symptoms secondary to transfusion reaction.

Situation 9: These are her vital signs at 9:15 P.M.: temperature 99.4°F, pulse 122, respirations 30, blood pressure 72/44. What should you do?

Author's Explanation: Immediately inform the nurse of these changes. The increased temperature could indicate a blood transfusion reaction, and the blood must be stopped immediately. Because she has been hemorrhaging, the volume of blood is low, and her blood pressure decreased and heart rate increased. These are signs of shock.

Situation 10: Mr. Byrd, seventy years old, is admitted to the hospital for abdominal surgery. He is 2 days post-op and is receiving an antibiotic medication intravenously. The IV is in his left lower arm. While you are assisting him with A.M. care, he complains of pain at the IV site. You look at the IV site and note that it is red and swollen; it feels warm to the touch. What should you do, and why?

Author's Explanation: You should report this immediately to the nurse because Mr. Byrd probably has phlebitis caused by the medication's irritating the vein. This IV catheter will have to be removed. A new vein will be selected for administering the medication.

Situation 11: Mr. Nyugen is a forty-five-year-old man who arrived at the ER complaining of weakness and shortness of breath. While you are taking his vital signs in the ER, waiting for the nurse to assess him, he complains of severe chest pain. His pulse is weak, rapid, and irregular. He is sweating and pale. What do you do?

Author's Explanation: Stay with Mr. Nyugen and call for the nurse stat via the intercom. Ask Mr. Nyugen if he can describe the pain and rate it on a scale from 1 to 10. The **pain scale** rates 1 as very mild pain and 10 as severe pain. Continue to monitor his pulse and blood pressure. Reassure him that help is on the way. When the nurse arrives, report your findings. Get the ECG machine and an oxygen hookup. While the nurse and doctor examine the patient, begin to take an ECG. Mr. Nyugen could be having a heart attack.

Examination Review Questions

1. The middle layer of the heart is called the
   a. endocardium   c. epicardium
   b. myocardium   d. pericardium

2. Which chamber of the heart carries oxygenated blood to the body?
   a. right atrium   c. right ventricle
   b. left atrium   d. left ventricle

3. The _____ valve separates the left atrium and left ventricle.
   a. pulmonic   c. mitral
   b. tricuspid   d. aortic

4. A heart rate over 100 beats a minute is termed
   a. tachycardia   c. myocardia
   b. bradycardia   d. brachycardia

5. Hypertrophy of the myocardium is called
   a. angina   c. arteriosclerosis
   b. cardiomegaly   d. fibrillation

6. Which of the following is the pacemaker of the heart?
   a. Purkinje fibers   c. SA node
   b. AV node   d. bundle of His

7. Blood vessels that exchange O_2 and CO_2 at the cellular levels are
   a. arteries   c. venules
   b. arterioles   d. capillaries

8. Which blood vessel contains valves?
   a. vein   c. artery
   b. capillary   d. aorta

9. Which blood cell carries oxygen?
   a. erythrocyte   c. thrombocyte
   b. leukocyte   d. lymphocyte

10. Another name for heart attack is
    a. angina pectoris   c. myocardial infarction
    b. cardiac arrest   d. ventricular fibrillation

Chapter 12

The Respiratory System

Breathing is life! When a newborn baby enters the world, the first breath taken signifies the start of an independent life—a life that is no longer dependent on the mother for oxygen. The respiratory system is vital to life; it is the system that controls the body's most basic need: oxygen.

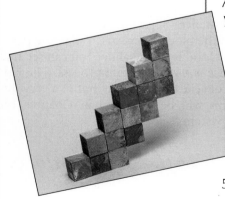

OBJECTIVES

After completing this chapter, you will be able to

1. Describe the functions of the respiratory system

2. Name the organs of the respiratory system

3. Describe the location of each organ

4. List the functions of each organ

5. Describe the conditions and diseases of the respiratory system

6. List the observations about the respiratory system that you should report to the nurse

7. Apply your knowledge of the respiratory system to problem-solving strategies in care delivery

8. Define and spell all key terms correctly

Airborne Precautions
alveolus
apnea
aspiration
aspiration pneumonia
asthma
atelectasis
auscultation
bronchi
bronchioles
Cheyne-Stokes
chronic bronchitis
chronic obstructive pulmonary
   disease (COPD)
cilia
dyspnea
emphysema

epiglottis
expiration
Heimlich maneuver
hemoptysis
hemothorax
inspiration
larynx
lungs
mediastinum
Mantoux test
nose
nostrils
orthopnea
pharynx
pleura
pleural
pneumonia (pneumonitis)

pneumothorax
PPD (Purified Protein Derivative)
   test
pulmonary edema
pulmonary embolism
respiration
septum
sinuses
stoma
tachycardia
tachypnea
thoracic
thrombophlebitis
trachea
tracheostomy
tuberculosis (TB)
vocal cords

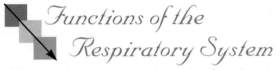

Functions of the Respiratory System

The respiratory system's main function is to exchange the gases, oxygen and carbon dioxide, with the external environment. This *external respiration* is accomplished in the lungs. With each breath (respiration), oxygen is breathed in, and carbon dioxide is breathed out. One respiration equals one **inspiration** (breathing in) and one **expiration** (breathing out). Every cell of the body absorbs oxygen, and every cell must remove carbon dioxide. The respiratory system exchanges these gases, and the blood transports oxygen from the lungs to the cells and carbon dioxide from the cells to the lungs. Respiration at the cellular level is considered to be *internal respiration*.

Another function of the respiratory system is to help balance the concentration of acid in the blood. When carbon dioxide combines with water in the blood, it creates a new compound, carbonic acid (H_2CO_3). Carbon dioxide (CO_2) and water (H_2O) molecules combine in this fashion:

$$CO_2 \text{ (carbon dioxide)} + H_2O \text{ (water)} = H_2CO_3 \text{ (carbonic acid)}.$$

Expressed another way,

$$\begin{array}{c} CO_2 \\ + H_2 \quad O \\ \hline H_2CO_3 = H_2CO_3 \end{array}$$

When the carbon dioxide level in the blood is high, the blood becomes acidic. And when the CO_2 level is low, the blood becomes alkaline (basic). To understand the difference between acids and bases, consider these two common substances. A common acid is acetic acid (vinegar). Common bases (alkaline examples) are baking soda, egg whites, and milk. Consider the difference between vinegar and milk. The blood should be more like milk than vinegar. Acid-base balance is measured in the blood, and the result is given in pH (Figure 12-1).

The average pH of blood is 7.4. The normal range is 7.35 to 7.45. The lower the pH, the more acidic the substance. The higher the pH, the more alkaline the substance. Slight variations in the acid-base balance of the blood alters pH. When the pH is 7.5 or 7.6, the blood is too alkaline. You can see that acid-base balance is a very delicate process. The kidneys also control acid-base balance, but in a very different way. This will be discussed in Chapter 14, "The Urinary System."

Structures of the Respiratory System

The organs of the respiratory system are the *nose, mouth, pharynx, larynx, trachea, bronchi,* and *lungs*. The organs that extend to the lungs are referred to as the *upper respiratory tract*. Within the lungs, the bronchi branch out to smaller bronchioles and end in microscopic air sacs called alveoli. This network of right and left bronchi and the tiny bronchioles is often referred to as the *respiratory tree*. Throughout the respiratory organs, a mucous membrane lines the inner surfaces. The diaphragm and the muscles between the ribs are responsible for the movement and

pH of Common Substances

Solution/Substance	pH
Gastric Juice	1.6
Lemon Juice	2.2
Vinegar	2.8
Coffee	5.0
Urine	5.5–6.0
Water	7.0
Blood	7.4
Bile	8.0
Detergents	8.0–9.0
Milk of Magnesia	10.5
Bleach	12.0

FIGURE 12-1   The pH scale and substances that fall along that scale.

mechanics of breathing air in and out of the lungs. The thoracic cavity, which contains the heart and lungs, is separated from the abdominal cavity by the large muscle, the diaphragm. The base, or bottom parts, of the lungs rests on the diaphragm.

The Thoracic Cavity

The **thoracic** (chest) cavity is subdivided into right and left **pleural** cavities. The right pleural cavity contains the right bronchus and the right lung. The left pleural cavity contains the left bronchus and the left lung. The center of the thorax is called the **mediastinum**. The sternum is the breastbone, which lies above the heart. The heart lies behind the sternum in the mediastinum slightly in the left pleural cavity. The thoracic cavity has a protective membrane called the **pleura**, which can be seen in Figure 12-2. This is a double-layered membrane. The outer pleura lines the cavity, and the inner pleura covers the outer surface of the lungs. Between these two layers is a small amount of fluid that serves as a lubricant. It prevents friction from the rubbing of these membranes during the process of breathing. When the pleura is irritated from inflammation, the condition is called *pleurisy*. With pleurisy, breathing is painful, and

when listening to breath sounds with a stethoscope, a "rub" can be heard.

The Nose

The **nose** is the first organ of breathing. The mouth is also able to breath air in and out of the respiratory tract. However, the nose is designed to filter, to moisten, and to warm air before it enters the lungs. The nose is divided into right and left **nostrils**, or nares, by the nasal **septum**. The septum is a wall or partition. What other organ has a septum?

The nose is lined with a mucous membrane and tiny hairlike structures called **cilia**. The cilia wave back and forth to "sweep" the air and to move mucus to the throat. Special nerve tissues containing olfactory cells are located in the uppermost part of the nasal cavity. These cells are the receptors for the sense of smell. Not only are the olfactory cells important for pleasurable smells and tastes, but they also warn the respiratory system of poisonous substances in the air.

The Paranasal Sinuses

There are four pairs of **sinuses** that are associated with the nose. These sinuses are cavities in the bones of the head and face. The sinuses are lined with a mucous membrane that is continuous with the lining of the nose. The sinuses affect the production of

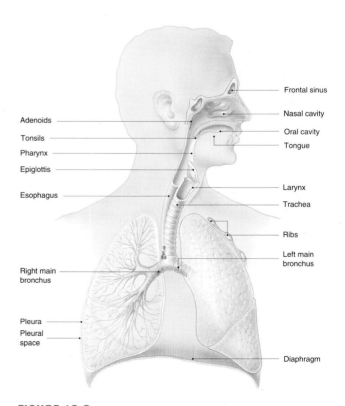

FIGURE 12-2   The respiratory tract.

sound when speaking. Their function is to produce mucus, which cleans and moistens the air.

The Pharynx

The **pharynx** (throat) is an organ of respiration and digestion. Air passes through the throat before it enters the larynx, and food passes through the pharynx enroute to the esophagus. The pharynx opens to the nose, mouth, larynx, and esophagus. It is a muscular organ that is lined with a mucous membrane. During breathing, the passageway to the larynx is open, and during swallowing, the passage to the larynx is closed. The structure that accomplishes this is called the *epiglottis*, a cartilage of the larynx. Figure 12-3 depicts the nasopharynx, oropharynx, and laryngopharynx.

The Larynx

The **larynx** is the voice box. It lies between the pharynx and the trachea. This organ is made of pieces of cartilage joined together by muscles and ligaments. The thyroid cartilage is known as the *Adam's apple*. During puberty, it becomes more pronounced in males. On top of the thyroid cartilage is the **epiglottis**, a cartilage shaped like a leaf. This structure acts like a lid when it closes the entrance to the larynx during swallowing. In the interior of the larynx are two fibrous bands called the **vocal cords**. The vocal cords open and close as air enters and exits the larynx. Speech is accomplished when exhaled air vibrates the vocal cords. The sound produced is low pitched when the vocal cords are loose and stretched. High-pitched sounds are produced by tight and short vocal cords. Figure 12-3 illustrates the larynx cartilages and vocal cords.

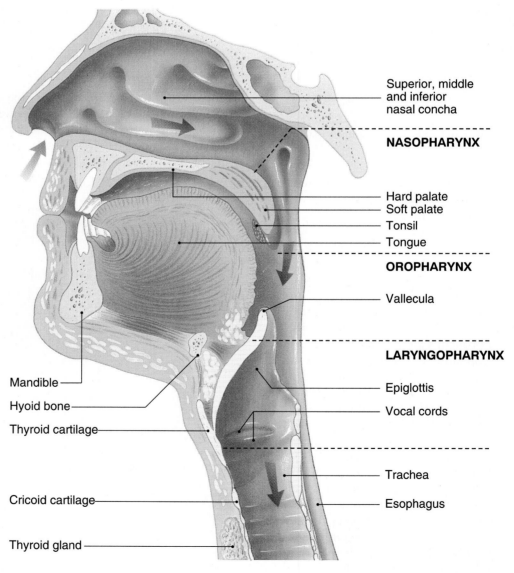

Superior, middle and inferior nasal concha

NASOPHARYNX

Hard palate
Soft palate
Tonsil
Tongue

OROPHARYNX

Vallecula

LARYNGOPHARYNX

Epiglottis
Vocal cords

Trachea
Esophagus

Mandible
Hyoid bone
Thyroid cartilage
Cricoid cartilage
Thyroid gland

FIGURE 12-3 The nasopharynx, oropharynx, and laryngopharynx.

The Trachea

The **trachea** (windpipe) is connected to the larynx and the bronchi. The trachea functions as a passageway for air to and from the lungs. It is made of C-shaped rings of cartilage with the closed side of the C facing the front surface of the trachea. If this passageway is blocked by food or some object, air cannot enter the lungs. When substances are accidentally sucked into the windpipe, it is called **aspiration**. The C-shaped rings of cartilage that form the trachea can be seen in Figure 12-3.

The Bronchi

The lower end of the trachea opens to two **bronchi**, the right bronchus and left bronchus, each leading to a lung. Each bronchus branches out through the lungs into smaller bronchial passageways that terminate in tiny **bronchioles** (*-oles* means "little"). These bronchioles support clusters of air cells throughout the entire surface of the lungs. A bronchiole is shown with alveolar sacs (clusters of air cells) in Figure 12-4a.

The Lungs

The **lungs** extend from the clavicles (collarbones) to the diaphragm. Entering each lung are the bronchi and the pulmonary arteries. The right lung has three lobes, and the left lung has two lobes. The heart occupies some of the space of the left pleural cavity. The lungs are spongy organs that contain millions of capillaries and alveoli.

The Alveoli

An **alveolus** is an air cell. There are millions of alveoli in the lungs. Alveoli are like clusters of tiny round balloons that expand when air is breathed into them. Alveolar sacs are clustered together at the twiglike endings of thousands of bronchioles; this increases the surface area throughout the lungs. The alveoli are surrounded by capillaries (Figure 12-4b). The capillaries and alveoli work together to exchange oxygen and carbon dioxide from the air and the blood. With each inspiration, oxygen enters the bronchial tree and passes to each alveolus. At this time, oxygen is absorbed into the capillary blood. At the point of expiration, carbon dioxide leaves the capillary blood and enters each alveolus to be breathed out into the atmosphere.

Respiration

Respiration is breathing. Inhaling is inspiration, and exhaling is expiration. Respirations are measured by counting the number of times in a minute that the chest rises and falls in the mechanics of breathing. The average respiratory rate is 12 to 20 per minute. The rate and depth of respiration is regulated by the respiratory center in the medulla. As blood flows through the medulla, special receptor cells detect the concentration of oxygen, carbon dioxide, and pH of the blood. If the carbon dioxide level is high, the respiratory rate increases. This prevents acidosis (an acid state) from developing in the blood. The rate of respiration changes with age. As the lungs mature, the respiratory rate decreases. An infant's rate is 30 to 40 per minute, while a small child breathes 20 to 30 times

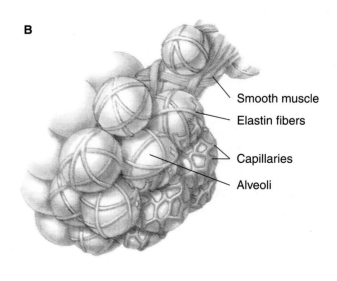

FIGURE 12-4   (a) Bronchiole, alveolar ducts, and sacs. (b) Alveoli with surrounding capillaries.

per minute. In older adults, respiratory rates may be more rapid than in younger adults due to a decreasing efficiency of the lungs. Observation of respiration includes the rate, depth, and effort of breathing. Depth is described as *shallow* or *deep*. Effort is described by terms such as *labored, difficult,* and *easy.* **Dyspnea** is the term used to describe difficulty breathing (*dys-* means "difficult," and *-pnea* is "breathing"). When a person needs to sit up to breath effectively, this is called **orthopnea** (*ortho-* means "straight"). **Tachypnea** means rapid breathing. **Apnea** literally means "without breathing"—in other words, breathing has stopped. **Cheyne-Stokes** respirations are usually observed when someone is near death. This type of breathing is characterized by alternating periods of dyspnea and apnea. To hear breath sounds, a stethoscope is used. The act of listening for sounds within the body is called **auscultation.** Wheezing caused by narrowing of the bronchial tubes can be heard on inspiration or expiration. Rubbing is heard with friction of the pleura. Crackles are heard with inflammation of the lungs, and rales are noisy, moist breath sounds due to fluid accumulation in the lungs or pleural cavity.

Conditions and Diseases of the Respiratory System

Emphysema results from chronic inflammatory and obstructive conditions of the bronchi and the lungs. Asthma and chronic bronchitis are frequently the underlying diseases. With emphysema, the alveoli are stretched, deteriorated, and thin. Smoking and pollutants cause destruction of the alveoli. During expiration, the person with emphysema often purses the lips to push air out. The chest cavity takes on a barrel shape, and the ends of the fingers may be broad and thickened.

Asthma is a condition caused by intermittent obstruction of the bronchial tubes. Allergies to food and pollen are often underlying causes. Symptoms include wheezing and prolonged expiration. The person with asthma has more difficulty exhaling than inhaling. During an asthma attack, the individual's breathing is labored.

Pneumonia (pneumonitis) is inflammation of the lungs. The alveoli become filled with fluid, and the lung tissue becomes edematous (filled with fluid). Pneumonia is often caused by a viral or bacterial infection. It can be caused by aspiration of fluids such as stomach contents that are breathed in during vomiting. This type of pneumonia is called **aspiration pneumonia.**

Tuberculosis (TB) is an infectious disease of the lungs. It is caused by the tubercle bacillus. This bacterium invades the lungs and produces a reaction that causes areas of infection to become walled off by fibrous connective tissue. The Latin word *tuber* means "swelling," and affected areas of the lungs are called *tubercles.* The fibrosis makes the lungs less able to expand and decreases the working surface of the lungs. This makes the lungs less effective in exchanging gases. The tubercle bacillus is transmitted through the air exchanged from a person with TB. A special mask called the *N-95 respirator* must be worn when caring for a person who has or is suspected of having TB. **Airborne precautions** are indicated, and the isolation room must have a separate air exchange. When the patient leaves the hospital room, it is the patient who wears the mask. Periodically, health care workers must be tested for TB. This interval may range from 3 months to a year. A **Mantoux** or **PPD** (Purified Protein Derivative) **test** (intradermal skin test) is used. If the individual cannot be skin tested, a chest x-ray is performed. The disease is treated with medications for approximately 6 months. The people at greatest risk for TB are those who are homeless, who have been exposed to someone with undiagnosed TB, and who are immunocompromised from acquired immunodeficiency syndrome (AIDS) or conditions causing neutropenia.

Chronic obstructive pulmonary disease (COPD) is a general term used to describe the diseases **chronic bronchitis**, asthma, and emphysema. The person with COPD is unable to exchange gases effectively and consequently has decreased O_2 and increased CO_2 in the blood. Figure 12-5 shows an x-ray of a normal lung and an x-ray of a patient with emphysema.

Tumors of the respiratory system, both benign and malignant (cancerous), cause obstruction of the respiratory tract or bronchial tree and impede the flow of air to and from the lungs. Lung cancer and tumors of the larynx and trachea are often the result of smoking. These tumors may require surgical removal of the affected organ. The person will require a surgically produced **stoma** (a new opening) to create an airway. **Tracheostomy** is the creation of a stoma and the placement of a tracheal tube to allow air to enter the respiratory system. The person with a tracheostomy no longer inhales air through the nose and mouth but through the new opening in the neck. With a laryngectomy, the person will no longer be able to speak since the vocal cords are removed. A vibrating device can be held on the throat to produce vocal sounds, or the person can learn esophageal speech. In this situation, the person swallows air and burps the air through the esophagus, causing vibrations, to produce vocalization. In either situation, the speech is distinctly different from normal vibration of the vocal cords.

Pulmonary edema is swelling of the lungs due to the accumulation of fluid in lung tissue. It can

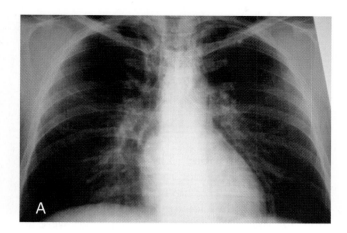

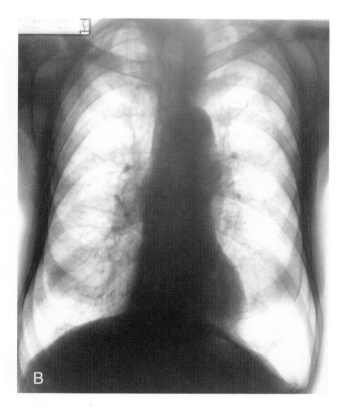

FIGURE 12-5   (a) Normal chest x-ray. (b) Chest x-ray of a patient with emphysema. (top) Charles Stewart, MD; (bottom) Scott Camazine, Photo Researchers, Inc.

result from chronic lung diseases or from congestive heart failure. The condition is characterized by severe dyspnea. This person will need treatment with diuretics, drugs that increase urinary output by increasing the amount of water removed by the kidneys or by attracting water from tissue spaces to eventually be excreted by the kidneys. The underlying cause must be treated to manage the edema of the lungs.

Pneumothorax and **hemothorax** are conditions that affect the thoracic cavity and are the result of air (*pneumo-*) or blood (*hemo-*) in the thorax (Figure 12-6). Pneumothorax can occur spontaneously,

without warning, but usually it results from injury to the pleura due to stab or puncture wounds. A rib that fractures can tear the pleural membrane and create pneumothorax and, subsequently, hemothorax. The presence of air in the thorax creates a negative pressure on the lungs and may cause a lung to collapse (**atelectasis**). The air, fluid, or blood must be removed from the pleural cavity. A chest tube is inserted to remove the air and blood, which allows the lung to inflate again. Drainage is collected in a special container called a *pleural seal*. The drainage is measured and examined for the presence of blood. The underlying cause of pneumothorax and hemothorax can be treated once the emergency is managed.

Pulmonary embolism results from a blood clot that is lodged in a pulmonary artery. A thrombus (clot) that travels to another area is called an *embolus* or *embolism*. Pulmonary embolism usually results from a clot in veins of the leg or the heart that become dislodged. The person experiences dyspnea, **tachycardia**, **hemoptysis** (coughing up blood), tachypnea (rapid respirations), and chest pain. Death can result. Emergency treatment includes surgical removal of the clot. Since most pulmonary emboli result from the **thrombophlebitis** (inflammation of veins due to blood clot) of the leg veins, prevention of emboli is managed with anticoagulant medications and bed rest.

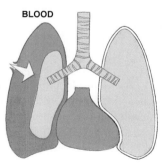

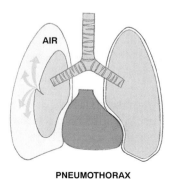

FIGURE 12-6   Hemothorax and pneumothorax.

application to practice

As a clinical care associate, you will be assisting with the activities of daily living (ADLs) of respiratory patients. Respiratory diseases and conditions vary in severity, but many patients require oxygen. It is important to continually monitor patients receiving oxygen or patients with severe respiratory conditions and to advise the nurse of any changes you observe. Consider the information you have just learned about the respiratory system, and apply this knowledge to the following situations.

Learning Activities

Situation 1: You are feeding a patient breakfast, and the patient begins to talk as he is chewing his toast. Suddenly, the patient chokes, and his face turns bright red. What actions will you take?

Author's Explanation: Immediately ask the patient if he can speak; determine if he is able to cough. If unable to speak or cough, the patient has complete airway obstruction. Perform the **Heimlich maneuver** to relieve the obstructed airway. Call for help, and continue to do abdominal thrusts until the obstruction is relieved. Once the obstruction is relieved, maintain an open airway if the patient has become unconscious. *Call a code, and get the crash cart.* Follow the steps for cardiopulmonary resuscitation (CPR) while awaiting the code team.

Situation 2: Mrs. Cruz is a seventy-year-old woman who has been admitted to the orthopedic unit following a left hip replacement. She is receiving 4L of O_2 via a mask. You are assigned to assist her with care 2 days post-op. When you enter the room, you see that she is washing her face and has removed the O_2 mask. Your first interventions involve taking vital signs. As you speak with her, you notice that she is short of breath and that she looks pale and sweaty. Her temperature is normal, but her pulse is a rapid 106, respirations 34, and blood pressure (BP) 160/90. What is your immediate action?

Author's Explanation: Return the O_2 mask to her face, and use the intercom to call the nurse stat to the patient's room. Do not leave Mrs. Cruz, and ensure her safety.

Situation 3: Two days later, Mrs. Cruz returns to your unit from the intensive care unit (ICU).

You are assigned to Mrs. Cruz again. Today you are told that she had a pulmonary embolism and that she is now receiving O_2 at 6L and intravenous heparin, an anticoagulant. Why do you think these treatment changes are indicated?

Author's Explanation: The pulmonary embolism means that a blood clot formed and traveled to a pulmonary artery. Her hip replacement surgery may have instigated the clot formation. She is receiving more O_2 than yesterday because her lungs were affected by this event.

Situation 4: As you assist Mrs. Cruz with A.M. care, you notice that when she rinses her mouth after brushing her teeth, there is blood in the emesis basin she is using. What could be causing this? What do you do?

Author's Explanation: The heparin she is receiving interferes with the blood-clotting mechanism. While it prevents clot formation, it also can cause bleeding. You should instruct Mrs. Cruz to stop brushing her teeth at this time, and immediately tell the nurse what you observed. Mrs. Cruz should be instructed to use a soft toothbrush to prevent bleeding of the gums.

Situation 5: Mr. Augustin is a forty-year-old man who is being admitted to your unit today. He has a diagnosis of AIDS and rule out (r/o) TB. You are assigned to set up his room. The unit clerk tells you he is assigned to isolation room 102. Why does he have a special isolation room? What supplies do you need to prepare for his admission?

Author's Explanation: Since Mr. Augustin might have tuberculosis, he will need a room with a separate air-exchange system. You should get a sign for his room door that says "Airborne Precautions" and get the correct respiratory mask indicated for TB. Your hospital will have instructed you on the correct mask used in the care of patients with TB, and the hospital will have taught you how to "fit test" the mask for correct application and use.

Situation 6: Mr. Augustin asks you why his door remains closed and why you are wearing a mask when you enter his room. What do you tell him? What special instructions does he need regarding his r/o TB?

Author's Explanation: You should tell Mr. Augustin that since the doctor indicated r/o tuberculosis, it is necessary to treat his condition as if he were diagnosed with TB. The risk of contracting TB is the reason for using the special mask. The procedure for this type of isolation requires a room with its own air-exchange system. Also, to protect others from possible TB, it is important to close the outer door. Tell him that when he leaves the room, he will need to wear a mask to prevent the possible spread of TB.

Situation 7: Mrs. Ramos is a patient in your rehabilitation unit. She was admitted following treatment in the hospital for multiple injuries from a MVA (motor vehicle accident). Today is the first day that you have been assigned to her. She has had a tracheostomy because of damage to her trachea from the crash. You have never had a patient with a tracheostomy. What do you expect to find when you meet Mrs. Ramos?

Author's Explanation: She will have an opening in her throat with a tracheostomy tube in place. There will be a small dressing around the opening of the stoma, and cotton strips of cloth will be attached to the outer part of the tube and will be tied in the back of her neck. She will breathe through the trach tube and not through her nose or mouth. She will only be able to speak when she blocks the opening of the tracheostomy tube as she exhales air. Remember that the voice box is above the trachea, and in order to speak, the exhaled air must vibrate the vocal cords. By placing her finger over the opening of the tube, she allows expired air to move into the larynx. When she coughs to expectorate mucous, it will be expelled from the trach tube, not from her mouth.

Situation 8: Jenny Smith is a twelve-year-old girl who had abdominal surgery two days ago. You are told in report to encourage her to cough and deep-breathe and to use the incentive spirometer. Why?

Author's Explanation: Following general anesthesia, there is a risk of pneumonia. The anesthetic drug immobilizes the lungs, and the effect of the surgery on the abdominal muscles make it difficult to fully expand the chest muscles and make it painful to cough and deep-breathe. As a result of these risks, mucous secretions build up in the lungs and increase the possibility of infection of the lungs. The incentive spirometer is used to promote deep inspiration and expiration. Jenny should splint her abdominal incision or hold a pillow over her abdomen to assist her with coughing and deep breathing.

Situation 9: Mr. Judas is a seventy-seven-year-old man who resides in your long-term care (LTC) facility. He has a medical history of congestive heart failure (CHF) and COPD. He is able to perform most of his care independently and uses a walker for ambulation. You are assigned to him when you return to work after a weekend off. When you enter his room, you can hear him breathing in his sleep. His respirations are labored, and you can hear crackling sounds as he inspires air. He is cool and clammy and does not wake up when you begin to take his vital signs. The veins in his neck are distended; his neck looks swollen. What will you do?

Author's Explanation: Try to awaken Mr. Judas to see if he is unconscious or asleep. Call for the nurse stat. Take his pulse, respirations, and BP, and immediately report the results to the nurse. Tell the nurse about your observations of his breathing and his skin. Report the observations about the swelling in his neck and his deep state of sleep.

Situation 10: The doctor comes to examine Mr. Judas and says that he is in a state of pulmonary edema and needs to be hospitalized for treatment with intravenous (IV) diuretics and acute care measures. What does the doctor's diagnosis and reason for hospitalization mean to you?

Author's Explanation: Mr. Judas has an accumulation of fluid in his lungs as a result of his lung and heart conditions. He will get medications intravenously that will increase the release of salt and water from his tissues and thereby reduce the accumulation of fluid in his lungs.

Examination Review Questions

1. The average pH of blood is
   a. 7.0   c. 7.35
   b. 7.45   d. 7.4

2. The respiratory organ called the *voice box* is the
   a. pharynx   c. larynx
   b. trachea   d. epiglottis

3. Abnormal respirations that indicate impending death are called
   a. dyspnea   c. tachypnea
   b. orthopnea   d. Cheyne-Stokes

4. An infectious disease of the lungs that poses a public threat is
   a. asthma
   b. pleurisy
   c. tuberculosis
   d. emphysema

5. During the act of swallowing, the epiglottis closes over which organ?
   a. pharynx
   b. larynx
   c. bronchus
   d. trachea

6. Stretching and loss of elasticity of the alveoli cause
   a. bronchitis
   b. pneumonia
   c. emphysema
   d. asthma

7. The serous lining of the thoracic cavity is called the
   a. pneumothorax
   b. pleura
   c. peritoneum
   d. alveoli

8. Blood clots lodged in the pulmonary arteries cause
   a. pulmonary embolism
   b. pulmonary edema
   c. COPD
   d. thrombosis

9. Breathing at the cellular level is termed
   a. aspiration
   b. internal respiration
   c. ventilation
   d. diaphragmatic respiration

10. Which is a fatal type of lung inflammation caused by breathing in vomitus?
   a. aspiration pneumonia
   b. pulmonary edema
   c. bronchitis
   d. pleurisy

Chapter 13

The Digestive System

The digestive system is often referred to as the **gastrointestinal (GI) system**. However, the organs of the GI system are described also as the *alimentary canal*. This chapters references will be made to the digestive system, the gastrointestinal system or tract, and the alimentary canal. The main organs of digestion form a continuous extension of muscular components that begin in the mouth and extend to the anus. Miraculously, a tortuous muscular canal of more than 20 feet of digestive organs provides the body human with all of its life-sustaining nutrients. Nonetheless, there are accessory organs vital to the processes of digestion and absorption of nutrients. These accessory organs are the *liver*, *gallbladder*, and *pancreas*. Without these accessory organs, the digestive system would simply be an alimentary canal incapable of sustaining human life.

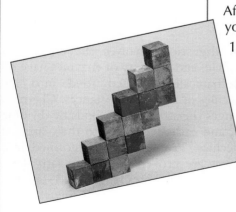

OBJECTIVES

After completing this chapter, you will be able to

1. Describe the functions of the digestive system
2. Name the organs of the alimentary canal
3. Describe the location and function of each organ
4. List and describe the functions of the accessory organs
5. Describe the conditions and diseases of the digestive system
6. List the observations about the digestive system that you should report to the nurse
7. Apply your knowledge of the digestive system to problem-solving strategies in care delivery
8. Define and spell all key terms correctly

key terms

absorption	esophagus	melena
acute gastritis	fecoliths	metabolism
alimentary canal	gallbladder	mouth
anus	gastritis	palate
appendicitis	gastrointestinal (GI) system	pancreas
appendix	gastrostomy	pancreatitis
ascending colon	glucagon	peptic ulcers
bile	glucometer	perforation
buccal cavity	heparin	peristalsis
chemical digestion	hepatitis	peritoneum
chronic gastritis	hyoid	pharyngitis
colitis	hyperglycemic	pharynx
colostomy	hypoglycemia	polyps
deciduous teeth	ileitis	rectum
descending colon	ileostomy	rugae
diabetes mellitus (DM)	ileum	secondary teeth
digestion	insulin	sigmoid colon
digestive system	islets of Langerhans	small intestine
diverticulitis	jaundice	sphincter
diverticulosis	jejunum	stomach
duodenum	ketoacidosis	stomatitis
elimination	ketones	tongue
enteritis	large intestine (colon)	transverse colon
enterostomal therapist	liver	ulcerative colitis
enzymes	mastication	villi
esophagitis	mechanical digestion	

Functions of the Digestive System

The **digestive system**, or **alimentary canal**, has three primary functions: *digestion*, *absorption*, and *elimination*. **Digestion** is derived from a Latin word meaning "to divide." The processes of digestion "divide," or break down, food substances into absorbable nutrient molecules. For example, a piece of steak, once digested, becomes thousands of amino acids, fatty acids, and glycerol. Potatoes, once digested fully, become a simple sugar molecule, glucose. Digestion is both a *mechanical* process and a *chemical* process.

Mechanical digestion involves the activities of chewing, swallowing, churning (mixing), peristalsis, and defecation. **Peristalsis** is the term used to describe the wavelike movement that pushes mechanically digested food through the alimentary canal (Figure 13-1). Peristalsis is stimulated by the autonomic nervous system. At times, there may be hyperactivity in the intestines, and you can feel the peristaltic motion. You may hear the rumbling of bowel sounds without the use of a stethoscope. Nurses and physicians listen for bowel sounds to assess the nervous and muscular activity of the intestines. This is a particularly important assessment following abdominal surgery or when there is disease of the GI system.

Chemical digestion involves the effect that stomach acid, bile, and a variety of enzymes have on changing mechanically digested food into absorbable molecules of nutrient substances. Chemical digestion changes the structure of foods by dividing proteins, fats, and carbohydrates into their smallest nutrient molecules. Proteins are transformed into amino acids; fats are broken down into fatty acids and glycerol. All carbohydrates (sugars and starches) become the simplest sugar, glucose. Glucose is the sugar that provides energy for cellular activities. At all costs, the cells must have glucose. Stored fat can be turned into glucose when the body has not ingested enough carbohydrates. When you diet, the process of changing fat into glucose is desired. You eat fewer calories and increase your body's demand for glucose by exercising.

Absorption is the process of transferring these nutrient molecules into the circulating blood so they can be distributed and used by the cells of the body. The amino acids from that juicy steak are absorbed by the small intestine. Once in the bloodstream,

The Mouth

The first organ of digestion is the **mouth**. The mouth is called the **buccal cavity**. This cavity is framed by the jaw bones and the **palate** and is lined with a mucous membrane. The structures of the mouth that are important for digestion are the tongue, salivary glands, and teeth.

The Tongue

The **tongue**, a skeletal muscle, lies on the floor of the mouth (Figure 13-2). It is attached to the **hyoid** bone, which is located below the pharynx. The tiny elevations on the surface of the tongue, the *papillae*, have nerve endings called *taste buds*. The tongue helps to move food in the mouth to be mixed with saliva. It propels food into the throat for swallowing. Of course, the tongue helps us to enjoy the taste of food. It is also an important organ for speech.

The Teeth

The adult mouth has an average of twenty-eight to thirty-two teeth called **secondary teeth**. A baby's full set of teeth are twenty in number. These baby teeth are called **deciduous teeth** because they are like deciduous trees that shed their leaves. The teeth tear, grind, chew, and mechanically digest food into smaller portions. This process is called **mastication**. Figure 13-2 shows the adult mouth and teeth.

The Salivary Glands

These exocrine glands produce saliva, which lubricates the mouth and assists with mechanical digestion (Figure 13-3). The three pairs of salivary glands release saliva, which has a digestive enzyme that begins the chemical digestion of starches. **Enzymes** are chemical substances that act as catalysts (necessary helpers) to produce a chemical reaction. For example, heat is a catalyst in many chemical reactions. The oven will not roast a chicken without heat.

The Pharynx

The **pharynx** is a tubelike structure made of muscle and lined with a mucous membrane. It serves as a passageway for food to enter the esophagus. It is also the passageway for air to enter the larynx. In swallowing, the epiglottis of the larynx closes the entrance to the respiratory system. The nerve that stimulates the action of swallowing also provides a necessary gag reflex. This protective gag reflex prevents the aspiration of food into the respiratory organs. When your mother told you not to talk with food in your mouth, it was to protect you. You cannot swallow and speak

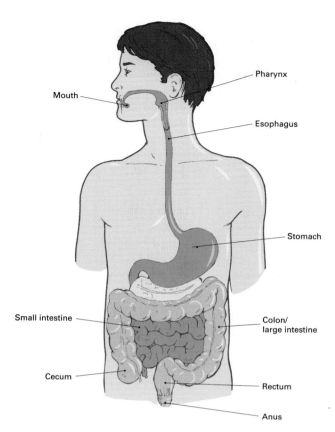

FIGURE 13-1   Mechanically digested food moves through the alimentary canal.

they are then transported across cell membranes to build new proteins of muscle cells.

Elimination is the process of ridding the body of unusable solid waste products. If you eat corn on the cob, your digestive organs will use all the nutrients that can be absorbed by microscopic cells. The cellulose waste (unusable fiber) will serve as an irritant in the colon and help you to eliminate other unusable substances in the form of feces.

Metabolism

Metabolism is the process of breaking down and building up foods in the body. Metabolism is controlled by many factors that influence the speed at which substances are broken or built in the body.

Structures of the Alimentary Canal

The structures of the alimentary canal include the following organs: *mouth, tongue, teeth, salivary glands, pharynx, esophagus, stomach, small intestine,* and *large intestine (colon)*. A description of each of these organs of the alimentary canal follows.

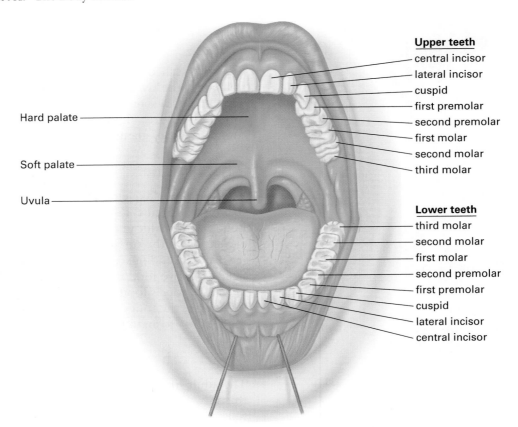

Upper teeth
- central incisor
- lateral incisor
- cuspid
- first premolar
- second premolar
- first molar
- second molar
- third molar

Hard palate

Soft palate

Uvula

Lower teeth
- third molar
- second molar
- first molar
- second premolar
- first premolar
- cuspid
- lateral incisor
- central incisor

FIGURE 13-2   The tongue and teeth.

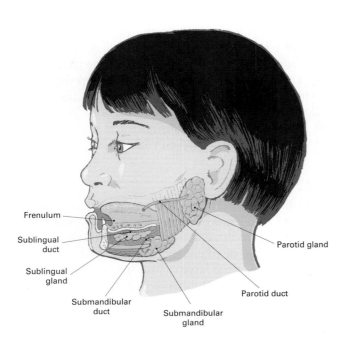

Frenulum

Sublingual duct

Sublingual gland

Submandibular duct

Submandibular gland

Parotid gland

Parotid duct

FIGURE 13-3   Salivary glands are important in the process of chemical digestion.

at the same time because the force of exhaled air keeps this lid, the epiglottis, held up.

The Esophagus

The **esophagus**, or food pipe, is a muscular organ lined with a mucous membrane. It connects the pharynx (throat) with the stomach. The esophagus is about 10 inches long. It passes through the chest cavity and exits through an opening in the diaphragm to the abdominal cavity, where it connects to the stomach.

The Stomach

The **stomach** is a strong muscular organ that lies in the upper left abdominal cavity just below the diaphragm. It is composed of three layers of muscular tissue and is capable of great expansion. It stretches after a meal has been consumed and empties into the small intestine. Figure 13-4 depicts the structure of the stomach. There are two sphincter muscles at either end of the stomach. The cardiac sphincter is the opening from the esophagus. The pylorus, or pyloric sphincter, opens into the duodenum, the first part of the small intestine. A **sphincter** is a round muscle that opens and closes. The mucous membrane that

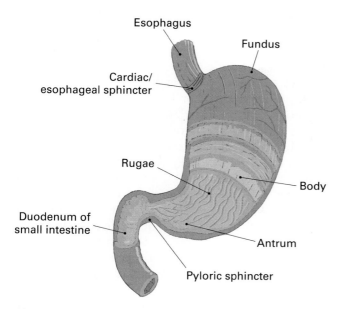

FIGURE 13-4 The structure of the stomach.

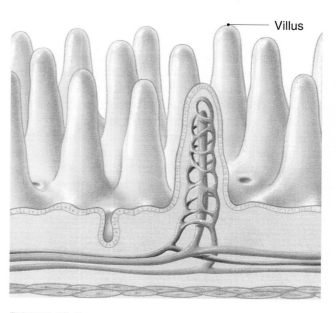

FIGURE 13-5 The villi of the small intestine.

lines the stomach lies in folds called **rugae**. This membrane is covered by thousands of microscopic glands that secrete hydrochloric acid and gastric juices rich with enzymes. The muscular contractions of the stomach start peristalsis to digest food mechanically, and the acid and gastric juices digest food chemically.

The Small Intestine

The **small intestine** is composed of three sections: the **duodenum**, **jejunum**, and **ileum**. This tube of smooth muscle is approximately 15 to 20 feet long and lies coiled within the abdominal cavity. The mucous membrane of the small intestine is rich with microscopic glands that secrete digestive juices rich in enzymes for chemical digestion. Within the mucous lining are millions of microscopic structures called **villi**, which under a microscope look like tiny fingers (Figure 13-5). The villi have lymph and vascular capillaries that absorb molecules of nutrients into the circulatory system. Blood then transports these nutrients to all the cells of the body. The first part of the small intestine receives digestive juices from the liver, gallbladder, and pancreas.

The Large Intestine (Colon)

The **large intestine (colon)** connects with the small intestine at the ileocecal valve. Undigested food substances mixed with the fluid of digestive juices enter the colon through this valve. Attached to the cecum is the appendix. The **appendix** has no known function in digestion. It can become inflamed, and a painful condition called, *appendicitis* results. The

colon is a muscular tube that is 5 feet long (Figure 13-6). It is larger in diameter than the small intestine. The large intestine lies in the lower portion of the abdominal cavity. Much of the small intestine lies coiled within its borders. The colon begins at the cecum in the lower right abdomen. The **ascending colon** travels up the right side and turns into the **transverse colon**. Then it turns left as the **descending colon** lies in the lower left abdominal cavity. The colon makes an S-shaped turn at the **sigmoid colon**, which connects to the rectum. The **rectum** is about 7 to 8 inches long and terminates at the internal anal

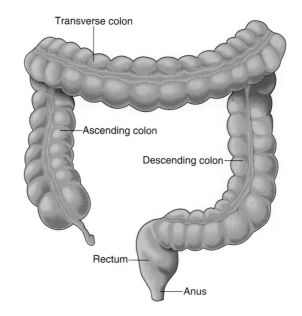

FIGURE 13-6 The colon, or large intestine, is a 5-foot-long muscular tube.

sphincter. The **anus** is a sphincter muscle with an inner involuntary muscle and an outer voluntary muscle that opens for defecation of solid waste. The colon compacts the solid waste products of digestion into feces. Water is absorbed by the mucous membrane of the colon. When there is hyperactivity in the colon, solid wastes and water are quickly moved into the rectum, and diarrhea results. A diet that is lacking water can lead to constipation (hard feces). The colon will absorb the water needed for the body, and if insufficient water has been ingested, the wastes are drier and harder to expel.

The Protective Membrane of the Abdominal Cavity

The abdomen is lined with a membrane called the **peritoneum**. This serous membrane is double-layered with a small amount of fluid and serves as a lubricant for the cavity and the abdominal organs. Much of the outer layer of the peritoneum is covered with adipose (fatty) tissue. As with any membrane, the peritoneum decreases irritation from friction as the organs move within the cavity.

Accessory Organs of the Gastrointestinal System

The liver, gallbladder, and pancreas are referred to as *accessory organs* of the gastrointestinal system because each organ performs a vital function in the digestive process. These organs are illustrated in Figure 13-7.

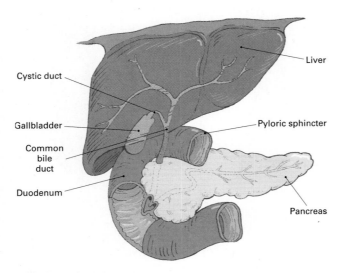

Cystic duct

Gallbladder

Common bile duct

Duodenum

Liver

Pyloric sphincter

Pancreas

FIGURE 13-7   The liver, gallbladder, and pancreas.

The Liver

The **liver** is a large organ that lies in the upper right abdominal cavity. It is an exocrine gland because it releases substances through ducts into another organ. This vital organ has many functions. One function is to produce **bile**, a green-yellow liquid that is alkaline. Bile is released by the liver and is stored in the gallbladder. Figure 13-7 shows the liver in relation to the gallbladder. Bile helps to neutralize acid, emulsify fats, and remove toxins from the liver. To emulsify fat means to break it up into globules like drops of oil that float when dropped into water. Other functions of the liver include the storage of excess glucose in the form of a starch, glycogen. This starch can be broken down into glucose when the supply in the blood is low. The liver also makes new glucose by a chemical process of changing fats and proteins into glucose. The liver detoxifies the blood, which means that it removes poisonous substances from the blood. Alcohol is detoxified by the liver. Also, many medications are detoxified by the liver. The liver stores blood and produces proteins needed in the processes of blood clotting. It is also rich in **heparin**, which is an anti-coagulant. It stores vitamins A, D, E, K, and B_{12}. It also stores iron.

The Gallbladder

The **gallbladder** is a hollow sac that lies behind the liver. After bile is produced in the liver it is stored in the gallbladder. The gallbladder has ducts that open from the liver and into the duodenum. The duct that opens into the duodenum is called the ampulla of Vater. When fats are present in the duodenum, the gallbladder releases bile through a duct to aid in the chemical digestion of fats. Bile has salts, water, and the pigment from old red blood cells. At times, the salts present in bile crystallize and form stones. Gall stones obstruct the flow of bile from the ducts of the gallbladder. The obstruction causes pain, especially after eating, when the gallbladder is attempting to release bile into the duodenum.

The Pancreas

The **pancreas** is both an exocrine gland and an endocrine gland (Figure 13-7). As an exocrine gland, it releases digestive juices rich in enzymes into the duodenum. Within the pancreas are special cells called the **islets of Langerhans**. These cells produce two hormones, hence the endocrine gland function of the pancreas. These hormones, **glucagon** and **insulin**, are involved in the metabolism of glucose. Glucagon is involved in the liver processes of manufacturing glucose from fats, proteins, and stored glycogen. Insulin is a necessary hormone for transporting glucose into cells. Insulin is like a key that opens the door to the cells to let glucose out of the bloodstream and into the cell. As glucose is circulated in the blood, it is transported across the cell membrane into the cytoplasm by insulin. Without insulin, glucose cannot unlock the cell membrane; therefore, it remains in the blood. A high level of glucose in the blood is a condition called *hyperglycemia.*

Diabetes mellitus, often referred to as *sugar diabetes*, is a disease that results from a lack of insulin production in the pancreas. Sometimes, the pancreas produces no insulin. When no insulin is produced, the person has insulin-dependent diabetes mellitus. This means that insulin injections are needed to control blood sugar levels. Sometimes, the pancreas does not produce enough insulin. These individuals may need medications that stimulate the islet cells to produce insulin; this is called *non-insulin-dependent diabetes mellitus.* Insulin is a hormone, and hormones are proteins. Since proteins are digested in the stomach and small intestine, insulin must be given through injection, or it would be digested before being useful.

Conditions and Diseases of the Digestive System

Inflammatory conditions affecting the mucous membrane of the gastrointestinal system can occur anywhere along this continuous tract. The terms that describe these conditions are related to the area of the inflammation or infection. The nature of the symptoms varies, but is generally consistent with the organ that is inflamed. **Stomatitis** is inflammation of the mouth; **pharyngitis** is inflammation of the throat, and **esophagitis** is inflammation of the esophagus. **Enteritis** is inflammation of the small intestine. **Colitis** is inflammation of the colon. **Pancreatitis** is inflammation of the pancreas. These conditions can be acute or chronic in nature, and most are related to an underlying disease that is causing the inflammation.

One of the more common inflammatory conditions of the GI system is gastritis. **Gastritis** refers to inflammation of the mucous membrane of the stomach. This condition can be acute or chronic in nature. **Acute gastritis** can be related to dietary intake of irritating food, medications, and alcohol, or it can be a sign of an infection that has affected the GI system. Symptoms may include nausea, heartburn, vomiting, coated tongue, and headache. Vomiting sometimes relieves the discomfort because the irritant is removed from the stomach. **Chronic gastritis** changes the mucous lining of the stomach. Even-

tually, the lining becomes thin, the gastric secretions decrease in quantity and quality, and the stomach contents consist of mostly mucous and water. Nausea, vomiting, gas, heartburn, and a bad taste in the mouth are common complaints.

Peptic ulcers involve the pyloric area of the stomach and generally include ulceration of the mucous membranes of the stomach and the duodenum. The mucous lining becomes eroded due to an excess of hydrochloric acid. Causes have been associated with severe stress and poor diet, excessive histamine release in the stomach, chronic infectious process of the stomach, and certain medications like steroids. The symptoms may include a burning, severe pain in the upper abdomen, heartburn, gas, swelling of the upper abdomen, nausea, vomiting, and diarrhea. If the ulcer penetrates the mucous lining and penetrates the muscle tissue, bleeding will occur. This will be manifested in two ways. If the ulcer causes hemorrhage, the person may vomit blood. If the blood is present in the stomach before vomiting, it will look like coffee grounds, or bright red blood may be vomited. If the ulcer is in the duodenum, the person may have stools (feces) that are black and tarlike. This is called **melena**. The complications of peptic ulcers include hemorrhage, perforation, and obstruction of the pyloric sphincter. **Perforation** means that the ulcer has eroded through the muscular layer, allowing the contents of the stomach and duodenum to escape into the peritoneal cavity. This penetration can cause massive infection and lead to death.

Appendicitis is an inflammation of the blind pouch in the right lower quadrant of the abdominopelvic cavity. When food substances accumulate in the appendix, it may become acutely inflamed. With this inflammation, there is associated severe abdominal pain, which becomes localized in the right lower quadrant of the abdomen. Other symptoms include nausea, anorexia, rigid abdomen, increased white blood cell count, and fever. The appendix can become filled with pus. The greatest danger of appendicitis is the rupture of the appendix. This can result in infection in the peritoneal cavity and can be fatal.

Ileitis (enteritis) is an inflammatory disease of the small intestine, usually in the area of the ileum. The mucous membrane swells, thickens, and later forms scar tissue. The person complains of cramping abdominal pains, especially after eating. This is because eating stimulates peristalsis, and the ileum is narrowed due to the chronic inflammation. As the ileum empties its contents into the large bowel, the pain increases; therefore, the person generally begins to eat small, nutritionally inadequate meals or begins to avoid food. The results are malnourishment, weight loss, and possible anemia. The small bowel may no longer absorb nutrients. Bleeding and melena may occur. There is a strong familial link to ileitis. Diet, anti-inflammatory medications, and medications to control anxiety are used for medical management. However, ileostomy may be necessary if medical interventions fail.

Ulcerative colitis is an inflammatory and ulcerative disease of the colon. The process usually begins in the rectum and sigmoid areas and progresses upward in the colon. The symptoms include frequent bouts of diarrhea, bloody stools, mucus or pus in the stool, cramping, and bloating. The complications include malnutrition, weight loss, skin ulcers, abscesses of the colon, and colon cancer. Diet therapy, emotional support, antibiotics, anti-inflammatory drugs, iron replacement, adequate fluid intake, and medications that slow down peristalsis are used to medically manage the disease. When medical treatment is unsuccessful, then surgical treatments are performed. Surgery will remove the ulcerated portions of the colon, and a colostomy will be formed. If the entire colon is inflamed, an ileostomy will be performed. This means that the entire colon will be removed.

Diverticulosis means "condition of little diversions." Along the colon wall, "outpouching" may occur due to weakened musculature. These *diverticula* (pouches) are prime targets for **fecoliths** (fecal stones) to form. When undigested particles get trapped in the pouches, inflammation can result. This is called **diverticulitis**. Symptoms include left lower quadrant pain, fever, nausea, bloated abdomen, and difficulty with defecation. Diverticulitis is treated with antibiotics, dietary restrictions, and, sometimes, surgical resection or colostomy. Compli-

cations include peritonitis if the diverticula burst. When this happens, the colon contents are released into the peritoneal cavity around the abdominal organs. Figure 13-8 depicts diverticulosis.

Surgical Treatments

When a **colostomy** is performed, a portion or all of the colon must first be removed; this is a colectomy. A new opening for intestinal waste (feces) is formed (Figure 13-9). This means that the person will no longer defecate through the anus. Now, the person will defecate through an opening on the abdomen. A piece of the intestine will be pulled through the abdominal wall, and a new opening called a *stoma* will be present on the surface of the abdomen. This individual will wear an appliance, a plastic bag that has a hard plastic circular opening on the plastic collection device. The opening is sized to fit the stoma. An adhesive and skin barrier paste is applied to the skin around the stoma. The plastic bag has an opening at the bottom that is used to empty the fecal contents. The opening is held closed by a plastic clip so that the fecal contents will be secured. The person controls the release of the contents by unlocking the plastic clip and emptying the fecal material from the bag into the toilet. The colostomy appliance is effective for several days; then it is removed, and a new appliance is applied. The location of the stoma and the consistency of the fecal contents will depend on the amount of colon that is removed. If the descending colon is removed, then the fecal contents will be more formed and the stoma will be on the left side of the abdomen. If a transverse colostomy is performed,

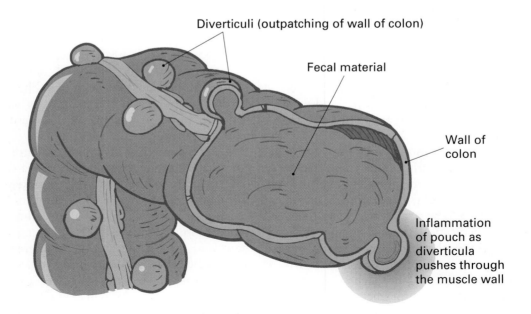

Diverticuli (outpatching of wall of colon)

Fecal material

Wall of colon

Inflammation of pouch as diverticula pushes through the muscle wall

FIGURE 13-8 Diverticulosis.

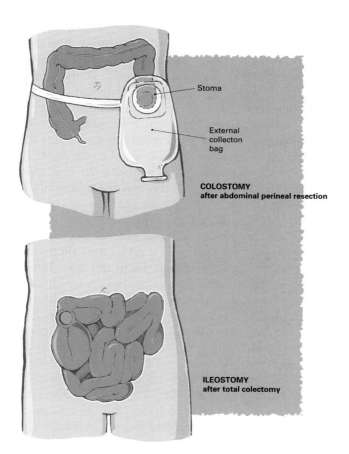

Stoma

External
collecton
bag

COLOSTOMY
after abdominal perineal resection

ILEOSTOMY
after total colectomy

FIGURE 13-9 Colostomy and ileostomy.

the stoma will be near the midline, and the fecal contents will be semiliquid to semiformed. The amount of colon remaining relates to the amount of water absorbed and the consistency of the stool. The timing of a bowel movement is more predictable if more colon remains. The procedure for colostomy care and the psychosocial considerations of the care for the colostomy patient are discussed in Chapter 26.

An **ileostomy** is a surgical procedure that is performed to create a new opening for the removal of fecal waste. The individual with an ileostomy does not have any colon remaining to absorb water and to compact solid waste products. As a result, stool is liquid and is more frequently produced. The stoma is formed from the ileum, the last section of the small intestine. This person also will wear an appliance that operates in the same manner as described for a colostomy. However, the appliance will require more frequent emptying.

At times, it is necessary to make a new opening into the stomach (**gastrostomy**) for the purpose of feeding and nutritional support. A surgical opening is made, and a tube called a *Peg tube* is placed in the stomach and leads to the surface of the abdomen. This is used to feed the person. Liquid nutrients,

such as Ensure and Sustacal, are instilled into the stomach through the Peg or gastrostomy tube. If a person has a disturbance in the esophagus, pharynx, or mouth and is unable to eat or swallow for any reason, this is the surgical remedy. The procedure for gastrostomy feedings will be discussed in Chapter 26.

Tumors of the GI System

Tumors may be benign or malignant in nature. **Polyps**, or outgrowths of the intestinal tract, are commonly benign; however, some polyps may be precancerous. Malignant tumors that tend to form in the GI system usually arise in connective and lymph tissue. They cause obstruction and hemorrhage. Malignant tumors of the large intestine are more common than those of the small intestine. Colorectal tumors generally arise in the epithelial tissue of the mucous membrane. Changes in bowel movements, ranging from constipation to diarrhea, are initial signs. Bleeding, anemia, obstruction, and perforation through the smooth muscle are symptoms. Warning signs of colorectal cancer include changes in bowel movements and blood in the stool. After the age of fifty, men and women should be checked by their physician for colorectal cancer.

Hepatitis

Because the liver is an organ of the digestive system, inflammation of the liver (**hepatitis**) is discussed here. There are several forms of hepatitis. *Hepatitis type A* is an infectious disease transmitted through the oral-fecal route. One of the most common means of spreading hepatitis A is through food handlers who do not wash their hands, especially after using the toilet. This is one reason the board of health mandates that restaurants post the sign in the bathroom, "Employees must wash their hands before returning to work." *Hepatitis type B* is caused by hepatitis B virus (HBV). It is a blood-borne pathogen that is transmitted by blood and body fluids. Sexual contact or sharing needles to inject drugs are ways in which it is spread. Health care employees must use standard precautions with all patients to control the spread of this disease as well as other blood-borne pathogens. There is another form of hepatitis that is Non-A (not type A) and Non-B (not type B). This is *hepatitis type C*, which is also spread through blood and body fluids. Hepatitis is a serious disease that can cause death. The initial symptoms take weeks to months to appear after infection with the virus. Consequently, people may transmit the virus because they do not know they are infected. The classic initial symptoms are flu-like symptoms, and then the skin and whites of the eyes become yellow. This is called jaundice and is a classic sign of liver disease. There is no cure for hepatitis. However, there is a vaccine that can prevent one from getting HBV. This vaccine is now given to children along with their other immunizations. Health care workers are encouraged to get the vaccine, and most organizations offer this as a free service to at-risk employees.

Diabetes Mellitus

The endocrine glands of the pancreas produce the hormone insulin, and because the pancreas is an accessory organ of the digestive system, **diabetes mellitus (DM)** is discussed here. When the pancreas fails to produce enough insulin or does not produce any insulin, diabetes mellitus results. Review the types of diabetes described earlier in the section "The Pancreas." Children and adults are victims of this disease. Obese adults are at greater risk for developing non-insulin-dependent diabetes mellitus (NIDDM). There is a strong familial link to diabetes.

People with diabetes experience hunger even though they have eaten. This is because their cells are not able to use the glucose. Their blood sugar is higher than normal levels—they are said to be **hyperglycemic**—and the breakdown of fats to make sugar occurs because the cells do not recognize the presence of glucose in the blood. This causes **ketoacidosis**. This is an acid state caused by the byproducts of fat metabolism, **ketones**.

When the blood sugar is high, the person may have a fruity smell to the breath, and glucose may be present in the urine. The kidneys will excrete excess glucose, and this causes excessive urination. The presence of excess sugar in the blood causes a water-pulling action in the kidneys. Along with the water will follow salts and glucose in the urine. The skin may be flushed and dry, and the person feels thirsty and hungry and urinates frequently. If the blood sugar level rises high enough, the person may become unconscious, go into a coma, and die. Sometimes, people with diabetes who have taken their oral medication or who have injected their dose of insulin do not eat properly, and their blood sugar drops or becomes very low. When this happens, the condition is called **hypoglycemia**. This is why the timing of the insulin dosage is regulated to the person's meals, food intake, and exercise. Increased exercise increases the body's demand for glucose because the glucose is used for energy. It is difficult to always detect the difference between high and low blood sugar, especially if the person becomes unconscious, because you cannot ask if he or she ate or took the medication. Initially, hypoglycemia (low blood glucose) will present with clammy, cool skin and complaints of (c/o) hunger.

People with diabetes mellitus need to follow a calculated, prescribed diet called the American Diabetes Association (ADA) diet. The diet prescribes the correct balance of carbohydrates, fats, and proteins needed to help to control blood sugar levels. The total calories depend on the individual's needs. Some people with NIDDM can be treated by diet alone.

Blood sugar levels can be checked with a simple bedside testing device called a **glucometer**. There are many different glucometers on the market. The principles of this procedure are discussed in Chapter 26. What is essential for the clinical care associate to know is the importance of performing the test on time and the importance of documenting the results and reporting them to the nurse.

application to practice

The overall health of the patient begins with adequate nutrition. Knowledge of the gastrointestinal system will increase your understanding about how assimilation of nutrients occurs. Understanding the GI diseases will promote effectiveness in assisting with eating adaptations and bowel regimens. Relate what you have learned about the GI system to the following clinical situations.

Learning Activities

Situation 1: Mr. Schnyder is a fifty-two-year-old man who comes to your emergency room (ER) complaining of abdominal pain, fever, and chills. The triage nurse asks you to take his vital signs. These are your results: temperature 102°F, pulse 102, respirations 28, blood pressure 140/88. Which of these results do you report to the nurse, and when do you tell the nurse?

Author's Explanation: Immediately tell the nurse that the patient's temperature is elevated and that his pulse and respirations are rapid.

Situation 2: Mr. Schnyder also tells you that he has had this severe pain on the right side for about three hours. Two hours ago, his wife gave him an enema because she thought he was constipated. The pain intensified after the enema. When the doctor comes into the room to obtain a history and physical, Mr. Schnyder does not tell him about the enema. Should you? The physician asks Mr. Schnyder to locate the pain, and he points to his left side. What is unusual about the difference in the patient's location of the pain? Is this important to tell the doctor, and why?

Author's Explanation: The enema could be very important because the patient reported that the pain got worse afterward. You should tell the doctor immediately. Mr. Schnyder also told you the pain was on the right side. When the doctor asked him, he pointed to the left side. Mr. Schnyder could have appendicitis, and his pain may cause him to be confused. He may not realize the importance of describing the location and significant events related to the pain. You might talk to the doctor immediately outside of the patient's room, or you might state the different reports to the doctor by discussing it with Mr. Schnyder in the physician's presence. "Mr. Schnyder, you described the pain to me as being on the right side. Has the pain moved?"

Situation 3: Ms. Jones is a forty-eight-year-old mother of three who is a familiar patient to you. She has a diagnosis of ulcerative colitis. She has been admitted to your medical unit several times over the past three years. In report, the nurse said, "She was admitted yesterday with a flare-up of the symptoms, and she is dehydrated." What does her diagnosis mean to you? What is the "flare-up" of symptoms to which the nurse is referring? Why would she be dehydrated?

Author's Explanation: Ms. Jones has a condition that causes ulcers in her colon. These ulcers are like sores that form in the mucous lining of the large intestine. She probably has had diarrhea that is watery, bloody, and filled with mucous. Roughage is not digested and causes hyperactivity of the colon, and water does not remain in the colon long enough to be absorbed into the blood stream. Therefore, she loses water and becomes dehydrated.

Situation 4: The doctors tell Ms. Jones that she needs a colostomy. When you go into her room, you find her crying. She tells you that she doesn't want to be disfigured. What is a colostomy? Why is she crying about this? What does she mean by "disfigured"?

Author's Explanation: When a colostomy is performed, a new opening for the passage of fecal waste is created on the abdomen. It can be temporary or permanent. A temporary colostomy rests the colon for a period of time so that the ulcers can heal. After

the ulcers heal, the portions of the large intestine are sewn back together again, and the person resumes normal bowel movements through the anus. When the colostomy is permanent, the person defecates through a stoma on the abdomen for the remainder of his or her life. Ms. Jones is sad and possibly angry that she will have to have a new opening for removing fecal wastes. She will feel "disfigured" because this is not physically appealing or attractive. It takes a long time to come to accept and to cope with a colostomy. There are many concerns about attractiveness to sexual partners. Most people worry about odor and are embarrassed by the collection of stool in a colostomy appliance. Just imagine that you were told that you would need a colostomy to save your life. How might you feel? What are your fears and worries?

Situation 5: Ms. Jones becomes angry when you ask her to explain why she is crying and what she means about being "disfigured." You did not mean any harm; you just wanted to clarify what she was feeling. Do you have any resources or people who can help Ms. Jones and you deal with her feelings?

Author's Explanation: Yes. Most hospitals and home care agencies have a resource nurse who specializes in this area. This nurse is called an **enterostomal therapist**. This is a nurse who specializes and is certified to care for patients who have an ileostomy or a colostomy. You should ask Ms. Jones's nurse to consult this nurse specialist. He or she will be able to assist Ms. Jones in many ways. One important thing the nurse might do is help her contact the Ostomy Society. People who have had similar colostomies may be able to help Ms. Jones learn how they coped with their situations and give practical advice that only a person with a colostomy would know.

Situation 6: Mrs. Avalon is a thirty-eight-year-old woman with insulin-dependent DM (IDDM). She was admitted to the ER at 2:00 A.M. in an unconscious state with an insulin reaction. What is her diagnosis, and why was she brought to the ER?

Author's Explanation: Mrs. Avalon has insulin-dependent diabetes mellitus. She requires insulin injections to control her blood glucose. An insulin reaction means that she had more insulin than her blood glucose required. There could be multiple causes for this reaction. She was brought to the ER because the paramedics or people who were with her were unable to help her regain consciousness.

Situation 7: The RN asks you to get a stat blood glucose on Mrs. Avalon. Why? How can you do this?

Author's Explanation: You were asked to immediately determine Mrs. Avalon's blood sugar level. You will use a glucometer or glucose machine to check her blood sugar level at the bedside. You will stick her finger, get a sample of capillary blood, and follow the procedure for the meter used in your ER. You will report the results immediately to the nurse. You or the nurse will also do a venipuncture to send a venous blood sample to the lab for stat glucose results. The nurse will base the actions to be taken on the results that you obtain from the bedside test and then from the lab results.

Situation 8: After Mrs. Avalon is given an intravenous (IV) solution that is high in dextrose (sugar), you will be asked to take another bedside glucose reading. Why? When you go into Mrs. Avalon's cubicle after she has been receiving the dextrose solution for about 15 minutes, she is awake and confused about how she got to the ER. Why is she now awake?

Author's Explanation: The nurse wants to know what the current blood sugar is. The nurse wants to see if it is within normal range and will regulate the amount of IV solution based on the results. Mrs. Avalon's blood glucose is probably returning to normal range, and this is allowing her brain cells to function effectively. That is why she is awake. She is confused because she came to the ER in an unconscious state. She was not awake, alert, and oriented when she was transported to the ER.

Situation 9: What organ is involved in diabetes mellitus? What is the hormone that is involved? Does an excess or a lack of this hormone cause diabetes mellitus?

Author's Explanation: The pancreas is the organ. The hormone is insulin. It is a lack of insulin that causes diabetes mellitus.

Situation 10: Mr. Aramingo is a forty-year-old man who was admitted to your unit yesterday. In a report, the nurse tells you that he has a GI bleed and must be closely monitored for bleeding. You are instructed to hemetest all stool and any emesis. What is a hemetest? What is emesis?

Author's Explanation: A hemetest is a measurement of the presence of any blood in a body fluid. You will follow the instructions for the specific hemetest that is used by your organization. You take a sample of the stool or emesis (vomit) and use the hemetest kit to see if there is any blood present.

Situation 11: While you are caring for Mr. Aramingo, he has an episode of vomiting. You look at the contents of the basin and find emesis that looks like wet coffee grinds. You cannot imagine what happened because the patient has been NPO since admission. What should you do?

Author's Explanation: You should report to the nurse immediately. Describe exactly what you saw, and let her see the emesis. You should also test the emesis. What you will find with the hemetest is the presence of blood. This is a classic sign of bleeding from the stomach or the duodenum.

Situation 12: The nurse asks you to check Mr. Aramingo's vital signs and to measure the contents of the emesis. These are your findings: temperature 99°F, pulse 110, respirations 30, blood pressure 98/58, emesis 350 cc. What do you do? What do you think is happening to this patient?

Author's Explanation: You should report the results to the nurse immediately. Mr. Aramingo's pulse and respirations are rapid, and his blood pressure is low. There is a considerable fluid loss from vomiting. He may be going into shock from the GI bleed. Immediately after reporting this, return to the patient and continue to monitor his vital signs at least every 15 minutes. Report the results immediately.

Situation 13: When you return to Mr. Aramingo, you find that his skin is moist and cool. He is lethargic and tells you he needs the bedpan. You give him the bedpan, and his stool is very dark and almost looks like tar. What do you do?

Author's Explanation: Call for the nurse stat. Hemetest the stool stat. Report the results. Tell the nurse exactly what the stool looked like, and check the patient's vitals stat. Mr. Aramingo's melena is another sign of a GI bleed.

Situation 14: Mrs. Jenge is a thirty-year-old woman whom you meet, for the first time, as you make your rounds before the nurse gives you the evening shift report. You find that Mrs. Jenge is a Caucasian woman whose skin is very yellow. What do you think is the cause of this yellow skin condition?

Author's Explanation: Yellow discoloration of the skin is called *jaundice*. This is a sign of liver disease, especially hepatitis. The yellow condition is caused by the accumulation of bile pigments absorbed by the skin.

Situation 15: The nurse tells you that Mrs. Jenge has hepatitis type A and that she was admitted because of dehydration. What is hepatitis A, and how could she have acquired this condition?

Author's Explanation: Hepatitis A is a viral infection transmitted by an infected person who handles food in a restaurant or cafeteria, by water contaminated by sewage, or by shellfish from sewage-contaminated waters. The liver is the organ affected by this virus.

Situation 16: You remember that you cared for another person with hepatitis. This man had skin discoloration like Mrs. Jenge, but you were told by the nurse at the time that he had HBV. What was that condition, and what was different about his hepatitis?

Author's Explanation: The other patient had hepatitis B, which is a viral infection of the liver transmitted through blood or other body fluids, including semen and vaginal secretions. This patient may have received a blood transfusion that was infected. This would have occurred before the American Red Cross began testing blood for the hepatitis virus. Or this man may have shared a needle for injection of drugs or had sex with a person who was infected. With either type of hepatitis, the patient will be jaundiced.

Situation 17: List the observations that the clinical care associate should make about a patient's digestive system.

Author's Explanation: Observe the mouth for dryness and sores of the lips and mucous membranes. Does the patient have teeth or wear dentures? Do the dentures fit properly? Does the patient have the dentures in when it is time to eat? Look at the condition of the tongue. Is it coated or cracked? Are there any ulcers or sores? Observe the throat by watching the patient swallow food and liquids. Does the patient have difficulty swallowing? Does the patient eat? What are the food preferences? When does the patient like to eat? Are there any complaints about the effects of certain foods after eating? Does the patient complain of indigestion, heartburn, belching, bloating, flatus? What is the patient's prescribed diet? Does the patient adhere to the diet? How does the patient tolerate his diet? What percentage of the meals does the patient eat? Have nutritional supplements or scheduled snacks been prescribed for the patient? Is the patient on any fluid restriction? Is the patient on measured intake of liquids? Does the patient need assistance with eating or need to be fed meals? Are there any cultural or religious dietary requirements or restrictions? What is the route of food or nutritional intake? Does the patient have a feeding tube, such as a Dubhoff or Peg tube (gastrostomy tube)? Is the patient receiving intravenous nutrition, hyperalimentation, or lipids? How often does the patient have a bowel movement? What is the color and consistency of the stool? Does the patient have bowel incontinence? Does the patient have a colostomy or an ileostomy? Does the patient care for this independently? What is the condition of the stoma? Is it pink, red, moist, or raised above the skin, or is it even with the skin surface? How does the patient cope with the alteration in bowel function? Has the patient had diarrhea, or is the patient constipated? Is there any nausea, vomiting, or loss of appetite? Is the abdomen distended or swollen? Does it feel hard or soft? Are there any complaints of difficulty with having a bowel movement, such as pain, burning, itching, bleeding, or straining to have a bowel movement?

Examination Review Questions

1. Wavelike motions of the intestinal muscle are called
   a. peristalsis
   b. rugae
   c. polyps
   d. villi

2. The process of transferring nutrients into circulating blood for distribution is
   a. digestion
   b. absorption
   c. elimination
   d. metabolism

3. What is another name for the large intestine?
   a. rectum
   b. anus
   c. borvel
   d. colon

4. Which of the following digestive organs is both an exocrine gland and an endocrine gland?
   a. liver
   b. gallbladder
   c. stomach
   d. pancreas

5. The process of chewing food is called
   a. metabolism
   b. digestion
   c. mastication
   d. salivation

6. Microscopic projections along the small intestine that increase absorption surfaces are
   a. cilia
   b. sphincters
   c. rugae
   d. villi

7. The colon connects to the small intestine at the terminal end of the
   a. ileum
   b. jejunum
   c. duodenum
   d. sigmoid

8. The main function of the liver is to
   a. detoxify medication
   b. store bile
   c. emulsify carbohydrates
   d. produce bile

9. Inflammation of the stomach is called
    a. stomatitis
    b. esophagitis
    c. gastritis
    d. enteritis

10. Outpouching of the bowel wall results in
    a. appendicitis
    b. polyps
    c. diverticulitis
    d. carcinoma

Chapter 14

The Urinary System

The urinary system, a sterile system of organs, is responsible for producing and eliminating urine from the body. What you may not know are the processes involved in urine formation and how the urinary system interacts with other body systems to maintain homeostasis (a state of balance).

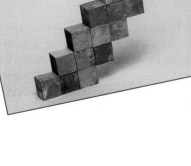

OBJECTIVES

After completing this chapter, you will be able to

1. Describe the functions of the urinary system
2. Name the organs of the urinary system
3. Describe the location of each organ
4. List the functions of each organ
5. Describe the conditions and diseases of the urinary system
6. List the observations about the urinary system that you should report to the nurse
7. Apply the knowledge of the urinary system to problem-solving strategies in care delivery
8. Define and spell all key terms correctly

key terms

antidiuretic hormone (ADH)	hilum	renal pelvis
adipose capsule	kidneys	renal tubule
aldosterone	laser	renal vein
ammonia	magnesium	retroperitoneal space
anuria	microorganisms	rugae
bladder	mucus	shunt
Bowman's capsule	nephrectomy	sodium
calcium	nephrons	specific gravity
chloride	oliguria	stoma
creatinine	organic wastes	sulfate
cystectomy	peritoneal dialysis	suprapubic cystostomy
cystitis	phosphate	urea
cystoscope	phosphorus	ureter
dialysis	plasma proteins	ureterostomy
diffusion	polycystic disease	urethra
electrolytes	potassium	uric acid
elimination	production	urinalysis
glomerulus	pyelonephritis	urine
glucose	renal artery	urosepsis
hematuria	renal calculi	
hemodialysis	renal failure	

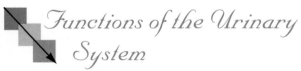 Functions of the Urinary System

The primary functions of the urinary system are the **production** and **elimination** of urine. What is urine, and how is it formed? **Urine** is formed from the blood by the kidneys. As blood flows through the kidneys, excess water and salts are removed from the blood. Urine is made of about 90 percent water, and concentrated in this water are the excess salts that the body does not need to function healthily. These salts include **sodium**, **potassium**, **calcium**, **chloride**, and **phosphoros**. Therefore, the urinary system helps to maintain a balance of water and salts or electrolytes in the body. The waste products from the breakdown of proteins in the body are also eliminated in urine. **Urea** and **uric acid** are two waste products of proteins. These products contain nitrogen, an element that is part of all amino acids (the building molecules of proteins). Some drugs and water-soluble vitamins are excreted in urine. The kidneys also help to balance the amount of acids and alkalines in the blood and work in conjunction with the lungs to achieve acid-base balance. The *bladder* stores urine that is formed in the kidneys. And when the bladder is full, the urge to urinate is realized by the nerve endings present in the bladder. Urine is passed to the outside through a muscular tube called the *urethra*.

Structures of the Urinary System

The *kidneys, ureters, bladder,* and *urethra* are the main organs of the urinary system. Each organ has unique structures and functions. The urethra functions as both a urinary organ and a reproductive organ in the male. Descriptions of these organs follow.

The Kidneys

There are two kidneys and both are shaped like beans, and that's why one type of bean is named for the kidneys (Figure 14-1). The kidneys lie in the back of the abdominal cavity, just above the waist area. Their location is referred to as the **retroperitoneal space**, the space in the back of the peritoneum. (The peritoneum is the lining of the abdominal cavity.) The kidneys are held in place by a capsule of fat called the **adipose capsule**. This fat supports and cushions the kidneys, which are located close to the posterior surface. Each kidney has a blood supply: The **renal artery** carries blood to the kidneys, and the **renal vein** takes blood away from the kidneys. These blood vessels, along with lymphatic vessels and nerves, enter and leave the kidneys at a notch called the **hilum**. Located at the hilum is the urine collection space called the **renal pelvis**. Located on top of each kidney is an adrenal (suprarenal) gland.

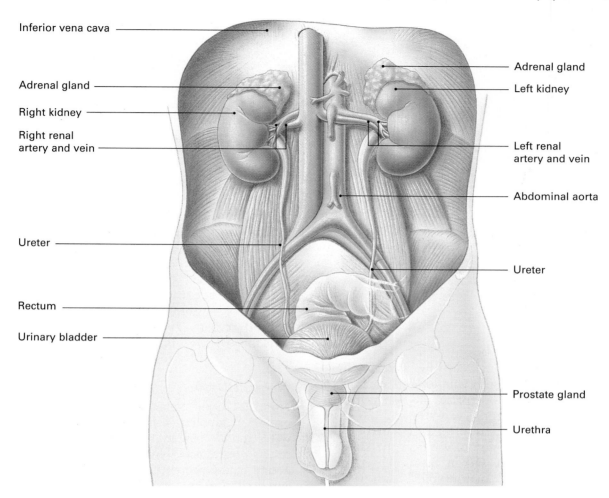

FIGURE 14-1 The urinary organs.

The Working Units of the Kidneys

The **nephrons** are the microscopic working cells of the kidneys (Figure 14-2). There are millions of nephrons in each kidney. These tiny structures have three sections: the *glomerulus, Bowman's capsule,* and *renal tubules.* (*Glomerulus* comes from the Latin *glomero,* which means "to wind into a ball.") The **glomerulus** is a tuft, or ball, of interwoven capillaries that are nestled in a cuplike structure called **Bowman's capsule**. Extending from this capsule is a twisted **renal tubule**. A tubule is a tiny tube.

The Work of the Nephrons

As blood flows through the renal artery, it is diverted into millions of arterioles (tiny arteries), each connected to the arterial ends of the glomerular capillaries. These capillaries filter blood as it flows through, and they filter out the plasma proteins. These plasma proteins create a water-pulling pressure that is essential to the return of water to the blood. All of the other contents of the blood (also known as the *fil-*

trate) pass into Bowman's capsule. Imagine the filtration of blood in the glomerulus as the process of making coffee with a drip-type coffeemaker. The ground coffee is placed into a lined container. Water is forced through the top of the coffeemaker and over the coffee grinds. As it passes over the grinds and through the filter, the water picks up elements from the coffee grinds. The coffee grinds remain behind in the filter. The coffee passes through the filter and is collected in the coffeepot.

After the filtrate enters Bowman's capsule, it then travels through the renal tubule. This tubule is convoluted (twisted). Along the entire length of this tubule are highly selective cells that reabsorb water and electrolytes and that secrete water and electrolytes. The tubule is sensitive to the amount of electrolytes, water, nitrogen, and acid-base present in the blood. It is selective of the substances reabsorbed and sent back to the bloodstream, and it is selective of the substances secreted (removed) in the final product produced by nephrons. When the body is in need of water, the tubule reabsorbs water. The same is true of electrolytes.

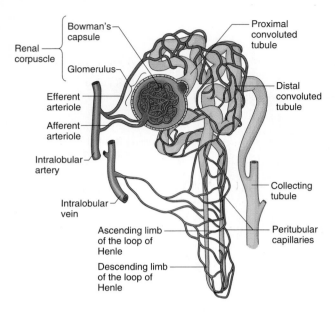

FIGURE 14-2   A nephron.

Consider a hot summer day when you are physically active and sweating. If you do not have time to drink enough fluids to replace the water lost in sweat, your nephrons conserve water, and less urine is formed. Fluid balance is maintained based on the reabsorption and secretion of water in the kidneys. Water is lost in sweat and in breathing. A small amount of water is released in your breath. (When you fog up the car windows, the vapor of your breath creates the moisture.) Acid-base balance is maintained by the kidneys in a slower, but greater amount than by the respiratory system. Remember that breathing rate increases when there is too much carbon dioxide in the blood. Carbon dioxide and water in the blood create carbonic acid. The kidneys are sensitive to the presence of acid in the blood and remove hydrogen to reduce the acidity in the blood. This makes the urine acidic. The pH of urine is about 5.5 which is acidic, but the acid state of urine is desirable to restrict the presence of acid in the blood.

Factors That Control Kidney Function

Blood pressure is important to kidney function. When blood pressure is too low, the amount of blood getting to the glomeruli of the kidneys is reduced. Each heart beat sends blood out to the arteries of the body, including the renal artery. The kidneys filter about 1,200 cubic centimeters (cc) of blood each minute. The amount of filtrate formed is about 125 cc per minute, and from this, about 1 cc per minute becomes urine. The rest of the filtrate is returned to the blood. When blood pressure drops or when cardiac output is decreased, the amount of

pressure in the glomerulus drops, and the kidneys are unable to produce urine.

Water and salt intake in the diet, as well as water and salt loss through sweat, affects the amount of urine produced. Hormones control the function of the kidneys as well. There are two hormones that regulate the kidneys. One is called **antidiuretic hormone (ADH)**. A diuretic is a substance that causes increased secretion of water and, therefore, increased urine production. ADH makes the kidneys retain water and is called the *water-retaining hormone*. When the intake of fluids is less than the body needs, this hormone is released, and it stimulates the renal tubules to reabsorb water. **Aldosterone** is another hormone that influences the kidneys. It helps them to retain sodium, an important electrolyte for the body. If you drank ample water, sweat profusely, and did not have adequate dietary intake of sodium, your renal tubules would be stimulated by aldosterone to reabsorb sodium. This is why aldosterone is referred to as the *salt-retaining hormone*.

Normal Urine

Normally, urine consists of the waste products of protein metabolism, called *organic wastes*, along with water and electrolytes. **Organic wastes** are the end results of the metabolism of all proteins that are ingested in the protein food sources eaten as well as any body proteins that are broken down in cellular activity. These organic wastes include urea, **creatinine**, **ammonia**, uric acid, and other substances containing nitrogen. The **electrolytes** (inorganic salts) present in normal urine are sodium, chloride, **sulfate**, **phosphorus**, potassium, and **magnesium**. Water is a major component of normal urine. A laboratory test called a **urinalysis** is performed to examine the components of urine. This test searches for the above substances and determines the amount of each present in a urine sample. This is a simple test for the clinical care associate to obtain. It requires securing a small container of at least 40 cc of urine. In this laboratory study, the lab technician also detects the presence of *abnormal* constituents in urine, such as **plasma proteins**, blood cells, blood, **glucose**, **mucus**, and **microorganisms**.

A test for **specific gravity** is included in the urinalysis. The specific gravity test will reveal the concentration of water in the urine. If the patient is dehydrated, the specific gravity is high. The opposite is true when the patient is overhydrated. A specific gravity of 1.025 with an absence of glucose and albumin usually indicates normal kidney function. Normal urine is thin, clear, and without any odor; it does not have any mucus, pus, crystals, or blood; and it is light to amber yellow in color. When urine is abnormal, it can be pink, tea-colored, or cloudy. It may contain crystals and mucous threads, or it may present as clear but may have an odor. There are simple tests that can be performed by patient care staff to examine urine with a Chemstick (a reagent strip that is dipped into a urine sample to reveal any abnormal contents). However, examining patient urine for any visible abnormal signs is within the role of all clinical patient care staff.

The Ureters

Extending from the renal basin of each kidney is a tube called the **ureter**. Figure 14-3 shows a cross section of a kidney with a ureter. Each ureter is made of smooth muscle and is lined with a mucous membrane. The ureters are about ¼ inch in diameter and about 10 to 12 inches long. The function of the ureter is to pass urine from the kidney to the bladder. This is achieved through peristalsis.

The Bladder

The **bladder** is a muscular organ that, when empty, lies in the pelvic cavity in an anterior position to the rectum. This expandable organ is lined with a mucous membrane, and, when empty, its interior lies in folds called **rugae**. The function of the urinary bladder is to act as a storage container for urine. When the bladder becomes full, the nerve cells in the walls of the bladder recognize the need to void (urinate). The muscles of the pelvis assist the bladder to release urine through the urethra. Figure 14-4 shows the interior of the bladder.

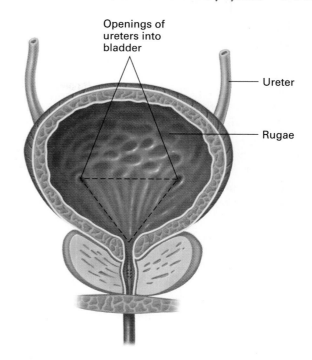

FIGURE 14-4   Interior of the bladder.

The Urethra

The **urethra** is a tube leading from the bladder to the outside of the body. The sphincter muscle of the urethra remains closed to keep urine in the bladder, and then it relaxes to let urine pass to the outside. In the female, the urethra is about 1 to 2 inches long, and the urethral opening is located just above the vagina and below the clitoris. In the male, the urethra is about 8 inches long, extending from the bladder through the center of the penis. In the male, the urethra is also the passageway for semen. Therefore, in the male, it is an organ of both the urinary and reproductive systems.

Conditions and Diseases of the Urinary System

Renal failure can be an acute or chronic condition. *Acute renal (kidney) failure* can be caused by a complication of poisoning from aspirin overdose, infections, impaired renal circulation, blood transfusion reactions, severe burns, or crushing injuries to the kidneys. The symptoms include **oliguria** (little amount of urine), **anuria** (absence of urine), nausea, vomiting, diarrhea, dry skin and mucous membranes, dehydration, a urine smell to the breath, and muscle twitching or convulsions. The objective of treatment is to remove the cause of the kidney failure and to correct the fluid imbalance and disturbance in releasing the waste

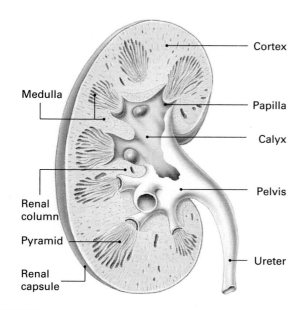

FIGURE 14-3   Cross section of a kidney with a ureter.

products from the body. Dialysis is performed when the kidneys are unable to remove the wastes of protein metabolism, electrolytes, water, and acid. **Dialysis** is an external means of compensating for loss of kidney function. It can be performed in two ways: *peritoneal dialysis* and *hemodialysis.* **Peritoneal dialysis** is accomplished by instilling a dialysis solution through a catheter into the peritoneal cavity. The dialysis solution draws out the waste products through diffusion. **Diffusion** is a process in which substances in greater amounts in one compartment travel across a semipermeable membrane to another solution with smaller amounts of the same substances. The dialysis solution draws the waste products from the peritoneal cavity into the solution, and it is drained by another catheter into a collection device.

Hemodialysis is the process of removing the waste products from the blood that are normally removed by the kidneys (Figure 14-5). A **shunt** is created between an artery and a vein—usually the radial artery and vein of the forearm—to remove and return the blood. The shunt is a plastic or Teflon catheter that is implanted permanently in the arm. This allows for easy access to perform the hemodialysis. A needle, usually 14-gauge, is inserted into the shunt to remove the blood, which is forced into an artificial kidney. The artificial kidney has dialysis fluid on one side of a cellophane membrane, and the blood is pushed through the inner fibers of the membrane. The dialysate fluid flows in the opposite direction of the blood on the other side of the membrane to draw the impurities from the blood. In this way, waste products are removed from the blood, and the cleansed blood returns to the venous side of the shunt. This is a continuous process that takes an average of 4 hours to complete.

In *chronic renal failure,* hemodialysis is performed two to three times a week. There are outpatient dialysis centers where the patient reports for this treatment. With chronic renal failure, the patient is placed on a kidney transplant list, depending on qualifications, as dialysis is not viewed as a permanent solution. It is taxing to the heart and vessels, and it can be restricting to a patient's normal lifestyle.

Infections of the Urinary System

Pyelonephritis is a bacterial infection of the renal tissue and the renal pelvis. It can affect one or both kidneys. The walls of the renal pelvis are lined with a mucous membrane that becomes infected. The membrane swells and is inflamed, and the cells of the membrane are discarded and travel to the rest of the urinary organs. The urine is cloudy and may contain pus. This infection can become chronic and cause kidney failure.

Cystitis is an infection of the bladder. Frequently, the infection is caused by an external source; however, it can be the result of kidney infection. Most often it is caused in the female by incorrect wiping of the genitalia after urinating. Females should always wipe from front to back because there are microorganisms in the stool (*E. coli*) that do not belong in the urinary system. The symptoms include burning and itching with urination, along with frequent and painful urination. Mucus, white blood cells, and traces of blood are found in the urine. The urine is usually cloudy. Antibiotics are used to treat cystitis, and the person is encouraged to force fluids to flush out the bladder.

Renal calculi (kidney stones) are formed in the urinary tract by crystalline deposits formed from calcium, from phosphate electrolytes, and from uric acid (Figure 14-6). The conditions that may lead to the formation of stones include kidney infection, dehydration, and immobility. Some people have a familial tendency to form stones. Renal calculi can be as fine as sand, the size of gravel, or much larger. There have been bladder stones the size of an orange. Needless to say, these calculi cause pain in the kidney area, and they can obstruct the flow of urine and lead to infection. Blood and pus may be found in the urine. Sometimes, the stone passes, causing intense pain and bleeding. Sometimes, the stones have to be crushed surgically. Usually, a **laser** instrument is used to dissolve the stone. The patient may need to have the urine strained to see if fine stones are passed. Fluid intake is increased, and the person may be treated with antibiotics for infections of the urinary organs.

Tumors of the urinary system, both benign and malignant, may develop in any urinary organ. Tumors of the kidney usually present with painless **hematuria** (blood in the urine). This may be the only warning sign. Radiation, chemotherapy, and

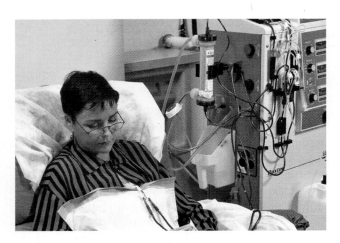

FIGURE 14-5 Hemodialysis machine.

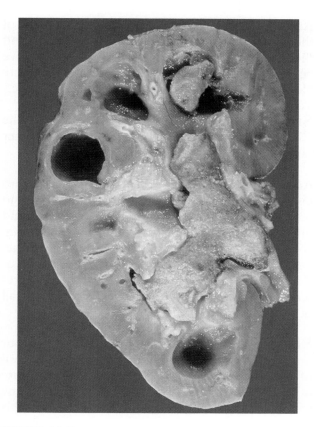

FIGURE 14-6 Renal calculi. Dr. E. Walker, Science Photo Library, Photo Researchers, Inc.

nephrectomy (surgical removal of the kidney) are the treatments used. Sometimes, the kidneys form cysts. It may be a single cyst or many cysts, which is called *polycystic disease*. **Polycystic disease** is usually congenital and is treated by surgery if infection occurs. A single cyst may grow to be very large, and it is removed to repair kidney functions.

Tumors of the bladder are usually seen as primary tumors in older persons. The tumors are usually cauliflower-like growths in the mucous membrane. The person experiences pain and hematuria with urination. Sometimes, a small tumor can be removed through a **cystoscope**. This is an instrument that is passed through the urethra into the bladder to examine the bladder, and it can be used for destruction of small tumors. If the tumor cannot be removed, the entire bladder is surgically removed. This surgical procedure is called a **cystectomy**.

Tumors may also form in the ureters. These cause obstruction of the flow of urine, hematuria, pain, and mucus in the urine. They may be detected because of the infection that results from the obstruction of urine flow. The ureters are surgically removed.

Surgical Procedures for Urinary Diversion

Suprapubic cystostomy is a surgical procedure performed to create a new opening above the pubic bone for the removal of urine. It is necessary for tumors of the bladder and for diseases that cause strictures of the urethra. A plastic collection device is used to collect the urine. This can be a permanent or temporary treatment.

Ureterostomy is a surgical procedure to create a diversion for the ureters. It is usually done in one of three ways: (1) The detached ureter is brought through the abdominal wall and attached to an opening in the skin. This stoma is about 1 millimeter (mm) above the skin level and is surrounded by periureteral tissue to supply it with blood. (2) The ureter is introduced into the sigmoid colon, and urine is diverted to the rectum for removal. (3) The ureters are diverted to the ileum and are brought to the skin surface, where a stoma is formed. The person will have a **stoma** as with an ileostomy. A collection device must be worn to collect the urine. A small drain is attached to the bottom of the plastic collection bag so that urine can be emptied. Excellent skin care is required to prevent excoriation of the abdominal skin. Care measures must also be effective to prevent infections.

application to practice

Knowledge of the structure and function of the urinary system prepares the clinical care associate (CCA) to assist the nurse in providing care to patients with urinary problems. Delivering activities of daily living (ADL) care to patients with ostomies and catheters provides an opportunity for the CCA to observe, report, and document changes. These changes may assist the nurse and physician in determining future care.

After studying the normal functions and structures of the urinary system, you should be able to respond to the following clinical situations by applying what you have learned.

Learning Activities

Situation 1: Mrs. Dell is a patient in your long-term care (LTC) facility. She has been a resident of this facility for 10 years. She has neurologic impairments of bladder functions due to multiple sclerosis, and as a result, she has an indwelling Foley catheter to drain urine. Yesterday, she was admitted to the intensive care unit (ICU) at the local suburban hospital with fever, nausea, and lower abdominal pain. The LTC administrator comes to a staff meeting on your unit to discuss the claims of nursing home neglect charged by the ICU nurses. You have not been assigned to Mrs. Dell for several months but are concerned about the report that the administrator reads to the staff. The patient is thought to have been grossly neglected because no competent care provider could empty the contents of her urine collection bag without seeing and smelling the state of her urine. The patient has multiple organisms infecting her bladder, kidneys, and ureters. The results of urine testing confirm pus, a gross amount of white blood cells (WBCs), mucus, albumin, blood, and brown-colored urine with a pungent odor. Discuss the accusation of neglect. What actions were "negligent" on the part of the nursing staff at the LTC? What were the abnormal findings of Mrs. Dell's urine?

Author's Explanation: Since this resident had an indwelling Foley catheter for urine drainage, it is obvious that staff failed to inspect, report, and respond to the contents in her urinary drainage bag. Each shift, some member of the nursing staff had to have emptied the bag, and a nurse should have changed the indwelling catheter at least monthly according to the orders. The presence of a foreign object in the bladder, which is a sterile organ, increases the risk of infection even when care is adequate.

The abnormal findings in her urine studies include pus, the presence of white blood cells, mucus, albumin, blood, brown-colored urine, and a pungent odor. Urine should not smell "foul" (pungent), have a brown color, or contain any of the elements described. The brown discoloration of the urine is indicative of the presence of blood and inadequate hydration. She was not receiving enough fluids. This patient did not receive adequate care.

Situation 2: Mrs. Dell's diagnosis was **urosepsis** resulting from pyelonephritis and cystitis. She was treated with intravenous (IV) antibiotics, and within three days, her WBC count of 18.9 was reduced to 10.7. Her temperature was normal. What does her diagnosis indicate about the organs that were infected? What is the significance of the WBC changes?

Author's Explanation: She had an infection of the urinary system that involved the renal pelvis and the bladder. Her antibiotic treatment was effective because her temperature was normal, and her white blood cell count was declining to the normal range.

Situation 3: When Mrs. Dell returns to the LTC, what factors will you consider in delivering her care?

Author's Explanation: You should be certain to inspect the contents of her urinary drainage bag and be sure that she has an adequate intake of water and other beverages. When you empty the Foley bag, you should measure the amount of urinary drainage, examine the color, look to see if the urine is clear or cloudy, examine the urine to see if any mucus is present, and check for any odor to the urine. Report all of your findings to the nurse.

Situation 4: Mr. Isreal is a patient on your oncology unit. He was admitted for surgical removal of his urinary bladder and prostate gland because of malignant tumors. Mr. Isreal had a cystectomy with prostatectomy. How will Mr. Isreal excrete his urine?

Author's Explanation: Mr. Isreal will have a urinary diversion, which probably will involve a ureterostomy. He will have his ureters brought through the ileum, and a stoma will be present on his lower abdomen. He will wear a urine-collection appliance that looks much like the colostomy appliance.

Situation 5: What considerations must you consider in your observation and care of Mr. Isreal concerning his ureterostomy?

Author's Explanation: Remember that urine is acidic and contains electrolytes and waste products. This means that any urine that comes into contact with his skin could cause skin breakdown. You should be sure that the collection device has a tight seal around the stoma. You should observe the condition of the skin on the abdomen and the condition of the stoma. Notice if it is raised above the surface of the skin or if it is level or indented. It should be pink and raised above the skin surface. Be sure to keep the skin dry, wash the area around the stoma with soap, and rinse well with water. Report any skin redness and the color and condition of the stoma. Empty the collection bag as necessary; do not allow it to become full.

Notice and discuss with Mr. Isreal his ability and willingness to care for his stoma and ostomy appliance. Report to the nurse his reaction to self-care of the stoma.

Situation 6:
Ms. Kim is a patient on the rehab unit. She has an indwelling urinary catheter. The nurse tells you that the patient has cystitis. Where is the catheter? What is cystitis? Why might she have cystitis?

Author's Explanation: Ms. Kim's catheter is in her urinary bladder. Cystitis is an inflammation of the bladder, generally caused by infection. In addition, the presence of a foreign object (the indwelling rubber tube that drains urine) creates irritation in the bladder, and this leads to inflammation or infection. Proper cleansing of the perineal (genital) area is very important for patients who have a Foley catheter. If Ms. Kim or the clinical care associate washes from the anal area to the genital area, this could bring the bacteria present in stool to the urethra and the Foley. Although *E. coli* is a normal bacterium in the bowel, it is an infectious bacterium in the bladder. Remember, the bladder is a sterile organ. It is very important for women to wipe and wash the perineal area from front to back (clean to dirty). Often, cystitis in women is due to improper cleaning of the perineal area. Also, the urine drainage tube should be cleansed with soap and water at least daily or more frequently if the person is incontinent of stool. Always keep the drainage bag below the level of the bladder. Research has shown that the most significant cause of infection with a urinary catheter is the backflow of urine from the collection bag.

Situation 7:
You are working on a pediatric rehabilitation unit in an LTC. You are assigned to John Kniezweski, an eight-year-old boy who has paraplegia. He has an indwelling Foley catheter, and he had a colostomy 3 months ago. At 8:00 A.M., John rings his call bell to tell you that his "tummy hurts." When you check his ostomy appliance, you see that it is full of liquid stool, so you empty it. At 9:00 A.M., you return to his room, and he complains of cramps in his tummy; once again, you find the colostomy appliance is full of liquid stool. John looks sad and tells you he did not eat yesterday, and he doesn't want to eat today. He refuses any liquids and just wants to stay in his room. At 3:00 P.M. you empty his urinary drainage bag, and it has only 100 cc of urine. His colostomy ap-

pliance is full of liquid stool. What do you do with this information? What do you think is the connection between a small amount of urine and a large amount of liquid stool (diarrhea)?

Author's Explanation: You should tell the nurse immediately what you measured in John's urinary drainage bag and the frequency and amount of diarrhea. (Always inform the nurse of each diarrhea event as it occurs.) You should also report that John refused to eat or drink and that he did the same yesterday. Also tell the nurse that you found John to be sad. The connection between a large amount of diarrhea and a small amount of urine is significant, especially because he has not had fluids. His kidneys are conserving water because of the fluid loss from the colon in his stool and because he has been without fluids for at least 24 hours.

Situation 8:
The nurse asks you to take his temperature and to report the results stat. You immediately take his temperature orally, and it is 101.4°F. You report it to the nurse. The nurse seems angry and tells you that you need to be more responsible and accountable for your patient care. Why? What could the nurse mean?

Author's Explanation: The nurse is concerned about your accountability and sense of responsibility because you failed to report stat the significant findings of diarrhea, a "stomachache," the scanty amount of urine in the drainage bag, and his sad mood and refusal of food and fluids. He now has an elevated temperature that might be the result of dehydration due to lack of fluids and diarrhea. The nurse should have been told of these findings when they occurred. His fever could be related to an infection in the GI system, which leads to abdominal pain, diarrhea, and loss of appetite. His mood could also be a sign that he is physically sick and, because of his age, he is unable to clearly express the symptoms. Or, his sadness might be depression due to his physical problems and his placement in an LTC. When a resident has an indwelling urinary catheter, the drainage should be observed throughout the shift for color and amount of urine and again before emptying and measuring at the end of shift rounds. The 100 cc of urine is not normal for an 8-hour period. None of these problems are normal, and the nurse needed to know stat so that a complete assessment and interventions could occur sooner. In the future, report any abnormal events as soon as they occur.

Examination Review Questions

1. Which of the following constituents of urine is abnormal?
   - a. urea
   - b. albumin
   - c. sodium
   - d. potassium

2. The cuplike network of kidney tissue inside the nephron is called the
   - a. adipose capsule
   - b. Bowman's capsule
   - c. glomerulus
   - d. hilum

3. Signs of cystitis may include all *but*
   - a. dysuria
   - b. hematuria
   - c. fever
   - d. anuria

4. What factor does *not* affect kidney function?
   - a. fat consumption
   - b. blood pressure
   - c. fluid intake
   - d. excessive sweating

5. The kidneys are protected by
   - a. Bowman's capsule
   - b. adipose tissue
   - c. the adrenal gland
   - d. the peritoneum

6. Urine is passed from the kidneys to the bladder by
   - a. gravity
   - b. peristalsis
   - c. rugae
   - d. filtration

7. A complication of drug overdose, infections, or transfusion reaction is
   - a. acute renal failure
   - b. pyelonephritis
   - c. cystitis
   - d. renal calculi

8. Kidney stones are formed from all but one of the following:
   - a. calcium
   - b. phosphate electrolytes
   - c. uric acid
   - d. infection

9. The surgical procedure to divert urine above the bladder is called
   - a. suprapubic cystotomy
   - b. ureterostomy
   - c. cystectomy
   - d. ileoconduit

10. Urine consists of waste products from the metabolism of
    - a. fats
    - b. proteins
    - c. sugar
    - d. starch

The Reproductive System

Throughout the ages, the reproduction of another life has been a marvel and a mystery. Philosophers and physicians alike theorized about the contribution of males, females, spirits, and gods in the conception of another living being. Animal and human sexual attraction and behavior have been and still remain a subject of discovery. What science has taught us is that males and females of all species each contribute a distinct and genetically identifiable cell to the conception of a new life. The power and beauty of reproducing a new living being will always astonish us with wonder and magnificence.

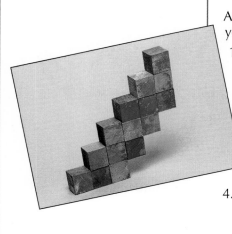

OBJECTIVES

After completing this chapter, you will be able to

1. Name the organs of the male and female reproductive systems
2. Describe the functions of the reproductive system
3. Describe the location and function of the male reproductive organs
4. Describe the location and function of the female reproductive organs
5. Describe conception
6. Describe the conditions and diseases of the male and female reproductive systems
7. List the observations about the reproductive system that you should report to the nurse
8. Apply your knowledge of the reproductive system to problem-solving strategies in care delivery
9. Define and spell all key terms correctly

key terms

antiprostaglandin/
  anti-inflammatory
areola
Bartholin's glands
breasts
bulbourethral glands
cervix
circumcision
clitoris
copulation
corpora cavernosa penes
corpus cavernosum urethra
corpus luteum
ductus deferens
dysmenorrhea
ectopic pregnancy
embryonic disk
endometriosis
endometrium
epididymis
fallopian tubes
fetus
fimbriae

foreskin
fundus
gonads
Graafian follicles
human chorionic gonadotropin
  (HCG)
hymen
labia majora
labia minora
labor
menarche
menopause
menorrhagia
menstruation (menses)
myometrium
orchidectomy
ovaries
ovulation
ovum
Pap test
pelvic inflammatory disease (PID)
penis
placenta

pregnancy
prepuce
primary amenorrhea
prostate
salipingectomy
scrotum
secondary amenorrhea
seminal vesicles
seminiferous tubules
sperm
spermatozoa
sterility
testes
testicles
testosterone
urethral orifice
vaginal orifice
vas deferens
vulva
womb
zygote

The Male Reproductive System

The male reproductive system has both external and internal organs.

■ The external genitalia, or the visible reproductive organs of men, are the *scrotum* and the *penis* (Figure 15-1). The *testes*, or *testicles*, are also located externally, but they are concealed in the scrotum.

■ The internal organs of the male can be divided into three categories: the *gonads*, the *ducts*, and the *glands*.

The structure, location, and function of each of these organs are described in the sections that follow.

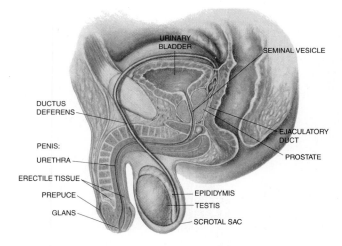

FIGURE 15-1 Male reproductive organs.

The Scrotum

The **scrotum** is a sac that hangs behind the penis. It is divided by a septum, and the tissue is a continuation of the abdominal wall. It is covered with skin, and within each divided section is a testis and a duct, the epididymis, that leads to the pelvic cavity. The function of the scrotum is to hold the testes outside the body. This is important because the testes must be kept at a constant temperature that is cooler than the internal temperature of the ab-

dominopelvic cavity. The scrotum draws the testes closer to the body when the body is exposed to cold temperatures to keep the testes warm. Its muscle tissue relaxes to suspend the testes lower in the groin when the body is exposed to heat or fever to keep the testes cool.

The Penis

The penis is made of three separate structures, which have Latin names. There are two **corpora cavernosa** penes and one **corpus cavernosum urethra**. What this means is there are three cylinders of tissues full of tiny cavities. These vascular cavernosa (caves) become engorged with blood during sexual stimulation. Normally, they are collapsed, but when sexual arousal occurs, the arteries that supply the penis with blood fill these tiny cavities, and an erection results. When ejaculation occurs or sexual arousal ceases, the blood that filled these caves returns to the circulation. Erection of the penis permits the penis to penetrate the vagina during intercourse. The urethra is surrounded by the cavernous tissue, and it is the organ through which semen passes during ejaculation and through which urine passes when emptying the bladder in urination. At the end of the penis is the **prepuce (foreskin)**. The foreskin is removed in the surgical procedure called **circumcision**. In some cultures, the foreskin is removed during a religious ritual. For thousands of years, it has been customary in some cultures to remove the foreskin of a male child soon after birth for the purpose of cleanliness. Today, physicians discuss the option of circumcision with parents.

The Testes: The Male Gonads

The **testes** (*testis* is the singular), or **testicles**, are the male **gonads**. (*Gonad* in Greek means "seed.") The testes produce **sperm (spermatozoa)**—the male seeds of reproduction. The testes also produce the male hormone, **testosterone**. Coiled within each testis are tubes called the **seminiferous tubules**, which are responsible for the production of spermatozoa. Throughout these tubules are cells that produce testosterone. This masculinizing hormone transforms a body into a man and is needed for the production of sperm.

The Ducts

At the upper end of each testis is a duct called the **epididymis**, which is about 16 feet of tube coiled around the surface of each testis. This duct leads to the **ductus deferens**. (*Defero-* is Latin for "carry down.") This duct is also called the **vas deferens**, and it carries sperm from the epididymis to the common ejaculatory duct. When males have a vasectomy for the purpose of sterilization (surgical birth control), the procedure involves the tying off or severing of this duct to prevent the passage of sperm. The vas deferens extends from the testes about 18 inches into the abdomen, where it forms the common ejaculatory duct. The common ejaculatory duct opens into the urethra. The urethra carries semen through the penis to the outside of the male body.

The Glands

These excretory glands produce the thick, white, alkaline fluid that is secreted during ejaculation. The glands that produce seminal fluid are the **seminal vesicles**, **prostate**, and **bulbourethral glands**. Seminal fluid is alkaline, and it is important for the fluid that carries sperm to be alkaline because sperm "swim" and thrive in an alkaline fluid. The prostate gland is an important gland, especially when it becomes enlarged and obstructs the passage of urine from the male bladder. The prostate gland is about the size of a chestnut, and it lies under the bladder and surrounds the urethra at this juncture. In one out of three older males, this gland becomes hypertrophied (overgrown), and it is difficult for the man to begin a stream of urine. The prostate is sometimes not only enlarged, but a site for cancerous growths in older males. Men can be screened for prostate cancer with a blood test that identifies this cancer. A digital examination of the prostate is performed by the physician to feel the size and shape of the prostate. This digital palpation (feeling) of the prostate is performed when the physician inserts a finger into the rectum, which lies posterior to the prostate.

Spermatozoa and Seminal Fluid

Each time a man ejaculates, millions of sperm are released from the epididymis and travel through the ducts. The glands release seminal fluid into the ducts to mix with the spermatozoa. (*Spermatozoa* is Greek and means "seeds of the animal.") Each microscopic sperm is a single cell with a head, neck, and tail. Figure 15-2 depicts sperm seen through an electron microscope. The tail allows the sperm to "swim" through the female's vaginal canal into the pelvic cavity and to penetrate the ovum (egg). Even though millions of sperm are released with each ejaculation, only one fertilizes the egg. Each sperm and each egg contain twenty-three pairs of chromosomes. Male sperm have either an X or a Y as the twenty-third chromosome. Female eggs have only an X chromosome. If the sperm

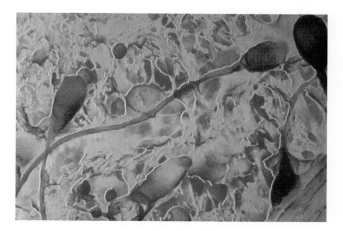

FIGURE 15-2 Sperm seen through a microscope. Kunkel CN, Phototake, NYC.

carries a Y on the twenty-third chromosome, the twenty-third pair when united with the female X will be XY, and the offspring will be male. If the sperm carries an X on the twenty-third chromosome, the twenty-third pair when united with the female X will be XX, and the child will be female. It is the male cell of reproduction on the twenty-third (sex) chromosome that determines the sex of the offspring. Henry the VIII had five wives beheaded because his queens did not give him a male heir. Neither the king nor the scientists knew then that the sex of a child was determined by the male.

Conditions and Diseases of the Male Reproductive System

Benign prostatic hypertrophy (BPH) results when the prostate gland becomes enlarged. It is common among men over the age of sixty. The enlargement of the prostate gland causes pressure on the bladder and restricts the flow of urine to the urethral opening. The BPH results in difficulty starting a stream of urine, pain on urination, and frequent urination. The man may, at some point, be unable to void. The retention of urine can lead to bladder infection, calculi, and potential infections of the ureters and kidneys.

Cancer of the prostate gland is the most common form of cancer in the United States among men over the age of fifty years. The symptoms are the same as those of BPH if the tumor is large enough to encroach on the urethra and bladder. The tumor may grow with no noted symptoms. Any man over fifty years should have an annual examination by a physician to screen for prostate cancer. A blood test called a PSA (Prostatic Specific Antigen) is performed to screen for the presence of the antigen that is found in the blood of men who have prostate cancer.

Treatment is based on the size and exact location of the tumor or the hypertrophy. Treatment usually involves surgical removal of the prostate gland. A transurethral prostatectomy (TURP) is typical. Following this surgery, the bladder is continuously irrigated with normal saline through a Foley catheter with three extensions of tubing instead of the usual two. This Foley Alcock has a third extension to connect with the large bag of irrigation fluid. Radiation may be the treatment of choice for some tumors of the prostate. Sometimes, the removal or radiation treatment may cause impotence in the man. This is, of course, an important concern for the patient and his partner. Counseling and emotional support are very important. The man may

also experience "dribbling" of urine when the catheter is removed. Exercises to strengthen the pelvic muscles will help the man to regain bladder control.

Sexually transmitted diseases (STDs) are those infectious diseases spread through sexual activities, such as anal intercourse, vaginal intercourse, oral sex, and any sexual activity in which semen or vaginal secretions are exchanged between partners.

Table 15-1 is a list of STDs with a brief summary of the causative microorganism, the associated symptoms, and treatment. AIDS is a disease that can be sexually transmitted. AIDS is discussed in the unit on conditions of the immune system.

Testicular cancer usually presents in men in their twenties to forties. Usually, there is an unknown congenital problem with the testis. The symptoms include nonpainful swelling of the testis, back pain, and abdominal pain. If the disease is advanced, weakness, weight loss, and possible metastasis of the cancer occur. The treatment is **orchidectomy** (removal of the testis).

Testicular Exams

Monthly testicular self-exams should be performed by men. The testes are palpated as in a breast self-exam to note any lumps on the surface of the testes. The fingertips should be used to inspect the entire surface of each testicle and the scrotum. The presence of a lump should be brought immediately to the attention of the physician for further examination.

Infertility

Infertility is the inability to conceive. The causes of infertility are numerous, and if the causes cannot be remedied, then the condition is referred to as **sterility**. The underlying cause that renders the couple infertile may be in the male or the female. The possible causes are numerous and include the following: structural abnormalities of reproductive organs, infections, tumors, low sperm counts, immotility of sperm, acid-alkaline imbalance of the semen or the vaginal or cervical mucosa, hormonal imbalances, disturbances of the menstrual cycle, and absence of ovulation. Investigation of the cause usually begins with the male because the tests for the female are more numerous and costly. In most cases the cause of infertility can be remedied.

The Female Reproductive System

The female reproductive system has both external and internal organs.

TABLE 15-1   Sexually Transmitted Diseases

Sexually Transmitted Diseases	Microorganism	Symptoms	Treatment
Gonorrhea	Gonococcus (bacterium)	Purulent (pus) discharge, painful discharge from the urethra in the male and the vagina in the female. Symptoms appear 2–7 days after infection.	Antibiotic therapy
Syphilis	*Treponema pallidum* (spirochete)	Presence of a chancre (sore) located on the lip, genitals, or wherever the spirochete entered the body. Usually painless, the ulcer is hard but has no discharge. Rash, fever, and swollen lymph nodes may occur. This disease will spread throughout the body and eventually cause destruction of brain and nervous tissue if not treated in the primary stage.	Antibiotic therapy
Herpes	Herpes simplex (virus)	Painful vesicles (ulcers) present at the site of entry: genitals, cervix, anus, mouth. Fever and swollen glands.	Symptomatic treatment of vesicles. Preventive measures to reduce number of outbreaks. *No cure.*
Chlamydia	Rickettsia	Asymptomatic or vague; possible purulent white discharge.	Early intervention with erythromycin.
Condylomata (venereal warts)	Human papilloma virus (HPV)	Genital warts, cauliflower-like growths outside or inside the genital area.	Cryosurgery, laser, electrosurgery, excisional biopsy of lesions, chemical therapy, podophyllin topically, and interferon.
Trichomonas vaginalis	*Trichomonas* (protozoan)	Inflamed vaginal tissue, burning, itching, green-yellow discharge. The male may be free of symptoms.	Antiprotozoal therapy (Flagyl)

- The **vulva** is the collective name for the female external genitals (Figure 15-3).
- The internal organs of the female include the *ovaries, fallopian tubes, uterus,* and *vagina.*

The structure, location, and function of each of these organs are described in the sections that follow.

The Vulva

The vulva is made up of a number of structures. They are the *labia majora, labia minora, vaginal orifice, urethral orifice, hymen, clitoris,* and *Bartholin's glands.* The **labia majora** (major lips) are the larger folds of skin, and between these lie the **labia minora** (minor lips). At the top of the labia lies the **clitoris**, a small projection of erectile tissue with nerves and blood vessels. The clitoris is usually partially covered by the prepuce, a structure that becomes engorged like the penis during sexual arousal. Between the labia minora is the **vaginal orifice** (the opening of the vagina). The **hymen** is a thin fold of mucous membrane that partially or completely covers the opening to the vagina. The hymen may be absent at birth; therefore, its presence is not an absolute sign of virginity. Just above the vagina is the **urethral orifice** (the opening of the urethra). The openings of the **Bartholin's glands** lie lateral to the

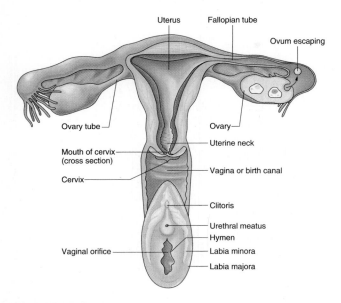

FIGURE 15-3   Female reproductive organs.

vaginal opening. These two exocrine glands secrete a lubricating fluid.

The Ovaries

The female gonads are the **ovaries**. These correspond to the male testes because they produce the female reproductive cells: the ova (eggs). There are two ovaries, which are oval-shaped organs. The ovaries are in the pelvic cavity, one on each side of the uterus. They are anchored to the uterus by the ovarian ligament. The inner surface of the ovaries contains thousands of microscopic follicles (sacs). These follicles, named after the anatomist who dis-

covered them, are called the **Graafian follicles** (sacs). Within each follicle is an **ovum** (egg). Each menstrual cycle, a follicle grows to a mature state. When the follicle ruptures, the ovum is released, ready to be fertilized by a sperm. **Ovulation** is the term that describes the rupturing of the follicle and the release of the egg. Once ovulation occurs, the follicle develops into a new structure called the **corpus luteum**, which means "golden body." The corpus luteum produces a hormone that readies the uterus (womb) for implantation of a fertilized ovum. When fertilization does not take place, the corpus luteum ceases to function and to produce the hormone, progesterone, and menstruation begins.

The activities of the ovaries are controlled by the pituitary and ovarian hormones. The interrelationship of the pituitary-stimulating hormones and the female hormones estrogen and progesterone is an excellent example of the chemical feedback mechanism of the endocrine system. Figure 15-4 is an illustration of an ovary and a fallopian tube.

The Fallopian Tubes

The uterine ducts, named for another anatomist, Gabriel Fallopius, are called the **fallopian tubes**. The fallopian tubes carry the ovum from the ovaries to the uterus. The fallopian tubes are not connected to the ovaries but have fingerlike projections called **fimbriae** that sweep the ovum into the ducts. When fertilization occurs, it takes place in the fallopian tubes, and then the fertilized ovum is transported to the uterus. Sometimes, fertilization takes place outside of the fallopian tubes, and then an ectopic ("out of place")

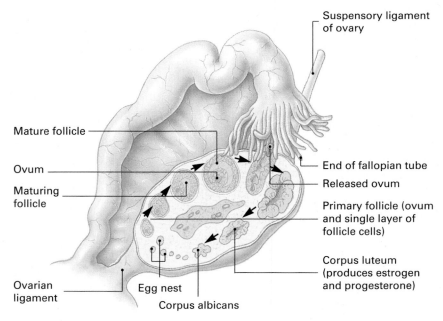

FIGURE 15-4   An ovary and a maturing ovum.

pregnancy results. The fertilized egg begins to develop in the pelvic cavity. A frequent site of ectopic pregnancy is in the fallopian tubes. This occurs because the fertilized egg does not migrate to the uterus.

The Uterus

The uterus is the **womb**. It is a pear-shaped organ composed of a thick muscular wall and is lined with a mucous membrane. It is situated behind the bladder and in front of the rectum. It is about three inches long and two inches wide. It is capable of great expansion, and the layers of muscular tissue stretch to the size of a watermelon during pregnancy. There are three portions that make up this organ: the **fundus** (bulging upper part), the body (middle section), and the **cervix** (neck), which opens into the vagina. The uterus has three functions: menstruation, pregnancy, and **labor**.

The uterus has three layers of tissue. The outer layer is continuous with the peritoneum (the outer covering of the abdominopelvic cavity) and the broad ligaments that suspend the uterus in the pelvic cavity. The middle layer is the **myometrium**, a thick, muscular layer that thickens and enlarges during pregnancy. The inner layer is the **endometrium**. This inner layer of epithelial and connective tissue is prepared each menstrual cycle for implantation of the fertilized ovum by the hormone progesterone, which is released by the corpus luteum. Progesterone causes the endometrium to thicken and decreases muscular contraction of the uterus. These actions of progesterone protect the uterus if the woman becomes pregnant until the placenta is developed. When pregnancy does not occur, the corpus luteum stops producing progesterone, and the endometrium is shed during menstruation. The bleeding is caused by the tearing away of the thickened endometrial tissue, which is released through the vagina along with blood during menstruation.

The Vagina

The vagina is a tubular organ that is about 5 to 6 inches long and is directed upward and backward toward the uterus. The vagina is the organ of **copulation** (sexual intercourse) and is part of the birth canal. It is made of a muscular layer in folds called *rugae*. These folds make it capable of expanding to allow the baby to pass during delivery. It is lined with a mucous membrane and is lubricated by cervical secretions.

The Mammary Glands

The mammary glands are the two **breasts**. The female breasts are designed to produce and release milk to nourish the infant child. The breasts lie over the pectoral muscles, and each contains about fifteen to twenty milk glands. These glands open to milk ducts, which are arranged like the spokes of a wheel. All of the ducts converge to the nipple, through which milk is released when the infant sucks. The size of the breast is not relevant to the breast's ability to produce milk. Most of the size of the breast is determined by the amount of adipose (fatty) tissue that surrounds the glandular tissue. The breast has a rich lymphatic supply, which is relevant to the metastasis (spread) of breast cancer cells to other parts of the female body. The lymph nodes in the axilla (armpit) are tested for the presence of cancer cells when a malignant tumor is discovered in a woman's breast.

The pigmented circular area around the nipple is called the **areola**. This tissue darkens when pregnancy occurs. In pregnant Caucasian women, it changes from pink to brown, and in women of darker races, it changes from pale brown to dark brown. This increase in pigmentation may be permanent after delivery.

The production of milk is related to the release of the lactogenic hormone, which is produced during pregnancy to stimulate the mammary glands to produce milk. The sucking of the nipple by the infant after pregnancy causes the posterior pituitary hormone, oxytocin, to release ("let down") the milk.

The Menstrual Cycle

Menstruation (menses) is the shedding of the endometrium and blood flow from the uterus through the vagina. The first menstrual cycle, called the **menarche**, usually starts at twelve to thirteen years. Menstruation continues until menopause. **Menopause** is the cessation or pausing of menstruation. Most women menstruate for about 35 years. The first day of the menstrual cycle is the first day of bleeding, and the last day of the cycle is the day before the next event of bleeding occurs. Usually, the cycle is about 28 days long, but in some women it is as short as 22 days, and in others as long as 35 days. Ovulation usually occurs at the midpoint of the menstrual cycle. This cycle is interrupted in the years between the menarche and menopause when fertilization takes place. Pregnancy stops the secretion of follicle-stimulating hormone (FSH), and luteinizing hormone (LH). During pregnancy ova will not reach maturity or be released.

Pregnancy

Within the nine months of **pregnancy**, the most rapid and diverse growth and developmental period of human life takes place. Never again in this person's life history will so many anatomical and physiological events unfold so quickly. Starting with a single cell that matched the twenty-three chromosomes from the female and the twenty-three chromosomes from the male, the newborn emerges after multiplying to a billion cells of human life. Pregnancy begins when fertilization takes place, and within a few days the **zygote** of about sixteen cells tumbles through the fallopian tubes and finds its way to the uterus. In a day or two, the zygote implants itself in the soft lining of the endometrium. In 15 days, the site of implantation is rich with a nest of blood vessels that will become the **placenta**. By the time the woman recognizes that she has missed her period, the three layers of cells that will become the organs and systems of the embryo have organized themselves into the **embryonic disk**. By the middle of the third week, the embryo has grown to one-eighth of an inch.

Pregnancy is confirmed by the presence of a hormone in the woman's urine and blood; this is **human chorionic gonadotropin (HCG)**. HCG stimulates the corpus luteum to secrete the hormones necessary to sustain the pregnancy. From the eighth week to the fortieth week, the **fetus** grows from less than an ounce to approximately 7 pounds, and from less than an inch to about 20 inches. By the eighth week, the fetus has developed all of the body organs; only the face and the external genitals need to mature. The fetus needs the next 32 weeks of pregnancy to allow these organs to grow and mature. Figure 15-5 illustrates fetal development and growth.

The female body undergoes numerous changes in this pregnant state. Some of the first signals of pregnancy might be confused with the sensations associated with menstruation. The breasts feel fuller and are tender at the nipples, the growing uterus feels full, and pressure on the bladder causes frequent urination. Other symptoms include extreme lethargy, mood swings, and nausea with or without vomiting. Upon physical examination, the physician can feel the softening of the cervix caused by an enriched blood supply. The cervix and vagina have a bluish color as a result of the swollen blood vessels.

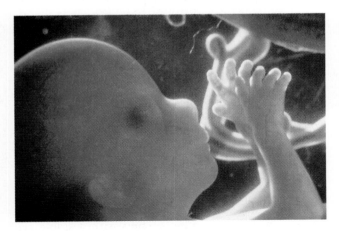

FIGURE 15-5 A fetus at 4 months. Petiti Format, Photo Researchers, Inc.

Estrogen causes the enlargement and softening of the pubic joints and ligaments. Estrogen and progesterone relax smooth muscle tissues and decrease the muscle tone of the colon and bladder. Some women experience constipation as a result. These hormones cause the kidneys to retain more water. They also cause the stomach to release small quantities of the digestive enzyme, pepsin. Along with these areas of change, the skin of the nipples darkens. For some women, a darkening of the skin of the nose and cheeks occurs. The volume of blood in a pregnant woman increases by 50 percent, which is a protective mechanism against blood loss during delivery. The retention of water and increase in blood volume usually causes some swelling of the feet during the late stages of pregnancy. When the edema is marked by excessive swelling in the fingers and hands and there is a significant rise in blood pressure, the woman must be carefully monitored by her physician.

Without a doubt, the presence of life within the womb is most apparent when the woman begins to feel "quickening" (the first movements of her baby). This occurs during the twentieth week.

Conditions and Diseases of the Female Reproductive System

Ectopic pregnancy literally means "a pregnancy that is out of place" (*ecto*- means "outside of"). The embryo fails to migrate to the uterus to implant on the wall of the uterine lining. Often, the ectopic pregnancy occurs in the fallopian tube where fertilization takes place. However, the ectopic pregnancy can be in the abdominopelvic cavity outside of the reproductive organs. If the ectopic pregnancy is in the fallopian tube, the tube becomes distended and may even rupture, discharging the fertilized ovum into the abdominal cavity. Symptoms usually begin with colicky abdominal pain or cramping. Bleeding occurs, and hemorrhage, shock, and death can result unless treatment is sought immediately. If the fallopian tube has ruptured, the tube will need to be removed surgically. This is called a **salpingectomy**.

Endometriosis literally means "condition of the uterine lining." This condition involves cells of the uterine lining growing in areas of the body other than the uterus. The cells may attach to the ovaries, fallopian tubes, bowel, and remotely in tissue such as the lungs or the ear. As hormonal changes build the lining of the uterus, these cells also change and grow, causing increased pressure to areas of involvement and surrounding structures. When the progesterone and estrogen levels drop off and menstruation occurs, these cells also "bleed." Symptoms depend on the area of involvement but generally include pelvic pain, masses involving fallopian tubes or ovaries, and infertility.

Pelvic inflammatory disease (PID) is the result of an infection that begins with the external genitalia and spreads from the uterus to the pelvic cavity or to the ovaries and fallopian tubes. The causative organisms may be *streptococcus, staphylococcus,* or any STD. The symptoms include abdominal pain, nausea, vomiting, fever, and vaginal discharge. Treatment includes antibiotic therapy. The importance of early treatment of vaginal infections can aid in the prevention of PID.

There are basically three menstrual dysfunctions. They are *amenorrhea* (primary and secondary), *dysmenorrhea,* and *menorrhagia.*

■ **Amenorrhea** literally means "without menstrual flow." **Primary amenorrhea** is the term used to describe a girl of sixteen to seventeen who has not reached her menarche (first period). Anatomical abnormalities may be the cause. A physician should be consulted to investigate and treat this amenorrhea. **Secondary amenorrhea** that occurs during pregnancy is normal and expected. However, women may have secondary amenorrhea resulting from extreme anxiety, anorexia nervosa, acute and chronic illnesses, anemia, or tumors of the ovaries. Treatment is directed to correct the underlying cause of the amenorrhea.

■ **Dysmenorrhea** (painful menstruation) is not uncommon and is more often found in women who have not had children. The causes may be narrowing of the cervix, endometriosis, or hormonal imbalances. The symptoms include cramplike pains in the lower abdomen, headache, nausea, vomiting, and frequent loose stools, usually on the first day of bleeding. For some women, dysmenorrhea is most severe on the second or third day of the menstrual cycle. Treatment of any structural or hormonal abnormalities is indicated if present. Generally, aspirin or another **antiprostaglandin/ anti-inflammatory,** such as ibuprofen, is used to reduce the effects of prostaglandin or tissue hormones. A routine exercise program of at least 20 minutes of aerobic exercise three times a week is helpful for some women.

■ **Menorrhagia** literally means "menstrual hemorrhage." What usually occurs is excessive bleeding at the time of menstruation. In girls and young women, the cause is usually hormonal. In older women, it is usually due to tumors of the uterus. A woman should see her physician to determine and treat the underlying cause. Blood tests should be performed to determine the presence of anemia due to the excessive loss of blood.

Tumors of the Female Reproductive Organs

Malignant tumors of the uterus or cancer of the uterus frequently involves the cervix. The **Pap test** is a routine screening test for the presence of abnormal cell growth. This test, a smear of the cervical cells, is the most effective means of preventing and providing early treatment of cancer of the cervix. For most women, it is recommended that the Pap test be done annually. The most common symptoms of cervical cancer are leukorrhea (white discharge) and irregular vaginal bleeding or spotting. The bleeding may occur between periods and may occur after menopause. Trauma may initiate the bleeding; the trauma may be normal activities like intercourse or defecation. The tumor may involve the fundus of the uterus, and this causes extreme pain in the back and legs. The Pap smear will indicate the extent of the involvement of the cancer in the uterus. The stages of 0 to 4 indicate the progression of uterine tissue involved, with 1 indicating involvement of the cervix and 4 indicating extension of cancer to the bladder, rectum, and pelvis. Treatment ranges from surgical removal of the cervix to complete hysterectomy. Radiation and chemotherapy are measures used to treat the cancer of the uterus and other organs involved in the metastases.

Fibroid tumors of the uterus are benign tumors that form in the muscular tissue of the uterus. They are common and occur in 40 percent of women. They develop slowly and usually begin between the ages of twenty-five and forty. The most common symptoms are menorrhagia and dysmenorrhea. The treatment is dependent upon the size and location of the tumors. If the woman is of childbearing age and wants children, the growth of the tumor is closely monitored. If the tumor is large and creates pressure on other structures, removal of the tumor is indicated.

Ovarian cysts and tumors are frequent. Cysts may be in the follicles, corpus luteum, or other ovarian tissue. They are considered benign. Cysts may cause pain and even rupture as the follicle grows to maturity in the menstrual cycle. They may require surgical removal. Malignant tumors of the ovaries necessitate surgical removal of the ovaries. Chemotherapy and radiation treatment are used as indicated to treat the cancer and prevent the metastasis. Hormonal supplements are needed to replace the hormones produced by the ovaries.

Fibrocystic disease appears as firm, smooth, round masses in the breast. These cysts are usually tender when touched or with pressure on the breast. The cysts become enlarged in the premenstrual phase and tend to decrease in size and are nontender after menses begins. These cysts generally are not indicative of the development of breast cancer.

Malignant tumors of the breast are the most common form of cancer among women in the United States. The most frequent site of the tumor is in the upper outer quadrant of the breast. The only symptom is the presence of a lump that is not painful to the touch. As the tumor grows, it becomes attached to the chest wall or the skin of the breast. If the tumor remains untreated, the lymph nodes in the armpit become infiltrated with the cancer. If the tumor is growing in the medial portion of the breast, the lymph nodes within the thoracic cavity may become involved. The sites of metastases are bone, lung, liver, and brain. As the untreated tumor grows, there will be pain, and the skin of the breast will become dimpled. This is referred to as *orange-peel skin*. The nipple may retract, and the breast may not be symmetrical in shape and location compared to the unaffected breast. Treatment depends on the extent of growth and lymph node involvement. A mammogram will be the initial screening test, followed by a biopsy of the tumor and the surrounding lymph nodes.

Surgical interventions range from lumpectomy or lumpectomy with lymph node excision to simple or radical mastectomy. The woman and her physician should discuss the options for treatment. Some studies show that a lumpectomy with radiation is as effective as a mastectomy. If lymph nodes are involved, they will be removed surgically at the time of the lumpectomy. Chemotherapy is required to decrease the potential for metastases to other organs. Mammography and breast self-examination are the keys to preventing and treating breast cancer.

Breast Self-Examination

Most tumors are detected by the woman herself; therefore, breast self-examination is essential to the detection and prevention of breast cancer. Women should perform this monthly self-examination after the menstrual period. This is when the breasts are less likely to feel "lumpy" because of hormonal breast changes. Figure 15-6 describes the steps for breast self-examination.

application to practice

Knowledge of the male and female reproductive structures, their functions, and the associated diseases is essential in the delivery of care to all patients. Your own level of comfort about patients' sexuality will determine your level of compassion and professional delivery of care. Any awkwardness about patients' bodies and sexual functioning will be lessened by gaining an understanding through your study of this chapter. Consider the information you have just learned about the male and female reproductive systems, and apply this knowledge to the clinical situations that follow.

Learning Activities

Situation 1: Mr. Clemens is a seventy-year-old man who is experiencing the following symptoms: difficulty starting a stream of urine and pain on urination. His diagnosis is BPH. He is scheduled for surgery for a TURP. You are the clinical care associate (CCA) working in the recovery room. What can you expect will be the status of this patient post-op?

Author's Explanation: Mr. Clemens is suffering from BPH. He was scheduled for a transurethral resection of the prostate. Post-op, he will return with a urinary drainage bag.

Situation 2: You notice 500 cubic centimeters (cc) of bright red urine in Mr. Clemens's drainage bag. Is this normal?

Author's Explanation: Post-op hematuria is normal after a TURP. The urine should change from frank red blood to a dark tea color then lighten to normal color within two to three days.

Situation 3: It is Mr. Clemens's third post-op day. You are expected to observe and measure the contents of the urinary drainage bag. When you make morning rounds, you find that there is no drainage in the bag. The night shift I & O (intake and output) accounts for 200 cc of output at 6 A.M. It is now 8 A.M. What action will you take?

Author's Explanation: Report this observation to the nurse stat. Check the Foley catheter for any kinks in the tubing, and make sure that the drainage bag is below the level of the bladder.

Situation 4: When the nurse arrives, Mr. Clemens is questioned about any discomfort. He replies, "Yes, I have some pain in my pelvis." The nurse palpates the bladder. Distention is noted. The nurse asks you to obtain a Foley irrigation setup and proceeds to irrigate the bladder with sterile water. Blood clots are

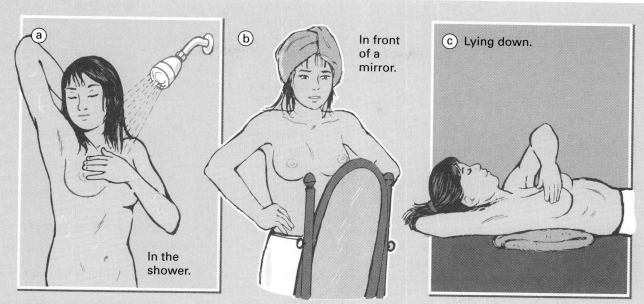

Raise one arm. With fingers flat, touch every part of each breast, gently feeling for a lump or thickening. Use the right hand to examine the left breast, and the left hand to examine the right breast.

With arms at your sides, and then with arms raised above your head, look carefully for changes in the size, shape, and contour of each breast. Look for puckering, dimpling, or changes in skin texture.

Gently squeeze both nipples and look for discharge.

Place a towel or pillow under the right shoulder and the right hand behind the head. Examine the right breast with your left hand.

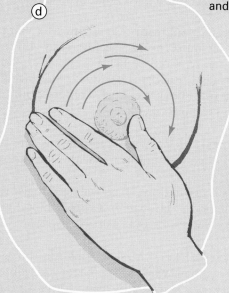

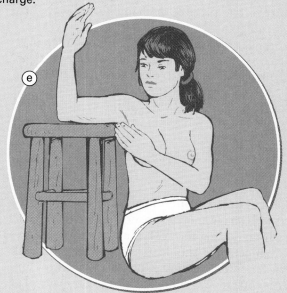

Fingers flat, press gently in small circles, starting at the outermost top edge of your breast and spiraling in toward the nipple. Examine every part of the breast. Repeat with left breast.

With the arm resting on a firm surface, use the same circular motion to examine the underarm area. This is breast tissue, too.

This self-examination is not a substitute for periodic examinations by a qualified physician.

FIGURE 15-6   Steps for breast self-examination from the American Cancer Society.

removed in the process. What was the cause of the distention?

Author's Explanation: The clots were obstructing the flow of urine through the urethra.

Situation 5:   You are the CCA working on the OB-GYN unit. A twenty-two-year-old female is admitted to your unit with severe abdominal pain and fever. Her last menstrual period (LMP) was 8 weeks ago. The initial diagnosis is rule out (r/o) ectopic pregnancy. What is an ectopic pregnancy? Why would the diagnosis of ectopic pregnancy be suspected?

Author's Explanation: Remember that an ectopic pregnancy is a pregnancy that is out of place. Since her LMP was 8 weeks ago, she might be pregnant. A pregnancy test will indicate the possibility of pregnancy.

Situation 6:   This twenty-two-year-old is not pregnant. She is diagnosed with PID. What are the causes and symptoms of PID?

Author's Explanation: The causes of PID are untreated vaginal or uterine infections that spread to the pelvic cavity. The symptoms include pain, fever, amenorrhea, and possible discharge from the vagina.

Situation 7:   Intravenous antibiotic therapy is initiated or started on a patient. What vital sign (VS) is particularly important to observe and report?

Author's Explanation: All of the vital signs are important, but the most important is temperature.

Situation 8:   Why is temperature of such value in this case?

Author's Explanation: The infection is being treated with an antibiotic that should destroy the microorganism causing the PID. If it is effective, the patient's temperature should decrease and return to normal. If her temperature is increasing, then the antibiotic is not effective and will need to be changed.

Situation 9:   Mrs. Shore is a forty-five-year-old mother of four children. She arrives in the emergency room (ER) with complaints of (c/o) a "very heavy period." She tells you that she has used seven pads in the past 2 hours. She has severe cramping and feels faint. What is the term for excessive menstrual flow?

Author's Explanation: *Menorrhagia* is the term to describe menstrual hemorrhage.

Situation 10:   The doctor orders an ultrasound of the uterus. And the nurse tells you to measure Mrs. Shore's VS and report the results stat. These are the VS: temperature 98°F, pulse 110 and thready, respirations 28, blood pressure (BP) 90/60 and faintly heard. Are these within normal limits?

Author's Explanation: No, these VS are not within normal limits. Her BP is low, her pulse is rapid and thready to the fingertips, and her respirations are rapid. Since she is bleeding heavily, her blood pressure is low, and her heart and lungs are working harder to compensate for the decreased blood volume. Her heart is pumping faster to circulate blood, and her lungs are breathing faster to absorb more oxygen to circulate.

Situation 11:   The nurse directs you to lower the head of the bed, to keep Mrs. Shore in bed, and to monitor her VS every 15 minutes. She increases the drip rate of the IV fluids. The ultrasound reveals a large growth in the uterus, and a computed tomography (CT) scan is ordered. Mrs. Shore continues to saturate the perineal pads at the rate of one pad every 30 minutes. Her pulse is thready, and her BP is not audible. She is not responsive when you try to check her perineal pad. What do you do?

Author's Explanation: Stay with Mrs. Shore and call for the nurse using the intercom. Ensure the patient's safety, monitor her VS and LOC (level of consciousness). Report the status of her bleeding. If directed, put the patient in Trendelenburg. Mrs. Shore is going into shock.

Situation 12:   How can you measure the patient's BP if you cannot hear it with the stethoscope?

Author's Explanation: You will need to use the palpation method to estimate her systolic blood pressure and report the results as a "palpable" systolic reading.

Situation 13:   Mrs. Jenkins is a thirty-eight-year-old woman who has a history of fibrocystic breast disease. She routinely performs breast self-exams. This month, she notes a nontender lump in the right upper quadrant (RUQ) of her right breast. In addition, she has lost 10 pounds in the past 3 months, which she attributed to the stress of her new job. Her last gynecology (gyn) exam was 6 months ago. Should she call her gynecologist? When is the best time to perform breast self-exams?

Author's Explanation: Yes, she should call her gynecologist. The best time for a woman to perform a monthly breast self-exam is after her period. Premenstrually, a woman may feel lumps if she has fibrocystic breasts. After menstruation, hormonal changes make the breast less likely to have cystic development.

Situation 14: At the gyn exam, the physician confirms Mrs. Jenkins' suspicions. She is scheduled for hospitalization. The surgical consult form on Mrs. Jenkins says "Breast Bx possible R mastectomy." Mrs. Jenkins asks you, the CCA, why the physician wrote this. What do you tell her? What is your next action?

Author's Explanation: You should explain to Mrs. Jenkins that she needs to speak with her physician about the statement written on the consult form. You are not qualified to interpret the surgeon's findings. Tell her that you will have the nurse call the surgeon to speak with her as soon as possible.

Situation 15: The pathologist confirms the presence of malignant cells in Mrs. Jenkins' frozen section. What does this mean?

Author's Explanation: This means that the cells in the growth are cancerous. The frozen section is a laboratory procedure for preserving the cells for examination by a pathologist.

Situation 16: Mrs. Jenkins has a right mastectomy. What is this procedure? She is 1 day post-op, and during report the nurse tells you not to take a BP or perform phlebotomy in her right arm. Why?

Author's Explanation: A mastectomy is the removal of a breast. Mrs. Jenkins lost her breast due to the cancerous growth, which required surgical removal. The surgical procedure usually includes the removal of lymph nodes in the axilla, and lymphatic tissue is removed when the breast is removed. This decreases the drainage of lymph fluid from the area. Swelling may be present in the arm, and there is usually a Jackson Prat drain inserted in the area to collect blood and lymph fluid from the operative site. You will be asked to measure the drainage from the collection device. Any pressure or disturbance to the venous or lymph vessels can cause increased swelling due to interference with the affected right arm. A sign should be posted over the head of the bed to remind staff members not to use the right arm for BP or venipuncture.

Situation 17: On the second day post-op, Mrs. Jenkins is tearful and very quiet when you go in to do morning care. As you check her surgical dressing, you notice blood on the outer dressing. It feels moist, and the Jackson Prat is full of bloody

fluid. Her hand is swollen, and she is having trouble moving her fingers. Mrs. Jenkins will not look at the dressing; she turns her head to the left, and you see tears rolling down her face. What should you do?

Author's Explanation: You should go to the nurse immediately and report the physical findings. You should also tell the nurse about Mrs. Jenkins' emotional state. Her sadness is to be expected. She is grieving over the loss of her breast. You should let Mrs. Jenkins know that you are there for her and that you are willing to listen to her fears. Allow her to cry; just stay quietly with her, and let her express her sadness. Your observations about her emotional response are important and should be reported along with any other observations that you note.

Situation 18: The surgeon comes to see Mrs. Jenkins and tells her that there is lymphedema in the arm. What is this?

Author's Explanation: Lymphedema is swelling caused by inadequate drainage of lymph fluid.

Situation 19: You have recently begun to work in an outpatient emergency facility. Mr. Blake, a twenty-eight-year-old male, comes to the facility with the following symptoms: dysuria and pyuria × 2 weeks (for two weeks). What do these symptoms mean? What questions should be included in the patient interview?

Author's Explanation: Dysuria is painful or difficult urination, and pyuria is pus in the urine. Questions that should be included in the history taking are sexual activity, use of prophylactic protection, color of drainage, and c/o fever.

Situation 20: Mr. Blake states that he has been sexually active with several partners. He says that he has not used condoms because the women with whom he has had sexual intercourse use other methods of birth control. He denies fever and states that the color of discharge from his penis is yellow. The doctor confirms the diagnosis of gonorrhea. What teaching should the nurse or doctor begin with Mr. Blake? What about the women with whom he has been sexually involved: Could they have gonorrhea also?

Author's Explanation: Mr. Blake needs to tell these women that he has gonorrhea, and they need to be checked for gonorrhea. If they are infected, they will be treated with penicillin or another antibiotic. Gonorrhea is an STD, and the patient needs education about protecting himself and his sexual partners. Condoms are used not only as a birth control method, but also for the prevention of STDs.

Examination Review Questions

1. An STD caused by a protozoan that produces green-yellow discharge is
   a. syphilis
   b. gonorrhea
   c. chlamydia
   d. trichomonas

2. What hormone is present in a woman's blood and urine when pregnancy occurs?
   a. HBV
   b. HIV
   c. HCG
   d. HPV

3. A nonmalignant enlargement of the prostate is
   a. carcinoma
   b. orchidectomy
   c. BPH
   d. TURP

4. The female exocrine gland that secretes lubricating fluid is the
   a. prepuce
   b. bulbourethral
   c. bartholin's
   d. vulvar

5. Which duct is severed, ligated, or cauterized in males for elective sterilization?
   a. epididymis
   b. vas deferens
   c. seminiferous tubules
   d. ejaculatory

6. Which chromosome determines the sex of the baby?
   a. 15
   b. 21
   c. 17
   d. 23

7. The most common cancer in women is
   a. uterine
   b. cervical
   c. ovarian
   d. breast

8. If left untreated, which bacterial STD will cause destruction of the brain and nervous system?
   a. gonorrhea
   b. syphilis
   c. herpes
   d. chlamydia

9. The thin fold of mucous membrane that covers the vaginal opening is the
   a. hymen
   b. prepuce
   c. clitoris
   d. labia

10. When cells of the uterine lining grow outside the uterus, the condition is called
    a. ectopic
    b. endometriosis
    c. PID
    d. menorrhagia

Chapter 16

The Endocrine System

The endocrine system is another system of communication for the body. But unlike the nervous system, which instantaneously transmits signals via nerves, the endocrine system uses chemical messengers to communicate with the organs of the body. These chemical messengers are hormones. Hormones are produced by ductless glands and are released directly into the bloodstream. The blood carries the hormonal message to the target organ. This signals the organ to perform in a specific way. The pituitary gland coordinates the activities of other endocrine glands, signaling and directing their activity. The hormones of the endocrine system play a part in physical appearance, reproduction, fight-or-flight reactions, growth, metabolism, and reproduction.

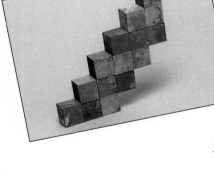

OBJECTIVES

After completing this chapter, you will be able to

1. Name the organs of the endocrine system

2. Contrast exocrine and endocrine glands

3. Describe the location of the endocrine glands

4. List the hormones produced by each endocrine gland

5. Describe the function of each hormone

6. Describe the conditions and diseases of the endocrine system

7. List the observations about the endocrine system that you should report to the nurse

8. Apply your knowledge of the endocrine system to problem-solving strategies in care delivery

9. Define and spell all key terms correctly

key terms

acromegaly
Addison's disease
adrenal glands
adrenocorticotrophic hormone
  (ACTH)
aldosterone
alpha cells
American Diabetes Association
  (ADA)
androgens
anterior lobe
antidiuretic hormone (ADH)
beta cells
calcitonin
corticosterone
cortisol
Cushing's syndrome
diabetes insipidus
ductless
dwarfism
epinephrine (adrenalin)

estrogen
follicle-stimulating hormone (FSH)
gigantism
glucagon
goiter
Graves' disease
growth hormone (GH)
hormones
hydrocortisone
hyperparathyroidism
hyperthyroidism
hypoparathyroidism
hypothyroidism
insulin
insulin-dependent diabetes
  mellitus (IDDM)
islets of Langerhans
luteinizing hormone (LH)
master gland
miscellaneous hormones
myxedema

negative feedback
non-insulin-dependent diabetes
  mellitus (NIDDM)
norepinephrine (noradrenalin)
oxytocin
pitocin
pituitary gland
posterior lobe
progesterone
prolactin (lactogenic hormone)
prostaglandins
protein
Simmond's disease
stat
steroids
suprarenal
tetany
thyroid-stimulating hormone
  (TSH)
thyroxine (T3)
triiodothyronine (T4)

The Endocrine Glands and Their Hormones

The endocrine glands are called **ductless** glands because, unlike the exocrine glands, they secrete substances directly into the blood rather than through a tube or duct into another organ. Remember that the exocrine glands are the salivary glands, the liver, the seminal glands, and so on. The pancreas is both an exocrine gland and an endocrine gland because it releases digestive juices via a duct into the duodenum and also releases a hormone, insulin, into the blood. The endocrine glands are scattered in places throughout the body, from the head to the pelvis (Figure 16-1). The hormones produced by endocrine glands are able to exert widespread effects on target organs far from the site of release from the gland. Positive and negative feedback mechanisms regulate the release of hormones from one gland to another. **Negative feedback** is the process of regulating the activity of an endocrine gland by directly or indirectly stopping or slowing its activity. Essentially, this means that the flow of one hormone is regulated by the rising and falling blood level of another hormone.

Consider your household heating system. The energy source (gas, oil, electricity) is discharged when the demand for increased heat is indicated by the thermostat. In the cold months of the year, you probably turn down the thermostat to a low setting when you will be out of the house for a period of

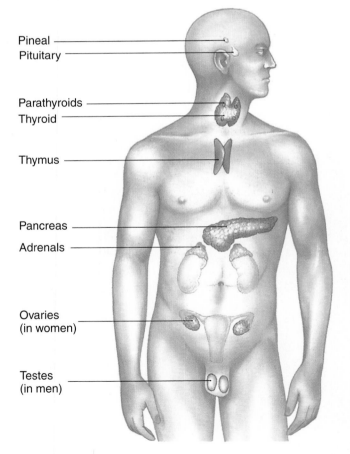

Pineal
Pituitary
Parathyroids
Thyroid
Thymus
Pancreas
Adrenals
Ovaries
(in women)
Testes
(in men)

FIGURE 16-1   Endocrine glands scattered throughout the body.

time. When you return home, you reset the thermostat to the desired temperature. If you reset the thermostat at 70° and the house temperature is 50°, then the heater will use the fuel to reach that 70° temperature. Once the thermostat registers 70°, the heater will stop using fuel. When the temperature begins to dip below the 70° setting, the heater will use more of the energy source to heat the house. In essence, it is a feedback mechanism that turns the heater off and on to regulate the household temperature. In a similar way, glands release hormones based on the demands of the body. Some glands are active or inactive in hormone secretion based on feedback messages. This will become clearer as we discuss the role of the master gland, the anterior pituitary gland.

Classes of Hormones

Hormones are the chemical messengers of the body. There are three classes of hormones, each based on the biochemical structure of the hormone. These are **protein**, made from amino acids, **steroids**, made from cholesterol, and **miscellaneous hormones**. Miscellaneous hormones act locally at the site where they are made. These local, or tissue, hormones are also called **prostaglandins**.

The responsibility of hormones is to maintain homeostasis (a balance in the cellular environment of the body). Hormones help the body to compensate for changes that may disrupt the body's harmony. If we compare the metabolic activities of the body to a war, then hormones are the soldiers that carry messages from the command post to the battlefield. Without these messengers, the command post would have no way to coordinate the battle. Chaos would result on the battlefield, and there would be no hope for winning the war.

Each endocrine gland manufactures its hormones and releases them directly into the blood. As blood flows through an endocrine gland, the absence or presence of specific substances, like glucose, triggers the gland to release or withhold a specific hormone, like insulin. The pancreas is the command center for the glucose battlefield. As blood rich in glucose flows through the pancreas, it signals the islet cells to send in the militia, insulin, to control the army of glucose molecules.

The Pituitary Gland

The **pituitary gland** is a pea-sized gland located in the midbrain below the hypothalamus. *Pituitary* is derived from the Greek word meaning "undergrowth," and the pituitary gland appears to be growing on a stalk under the hypothalamus. The pituitary gland is under the control of the hypothala-

mus, which receives messages from the body's organs and relates the messages to the pituitary gland.

There are two separate portions of this tiny gland: the **anterior lobe** and the **posterior lobe**. Each have separate and distinct functions. Figure 16-2 depicts the lobe of the anterior pituitary and the target glands.

The Anterior Pituitary Gland

The anterior pituitary gland is called the **master gland** because it controls the growth and secretions of other endocrine glands. The anterior pituitary's

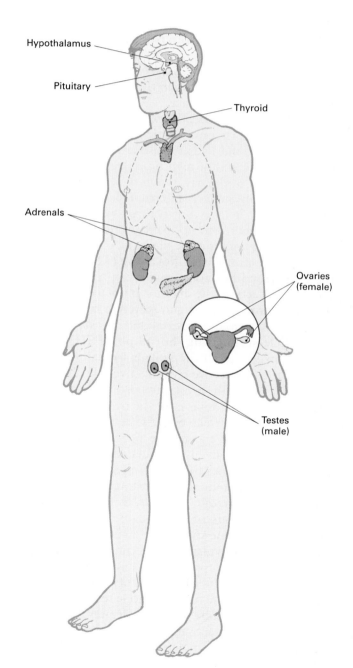

FIGURE 16-2 Anterior pituitary and target glands.

"stimulating" hormones stimulate the activities of these glands: the ovaries, testes, adrenal glands, and thyroid gland. The stimulating hormones also affect bone growth and skin pigmentation. The hormones produced by the anterior pituitary are referred to by the name of the gland or hormone that they stimulate and also by the initials that abbreviate their names. As you study these hormones, concentrate on the actual term describing the hormone, and then it will be easy to remember the abbreviation.

There are six main hormones produced by the anterior pituitary. Descriptions of each follow.

Adrenocorticotrophic hormone (ACTH) regulates the growth and secretion of the outer portion (cortex) of the adrenal glands. The **adrenal glands** are sometimes called **suprarenal** glands because they are located on top of the kidneys. ACTH is called a trophic hormone because *tropho-* means "to grow or to act." ACTH is a hormone that helps the adrenal cortex "to grow and to act." ACTH stimulates the adrenal glands to synthesize and to secrete these hormones: **hydrocortisone**, **corticosterone**, and *aldosterone*. ACTH and hydrocortisone are secreted at a high rate at the end of nighttime sleep and at a low rate at the end of the day. When the usual day-night and awake-sleep cycle is interrupted by changes in sleep patterns, it takes up to three weeks for these hormones to return to normal patterns of secretion. This effect is thought to be the cause of jet lag.

Thyroid-stimulating hormone (TSH) controls the growth and hormone production of the thyroid gland. TSH acts as the anterior pituitary messenger to regulate the synthesis and secretion of these thyroid gland hormones: *thyroxine* and *triiodothyronine*.

Follicle-stimulating hormone (FSH) stimulates the male and female gonads to mature and to produce their respective reproductive cells. In the female, every month from puberty to menopause, FSH stimulates the follicles of the ovaries to grow to maturity and to ripen an egg. As the follicle matures, the production of the female hormones, estrogen and progesterone, are also stimulated by FSH. In the male, FSH stimulates the testes to produce sperm.

Like FSH, **luteinizing hormone (LH)** is a gonadotrophic hormone because it stimulates the growth and actions of the gonads. In the female, luteinizing hormone stimulates the mature follicle to rupture, causing ovulation to occur. Once the follicle ruptures, the corpus luteum develops under the influence of LH. In the male, LH stimulates the testes to produce the male hormone testosterone.

Growth hormone (GH) accelerates the growth of the body. The exact mechanism of how it accelerates growth is not completely understood. It seems to work by increasing the cell's production of proteins, increasing the use of fats, and decreasing the cellular intake of glucose. When growth hormone is produced in excess during adolescence, **gigantism** results. While the individual may grow to over 7 feet tall, extreme weakness is experienced even to stand. When GH is overproduced in adults, it causes **acromegaly** (enlargement of the extremities). The jaw, hands, and feet are abnormally enlarged in individuals with acromegaly. Hyposecretion of GH, TSH, and ACTH in adults causes wasting of adipose and muscle tissues. This rare disease is called **Simmond's disease**. Metabolism is accelerated and the individual is extremely thin and malnourished. Hyposecretion of GH in children causes a condition known as **dwarfism**. The child with pituitary dwarfism is very short in stature, but arms, legs, and face are proportioned to body size.

Prolactin (lactogenic hormone) promotes breast tissue growth during pregnancy and lactation (milk production) after the birth of the baby. (The term *lactogenic* is derived from Latin; *lacto-* means "milk," and *-genic* means "to produce or make.") It is actually the sucking of the infant at the breast that stimulates the anterior pituitary to increase prolactin production and, therefore, milk production. The continued high blood level of prolactin is stimulated as long as the woman breast-feeds. High prolactin levels inhibit the menstrual cycle, and this is why breast-feeding has been called *nature's contraceptive*. Some women, though, have become pregnant during breast-feeding. Women are encouraged to use a birth control method while breast-feeding to prevent conception.

The Posterior Pituitary Gland

The posterior pituitary produces two hormones: *oxytocin* and *antidiuretic hormone (ADH)*.

Oxytocin is a hormone that operates to affect labor and delivery and to prevent hemorrhage after delivery of the baby. Oxytocin strengthens the contraction of the muscles of the uterus. It is vital to the natural inducing of labor. (In Greek, *oxys-* means "swift," and *tokos* means "childbirth.") It is also essential to the letdown (release) of milk from the mammary ducts. It is the infant's sucking at the breast that increases the release of oxytocin and the letdown of milk. This, in turn, increases contractions of the uterus and helps the uterus to return to normal size if the mother breast-feeds the infant. In emergency childbirth situations, the infant is put to the breast to suck to increase the release of oxytocin and contractions of the uterus. This is done to reduce the risk of hemorrhage of the uterus. Many women are given **pitocin** (synthetic oxytocin) during labor. It is usually given intravenously, and it helps to hasten the delivery by increasing the contractions of the uterus.

Antidiuretic hormone (ADH) stimulates the tubules of the kidneys to reabsorb water from the filtrate that will become urine. The action of ADH decreases the volume of water in urine and increases the volume of water in the bloodstream. (The word *antidiuretic* means "against"—*anti*—"excretion of urine"—(diuretic.) When the volume of water in the blood is high, the level of ADH decreases in an effort to increase water excretion from the kidneys. And when the volume of water in the blood is low, the amount of ADH produced increases to preserve water loss from the kidney tubules. When you have a large volume of fluid intake and you are not losing much water from perspiration, you tend to produce a large amount of urine and have frequent urination. The condition that results from an abnormally low production of ADH is called *diabetes insipidus*. People with diabetes insipidus may urinate up to 20 liters of urine a day. They tend to drink large amounts of fluids to compensate for the excessive loss of water in urine.

The Thyroid Gland

The thyroid gland is located in the neck and below the thyroid cartilage of the larynx, superior to the trachea. The thyroid gland produces these hormones: *thyroxin, triiodothyronine*, and *calcitonin*.

Thyroxin and Triiodothyronine

Thyroxin (T4) and **triiodothyronine (T3)** are hormones that accelerate metabolism in every cell of the body. These hormones increase the level of energy expended by the cells in the actions of breaking down or building up fats, proteins, and carbohydrates. The production and secretion of thyroid hormones are regulated by TSH from the anterior pituitary gland. TSH levels increase when T3 and T4 levels decrease. TSH stimulates the thyroid gland to secrete more thyroid hormones. When thyroid hormone levels are increased, the TSH level decreases. This is a classic example of the feedback mechanisms of the endocrine system. The thyroid gland uses iodine to manufacture these hormones. Iodine is supplied to the thyroid by dietary intake of this mineral. The thyroid cells use iodine and amino acids to form T3 and T4. An iodine deficiency in the diet renders the gland unable to manufacture these hormones, and hypothyroidism results. When the thyroid gland is enlarged due to overstimulation by TSH, a toxic goiter results. **Goiter** is the enlargement of the gland, and it is a visible swelling in the neck. Iodine is added to table salt to prevent a dietary deficiency of this mineral for people who live in areas of the world with iodine-poor soil.

Calcitonin

Calcitonin is involved in the regulation of blood calcium levels. When blood calcium levels are high, calcitonin is secreted by the thyroid gland to decrease the calcium level in the blood. The bones then increase the absorption of calcium, or the calcium is excreted in urine. This hormone works in opposition to the parathyroid hormone.

The Parathyroid Glands

There are four parathyroid glands, which are pea-sized structures located on the back of the thyroid gland. These glands produce a hormone called *parathyroid hormone (parathormone)*.

Parathyroid Hormone (Parathormone)

This hormone works to maintain blood calcium levels and to prevent an abnormally low blood calcium level. It is secreted when blood levels of calcium are low or decreasing. It also regulates the blood level of phosphorus by reducing the level of phosphorus in the blood. Both calcium and phosphorus are essential for maintaining the normal strength and health of the bones. The thyroid hormone, calcitonin and parathormone work in opposite ways to maintain normal blood levels of calcium.

The Adrenal Glands

The adrenal, or suprarenal, glands are two triangular glands. One is located on the top surface of each kidney. There are two distinct parts of the adrenal glands. The outer surface is the cortex, and the inner surface is the medulla. The adrenal cortex is stimulated to synthesize and secrete its hormones by the anterior pituitary hormone ACTH. The hormones of the cortex include *mineralcorticoids, glucocorticoids*, and *adrenal sex hormones*. The adrenal medulla is stimulated by the nervous system to secrete the hormones *epinephrine* and *norepinephrine*. The adrenal cortex and medulla are critical to the body's response to stress.

Mineralcorticoids

The adrenal cortex manufactures mineralcorticoids. Mineralcorticoids are hormones that help to regulate the concentration of minerals in the body, such as sodium and potassium. The chief mineralcorticoid is **aldosterone**. This hormone is sometimes referred to as the *salt-retaining hormone* because it works in the tubules of the kidneys to conserve sodium and to excrete potassium. At the same time, this conserves water and, therefore, reduces the amount of urinary output. Aldosterone is secreted by the adrenal cortex when the circulating blood level of sodium is low or when the level of potassium is high.

Glucocorticoids

The adrenal cortex also manufactures hormones called *glucocorticoids*. These hormones affect the metabolism of the sugar glucose. The chief glucocorticoid is **cortisol**, a natural cortisone for the body. Cortisol helps to maintain the necessary blood level of glucose to meet the energy demands of the body. During times of stress, the amount of circulating cortisol increases. The increased cortisol level stimulates a variety of metabolic actions, all of which produce more glucose for energy. The brain interprets the signals of stress and increases the amount of ACTH, which stimulates the adrenal cortex to secrete more cortisol. This hormone, like the drug cortisone, helps to decrease inflammation. It is a natural anti-inflammatory for the body.

Adrenal Sex Hormones

The cortex of the adrenal glands also produces **androgens**, or male sex hormones, like testosterone. The cortex also produces in smaller amounts the female hormones estrogen and progesterone. The amount of sex hormones produced by the adrenal glands is small, but these hormones may supplement the development of reproductive organs. And, in females, these hormones are believed to stimulate sex drive.

Epinephrine and Norepinephrine

The adrenal medulla (the inner portion of the adrenal glands) produces two hormones called **epinephrine (adrenalin)** and **norepinephrine (noradrenalin)**. These hormones are the chemicals released at the synapses of sympathetic nerves. If you remember, the sympathetic division of the autonomic nervous system prepares the body for fight-or-flight reactions. When a stressful situation is perceived by an individual, the sympathetic nerves trigger the rapid release of epinephrine and norepinephrine from the adrenal medulla. These hormones stimulate heart rate, increase the force of the heart's contractions, increase blood flow to muscles, increase breathing rate, and dilate the airway. All of these responses of the organs help to prepare the body to react swiftly to stressful situations.

The Pancreas

The pancreas is an organ that was discussed in Chapter 13, "The Digestive System," because it is both an endocrine gland and an exocrine gland. In this unit, we will discuss the endocrine gland functions of the pancreas.

The hormones of the pancreas are produced in special cells called the **islets of Langerhans**. There are two types of islet cells: **beta cells** and **alpha cells**. Alpha cells produce the hormone, glucagon. Beta cells produce the hormone, insulin.

Insulin

Insulin works to decrease the amount of glucose (sugar) that is present in the circulating blood. Insulin regulates the uptake of glucose into the cells. It acts like a key that unlocks the cell membrane to allow glucose to enter the interior of the cell. After eating, insulin is secreted most heavily. And the amount secreted decreases when the blood level of glucose decreases. When the beta cells fail to produce insulin, a condition called *diabetes mellitus* results. Sometimes, people refer to this as "sugar diabetes," or they may say, "I have sugar." A normal blood level for glucose is 60 to 120 mg percent. The glucose meter used at your facility will indicate the specific normal value for blood glucose for that particular instrument. The normal value can vary by ±5 to 10 mg percent.

Glucagon

Glucagon has the opposite effect of insulin on blood glucose. Glucagon works to increase the amount of circulating glucose. The alpha islet cells are stimulated to secrete glucagon when the level of circulating sugar (glucose) is low. Glucagon works on liver cells to make new glucose from stored starch.

The Ovaries

The structure and function of the ovaries are discussed in Chapter 15, "The Reproductive System." The ovaries produce two female hormones called *estrogen* and *progesterone*.

Estrogen

Estrogen is produced by the follicle cells of the ovaries. The follicles are stimulated by FSH to mature the ovum (egg). They also produce estrogen. Estrogen is called the *feminizing hormone* because it changes a girl into a woman. It helps the female to maintain her feminine characteristics and to continue reproductive functions. Estrogen causes breast development, genitalia development, growth of pubic hair, softening of the skin, rounding of the hips, and a round shaped pelvic basin.

Progesterone

Progesterone is secreted by the corpus luteum, the structure that is formed after LH causes the ovum to be released from the follicle (ovulation). Progesterone is also produced by the placenta. Progesterone prepares the inner lining of the uterus for pregnancy, maintains the development of the placenta, prevents the ovaries from producing ova during pregnancy, and decreases the contractions of the uterus during pregnancy. It also prepares the mammary glands for milk production during pregnancy. When progesterone levels are below normal, a woman may suffer from menstrual cramps and spontaneous abortion or miscarriage during pregnancy. Following menopause, the production of both estrogen and progesterone by the ovaries ceases.

The Testes

The testes produce the masculinizing hormone, testosterone.

Testosterone

Testosterone is produced in the testes. This hormone changes a boy into a man. Testosterone is needed for the following: production of sperm, growth of body hair, increase in muscle development, increase in the size and density of bones, increase in the size of the genitals, and thickening of the vocal cords, which causes the deepening of the male voice. In some men, testosterone continues to be produced by the testes well into a man's late seventies.

Conditions and Diseases of the Endocrine System

The disease processes of the endocrine system are caused by excessive or deficient production and secretion of hormones. These are either *hyper* or *hypo* conditions. The following sections present information about disorders of the thyroid, parathyroid, adrenal, pancreas, and pituitary glands.

Disorders of the Thyroid Gland

Hypothyroidism, or myxedema, results from the removal or destruction of the thyroid gland. The person's metabolism is slowed in proportion to the decrease or absence of thyroid hormones. The pulse rate is below normal, the temperature is low, and the person gains weight easily. The skin is thickened. There is hair loss, and, in women, menorrhagia. Emotional and mental responses are dulled, and the person feels a total lack of energy. Treatment involves replacement of the thyroid hormone. If the thyroid gland has been surgically removed because

of tumor or another cause, the person will also need thyroid medication.

The exact cause of **hyperthyroidism**, or **Graves' disease**, is not always clear because it may appear spontaneously after emotional shock or infection, especially a respiratory infection. Usually, the cause of hyperthyroidism, also referred to as *exophthalmic goiter*, is the result of overstimulation by the anterior pituitary hormone TSH. The symptoms are very much the opposite of hypothyroidism. The person has an accelerated metabolism, feels nervous, and often looks startled because of the exophthalmic goiter (bulging eyes). The heart rate is rapid, even at rest. There is a fine tremor of the hands and extreme restlessness. The person usually has a hearty appetite and weight loss despite eating large amounts of food. The increased heart rate can cause palpitations and atrial fibrillation. For some individuals, the disease resolves itself in a few months or years, but in others, it continues throughout life. Treatment involves the administration of drugs that block the use of iodine by the thyroid or the administration of radioactive iodine, which irradiates the thyroid gland. Surgical intervention usually involves removing five-sixths of the thyroid gland.

Disorders of the Parathyroid Gland

Hyperparathyroidism is the result of overgrowth of the parathyroid gland. It is characterized by the demineralization of bones (loss of calcium from bones), high blood calcium levels, and the formation of kidney stones. The demineralization of bones results in the softening of bones with spontaneous fractures, pain with weight bearing, formation of bony cysts, and, sometimes, bone tumors. The excess of blood calcium causes abnormalities of nervous and muscle tissues, including the heart. The treatment involves surgical removal of most of the parathyroid tissue to return the balance of calcium in the blood.

Hypoparathyroidism is the result of removal of too much parathyroid tissue in the surgical treatment of hyperthyroidism. It can also result from unexplained atrophy (wasting or shrinkage) of the gland. The blood calcium level is low, and the phosphorus level is high. The chief symptom is tetany. **Tetany** is hyperactivity of the muscles. The muscles are spasmodic, uncoordinated, and easily stimulated by touch. The arms and hands may be in a state of flexion from the stimulation of touch. The laryngeal muscle may spasm, causing difficulty breathing and speaking. Seizures may occur. The treatment in crisis is intravenous (IV) administration of calcium. Oral supplements of calcium and vitamin D are needed, and injections of parathormone solution are given to return the blood calcium levels to normal.

Disorders of the Adrenal Glands

Addison's disease results from deficient secretion of the cortisol hormones from the adrenal cortex. The chief symptoms of Addison's disease are low blood levels of sodium and glucose and high blood levels of potassium. The individual feels weak and anorectic. The skin darkens and is described as "bronze," and the blood pressure is low. The disturbance in sodium and potassium may cause cardiac irregularities and seizures. Treatment involves restoring sodium, potassium, and glucose levels to normal with diet and with administration of the electrolytes. Management of Addison's disease involves the administration of hydrocortisone and aldosterone.

Cushing's syndrome results from a tumor of the adrenal cortex or a tumor of the pituitary gland causing excessive secretion of ACTH (Figure 16-3). The prolonged administration of ACTH or hydrocortisone is treatment for diseases or conditions that require such medications. The symptoms include a "moon" face and "buffalo hump" due to excessive fat accumulation in the face and back. Weight gain is also apparent in the trunk, and the limbs seem thin. The person feels lazy and weak. Hypertension, congestive heart failure, and compression fractures of the vertebrae also accompany Cushing's syndrome. Women experience decreased menstrual flow, irregular periods, and growth of facial hair. Treatment involves removal of any tumor of the adrenal or pituitary glands. If the cause is overgrowth of the adrenal cortex, the affected adrenals are removed surgically.

Disorders of the Pituitary Gland

Diabetes insipidus is caused by a deficiency of the antidiuretic hormone. Tumors near the pituitary gland may cause this disease. The chief symptom is polyuria, or excessive urination of up to 40 liters a day. This cannot be controlled by restricting the intake of fluids. Doing so results in excessive thirst (polydipsia). Treatment involves the administration of vasopressin, the antidiuretic hormone.

Simmond's disease is a condition that results from the removal of the pituitary gland, a lesion in the blood vessels of the pituitary, or a tumor of the pituitary. The thyroid and adrenal glands are unable to function because the stimulating hormones are absent. In addition to the symptoms noted in the discussion on growth hormone under "The Anterior Pituitary Gland" earlier in this chapter, the person will have atrophy of all organs, hair loss, amenorrhea, slow metabolism, hypoglycemia, and, eventually, coma and death.

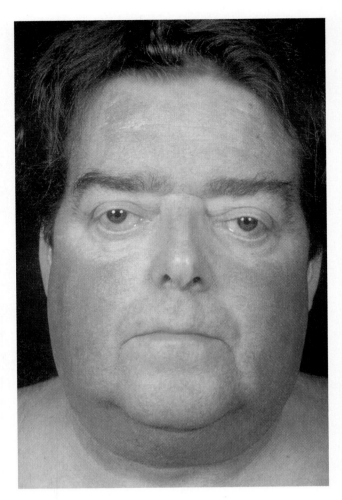

FIGURE 16-3 Cushing's syndrome. BioPhoto Association, Photo Researchers, Inc.

Review the discussion on growth hormone under "The Anterior Pituitary Gland" earlier in this chapter for a discussion of gigantism, acromegaly, and dwarfism.

Diabetes Mellitus

Insulin-dependent diabetes mellitus (IDDM) is the type of diabetes mellitus for which the patient requires insulin injections. **Non-insulin-dependent diabetes mellitus (NIDDM)** is the type of diabetes mellitus for which the patient does not require insulin injections. This person takes an oral medication that is categorized as a hypoglycemic agent.

The **American Diabetes Association (ADA)** dietary guidelines are used to prescribe the diabetic diet. The specific number of calories are prescribed with an ADA diet.

Information on diabetes mellitus is included in Chapter 13, under "Conditions and Diseases of the Digestive System."

application to practice

The usefulness of understanding the structures and functions of the endocrine system is in the application of this knowledge to your work with patients or clients. As a clinical care associate, you can utilize your skills in providing effective nursing care. Consider the following situations, and use the information that you have learned about the endocrine system.

Learning Activities

Situation 1: Mrs. Bickel is a sixty-three-year-old woman with diabetes mellitus. She has been on insulin for 2 years. What type of diabetes does she have?

Author's Explanation: Mrs. Bickel has insulin-dependent diabetes mellitus (IDDM).

Situation 2: Mrs. Bickel self-administers "40 u of NPH q.d." What does this mean?

Author's Explanation: Mrs. Bickel injects herself with 40 units of insulin every day. This type of insulin is intermediate-acting. This means that it is not an immediate-acting form of insulin like regular insulin. Insulin can be immediate-acting, intermediate-acting, or long-acting.

Situation 3: Mrs. Bickel is admitted to your medical unit. She has complaints of (c/o) "not feeling right." Her physician's note reads, "Pt. has been experiencing polyuria, polydipsia, and polyphagia." What do these terms mean to you?

Author's Explanation: Mrs. Bickel is experiencing excessive urination, excessive thirst, and excessive hunger. These are hallmark signs of diabetes mellitus (DM).

Situation 4: Her physician's admission note also indicates that she has a small ulceration on her right big toe. Her fasting blood sugar (FBS) today was 310. What does this mean to you?

Author's Explanation: Her fasting blood sugar is very elevated. Her ulcer on her right big toe is also a complication of her diabetes. When blood sugar is high, the environment for the growth of infections is ripe; people with DM are often plagued with slow healing. That is why it is particularly important to use extreme caution when handling the skin and nail care of a diabetic patient. The accumulation of sugar in the blood produces many long-range complications of the blood vessels. The blood vessels of the periphery of the body, like the feet and lower legs, are especially vulnerable. Diabetes can wreak havoc on the blood vessels of the eyes and cause blindness. The kidneys are especially at risk. One cardinal rule with diabetic patients is *do not risk injury* because their injuries are slow to heal and easily infected.

Situation 5: The Kardex states, "Never cut this patient's toenails." Why?

Author's Explanation: Never cut a patient's toenails because of the risk of injury with incorrect cutting and the potential for infection.

Situation 6: Mrs. Bickel's physician increased her insulin dose to 55 units of NPH with a sliding scale for regular insulin based on blood glucose monitoring, which will be conducted every 6 hours. What does this mean?

Author's Explanation: The physician has increased the intermediate-acting insulin. In addition, he will control continued high sugars with a short-acting insulin based on the findings of the fingerstick test. Dosage is precalculated according to the results.

Situation 7: You enter Mrs. Bickel's room this afternoon and find her unresponsive. Her skin feels hot and dry, and her respirations are slow and deep. What do you do? What could have happened to her?

Author's Explanation: You should call the nurse **stat**. Stay with Mrs. Bickel, check her pulse, respirations, and blood pressure, and report the results to the nurse. Mrs. Bickel is probably having a hyperglycemic reaction. You should get the glucose meter when the nurse arrives and should check her blood glucose stat.

Situation 8: The next morning before breakfast, Mrs. Bickel rings the call bell. You enter her room and find her sweating. Her hands are shaking, and she says, "I am starving. The nurse gave me my insulin and I need to eat." Why do you think that Mrs. Bickel is so hungry, sweating, and shaky? What will you do?

Author's Explanation: Mrs. Bickel may be hypoglycemic at this point. That is why she is sweating, hungry, and shaky. This can be life-threatening. Immediate action is necessary. You should call for the nurse, report your observations, and while the nurse remains with the patient, get the glucose meter and check her blood sugar. Liquid CHO (carbohydrates) may need to be administered, but the nurse (or physician) will make this decision. Check with the nurse and the dietary department about her breakfast tray.

Situation 9: Mr. Pepino is a twenty-four-year-old man who is admitted to the emergency room (ER) with rapid heart rate, nervousness, insomnia, and extreme restlessness. He states that these symptoms began about a week ago. He has been unable to sleep more than an hour at a time, and wakes up feeling "not rested and nervous." The physician reports that he has atrial fibrillation and a heart rate of 120. You note that Mr. Pepino has a startled expression and appears hyperalert; his eyes are bulging. You are directed to draw a blood sample for T3, T4, PBI, and TSH. What are T3, T4, and TSH? And based on your knowledge of these studies, what can a PBI test represent?

Author's Explanation: T3 and T4 are thyroid hormone tests to measure the amount of thyroxine and triiodothyronine hormones present in the circulating blood. TSH will measure the amount of thyroid-stimulating hormone secreted by the pituitary gland. PBI is a test to reveal the amount of protein-bound iodine. Remember that the thyroid gland absorbs most of the iodine intake and uses it to manufacture thyroid hormones.

Situation 10: What symptoms led the physician to request these studies?

Author's Explanation: Mr. Pepino had all the symptoms of hyperthyroidism, or Graves' disease. These include increased heart rate, irregular heart rhythm, nervousness, restlessness, insomnia, and exophthalmos.

Situation 11: The nurse asks you to get a set of vital signs (VS) and to measure his weight and height. You measure Mr. Pepino and find that he is 6'2" tall and weighs 170 lb. He is surprised at the weight and states, "Last week, I weighed 180 pounds." What would account for this weight loss?

Author's Explanation: If the patient has hyperthyroidism, his metabolic rate is accelerated. Every symptom he presented indicated increased metabolic demands.

Situation 12: Mr. Clinton is a forty-seven-year-old male who is admitted to your patient care unit. He has been treated with ACTH recently for his multiple sclerosis (MS) and has been prescribed oral hydrocortisone to decrease the inflammation of the nerves. He now has uncontrolled hyperglycemia and has been on insulin to control his high blood sugar levels. His face is puffy, and his legs are very thin in proportion to his trunk, which seems bloated. What could have caused these symptoms?

Author's Explanation: Mr. Clinton probably has an induced diabetes mellitus that resulted from the IV ACTH and the oral hydrocortisone used to manage the inflammatory process of MS. Remember that the adrenal glands are stimulated by the anterior pituitary hormone ACTH and that the oral hydrocortisone acts like natural cortisone. This increases the blood glucose level.

Situation 13: Mr. Clinton is diagnosed with Cushing's syndrome. What caused this to happen? What gland is involved in this condition?

Author's Explanation: The adrenal glands are involved, and the use of IV ACTH and oral hydrocortisone caused the Cushing's syndrome.

Situation 14: Ms. March is a fifty-six-year-old woman who was admitted from the ER to the MICU because of delirium, bradycardia, and hypotonic muscle and nervous responses. You are assigned to her, and the nurse asks you to draw an ionized calcium. She reminds you to wrap the Vacutainer tube for the blood sample in aluminum foil to protect it from exposure to light. Why would you be directed to draw an ionized calcium?

Author's Explanation: Ms. March has symptoms that indicate a generalized slowing of neuromuscular activity, including that of the heart. Calcium has a direct impact on the speed of neuromuscular response.

Situation 15: Ms. March has an increased blood calcium level which caused her symptoms. What gland(s) affect calcium levels in the body?

Author's Explanation: There are two glands that affect blood calcium: the thyroid and parathyroids. Usually, the thyroid gland is not the culprit of calcium dysfunctions. The parathyroid is responsible and usually indicated in abnormal blood calcium levels.

Situation 16: If Ms. March had a disease that caused demineralization of bones, such as cancer of the bones, then this would be an underlying cause of increased blood calcium. Yet, there is no sign of this in her H&P. Why is she delirious?

Author's Explanation: Elevated blood calcium affects the nerves of the central nervous system (CNS) and causes disturbances of brain functions. The delirium produces false perceptions of the environment. The person misinterprets sensory information and is often frightened, confused, disoriented, and unable to interpret visual, auditory, and other sensory messages from the environment.

Examination Review Questions

1. The chemical messenger that initiates labor is
   a. estrogen
   b. progesterone
   c. oxytocin
   d. prolactin

2. The "master gland" is the
   a. adrenal
   b. pituitary
   c. thyroid
   d. gonad

3. Excessive secretion of ACTH causes
   a. myxedema
   b. Cushing's syndrome
   c. Addison's disease
   d. hypoparathyroidism

4. Which hormone stimulates the male and female gonads to mature?
   a. ACTH
   b. FSH
   c. TSH
   d. LH

5. A toxic goiter results from oversecretion of which hormone?
   a. thyroxin
   b. triiodothyronine
   c. TSH
   d. LSH

6. The "fight-or-flight hormone" is secreted by which endocrine gland?
   a. adrenal
   b. thyroid
   c. parathyroid
   d. pituitary

7. The "feminizing hormone" responsible for reproductive functioning in women is
   a. oxytocin
   b. progesterone
   c. estrogen
   d. prolactin

8. Testosterone is responsible for all of the following *except*
   a. thickening of the vocal cords
   b. production of sperm
   c. increase in muscle development
   d. decrease in bone density

9. Which endocrine disorder causes bronzing of the skin and dangerously low blood pressure?
   a. myxedema
   b. Addison's disease
   c. Cushing's syndrome
   d. Simmond's disease

10. Acromegaly results from oversecretion of which hormone?
    a. LH
    b. GH
    c. FSH
    d. TSH

Problem Solving and the Fundamentals of Patient Care

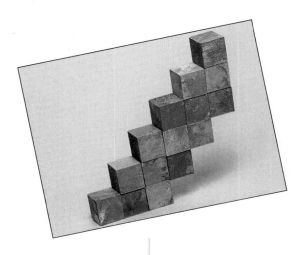

In this unit, the nursing-process method, a nursing method of approaching patient care problems, will be detailed. The sequential steps in this process underlie all of the clinical care assistant's actions in assisting the nurse to care for clients. The nurse depends on the clinical assistant to deliver aspects of planned care and to provide feedback about the patient's response to that care.

In all aspects of patient care, there are fundamentals that serve as guidelines for troubleshooting problems, responding to patient needs, and working effectively as a team member. Because these fundamentals serve to guide the actions of all team members, an understanding of them is essential to your role. These fundamentals are based on concepts, methods, and scientific and ethical principles. Quality care and the measurement of quality outcomes will provide a framework that unites the current issues that shape patient care delivery models.

Chapter 17

A Nursing-Process Approach to Care Delivery

In this chapter, the nursing process will be introduced as a method of problem solving in all aspects of patient care. Scope of practice and licensure will be discussed, along with concepts and trends in the delivery of patient care.

The fundamentals of patient care presented here include a discussion of teamwork, ethical principles, patient-centered care, and clients'/patients' rights. These fundamentals will help you to form the foundation on which to build a career as a clinical care associate. Without an understanding of these fundamentals, patient care becomes minimal, one-dimensional, and rote at best. The application of these fundamentals will strengthen your contributions in patient care. If you choose to pursue a professional nursing career, you will be able to build on this foundation with continued education.

OBJECTIVES

After completing this chapter, you will be able to

1. Describe the nursing process as a method of problem solving
2. List and describe the four parts of the nursing process and describe your role in each
3. Define the term *scope of practice*
4. Describe scope of practice as it applies to the role of the clinical care associate
5. Define *ethics*
6. Describe the fundamental ethical principles that relate to the health care environment
7. Define *teamwork* and list the five Cs of effective teamwork
8. Define *communication*
9. Distinguish between verbal and nonverbal messages
10. Describe patient-centered care
11. List the clients'/patients' rights
12. Apply the fundamentals of patient care to the problem-solving process
13. Define and spell all key terms correctly

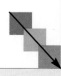

key terms

assessing	delegation	nonverbal
beneficence	ethics	objective data
collaboration	ethics committee	planning
commitment	evaluating	respect for autonomy
communication	implementing	scope of practice
contraband	justice	teamwork
contribution	licensure	verbal
cooperation	nonmaleficence	

Problem Solving

Throughout this text, the nursing-process model of problem solving is used to guide your learning. There is no intent to infringe on the cornerstone of professional nursing practice. Since the nursing process is the cornerstone of nursing and since, as a clinical assistant, you will work under the direct supervision of the professional nurse, what would be a better model to follow? Of course, the nursing process will not be presented at the professional nursing level, nor are you expected to apply it at that level. Nor will the nursing process defy the boundaries of the clinical assistant's role. It will serve merely to provide a means of developing critical thinking skills, which not only are desirable, but also are necessary for the continuity of patient care.

The Nursing Process

The four concepts of the nursing process, in sequence, are **assessing**, **planning**, **implementing**, and **evaluating** (Figures 17-1 and 17-2). Let's look at how the professional nurse uses this process. The nurse must first assess the patient and identify the problem that the patient is presenting. Next, a plan for solving the problem is established. After formulating a plan, the actions to resolve the problem must be implemented by the nurse or by a designated team member. Finally, the result of delivered care must be evaluated to determine its effectiveness. If the care has failed to resolve the problem, the

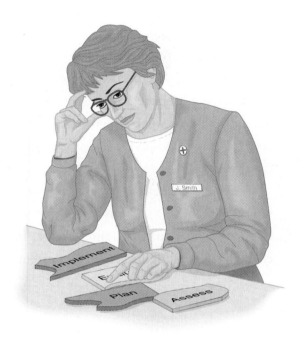

FIGURE 17-2 Ordering the steps of the nursing process.

nurse must reassess the situation and determine a new course of action or redefine the problem.

We use a method of problem solving daily to manage our activities of daily living. Think about your method of solving a problem. You may not use the terms *assessing, planning, implementing,* and *evaluating,* but you probably apply these concepts in your approach to problems. First, you recognize that there is a problem. You assess the situation. Next, you decide what to do about it. You plan. You follow your plan. You implement. Finally, you decide if your plan worked to resolve the problem. You evaluate.

In your work as a clinical assistant, you will encounter situations throughout the day that require problem solving on your part. You will not be assessing patients, determining the plan of care, implementing all the actions in the plan, or evaluating the results in the same way that the professional nurse will. However, you will be assisting the nurse in assessing, planning, implementing, and evaluating your part in the care of patients. Every time you give

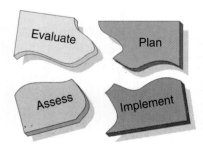

FIGURE 17-1 Concepts of the nursing process.

a bed bath, you assess the patient's readiness and ability to participate in the bath. You plan your actions and approach to the patient and the bath, you implement your plan to complete the task, and you evaluate the effectiveness of the bath. Throughout the procedure of bathing the patient, you observe the patient's skin, mobility, and participation. You listen to what the patient is saying, noting the emotional tone. You adapt your actions to the patient's needs, adjusting your plan as you proceed through the bathing process. You evaluate the results of the bath. Your evaluation will direct the approach that you will take the next time you are assigned to bathe this patient. You report your observations about the patient's physical and emotional condition to the nurse so that the patient's needs can be addressed in the plan of care. If you notice a rash, the nurse will need to assess it, so that a nursing plan can be developed to treat it.

It is the role of the professional nurse to assess the whole patient and his or her problems, as well as to determine the plan of care that will be implemented. But those who assist the professional nurse are responsible for completing patient care tasks and for providing **objective data** to help the nurse in all phases of this process. Objective data is a term used to describe measurable patient information, such as vital sign results, height, weight, and intake and output measurements. Objective information is not subject to interpretation, it is factual information. The clinical assistant plays a vital role in the implementation phase because the assistant is responsible for carrying out actions as part of the plan of care that are within his or her scope of practice.

Scope of Practice

Scope is defined as the range or extent of an action, observation, or inquiry. **Scope of practice** is the framework of boundaries and expectations from which one is presumed to function. To grasp the concept, let's consider a journeyman plumber. Licensed by the state, the journeyman plumber is knowledgeable and competent to handle all basic plumbing repairs. When the journeyman plumber sends an apprentice to a home for a repair, the journeyman assumes ultimate responsibility. Therefore, the journeyman will ensure that the apprentice is competent to execute the task and understands his or her scope of practice. What happens if the repair is not simple and straightforward? The apprentice will most likely need to call the journeyman for further directions before proceeding. However, to know when to call, the apprentice must comprehend the fundamentals involved in completing the task, the problem-solving method, and the scope of practice.

If the problem is a simple one, the apprentice may solve it without the journeyman's intervention. The journeyman plumber needs an assistant who can think through the situation and handle simple deviations from standard procedure. Knowing when to call for help is critical. This can only be achieved when the apprentice understands the standard plumbing procedures and codes and scope of practice. This is why it is imperative for the apprentice to know all the standard procedures that a journeyman executes that may be delegated to the apprentice. It is also important to know the scope of practice in which the apprentice may function.

The scope of practice for clinical assistants has been shaped by several sources. To understand, let's first examine the scope of practice for professional nurses. First, the legal definition of nursing practice is determined by each state, which defines the scope of nursing practice in that state. Therefore, what a nurse is able to do in California may not be legal in Maine. The primary purpose of the nurse practice acts is to protect the health and safety of the public. In addition to the state practice acts, each health care institution defines the scope of nursing practice with job descriptions and policies. Finally, organizations such as the American Nurses Association (ANA) govern the scope of nursing practice and refine it as necessary.

The scope of nursing practice as described by the American Nurses Association is the framework within which the registered nurse (RN) practices nursing. Registered nurses are held accountable to the public by these standards of practice. They supervise, delegate, and assign patient care activities. These actions must occur in the context of the profession's responsibility to the public. There are separate nurse practice acts for RNs and licensed practical nurses (LPNs). Each practice act defines the expected responsibilities and limitations of the nurse. Because each institution further defines the scope of practice with policies and job descriptions, it is essential for the RN or LPN to adhere to the institution's established standards. The same is applicable to the clinical care associate (CCA). Figure 17-3 defines the boundaries of the RN, LPN, and CCA.

Delegating Tasks

In some institutions, clinical assistants are permitted to administer cleansing enemas. In others, this is not a procedure that assistants are permitted to perform. Finally, even if the institution permits the assistant to perform this procedure, it is the nurse's assessment of the patient, the personnel, and the circumstances that dictates who will perform the procedure. In some cases, problems may necessitate the skills of the

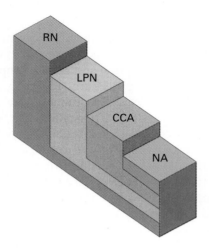

FIGURE 17-3 Scope of practice boundaries of the RN, LPN, and CCA.

RN. Can you think of a patient problem that would require a nurse rather than a clinical assistant to administer an enema? One example is a patient who has abnormal heart rate and rhythm and who is being monitored by telemetry. The enema may cause changes in cardiac status, and the nurse would need to assess the heart rate and rhythm throughout the procedure. The nurse would need to interpret the cardiac status by watching the monitor while administering the enema. There are many other patient situations that affect the nurse's decision to delegate this task. Most important, the nurse needs to assess the patient's status, the task, the need for problem solving, and intervention beyond the clinical associate's scope of practice.

There is no state practice act for clinical associates. Clinical associates are delegated aspects of patient care based on the premise that the professional nurse supervises this care. Before delegating tasks, the nurse must evaluate the tasks to be performed, the clinical associate's competence, the associate's job description, and the patient's condition. The nurse's license permits the delegation of certain tasks to the clinical assistant based on the nurse's professional judgment. As discussed in Chapter 4, "Health Care Employment," in home care agencies and long-term care facilities, the title *nurse aide* is defined by federal statute. Therefore, the role limits of clinical assistants are developed through the combination of legal and professional regulation of nursing practice. In other words, the tasks, duties, and responsibilities of clinical assistants are determined by state law under the nurse practice act. It is the ANA's position that the RN determines the utilization of clinical assistants. It is also the ANA's position that the clinical assistant is to assist the RN in providing patient care. This is important for safe patient care.

How do you, as a clinical assistant, determine your scope of practice? Each clinical assistant is responsible for knowing the assistant's role limits and job expectations. Each must know the reporting supervisor who gives assignments. Finally, each must have the competence to perform assigned tasks safely. Become familiar with the policy and procedure manual of your organization, and refer to it when you are unsure. These manuals exist as reference information and a source of guidance. You are not expected to know all the answers, but you are expected to know where to find the answers you seek. It is irresponsible and dangerous to perform any task with which you are unfamiliar that is delegated by the nurse.

Although the RN is responsible ultimately for patient care delivery, it is your responsibility as a clinical assistant to perform any task listed in your job description according to policy and procedure. It is not the nurse's responsibility if you perform delegated tasks negligently. You are responsible for your actions. You, the clinical assistant, must identify your own personal limitations and abilities. You must seek guidance and assistance when unsure or unfamiliar with any aspect of your job. Never hesitate to admit that to perform a skill safely, you might need assistance or guidance. Never try to conceal your uncertainty, and never permit a lack of knowledge and skill to jeopardize safe practice. Ask for help, read, and learn the knowledge and skills that are expected of you.

Deciding When to Delegate

In deciding when to delegate care tasks, there are factors that must always be considered. These factors are

- Potential for harm
- Complexity of the task
- Problem solving and innovation required
- Unpredictability of outcome
- Level of interaction required with patient

Think of an example of how a decision to delegate or not to delegate should be solved. Review the following scenario, and use the chart in Table 17-1 to determine the risk factors involved in delegating the patient care tasks.

Consider the five factors in column 1 of Table 17-1 in combination with each patient. Score each risk factor on a scale of 0 to 3 (0 = none, 1 = low, 2 = moderate, 3 = high). The higher the score, the less likely the task should be delegated to you. Score each factor separately. Then add them together for a total score for each patient.

For which of the patients should the nurse delegate to you the task of administering the tube feeding?

You are working as a clinical assistant on a surgical unit in a university hospital. In this hospital, you are permitted to administer gastrostomy tube feedings with the use of an IVAC pump that controls the rate of infusion of the feeding. You were taught to perform this procedure, and you have demonstrated your competence with this procedure on numerous patients. The RN that you are assisting is familiar with the quality of your work and trusts you and your ability to perform this procedure. Today, there are two patients on your unit who will need Peg (gastrostomy tube) feedings.

Patient 1: Mrs. Frost was admitted to your unit 5 days ago, and she has had a Peg tube in place for 3 years. When she is at home, she does her tube feedings by herself. Yesterday, you administered her tube feedings, and no unusual events occurred.

Patient 2: Mrs. Haley was admitted to your unit last night after surgery to insert a Peg tube. This morning she is to receive her first tube feeding.

The potential for harm, problem solving required, unpredictability of outcome, and level of interaction required with Mrs. Frost are much lower than with Mrs. Haley. The task is no more complex with either patient, but the response of the patient and the problem solving necessary are key factors in this delegation decision. Mrs. Frost knows this procedure and performs it independently. Mrs. Haley has never had a gastrostomy tube feeding, and she will need

TABLE 17-1 Delegation: Determining Risk Factors

Factor	Mrs. Frost	Mrs. Haley
Potential for harm		
Complexity of the task		
Problem solving and innovation necessary		
Unpredictability of outcome		
Level of interaction required with patient		
Total Score		

teaching. Therefore, the level of interaction required with Mrs. Haley will be high.

The nurse assigns you to do the tube feedings for both patients. She indicates that she is very busy with a fresh post-op patient and that she really needs your help. The nurse also says that she knows you can do it, and in addition she will be available if any problems arise. However, you do not feel comfortable with the idea of doing the tube feeding for Mrs. Haley.

■ What rationale will you use when you explain to the nurse what you feel you can and can't do?

■ What are your options in this situation?

■ What are your concerns?

You should tell the nurse that you do not feel that it would be safe for you to administer Mrs. Haley's tube feeding. Describe your rationale based on the combination of factors discussed above. Since the nurse is so busy with other patients, ask if there is anything else that you could do to assist. You should be concerned about Mrs. Haley's emotional response to the presence of a Peg tube and her physical response to the first tube feeding. You should also be concerned about the teaching that Mrs. Haley needs at this time. You should not administer the tube feeding, and you should present your position to the nurse based on your mutual concern for the safety of this patient. It would not be ethical to perform a procedure that you know requires more knowledge, skill, and problem-solving ability than you have to offer. The patient's well-being should be foremost to you and the nurse.

Licensure

Licensure refers to the granting of licenses, especially to practice a profession. It is assumed that the person who holds the license is trustworthy, has met certain educational requirements, and through examination has demonstrated competence to possess that particular license. Through licensure, RNs are permitted to perform procedures and planned patient care that LPNs are not permitted to perform. Sometimes, you will hear people say that a particular LPN is better than some RNs and should be permitted to function as an RN. The important element here is licensure. The LPN may be highly competent and knowledgeable but cannot operate outside the LPN's scope of practice. To function as an RN, the LPN needs to meet the same educational requirements and pass the same state boards as the RN. The same is true of the clinical assistant. Some clinical assistants will be mentally and physically capable of learning and performing tasks that an RN or LPN performs. However, practicing beyond one's scope of practice—without the proper educational credentials and the license—is not legal or safe. The American Nurses Association has stated very clearly its position on the use of unlicensed personnel. The ANA's position is based on the concepts described earlier.

The problems encountered by clinical assistants are narrower in scope than those faced by licensed practitioners because the assistant's scope of practice is not as broad. Therefore, the problem solving required of a CCA is on a smaller scale than that required of a nurse. This is not to say, however, that the CCA's problem solving is not valuable. Remember, the problem-solving method is utilized at the level of the assistant's scope of practice.

Fundamentals of Patient Care

An analysis of the fundamentals of teamwork, effective communication, delegation, and collaboration will help to provide a framework for a cooperative approach for working with other team members and will introduce you to standards of professional behavior in the workplace. Your understanding of patient's rights and the assurance of these rights is essential to the development of competent safe practice attributes. The ethical principles reviewed in this chapter will guide your actions and your purpose in doing what is best for the patient. You will develop a greater appreciation for the behavior that reflects a belief in the individual worth of all people.

Ethics

Keep in mind the *golden rule*: Do unto others as you would have them do unto you. This saying is one fundamental that most people hold as a truth in their belief system about human relations. People do not always abide by this rule when they interpret it to mean "do to others as they *do* to you." Think of a time when you stopped treating someone with respect because he or she stopped treating you respectfully. How did you feel about yourself after you broke the golden rule? Did you feel justified and proud of yourself, or did you struggle emotionally with your actions because you did not behave in a manner that you would have expected of yourself or others would have expected of you?

The term **ethics** refers to a moral code and standards of conduct that guide the behavior of people in a particular profession. Medical ethics guide the actions of people who work in health care. These standards of conduct are not necessarily dictated by a law but are established by a professional group as the code of behavior that is expected of everyone who works in a particular field. Think of the behavior that

you expect of a police officer, a lawyer, or a priest. There are certain standards that you expect of a priest that you do not expect of a police officer or a doctor. If you heard that a priest violated the confidentiality of a person who came to him seeking absolution, you would question the ethics of this behavior. People know and believe that a priest would not violate the confidentiality of someone who confesses a sin, even if this sin were a crime—even murder. Everything told to a priest in confession is protected by the confidentiality of the priest, and the priest is not expected, even by law, to report a confession of a crime to the police. Journalists hold as a basic truth of their profession the right to protect the confidentiality of their sources of information for stories that are published in newspapers. Once again, the law protects the confidentiality of the source of information for the journalist. The ethical code of the medical profession does include confidentiality, but this patient right is applied differently under the law.

The Issue of Confidentiality

Consider the issue of confidentiality in the following situation. A woman goes to confession and tells her parish priest that she wants forgiveness for a sin. She explains that she has beaten her son and that she is sorry for this. The priest counsels the woman. Will he contact the protective services agency to report child abuse? The woman's next-door neighbor contacts the local newspaper and asks to talk anonymously to a journalist who is doing a report on child abusers. The journalist prints the story, which describes the behavior that the neighbor has witnessed at the woman's house. The police ask the journalist to help them in a case connected with this newspaper article. Will the reporter reveal the name of his source? One day, the neighbor is baby-sitting for the son, and she sees bruises on the child and notices that he is limping. She brings the child to the emergency room (ER), and the mother is called to the ER to give permission for treatment of her son. The nurse in the ER suspects child abuse because of the child's current injuries and evidence of old injuries on the radiology reports. The neighbor says to the nurse, "Please don't tell anybody, but I have seen this child beaten by his mother." What will the nurse do? Table 17-2 addresses issues of confidentiality and responsibility in this situation.

Basic Ethical Principles

In medicine and health care, there are some basic ethical principles that guide behavior. These include

■ **Beneficence**—the assumption that the professional training and judgment of health care

TABLE 17-2   Issues of Confidentiality and Responsibility

Issue	Responsible Person
1. In this situation, who is obligated by law to report the case of suspected abuse to the authorities?	The nurse.
2. Who is protected under the law by his or her code of ethics for not reporting the abuse?	The priest.
3. Whose confidentiality is protected by the priest, and whose confidentiality is protected by the journalist?	The confidentiality of the mother in confession is protected by the priest. The journalist's source of information (the neighbor) is protected by the journalist.
4. Why must the nurse report this suspected abuse?	The nurse is ethically and legally responsible for reporting any suspected child abuse. All suspected child abuse must be reported by nurses, physicians, health care professionals, and teachers.
5. Doesn't the nurse have to respect the right of confidentiality?	The nurse should not discuss this case or any other case with those who are not involved in the care of this child. However, the local department of youth services legally must become involved in this case.
6. How do the ethical standards of the priest, the journalist, and the nurse differ?	Each person is guided by a different code of ethics for his or her profession.
7. Is there a code of ethics for neighbors? Why or why not? What do you expect as a moral code for neighbors?	There is no code of ethics for neighbors. Most people expect that their neighbors will not inflict harm on them or their property. Most people expect neighbors to "mind their own business." This neighbor was witness to the child's injuries, and the mother entrusted the neighbor with the responsibility of caring for her son. The neighbor felt that the child could not be protected from the abuse. Being a neighbor is not a "profession"; therefore, there is no code of ethics. Each of us has a unique expectation and relationship with different neighbors.

professionals will direct them to act in the best interests of the patient because they know what is good for the patient. Decisions about patient treatment are made in an objective manner, and the results will produce greater good than harm.

- **Respect for autonomy**—the assumption that it is of the utmost importance to act in accordance with the values and beliefs of the patient. Decisions are made based on the patient's individual preferences.
- **Justice**—the assumption that by the distribution of costs and benefits to the individual, family, and society, fairness and equity will be achieved.
- **Nonmaleficence**—the assumption that health care professionals will not knowingly act in a manner that is harmful to the patient.

Many situations in health care generate ethical dilemmas requiring the careful consideration of the patient, family, and health care team. These four ethical principles must be employed in determining the course of action in situations that present ethical dilemmas.

Ethical Dilemmas for Consideration

1. Your son is ill and asks you to stay home with him instead of having the baby-sitter care for him. Two clinical assistants have resigned in the past two weeks, and the unit is short-staffed already.

   This is a difficult situation for you. You must weigh your son's needs, and you should discuss the situation honestly with your supervisor. Your supervisor's response to your request for the day off, the ability of your baby-sitter to handle your son's illness, and the nature of his illness all need to be considered.

2. Your client is terminally ill and an atheist. You do not relate to this philosophy. What are your ethical boundaries?

It is the autonomy of your client that is most important in this situation. Each person has the right to choose his or her own beliefs. You cannot impose your beliefs on your clients. It is your ethical duty to respect this client's personal beliefs.

Table 17-3 presents two patient cases and describes the ethical fundamentals involved. Consider each case, and discuss the ethical fundamentals involved with your classmates.

In many ethical dilemmas, there are no right or wrong answers. That is why they are dilemmas.

These types of situations prompt questions and debates among professionals who understand ethical principles. These professionals try to balance the importance of each principle.

Most health care institutions have an **ethics committee**. This committee is consulted when these ethical dilemmas arise. Sometimes, the ethics committee is consulted because of a dilemma that involves patients, families, and staff. The committee helps the parties to weigh the benefits and the risks for the individual, for the family and also for the greater good of society. There is often no absolute or correct answer to these dilemmas. There are many other ethical principles that are employed by individuals who have studied ethics that are not discussed in

---

TABLE 17-3   Ethical Fundamentals

Case 1	Respect for Autonomy
A ninety-year-old woman who lives in a nursing home is unsteady on her feet. The nurse decides that restraints are necessary to prevent against injuries sustained from falling. The resident does not want to be restrained. She understands the risk of falling if she walks without assistance, but she wants the freedom to get up and walk around. She doesn't want to be "tied down."	The ethical principle involved in this situation is respect for the resident's autonomy. She is able to identify her risk of falling, and in any health care facility, the resident, client, or patient has the right to be free from restraints. It is the nurse's assumption of beneficence that motivates the use of restraints. Restraints do not prevent people from falling. In fact, there is a higher incidence of injury associated with the use of restraints for people who are at risk of falling. It has been proven that people do fall more frequently without restraints, but the injuries they suffer are less severe than those of people who are restrained and fall. The use of restraints is associated with more significant emotional and physical harm than not using restraints. A plan of care should be established to promote this resident's autonomy and the beneficent actions of the nurse. The resident should be ensured the freedom to move about the nursing home with assistance at specific times of the day.
Case 2	Nonmaleficence and Autonomy
A newborn infant is born with severe impairments. He is blind and deaf and has brain, heart, and other vital organ defects. The parents have been told that he will be profoundly mentally retarded and will probably need to be on a respirator for as long as he lives. The infant must be fed via a tube because of abnormal gastrointestinal (GI) organ development. Each time the infant is fed, it is stressful for him because of the pain of inserting a feeding tube and the vomiting that results. Even with the respirator, the doctors cannot predict that the infant will live. The parents have decided to withhold feeding, but the nursing staff is uncomfortable with their decision.	The ethical principles involved in this situation are nonmaleficence and autonomy. While the nurses know that withholding feeding means that the infant will ultimately die, they also realize that each feeding causes the infant pain and discomfort. Furthermore, the feedings may not save the infant's life. The nurses also know that it is the parents who must decide autonomously the care that their infant receives. It is not easy to weigh the "quality of life" issue based on the infant's potential for survival, his mental status, and the need to live on a respirator. Some people may also consider the issue of justice. For example, the cost of maintaining life "at all costs" without consideration of the care that may be denied to others is an issue of fairness. Other patients may need life-saving measures but may not be able to afford the cost of such measures.

this unit. The discussion of ethical principles and dilemmas continues in Chapter 20, "Care Delivery for the Dying Patient."

Why is it important for the health care assistant to employ a high standard of conduct or ethical behavior? When you are entrusted with the responsibility of providing care for other human beings, you must understand and appreciate the trust that others place in your sense of ethical behavior. You are expected to employ more than the golden rule; you are expected to act in the best interests of your patients. You are expected not only to do what is generally considered beneficent, but also to consider the wishes of the individuals for whom you provide care. You are given the great privilege and responsibility of "caring." This privilege should not be casually based on your personal beliefs, but it should be based on an awareness of the principles of ethics that guide your actions in the responsibility of caring for others.

Teamwork

A health care team can be equated to a wheel. The client is the hub, and the professionals are the spokes. Note that a wheel is circular. Where does it begin or end? The circular nature of the wheel represents continuity of care and continuous motion as the client moves to a positive health goal. Each spoke of the wheel strengthens the wheel and balances the circular structure. Each spoke must be equal in length, just as each member of the team must contribute equally in the provision of continuity of care (Figure 17-4); this is what **teamwork** means. Each member contributes uniquely to this continuity. How does the clinical assistant contribute to this team?

The Role of the Clinical Assistant

The clinical assistant is a vital member of the health care team. As an assistant in the care of patients, you should be ready to contribute your part in providing care. Each member of the team should be prepared to do her or his part in ensuring quality care and excellent service to the people who come to your facility for treatment. Every member of the team should appreciate the commitment and contribution of every other member.

Imagine a foundation of a high-rise building. If the foundation is built on sand, then the structure will not withstand the pressures of the environment or the weight of the building. The structure will fall. The clinical care associate is often a team member who contributes a foundation to the team for the provision of patient care. Relationships, including

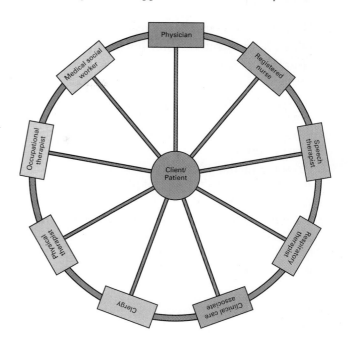

FIGURE 17-4 Teamwork model.

professional ones, require a strong foundation to withstand the pressures of health care delivery and the weight of responsibility.

The foundation of teamwork includes the five Cs: **collaboration, contribution, communication, cooperation,** and **commitment.** Working as a team means that each member of the team works together to get the job done. It is the responsibility of each team member to communicate to one another the needs and goals of the team and of the individual team members. Teams collaborate on the strategies and role responsibilities needed to achieve their goals. Members cooperate with one another by contributing their best efforts to accomplish the team's goals. Finally, they make a commitment to help one another meet the goals. It is the respect for the foundation of teamwork that builds a team among people who work together. People can work in the same institution on the same patient care unit and never form a team because they do not value teamwork or do not value the team members. In health care, it takes many workers to provide patient care. Even though people may feel that they are working alone, they are not. Other staff members are participating and contributing to patient care.

Since most people think of sports when they think of teams, consider your answers to the following questions about sports teams, and then discuss them with your team of classmates. Choose a team sport that you have watched or that you have played. Whatever the sport, the team's goal is usually winning the game, isn't it?

- How does the team accomplish this goal?
- Which team members contribute?
- How do the team players communicate with one another?
- What behaviors of the players show you their collaboration?
- How do the players cooperate with one another to score points?
- Do some members contribute more than others at times during the course of play?
- Who leads the team?
- How does the coach contribute, communicate, collaborate, and cooperate to achieve the committed goal of the team to win?
- What do team members do when other team members score points?

Discuss each of these questions with a classmate.

Now contrast your answers to these questions with the answers provided by another health care team member. What are the similarities and differences between a sports team and a health care team?

Most of the time, health care team members do not praise or high-five one another for a job well done, but when they *are* praised or recognized, they feel special and valued for their contribution. Often, some team members are so self-absorbed with their need for recognition for the team's efforts that they fail to see and appreciate the contributions of the other team members. In health care, team members are confronted with life-and-death issues, not scoring points. Health care is serious work aimed at achieving one goal: a positive patient outcome. When patients are discharged or make improvements, team members should reflect on this achievement and praise the patient and themselves. People may not tell you that you are doing a good job because nobody (including you) tells them that they are doing a good job. Try telling one person today that you appreciate the contribution he or she made for the "team." You might find that somebody tells you the same thing.

Remember, team building takes acceptance and trust among team members. Each member of the team must share in accomplishing team goals. When the goal is achieved, the team provides quality care to the patients.

Teamwork also involves knowing when and how to lead and when and how to follow. What are some situations in which a clinical associate leads? List some areas in which a clinical associate follows. Clinical associates lead when they identify patient needs and when they help other team members with the work of the team. The clinical associate may also lead by demonstrating emotional maturity and sensitivity to the needs of other team members. When you pitch in to help someone, you lead. When you help a new clinical associate in orientation, you lead. You follow when you accept the direction and constructive feedback of team members. You follow when you are directed by the nurse to perform planned patient care activities.

Consider the following scenarios and responses:

1. A new clinical assistant arrives on the floor and has completed orientation. You detect a hesitancy on her part to execute certain skills. Using the concept of teamwork, what could you do to lead in this situation?

   You should take the time to ask the assistant if she has performed these skills before or if she has reviewed the policy and procedure of the institution. You could also help the new clinical assistant to find the needed materials and show her any supplies that may be different in your facility. You could also ask the nurse to talk with the clinical assistant about the differences between procedures and equipment in this institution and the assistant's previous institution.

2. As a senior clinical assistant on the floor, you are frequently asked to perform leadership tasks. What could you do to demonstrate your leadership?

   You should always follow the plan of care and inform the nurse of problems that prevent you from doing so. You could ask other assistants and nurses how to do tasks in a more efficient way. You could ask for help when you need it, and you could accept constructive feedback to improve your skills and abilities.

Basing your work on the concept of teamwork, construct a daily assignment sheet using the following data:

A staff of 3 clinical assistants, one of whom is new to the floor

32 clients in a skilled nursing facility (SNF)

16 complete baths in a Century Tub

 8 showers with full assist

 8 showers with partial assist

 8 sets of vital signs

16 complete feeds

 8 feeds with supervision

 8 intake-and-output (I&O) reports

The three clinical associates should consult with the team leader to determine the specific needs of each resident of the SNF. You could work in pairs to care for residents in the tub and shower. It may be easier if you work in pairs to accomplish these tasks.

It might seem fair to say that each assistant will provide care to ten to eleven residents. However, the acuity and needs of each resident are unique; therefore, an equal number of residents per assistant may not mean an equal workload. The physical ability of each assistant to move and to transfer residents requires consideration. The physical layout of the SNF and the unique resident needs, wishes, routines, and schedules should help the three clinical assistants in determining a team plan of action. Foremost in this process of assignment is following the direction of the team leader. The leader of the team should make the assignments for the three clinical care associates. The associates can then assist one another to complete the assigned duties. The main idea here is to provide each resident with the best possible care. As a true team, you would work together to complete all necessary provisions of care.

Communication

Communication is a complex process that involves verbal and nonverbal messages. Verbal messages include not only the words spoken, but also voice tone. Medical terminology is needed in communicating with other professionals in the medical field. However, clients and their families often do not understand the vocabulary of the medical world. It is vital to consider the message and to whom the message is being given.

Verbal messages are communicated in spoken language, either face-to-face or via the telephone (Figure 17-5). Written language is another form of verbal communication. When we communicate in writing or by the telephone, the nonverbal aspect of communication is unavailable. As you read this textbook, you are unaware of the authors' facial expressions, body language, and so forth. The same is true when you communicate through the phone or computer e-mail. While the sender of the message chooses the words, style of writing, and word emphasis by boldfacing or capitalizing text to carefully create an emotional tone for the receiver of the message, the receiver's response cannot be read by the sender. The telephone provides some nonverbal clues to the emotional tone of the people communicating. It does not afford the opportunity to see the outward expressions conveyed in face-to-face dialogue.

Consider a time when you wanted to deliver a message to someone, but you were uncomfortable facing the person. Most probably, you wrote a letter, sent e-mail, or telephoned the person involved. It was easier to avoid witnessing the person's physical reaction to the message and to disguise your emotional tone, which would be conveyed in your nonverbal behaviors. Nonverbal behaviors are more revealing; they are "the picture worth a thousand words."

Nonverbal messages represent a larger segment of communication than verbal messages (Figure 17-6). These include

- Appearance
- Professional image
- Body language
- Eye contact
- Facial expressions
- Physical distance or personal space
- Touch

Touch, distance, and eye contact can be affected by one's culture. In some cultures, people are comfortable touching one another, standing close to one another while speaking, and making direct eye contact. The nature of the relationship also affects the level of comfort with these nonverbal behaviors. Have you ever observed people in conversation but not been able to hear their words or understand

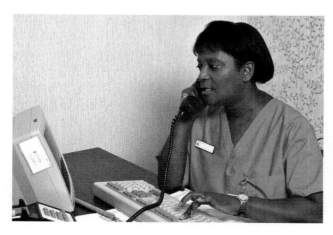

FIGURE 17-5   Example of verbal communication.

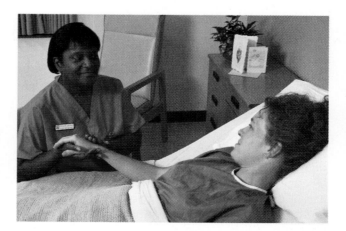

FIGURE 17-6   Example of nonverbal communication.

their language? Through nonverbal responses, however, you might have been able to assimilate the nature of the conversation or even the relationship!

Boundaries, territorial space, and touch are used unconsciously between people in the act of communicating. These are related to the sense of safety and comfort between the people involved in dialogue and the message that is being communicated. Consider the distance that is comfortable for you when you speak with your spouse, mother, friend, stranger, and coworker. Is it different depending on the person? Whom do you feel comfortable touching when engaged in conversation?

Imagine a depressed patient who says softly, "Don't touch me." Now imagine a patient who yells, "Get away from me! Don't touch me! I'll scream if you come near me!" Which one has told you that touching is inappropriate? Well, you should assume that neither wants to be touched, but the second patient is definitely sending you the message to stay away. While you may not touch either patient, the second patient is clearly stating that touch is a threat. You touch patients all the time as you perform your work. Patients are aware of the way you feel about them and the task you are performing with them based on the way you touch. They can tell when you are in a hurry, when you are concerned about their feelings, and so forth.

Perhaps you have not thought about the importance of touch in your daily work as an assistant. It is important to recognize when to touch and when not to touch. What are some nonverbal cues that let you know when a patient needs a hug, wants a hand held, or is afraid of being touched?

The ability to make and maintain eye contact is a vital component in communication. Sometimes, it is the singular act of making eye contact that sends a message. Remember how a parent or teacher could let you know that you were displeasing them with a single glance? Some people avoid eye contact; others seem to have such intense and prolonged eye contact that they stare. Both situations are extreme. How do you feel when someone speaks to you but doesn't look at you?

Eye contact, or its avoidance, is sometimes controlled consciously. Consider what you do with your eyes when you are on a bus, in an elevator, or walking down the street. Think about what you do with your eyes when you want to get someone's attention. People who use a wheelchair to travel often feel that others forget about making eye contact with them. They stand over the wheelchair, which creates inequality in the conversation and puts both individuals at a disadvantage. The person sitting must look up to the other person, which puts him or her in an inferior position and places the one standing in a position of authority.

Children are usually in the position of having to look up to adults to communicate with them. This intensifies the feeling of the adult as an authority. At times, it makes children feel vulnerable. When you really want to get your point across to a child, you either sit or squat to get their attention and to let them know that they have yours. Often, patients are sitting in a chair or lying in bed when we communicate with them. Sometimes, patients report that physicians stand at the foot of the bed to ask how they feel or to give them important information about their condition. They perceive the doctor as an authority figure who is in such a hurry that to sit down at eye level and communicate is unnecessary. When you feed patients, do you stand over them, or do you sit down at eye level? The position you choose as you feed someone affects the patient's satisfaction with the meal. You may have many patients to feed at mealtime, but it doesn't take any longer to sit and feed a patient than it does to stand. Both you and the patient will benefit from this experience. The patient won't feel that you are in a hurry. The patient can enjoy the food, and you can rest your weary feet. Most important, it will improve your relationship with this person.

Communication Role Play   To get some personal experience, set time aside to complete the following role play with two other classmates. Then discuss the feelings you experienced.

- Feed two classmates. Stand to feed one; sit to feed the other.
- Let two classmates take turns feeding you. One stands to feed you; the other sits and faces you while you are being fed.

Discuss your feelings about this role play. How did you feel about the food each time you were fed? How did you feel about the communication between you and the person you fed and between you and the two people who fed you?

Posture and stance speak for themselves. Slouched posture, crossed arms, clenched fists, and outstretched arms all tell you something about how the person feels regarding the message being communicated. Observe the body language of others as you communicate today.

- Do some people gesture with their hands frequently? Do others communicate with little movement?
- Do some people shake a foot or a crossed leg as they speak or listen to others?
- Do you notice that some people pace frequently, whereas others rarely move about?

Read and then discuss the scenario, "First Encounter," with a classmate. As you read the scenario,

SCENARIO First Encounter

The clinical care assistant enters the room clad in a dirty, wrinkled uniform. You can't see well, but you can see her printed underwear through the expanse of her tight pants. She is bejeweled in twenty gold chains that dangle from her neck. She bends over to talk loudly in your diseased ears, and you feel nauseated. You are not sure if it is the strong, pungent scent of her cologne mixed with sweat or her breath, which reminds you of your poor dog, Winston. You wonder if she has ever flossed her teeth. Her long red claws tell you that bath time won't be much fun. You wonder how particular she will be with *your* hygiene. You suddenly feel embarrassed and resistant to endure your personal care, and all the time you wonder why she doesn't introduce herself. You suppose she'll call you "Dearie." She doesn't tell you what she's doing next. You guess she's fed up with you because you can't hear well. Suddenly, you are reminded of a former experience in which you were mistreated, and you panic and fight back. What would you do?

the message from entering at all or misinterpret the communication. Other emotional barriers to communication are depression, euphoria, distrust, anger, impatience, and shame.

To enhance the reception of communication, it is important to provide an environment that reduces emotional barriers and adjusts to the physical and mental barriers encountered. Consider the following case of Mr. Levin, and identify the barriers to effective communication:

Mr. Levin is an eighty-six-year-old CVA client who is slightly hard-of-hearing (HOH). He is new to your SNF. Assistance with activities of daily living (ADLs) is difficult because he fights the nursing staff. His family states that ever since he fell and fractured his hip two years ago, he has been agitated, resistant, and defiant in the A.M. care and transfers. What are the physical barriers to communication in this case? The mental barriers? The emotional ones?

imagine you are a resident in a nursing home encountering a clinical assistant for the first time. As you discuss "First Encounter" with a classmate, share your responses to the clinical assistant's behavior, dress, hygiene, and treatment of the resident.

Remember, health care workers should practice good hygiene daily and use nonscented deodorants out of respect for patients. A soft voice and an unhurried manner are beneficial to patients. It gives the impression of orderliness and safety, which can be reassuring to patients.

Barriers to Communication and Ways to Overcome Them Barriers to effective communication—sending and receiving messages—can be *physical*, *mental*, or *emotional*. Physical barriers to communication include hearing impairment, impaired vision, and language (your native language, which the listener doesn't understand, or the speaker's foreign language, which you don't understand). There are many other barriers; these are some common communication barriers.

Mental barriers to communication include receptive aphasia resulting from a cerebral vascular accident (CVA). Some other mental barriers include confusion, distorted patterns of speech or thought, and lack of knowledge or understanding of the subject.

Emotional barriers to communication pose the largest problem. Emotional barriers are often hard to identify, and sometimes the environment in which the message is communicated actually triggers the barrier. Fear is one emotional barrier. In the presence of fear, some clients close down and prohibit

Mr. Levin is hard-of-hearing; this is the physical barrier. Mr. Levin may not be able to understand everything that you tell him because of his CVA; this could be a mental barrier to communication. Another mental barrier is that Mr. Levin is new to the SNF, and he does not know the staff and the routine of the facility. Mr. Levin's emotional barriers may include his fear of falling and the assistants' fear of his emotional agitation and resistance. When you and other assistants approach Mr. Levin, you may be expecting his resistance and agitated behavior, and you may be responding defensively to this. You may not be considerate of his hearing, speech, and physical disabilities, which make the world a frightening place for Mr. Levin.

Techniques for improving communication include using "I" messages when expressing feelings about a message, standing directly in front of the person, speaking slowly and distinctly, asking for feedback, and repeating the message from the receiver. "I" messages state what you feel and think. "I" messages do not tell the other person what you think he or she is saying. These "I" messages communicate what you think or feel about the verbal and nonverbal messages to which you are responding. "I" messages allow you to communicate what you think you heard and what you feel in response to the communication. These "I" messages do not threaten or elicit defensive reactions from the other party in the communication sequence. Examples of "I" messages follow:

"I think I heard you say . . . "

"When I heard . . . "

"I felt . . . "

Practice using "I" messages and other methods of improving communication with a lab partner. As you practice using "I" messages, remember that the purpose of "I" messages is to communicate what you feel and perceive. When you say, "I feel this way because . . .," it is different from saying, "You make me feel . . . " "I" messages simply state what you feel, think, and perceive. These messages do not imply the other person's intent, but the way the person's communication style affects you.

Collaboration

Collaboration in health care is vital to a holistic approach to quality care. Look carefully at the word *collaboration*. In it is the word *labor*. *Collaboration* comes from Latin and means "working or laboring together" (Figure 17-7). It is important to understand the concept of working together for the good of all.

Later in this book, you will learn about the therapeutic, or professional, relationship and how this relationship differs from friendship. Sometimes, there are stumbling blocks to working together. Time is one factor. Other stumbling blocks to collaboration are

- Lack of teamwork
- No sense of empowerment to voice ideas
- Unequal contribution of team members

At times, you will work with people whose personality style challenges you. Working with a person whose style of communication is challenging for you is probably one of the hardest barriers to collaboration to overcome. However, this should not deter you from working as part of a team. Each of us has a unique personality style. There are personality styles that you find comfortable and can accept easily in an individual, and there are others that are a challenge for you. Your personality also presents people with a level of comfort and challenge. It is important to distinguish between a "difficult" personality style that affects you personally and a "difficult" style or behavior that is unacceptable and inappropriate for a given situation. Is it just that you don't like the person, or is it that the person is using mechanisms that manipulate you and others on the team? When we work in collaborative relationships, we have to learn to work together, regardless of differences in style. Actually, different personality styles can enhance the team's work if we take the time to consider how each team member can best contribute to the team. When we learn to use our differences to balance the efforts of the team, we collaborate successfully.

A personality inventory can be used by your instructor to help you and others in your class to learn more about different styles and how to manage conflicts due to similar or opposite styles. You must keep in mind that a personality style is not right or wrong; what's important is how we use our style in our interactions with others. Regardless of style differences, a team must be able to communicate and collaborate to labor together.

Collaborative relationships imply that people in the relationship feel empowered. Feeling empowered means that you believe that your opinion matters, that your opinion or ideas are valued, that you have a position of authority, and that those in authority do not feel threatened or devalued by your empowerment.

Delegation

Delegation is the act of appointing certain tasks and duties to others (Figure 17-8). Delegation can occur *vertically* or *laterally*. Vertical delegation means that someone delegates a task to a person who possesses less authority. Lateral delegation means that someone delegates to a person of equal knowledge or authority. It is imperative to remember that when tasks or duties are delegated, the responsibility rests ultimately with the one who is delegating. The professional nurse delegates with this thought in mind, and as a clinical assistant, you should recognize and respect this professional's responsibility. Therefore, as a clinical assistant, it is your responsibility to perform an assigned duty or task to the best of your ability, in a timely fashion, and in accordance with policy and procedure.

As a clinical assistant, you are

- Responsible and accountable for your actions and for reporting the completion of the task and the results

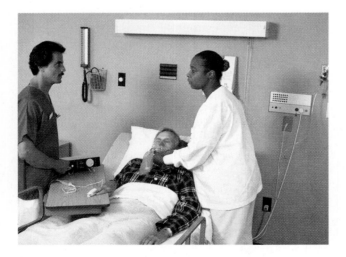

FIGURE 17-7   Collaboration.

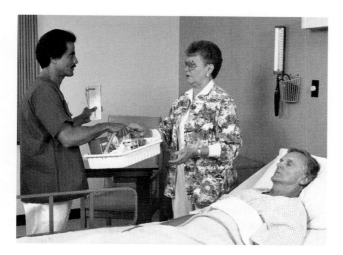

FIGURE 17-8   Delegation.

■ Responsible and accountable for the performance of any delegated tasks that are expected in your job performance

If a delegated duty or task falls outside your scope of practice as a clinical associate, what should you do? You should tell the nurse that the duty or task is not one that can be safely or legally performed by an assistant. Let the nurse who is delegating the task know that you are not rejecting the work and that you will gladly perform another task that is within your scope of practice.

If, as a clinical assistant, you are unable to perform a delegated task because the client refuses, tell the nurse that the patient refused. If you are unsure of any task, you should not perform it without further direction from the nurse, without reviewing the policy and procedure manual, or both.

The manner in which a nurse delegates tasks has an effect on clinical assistants, but this should not interfere with carrying out assigned duties in the best interests of the patients. If you feel uncomfortable with the manner in which the nurse delegates, you need to communicate this to the nurse in a constructive fashion. Use "I" messages to let the nurse know how you feel when you are uncomfortable with the delegation process. There will be times when you feel that the nurse delegates everything to you, even when it seems there is time for the nurse to do some of the delegated tasks. You may also feel that there are times when you are assigned tasks because the nurse is more comfortable delegating to you rather than to another assistant. It may seem that you do more work than the other assistants, and it feels unfair.

Nurses approach delegation in a variety of ways. Some ask, some plead, some direct, some order. Sometimes, all of these methods are used by a nurse, depending on the situation at hand. In the middle of a crisis, the nurse needs you to carry out orders and is focused on the crisis, not the delegation style. Nurses may not be comfortable delegating to others because they have difficulty asking for help or because they do not trust that the task will be performed adequately by the assistant. There are assistants who do not act with a sense of responsibility and accountability, and assistants who are disorganized and unable to prioritize tasks. Nurses fear delegating when they realize their ultimate responsibility for assuring the results of a procedure. Trust is a key factor in delegation. It takes time to build trust, and trust is built based on the ingredients of teamwork and honest communication. The personality styles of all the team members affect the issues involved in delegation. When nurses delegate, they often consider the person who is capable and the one who will carry out the assignment willingly, without resistance or complaints.

Delegation Conflicts   Imagine that Nurse Hakeem and Assistant Barrett work together in a SNF. It seems to Assistant Barrett that Nurse Hakeem does not trust her and is always checking up on her completion of assignments. Assistant Barrett considers herself a good worker who always completes assigned tasks carefully and efficiently. She has a habit of recording her vital signs (VS) results on her assignment sheet, which she carries in her uniform pocket. She sometimes forgets to document these on the clinical data sheet, and when Nurse Hakeem checks the data sheet for a blood pressure (BP) before administering blood pressure medication, she finds that the BP is not documented. Nurse Hakeem assumes that the assistant did not take the BP and retakes it herself. She learns in report that a patient had an elevated temperature that was not documented when she checked the clinical data sheet during rounds. Assistant Barrett and Nurse Hakeem are now in conflict. What events led to this conflict?

The two events that led to this conflict are given here:

1. Assistant Barrett failed to record VS results on the clinical data sheet.
2. Nurse Hakeem failed to communicate the need for Assistant Barrett to verbally report to her any abnormal VS results.

Nurse Hakeem did not discuss her issues with Assistant Barrett; instead, she conveyed a message of distrust and "checked up" on the assistant. Assistant Barrett did not communicate the distrust she sensed from the nurse and continued to record VS results on an assignment sheet rather than on the clinical data sheet.

■ How can the nurse and assistant resolve this conflict?

■ What will make Nurse Hakeem trust Assistant Barrett?

■ What will help the assistant believe that the nurse values her performance?

Nurse Hakeem and Assistant Barrett need to communicate their needs and feelings to one another. It is not fair to assume that someone knows how you feel. It is also important to communicate the parameters of a delegated task: "Come and tell me if the temperature is above or below . . ." When feelings of distrust are communicated between individuals, then faulty communication and expectations result. Nurse Hakeem and Assistant Barrett need to communicate their needs and feelings. They also need to communicate the positive aspects of their working relationship to one another. They need to let each other know what they value in one another.

Now imagine that Nurse Lewis has been a nurse for a year, and you have enjoyed working with him because he makes you and the other assistants feel useful and appreciated. He worked as an assistant while in nursing school. You have been working as an assistant for 10 years, and you know that some nurses do not seem to have the same attitude of respect for the assistant's role as Nurse Lewis does. He seems to understand how busy you are carrying out your assignments, and he tries to help with your patient care whenever he can. You notice that he often stays late to finish his work, calling doctors, writing progress notes, and doing other tasks that only an RN can do. At times, he answers patient call bells and performs tasks that he could delegate to one of the assistants sitting at the desk. You like that Nurse Lewis pitches in, and you don't want him to change this, but you have watched other new nurses who were like him burn out and leave the job. You feel that he could learn something from you about delegation.

■ How will you handle this situation?

■ Do you feel comfortable approaching Nurse Lewis with your observations of his delegation skills?

■ What will you tell him when he asks for your opinion about his ability to delegate effectively?

You should be honest with Nurse Lewis and tell him that you value his fairness and willingness to perform activities that assistants could do for him. Since you have 10 years of experience and have seen nurses come and go, you should share your life experiences with him. It is not easy to tell a professional nurse that you see ways in which he or she could improve their delegation skills. However, you are observing a process that you understand as an assistant in patient care, and this might benefit Nurse Lewis.

Be honest, and ask him if he wants you to help him analyze his delegation style.

Some nurses seem to request that you interrupt a patient's care to complete other tasks. Assistants often say, "I was called from my work in room 430 to put the patient in room 401 on the bedpan, when the nurse was closer to room 401."

What are some situations that might necessitate the nurse asking you to go to one room when you are in another? With a small group of clinical assistant classmates, make a complete list of possibilities.

■ Which of the possible situations seem fair to you as an individual? Which seem fair to the group as a whole?

■ How would you handle these situations?

■ Which situations seem unfair?

■ How would you handle these?

Remember that there are tasks that only the nurse can perform, and these are essential to patient care. The patient caseload necessitates nurses for multiple intravenous (IV) medications, physical assessments, dressing changes, communication with physicians, admissions and discharges, and multiple problems that require documentation. There will be days when the nurse cannot assist with baths and feedings because of these role requirements, and so it might feel as though you are alone in the care of the patients. The nurse may need to delegate as much as possible to manage the caseload of patients safely and efficiently.

As a learning experience, it would be valuable for clinical assistants to spend a day "shadowing" an RN. This would help strengthen their understanding the role of the professional nurse in delegating to others.

Patient-Centered Care

Patients have always been the reason for the existence of health care organizations. Old models of health care delivery always had the patient as the center of care. However, it was a very passive relationship. The health care team delivered care, and the patient entrusted the restoration of health and wellness to this team. Several factors caused the shift to the more active client involvement of the patient-focused model.

One factor was the demand for the patient to be informed and educated as a consumer. Patients enter the health care system with more education about disease, treatments, and health than before. In addition, studies have proven that recovery is better achieved when the patient plays an active role in goal setting, treatment, and care. However, the most critical factor in engaging the patient's participation in health and wellness has been cost containment. It has been recognized that a better way to approach health care is to focus on the prevention of illness and to use patient resources in the treatment and the cure of disease. Consumers, the health care industry, and the insurance companies all realize that services cannot be provided without regard to efficiency and the balance between quantity and quality. Health care institutions must operate in the same way that businesses are run. Consumers are the customers of the health care system just as they are the customers of the auto industry. Customers shop around for the best product at the best buy. In addition, they expect quality service from a dealer who meets their expectations and attends to their needs.

Insurance agencies, the third-party payers, have also told health care institutions what they expect and how much they will pay for provided services. Insurance agencies drove the concept of diagnostic related groups (DRGs) back in the late 1970s when health care costs escalated to uncontrolled heights. The formulation of DRGs occurred after careful examination of the trends in methods of treatment, diagnostic tests, and the management of care for specific diagnoses. The results were compiled, reasonable, necessary treatments were established, and cost guidelines for each diagnosis were compiled. Health care institutions now are reimbursed for services based on reasonable and customary measures according to these guidelines. Today, when entering a hospital, the patient, nurse, and physician can receive an outline of the expected care to be provided and reimbursed. This outline of care is called a *clinical pathway*. The expected tests, treatments, and days of patient care are predetermined. Also, the outcome of the treatment is predicted based on the study of the DRGs. An increasing number of pathways are used in patient care planning.

One emerging feature of the patient-centered model is the multiskilled worker. This worker is vital to the concept of efficient, consistent delivery. The multiskilled worker, or clinical assistant, can perform a variety of tasks, which might include basic bedside nursing care, phlebotomy, electrocardiograms (ECGs), respiratory treatments, and restorative care measures. The idea of the multiskilled worker arose in response to patient satisfaction surveys. These revealed the patient's request for fewer care providers—people with whom they were familiar—at the bedside. This decreased the number of health care workers entering the room to perform tests and treatments throughout the day. As a result, patients do not have to wait for technicians, and technicians do not spend needless time traveling to patients. Time wasted waiting for patients to become available is no longer an issue, and personnel are used efficiently.

Today, a service partner or associate typically provides the services of three individuals. Service associates usually clean the patient's room, transport the patient, and deliver the menus and meal trays. Before the reengineering of health care, there may have been three to six people who entered the patient's room to provide the services that one individual now provides. As a patient in a hospital, you encounter many individuals in the course of one hospital day, and limiting the number of unfamiliar people who enter your room is desirable. Seeing a familiar face enter your room feels much safer than encountering a number of unfamiliar faces.

Clients'/Patients' Rights

Clients'/patients' rights are vital, and they are protected by law. These rights are discussed here, along with the responsibilities that the patient has in the various circumstances of care.

Respect and Dignity

All individuals, regardless of personal characteristics and circumstances in life, are entitled to be treated with dignity and respect. Patients should be called by polite title and last name unless the patient requests otherwise. Young children, adolescents, and elders deserve the same respect and dignity. Age is not a deciding factor in the amount of respect that is given. In turn, the service partner should be treated with respect by patients. At times, people who are sick are unable to focus on anything except their own condition and fears. If you are treated disrespectfully by a patient or family member, you should try to find out what the issue is surrounding this situation. It is easiest to approach this by asking, "Is there something that I have done to upset you?" Avoid accusing the patient of being disrespectful. Rather, have the patient reflect on your question.

Patients of all cultures deserve dignity and respect. It is important to recognize that different cultures demonstrate respect and interest in others differently. Do not expect that everyone has the same set of personal or cultural values. The amount of eye contact, touching, and gesturing varies among cultures. You may not be aware that making direct eye contact with someone of a different culture makes them feel uncomfortable or uneasy with you. That is why it is important to ask if there is something that you have done rather than assume the patient is intentionally being disrespectful to you.

Hearing and vision problems can create difficulty in communicating respect and dignity. Do not yell or make facial expressions or gestures that demonstrate your frustration with language or communication barriers. Be aware of yourself at all times.

Privacy and Confidentiality

Patients have the right to privacy whether the door to their room is closed or open. You should knock before you enter the room. If the curtain is closed, find out if it is okay to open it to perform any task with the patient in the room. If you are assisting a patient to walk to the bathroom or go to another department, be sure that the patient is covered properly. When patients disrobe, the curtain should be closed. Read and follow the Guidelines to Protect Patient Privacy and Confidentiality presented here.

Guidelines: To Protect Patient Privacy and Confidentiality

1. Never expose a patient for others to see. If a doctor or nurse forgets to close the curtain and the patient is uncovered or exposed in any way, simply pull the curtain closed.

2. Never discuss a patient or a patient's condition with people who are not on the team caring for the patient. Do not talk about a patient on your unit with other hospital personnel. Patient information is to be shared *only* with staff who are directly involved in the patient's care.

3. Never discuss one patient with another. Explain that you want to respect the other patient's privacy and confidentiality if one patient asks questions about another.

4. Never talk about patients in public areas, even with treatment team members. Be sure that you cannot be overheard by patients, visitors, or other staff. Elevators and cafeterias are not appropriate places to discuss patient issues (Figure 17-9).

5. Never give out any patient information over the telephone.

6. Never leave a patient's chart unattended in another department or on the patient care unit. Be sure to give the chart to the appropriate person when you transport a patient with a chart. When you transport a patient back to the unit, put the chart in the appropriate place, or give it to the unit secretary or the patient's nurse.

7. Never give a patient's chart to people who come to the patient unit. Direct them to the unit secretary or to the nurse. Patients do have the right to read their chart. However, you should never hand the chart to the patient to read. If a patient asks to read the chart, inform the nurse, and arrangements can be made for the doctor to review it with the patient.

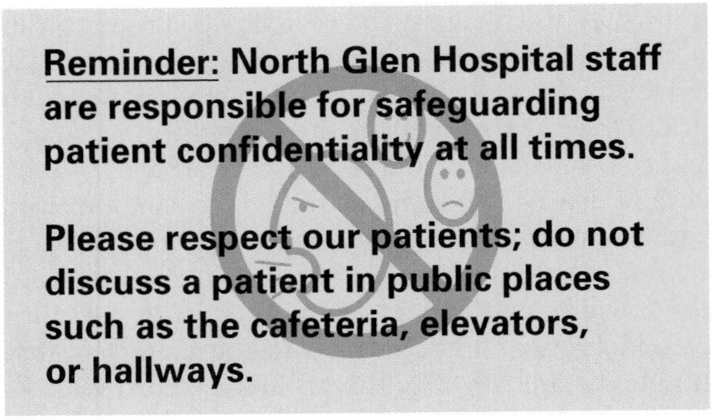

Reminder: North Glen Hospital staff are responsible for safeguarding patient confidentiality at all times.

Please respect our patients; do not discuss a patient in public places such as the cafeteria, elevators, or hallways.

FIGURE 17-9   Patient issues should not be discussed in public areas.

Identity

Patients should always know who you are and what your role is on the team (Figure 17-10). Wear your ID and name badge at all times. Always introduce yourself before executing any skill. Patients have the right to know the names and titles of everyone who is involved in their care.

Also, you must identify the patient correctly. Never perform any skill on a patient unless you have checked the patient's identification bracelet. If the patient does not have an identification bracelet, tell the nurse, have the patient correctly identified, and put an identification bracelet on the patient. Never refer to the patient as "the patient in room _____." Use both the patient's name and room number to decrease the chances of misidentifying the patient.

When the patient is a child or an adult who is confused, always identify yourself and call the patient by name to ensure proper identification. Even when patients are unconscious, tell them who you are and what you are doing with them.

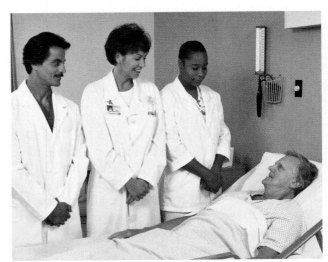

FIGURE 17-10   All personnel should wear visible ID badges. Notice that two of the staff members in this photo do not have visible identification.

Information

Patients have the right to explanations about conditions and treatments in language they can understand. You will not be explaining diagnoses or treatments, but you will have to provide information about tasks and procedures that you perform.

The patient must give permission to the doctor or nurse before family members or visitors are given any information about the patient. This is an issue of confidentiality.

When children or adolescents ask for information, tell them what you are permitted to discuss. If they ask questions about what you are doing with respect to your job responsibilities, you can discuss this with them. When children or teenagers ask you to explain what the doctor or nurse told them about their diagnosis or treatment, tell the doctor or nurse of this request. They will need to explain this again.

If you are asked to interpret for a patient who speaks a foreign language, you should do so in the presence of the doctor, nurse, or other person who asks you to interpret. Be sure to ask the patient if it is acceptable for you to interpret.

Communication

Patients have the right to communicate with others. Telephone and face-to-face communication with others is the patient's right, and you should not interfere with this. If you notice that a visitor is interfering with the patient's right to safety or communication or is threatening the patient in any way, you should report this to the nurse immediately.

Children and elders are most vulnerable to physical and emotional abuse. If you notice any person communicating with a patient in a way that is threatening or abusive or seems questionable, immediately inform the nurse. While it is the patient's right to communicate with others, it is your responsibility to protect the patient. Do not try to interfere. Quickly locate the nurse for swift professional intervention.

When patients speak a foreign language and require an interpreter, they should have one. If there are language barriers or physical disability barriers to communication, discuss this with the patient's nurse. Find out what measures can be taken to help to improve communication with the patient.

When you communicate with children, adolescents, young adults, or elders, remember to be respectful of their age and communicate in language that they understand and in a manner that is appropriate for their age. For example, you should not talk with an elder as though he or she were a child, and you should not talk with a person who speaks a different language as though he or she were stupid.

Consent

You should never touch a patient or perform any skill or procedure without the patient's consent. Do not assume that because the patient is part of the health care setting, consent is given for everything and anything. If you are going to perform or assist a patient with a task, ask the patient if this is okay. If you are to transport a patient for a test or treatment and the patient refuses, tell the nurse. You cannot force the patient to do anything.

If the patient does not want you to be the person who performs a certain task, ask for the reason and assure the patient that you will do your best to get someone else assigned by the nurse. Perhaps the nurse will want to talk with the patient about this concern.

Patients give permission by signing consent forms for tests, treatments, or operations. Consent forms are signed to receive blood or blood products and to have certain blood studies. You will not have to get these consents signed. You will not have to explain the surgical procedures, and so on. You may have to witness the patients' signing a consent form. Do this only if the nurse says that it is appropriate for you to witness the consent. Witnessing a consent means that you saw the person sign the form. It does not mean that you know if the patient understands what is being signed. You would simply witness that John Doe signed "John Doe" to the form.

Refusal of Treatment

As noted, the patient can refuse any treatment or medication or diagnostic test. The manner in which the refusal of treatment is managed is between the doctor and the patient or the patient's surrogate decision maker.

Consultation

Patients may want a second opinion or a consultation with another doctor. The patient and the doctor will arrange for consultation.

Transfer and Continuity of Care

Sometimes, patients are transferred to another facility for continued treatment. Often, patients are transferred from one inpatient unit to another. The patient has the right to know the reason for the transfer. The doctor and nurse usually explain these details. You may be responsible for escorting the patient to the new unit or for assisting ambulance transporters in preparing the patient for the transport. If a patient or family member wants to know more about the transfer and the other facility or patient unit, ask the nurse to answer these questions.

When patients are discharged from the hospital to home, they are given discharge instructions. Before you escort a patient to the discharge area, you should be sure that the patient has discharge instructions, his or her belongings, and any supplies or meds that were prescribed. The nurse should double-check any discharge instructions, meds, or supplies.

Hospital Charges

Patients have the right to know what things cost, what items are paid by insurance, and what items must be paid out-of-pocket. This is not information that you can provide. The nurse will call the appropriate department and have someone who can explain or can prepare a written document detailing financial responsibilities and charges.

Hospital Rules and Regulations

Patients have responsibilities, too! Hospital rules are in place for good reasons, and patients should be informed of the rules. Sometimes, there are restrictions on visitors, flowers, fresh fruit, and so on. There is a reason for these restrictions. Visitors should speak to the nurse or doctor about any restrictions so that explanations can be provided. **Contraband** (restricted items) is always prohibited. Patients with weapons, illegal drugs, or alcohol or patients who are smoking in their room should be reported immediately to the nurse.

Children and adolescents should have rules explained to them so that they will understand why they are not permitted to do certain things or why they can't have certain objects or foods. The nurse should discuss this with the children and their parents or guardians.

Collaborative Problem-Solving Exercises

Break into small groups to discuss the following cases. For each of the following situations, work with your group to determine the patients' right that is threatened or violated, and determine the acceptable actions that the service partner should take to manage the situation. Then, with your group, decide the answers to the additional exercises.

Case 1 Mary Jones and Iesha Mallory are care partners. Mary works on your patient care unit, and Iesha works on Ravdin 9. You are transporting a patient to radiology, and Mary and Iesha are on the elevator with you. Mary tells Iesha about patient Har-

vey Cytell, who has had testicular cancer and has had a testis surgically removed. You and the patient that you are transporting overhear this conversation. When you get off the elevator, the patient says, "I think the guy they were talking about is my next-door neighbor. I can't believe it! He is only twenty-five years old. I have to call my son and tell him about this."

Case 2 Frank Abdul is a fifteen-year-old whose family is from Iran. He speaks English well, but his parents speak limited English. The doctor talks to Frank Abdul and his parents about the need for surgery. Frank immediately refuses, and you hear him say, "You don't know what they are going to do to me. I refuse this surgery." His parents tell him, "Keep quiet in front of the doctor." Because this patient is a minor, his parents will sign a consent form for the surgery, and they will do this at the nurses' station. Frank is to be transported immediately to the operating room (OR), and you are to transport him on a stretcher. When you get to the room, Frank Abdul is in the bathroom and refuses to come out.

Case 3 Margaret McCullough is eighty-nine years old. She is always pleasant and friendly. She is hard-of-hearing, appears to be confused at times, and forgets her room number. She usually doesn't remember your first name. You observe Mrs. McCullough and another staff member performing a procedure in her room. The curtain is opened, and Mrs. McCullough's buttocks are exposed. The staff member is talking very loudly and telling the patient about the need to ring the call bell "when you need to use the toilet." The staff member also says, "Nobody wants to clean up this mess, Granny. It would be a lot easier on everyone, Honey, if you'd just use the call bell."

Additional Exercises Identify which of the following situations involve a violation of patient rights. Then identify what patient rights are being violated.

- The nurse asks the clinical care associate to put 549 on the bedpan. What's wrong with this?

    The patient has the right to be treated with dignity and respect—to be identified by name and not by room number.

- An eighteen-year-old female patient is newly admitted to your unit. Her name is Jane Samurai. You are to help the patient get settled into her room. What do you call this teenager? What right should you assure a patient of any age?

You should call her Ms. Samurai, unless she tells you otherwise. This is the right to be treated with dignity and respect.

- You are to transport a patient to nuclear medicine for a KUB. The patient says, "What kind of test is that? I don't think I gave consent for this test. I refuse to go until someone explains this to me."

  Patients have the right to be given information in language that they understand. Patients have the right to refuse. Patients must give consent for special studies. Get the nurse, and ask him to explain the procedure and check the chart for the consent form.

- You are to transport a pregnant patient for a test in the GI department. The woman says, "Don't take it personally, but I want someone else to take me."

  The patient has to give consent for you to transport her. You should simply ask if there is a particular reason that she wants someone else. It is important to respect the patient's right to privacy and confidentiality. If the patient is unsure of your ability to assist her, you may be able to reassure her of your competence. If the patient is concerned that you will see her in a compromising position or situation, you should reassure her of her right to privacy and let her know your respect for the dignity of your patients.

- You are assisting a patient to dress. A group of medical students and a resident have just finished rounds in this room. The patient says to you, "Who were those people?"

  The patient has the right to know the identity and title of everyone who is involved in his or her care. You should tell the patient their names if you know them, or simply tell the patient that they were medical students and the resident. Later, tell the resident about the patient's question, or ask the nurse to speak with the resident about this issue.

- While you are assisting Mrs. Morganstern to walk to the bathroom, she asks you, "What does it cost for one day in this lovely hospital room? No one ever mentions what things cost in the hospital. Do I have to pay for every pill that I take?"

  The patient has the right to know the charges for the room, medications, and so on. Most of the care team will not necessarily know the individual charges. You should ask the manager or a representative from patient accounts to talk with the patient regarding costs.

- You are in the cafeteria eating lunch, and you overhear a group of nursing students discussing Makita Joslin, a seventeen-year-old patient in maternity.

  This is a breach of confidentiality and privacy. If you feel comfortable, you might quietly tell the group of student nurses that you can hear what they are saying about a patient in the hospital. It may be enough to just let them know that you can hear them; they know what patients' rights are about, too.

- Marvin Mead is a nineteen-year-old patient who needs crutches to walk. His room is full of equipment, and he spilled a lot of water during his sponge bath at the sink. You are assigned to assist in the stat transport of another patient to the intensive care unit (ICU).

  The right to personal safety is threatened. Tell another team member that the room is unsafe for Mr. Mead. You are concerned that the patient could fall and be injured. Ask your coworker to dry the floor and move some of the equipment until the room can be cleaned.

- Does a resident in a nursing home have the right to return to his bedroom and lie down an hour after the assistant gets him up and into a wheelchair? Mr. Blackstone asks to do this every day. He argues, "It hurts to sit up for long periods. It's more comfortable lying down." This client is generally not sociable and has periods of confusion and lucidity. The family insists on seeing him up and out of bed and claims that he is depressed. The administration's rule is that all clients are to be out of bed from morning bath until bedtime. Picture yourself in this client's position. What is your course of action? Substantiate your answer based on the resident's bill of rights.

  This resident has the right to choose daily activities. It may be possible to establish a schedule both of activity and rest for this resident. Since this resident is suffering from depression, it is essential to plan care to improve his mood and decrease his isolation from others. Perhaps a daily plan could be established that gradually increases the amount of time spent out of bed and with others. The family and the resident need to be included in a plan-of-care conference. Remember that residents in a nursing home live in this facility as a home. While it is important to respect the resident's rights, it is also important to provide care for his depression.

application to practice

The nursing process is a complex concept that requires consideration of many factors. Your use of the sequential steps of the nursing process will serve as a strong model in the role of clinical assistant. You will use this problem-solving methodology to guide your actions in delivering patient care. Based on what you've learned in this chapter, respond to the situations described below. List your ideas first, and then discuss these with your instructor, your peers, and the nurses with whom you work.

Learning Activities

Situation 1: Mr. Smith is an eighty-year-old man who resides in your nursing home. He has lived there for 5 years, and you have been involved in his care for 4 years. He has been diagnosed with diabetes mellitus, hypertension, and recently a kidney infection. He will need a Foley catheter and an IV to manage his condition. Who will be permitted to insert the Foley catheter, and who will insert the IV?

Author's Explanation: The LPN or the RN will insert the Foley catheter and the IV. It is not acceptable to delegate these tasks to an assistant unless he or she has been trained and certified to perform these skills. There are hospitals that permit assistants who are trained in bladder catheterization to insert Foley catheters. In long-term care (LTC) facilities, however, nursing assistants cannot perform sterile procedures, and IV insertion must be performed by a licensed nurse or physician.

Situation 2: What are your responsibilities in maintaining Mr. Smith's IV and urinary catheter?

Author's Explanation: You should report any malfunctions regarding either. You should report any unusual observations of the IV site, the failure of the IV to run, the presence of inflammation at the IV site, and blood in the IV tubing. You should know the proper height of the IV fluid bag and should not readjust the height of the bag or the rate of fluid infusion. An IV should never be placed below the set height or rate. With the Foley catheter, you should observe the amount of urinary drainage, the color of the urine, the presence of any blood or sediment in the urine, the presence of any odor to the urine, and the failure of the catheter to drain urine. The clinical care associate is generally expected to make these observations, to report to the nurse observations of the quantity and quality of the urine, and to measure the contents in the drainage device.

Situation 3: Mr. Smith has always been able to perform some of his personal care and ADLs with assistance. He ambulates with the use of a walker, is alert, and is socially active with other residents. He likes to play checkers, and he reads the paper daily. He also discusses with you what he reads. Today, Monday, you are assigned to Mr. Smith after being off for the weekend. As you make your rounds, you expect to find him sitting in a chair eating his breakfast and reading his paper. When you enter the room, he is in bed, and he is waiting for you to assist him with his breakfast. He tells you, "I feel weak and don't have much of an appetite. I'll just have the juice and coffee." You notice that his urinary drainage bag contains a small amount of very dark, reddish brown urine. He complains of a backache when you raise the head of his bed to a sitting position. He appears sleepy and is slow to respond to your questions.

After you assist him with drinking his juice and coffee, you receive a report from the nurse. She directs you to provide A.M. care and to get Mr. Smith ready to attend a recreational activity at 10:00. She tells you he has a Heplock in his left arm for the administration of intravenous antibiotics and a Foley for accurate urinary measurement. He has been placed on I&O and was given Tylenol for pain during the night. During the report, you relate to the nurse the objective data collected on your rounds about Mr. Smith. What are the data that you report?

Author's Explanation: You should report Mr. Smith's lack of energy and his lack of appetite. You must report the color of his urine and his complaints of pain. Tell the nurse that he is sleepy and responding slowly to your questions.

Situation 4: Why is it important to report these data now?

Author's Explanation: These data reveal a change in Mr. Smith's usual behavior, activity, and mood. The reddish brown color of the urine is not normal, and the nurse needs to know this observation. A decreased level of energy and appetite are significant pieces of information in the nurse's assessment of his emotional and physical status. Your observations include the physical, emotional, and behavioral changes that you noticed in Mr. Smith since you last saw him.

Situation 5: What are the changes you have noticed in Mr. Smith?

Author's Explanation: You have noticed a change in his desire to eat and read the paper. He is sleepy and not mentally as sharp and alert as you have known him. He is complaining of pain and is asking for assistance to complete the task of eating, which he normally performs independently.

Situation 6: Describe your reasons for reporting each of these observations. Should your observations be assessed by the nurse?

Author's Explanation: Your reasons for reporting these observations are based on your knowledge of Mr. Smith's usual routine and the deviation from this routine. Without the other physical and emotional changes, these are significant differences in this resident. The color of his urine is not normal. Urine should be clear, yellow, or amber. Pain is not normal, nor is sleepiness or slow responses. The nurse needs to see Mr. Smith before you continue to care for him. The nurse needs to use her professional knowledge and judgment to determine the problem and plan for his care.

Situation 7: How will your observations and the nurse's assessment affect the way you plan to carry out your assignment?

Author's Explanation: The observations you provided should alert the nurse to assess Mr. Smith and to plan for a course of care based on the assessment. You may not be preparing Mr. Smith for a 10:00 activity; the nurse will determine the new priorities of care for you to implement.

Situation 8: The nurse contacts the physician to report the scanty amount and the color of the urine and her results of the chemstick test, which revealed the presence of blood (hematuria) and protein (proteinuria) and a high specific gravity (concentration of water in the urine). The physician orders continuous IV fluids in addition to IV antibiotics and vital signs taken every four hours. You take Mr. Smith's vital signs at 8 A.M., and these are your findings: temperature 100°F, pulse 98, respirations 28, blood pressure 180/100. Which of these VS is not within normal limits? When do you report these results to the nurse?

Author's Explanation: The pulse is high, even though it is the upper limit of normal heart rate. His temperature indicates fever. It is 1.4° higher than a normal temperature. His respirations are

rapid. His blood pressure is very high and could be dangerous even though he has a diagnosis of hypertension. You should report these results to the nurse immediately.

Situation 9: Why should you report his VS immediately?

Author's Explanation: Because every one of Mr. Smith's vital signs is above the normal range. You know that fever and pain increase pulse, respiration, and blood pressure. Also, you know that the color and amount of urine are not normal. You realize that Mr. Smith needs the RN's assessment and intervention.

Situation 10: The nurse tells you to increase his oral intake of fluids. You encourage Mr. Smith to drink more water. No instructions were given regarding a modification or alteration in A.M. care. Will you alter your usual approach to Mr. Smith's A.M. care? What will influence this alteration? For what reasons will you alter your plan?

Author's Explanation: You will alter your plan of usual care because you need to assist Mr. Smith with ADLs that he normally completes independently. You need to adjust his fluid intake and need to recognize his pain and change in mental status. Mr. Smith cannot attend the social activity if he is asleep and unable to participate in the activity.

Situation 11: You find that in performing Mr. Smith's A.M. care he can barely assist you because he is so lethargic. He does not want to get out of bed, and he refuses to attend the recreational activity because he is too weak. He also "does not want to be seen by other residents with a Foley." He has taken about 300 cubic centimeters (cc) of fluids by mouth (PO), and at 11 A.M., you decide to measure the contents of the drainage bag. The output is 50 cc.

At noon, you take vital signs again because of the q4° order. The results are temperature 100°F, pulse 110, respirations 28, blood pressure 180/100. Blood glucose measured via a fingerstick is 233 (normal range is 84–126). You are surprised because he hasn't eaten anything.

During the bath, you noticed that his feet are swollen, and when you touch them, you leave finger marks in his skin. His IV of 1,000 cc of Dextrose 5% and ½% normal saline solution has infused about 75% of the bag. His breathing is labored; it seems to take much effort for him to wash his face. What are the objective data (measurements and observations) about Mr. Smith's condition that you have gathered?

Author's Explanation: The objective data are the data that you found on measurement of vital signs, urinary output, PO intake, his swollen feet, his labored breathing, and the blood glucose. The signs and symptoms that you observed that are subjective, but are significant, are his lethargy (weakness and tiredness) and the amount of effort it took for him to wash his face.

Situation 12: What do you do with these data and when?

Author's Explanation: You should immediately tell the nurse your findings.

Situation 13: Will this clinical data influence the nurse's plan of care and your assignment?

Author's Explanation: Absolutely. These data are indicating a worsening of his condition and need to be reported stat to the nurse. The nurse will call the physician and report the changes in Mr. Smith's status after assessing the resident.

Situation 14: What do you expect you will be assigned to do next for Mr. Smith?

Author's Explanation: You probably will be assigned to increase the frequency of VS, I&O, and blood glucose measurement. The nurse will assess the status of the edema (fluid accumulation) in his extremities and his mental and neurological status. You will not be escorting Mr. Smith to any recreational activity; he may be placed on bed rest with the head of the bed elevated to ease his labored breathing. Oxygen may be administered, and the physician will need to come to evaluate his status and to determine his need for hospitalization. Mr. Smith's kidney infection has worsened and may be life-threatening.

Situation 15: In your own words, describe what you contributed to the nurse's assessment. What changes were made in the nurse's plan of care? What tasks were you assigned to implement? What data did you provide to assist the nurse in evaluating Mr. Smith's response to the plan of care?

Author's Explanation: You contributed a great deal of information to the nurse's assessment of this resident. If you did not alert her to the changes that you noted on your A.M. rounds before report, the nurse would not have assessed and altered the plan of care for Mr. Smith. You followed the nurse's directions and reported your findings

promptly. You also made Mr. Smith feel cared for by recognizing his change in status.

The nurse's plan was changed by an increased need to more frequently assess this resident and to call for the direction of his physician. Intravenous and PO fluids were increased as well as the frequency of vital sign measurement.

You were assigned the tasks of blood glucose monitoring, q4h VS, and output measurements. You increased the amount of PO intake and reported all noted changes to the nurse stat.

You provided the initial observations of change that you saw in Mr. Smith. These alerted the nurse for the need to assess him immediately. As a result of your observations and measurements of objective data, Mr. Smith received a timely change in his plan of care. The nurse listened to your report and responded, as did the physician. You did a great job in caring for Mr. Smith. Thank you!

At this point, you should begin to see the nursing process unfold and should begin to understand the role that an assistant plays in this problem-solving method. If you had not shared with the nurse in the A.M. report the changes that you noticed in Mr. Smith when you encountered him on your A.M. rounds, his treatment would have been delayed.

The role of the clinical assistant in patient care is a vital one. You are the frontline link in the nurse's assessment and evaluation when assigning certain aspects of the patient's plan of care. The clinical assistant is responsible and accountable for actions in all aspects of patient care. One of the responsibilities is to gather objective data that the nurse will use in the nursing process. Objective data are factual, including descriptive and accurate observations, results, and measurements. *Objective* means that it is not an opinion, an approximation, a guess, or a hunch. Objective data are gathered through observation of the senses and through accurate measurement. You observe through your sense of touch, sight, hearing, and smell. You measure and compare using scales, rulers, or tape measures and your knowledge of normal versus abnormal results. Sphygmomanometers, thermometers, fluid-measuring cylinders, glucose meters, pulse oximeters, ECG machines, and stethoscopes are the instruments that assist you in providing measurable or objective data to the nurse.

Situation 16: What data did you gather through your senses?

Author's Explanation: You gathered data through your sense of touch when you felt Mr. Smith's swollen feet. You visually inspected the depressions in the skin that resulted from touching his feet. You listened to his complaints, and you saw the amount and color of his urine. You heard his labored breathing and saw his lack of energy and slowness to respond.

Situation 17: What data did you gather through measurement?

Author's Explanation: The data that you gathered through measurement were increased temperature, pulse, respiration, and blood pressure. You also noted the elevated blood glucose.

Situation 18: Did you compare any of this data to previous findings and observations of Mr. Smith?

Author's Explanation: You compared his normal emotional and mental status with his emotional and mental tone and response to you on A.M. rounds. You know the color and amount of normal urinary drainage. You know normal vital signs and blood glucose. Most of all, you know your resident and his typical behavior.

Situation 19: How did you and the nurse work as a team in caring for Mr. Smith?

Author's Explanation: You and the nurse worked together to respond to the changes in Mr. Smith. You reported your observations and measurements to the nurse, and the nurse responded. You each worked within the scope of your defined roles in the nursing process. The nurse assessed, planned, and evaluated Mr. Smith. Each of you implemented care measures. You also assessed, planned, and implemented within your scope of practice. Had you failed to notice any changes in your resident's status and also failed to report these changes, the nurse may not have assessed and intervened promptly. The nurse delegated tasks that you could perform and completed the interventions that only the nurse could or should perform. Together, you worked as an efficient and responsible team. Congratulations!

Examination Review Questions

1. Gathering your equipment is which step in the nursing process?
   a. assessing
   b. planning
   c. implementing
   d. evaluating

2. Which of the following is *not* ethical?
   a. discussing dietary restrictions
   b. accepting tips from the patient
   c. reading mail to the patient
   d. refusing to give the patient information

3. Health care workers must act in accordance with the values and beliefs of their patients. This demonstrates
   a. benevolence
   b. justice
   c. respect
   d. nonmaleficence

4. Positive, abuse-free body language falls into what fundamental category?
   a. communication
   b. cooperation
   c. commitment
   d. contribution

5. A patient cannot communicate because of receptive aphasia. Which barrier is this?
   a. physical inability
   b. mental incapacity
   c. emotional instability
   d. nonverbal language

6. Which is hampered when there is no sense of empowerment to voice ideas?
   a. contribution
   b. commitment
   c. communication
   d. collaboration

7. When transporting a patient to another department, such as x-ray, what should be done with the chart?
   a. place it at the desk
   b. keep it with the patient
   c. leave it on the unit
   d. give it to the unit clerk

8. The nurse delegates the task of checking an abdominal dressing. Which of the following is *not* necessary?
   a. consent
   b. identification
   c. maleficence
   d. confidentiality

9. The patient adamantly refuses to get out of bed despite your orders. What should you do next?
   a. insist and proceed
   b. report and record
   c. encourage and continue
   d. explain and suggest

10. Privacy is a right and can be protected by all of the following *except*
    a. closing the door
    b. knocking before entering
    c. screening the unit
    d. asking for permission

Nutrition

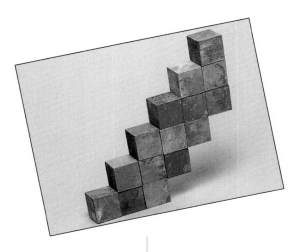

Ah, food! Weddings are celebrated with it. Life events are discussed over it. Friendships are strengthened by it, and business deals are sealed around it. You can't help but notice that food is more than our body's warehouse of supplies. In many cases, food often provides pleasure and when balanced properly, food helps to provide health. But for many, the balancing act remains a mystery, while the rewards of proper nutrition are neglected. Because food is an essential key in the restoration and rehabilitation of the illness-health process, it is important for the clinical care associate to promote and practice sound nutritional habits.

Chapter 18

Elementary Nutrition

Nutrition serves as one determinant of our physical, mental, and emotional well-being. It affects our height, weight, strength, musculoskeletal development, mobility, immune response, and skin tone and texture. In addition, it affects our sleep, bowel function, energy, mood, and mental function. Sound nutrition also plays a role in preventing or deterring the degenerative illnesses, such as osteoporosis, atherosclerosis, hypertension, and malnutrition.

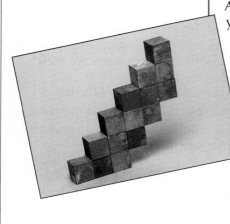

OBJECTIVES

After completing this chapter, you will be able to

1. Define *nutrition*
2. List the five processes involved in nutrition
3. List the seven essential nutrients
4. Describe the functions of each nutrient
5. List the vitamins
6. Describe the functions of each vitamin
7. List the major minerals
8. Describe the functions of each major mineral
9. Develop a twenty-four-hour menu for a regular diet using the food pyramid
10. Name the therapeutic diets
11. Correlate the therapeutic diets and the associated conditions or diseases for which each is prescribed
12. Apply the principles of nutrition as they relate to the role of the clinical care associate
13. Define and spell all key terms correctly

key terms

absorption	fat-soluble	nutrition
amino acids	fiber	proteins
assimilation	high-density lipoproteins (HDLs)	saturated fat
basal metabolic rate (BMR)	hypervitaminosis	therapeutic diets
carbohydrates	incomplete proteins	total parenteral nutrition (TPN)
cholesterol	ingestion	tube feedings
colostrum	irritable bowel syndrome	unsaturated fat
complete proteins	low-density lipoproteins (LDLs)	very low-density lipoproteins
diaphoresis	menarche	(VLDLs)
digestion	minerals	vitamins
elimination	monosodium glutamate (MSG)	water-soluble
empty calories	nasogastric tube	
fats	nutrients	

The Process of Nutrition

Nutrition is the process of taking in food and using it for proper body function, including growth, repair, and maintenance. The processes involved in nutrition are *ingestion, digestion, absorption, assimilation,* and *elimination.* **Ingestion** is the act of taking in food and fluid by mouth. **Digestion** is the breakdown of food. Digestion is achieved mechanically and chemically. Mechanically, digestion occurs through mastication. Chemical digestion occurs through the mixing of food with saliva and gastric enzymes. Once food is digested, the broken down nutrients pass into the bloodstream through the capillaries of the small intestine to be used as necessary. **Absorption** is the process of taking into the blood, the end-products of chemical digestion. **Assimilation**, or metabolism, is the sum of all physical and chemical changes and all energy and material transformations that take place within the body. (*Metabolism* is derived from the Greek *metaballein*, which means "to change," and *-ismos* means "the state of.") The rate at which this process occurs is referred to as the *metabolic rate.* The **basal metabolic rate (BMR)** is the resting rate of a person's metabolism when no voluntary work is being performed. **Elimination** is the process through which unusable nutrients are excreted or eliminated from the body.

Seven Essential Nutrients

A **nutrient** is a substance that nourishes the cells of the body. Nutrients are needed for the metabolic processes of the cells, tissues, and organs of the body. There are seven major and essential nutrients. Each essential nutrient is chemically different because each provides specific body functions. The seven essential nutrients are

- Water
- Carbohydrates
- Fats
- Proteins
- Vitamins
- Minerals
- Fiber

Let's examine each of these nutrients in turn (Figure 18-1).

The body is made up of 80 percent water. Without water, the cells are unable to function and the body dehydrates. In 3 to 4 days, the person dies. The ingestion of water should be approximately 1,800 cubic centimeters (cc) per day. Water is made of hydrogen and oxygen. Its chemical symbol is H_2O. Water performs three essential life functions. The three essential functions of water are these:

1. It contributes to the structure of the body.
2. It aids in the regulation of body temperature.
3. It provides a cellular environment conducive to proper cellular activities.

In addition to the water and fluids we drink, certain fruits and vegetables provide the body with water. Intake of water should match output of fluids to assure a daily supply of fresh fluids. This means that if a healthy person takes in the normal amount of 1,800 cc per day, he or she should excrete 1,800 cc per day, almost all of which will be urinary output. Certain factors may reduce urinary output but still reflect a normal intake-output balance. For example, profuse sweating, called **diaphoresis**, can account for some of the body's fluid output. Other ways to lose fluid include diarrhea, vomiting, wound drainage, and blood loss. If there is any question of fluid imbalance, the patient may be placed on intake-and-output

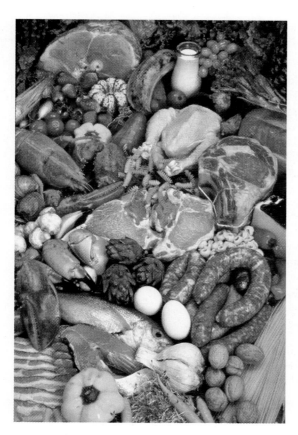

FIGURE 18-1 The seven essential nutrients. Lee Snyder, Photo Researchers, Inc.

(I&O) records. This will be discussed in detail in the essential skills and procedures unit.

Carbohydrates are made of carbon, hydrogen, and oxygen. The chemical symbol is CHO. Current recommendations are that 55 to 60 percent of a healthy person's daily caloric intake should come from carbohydrates. The main sources of CHO are grains, cereals, legumes, nuts, vegetables, and fruits. Carbohydrates provide 4 calories of energy per gram weight. In two forms, *simple* and *complex*, carbohydrates are broken down to glucose, a simple sugar, which is necessary for energy to the cells.

Fats are also made from carbon, hydrogen, and oxygen. They contain more oxygen and therefore are a concentrated form of energy. Fats, in combination with other nutrients, form important compounds, such as blood lipids, steroids, cell membranes, bile, and vitamin D. Stored fat insulates the body and therefore assists in the regulation of body temperature. The other functions of fats are cushioning the bones and internal organs and adding flavor to meals. Fats provide 9 calories per gram weight. The main sources of fats are butter and margarine, oil, cream, fatty meat, and egg yolks. All fats

are water-insoluble. Sometimes, they are called *lipids*.

Lipids can be divided into two major categories: *saturated* and *unsaturated*. The identification of a **saturated fat** is easy because it is solid at room temperature. All animal fat is generally saturated. Saturated fat is also a source of cholesterol in food. **Cholesterol** is a fatlike substance that circulates in the blood as lipoproteins. There are three types of circulating lipoproteins.

1. **Very low-density lipoproteins (VLDLs)**
2. **Low-density lipoproteins (LDLs)**
3. **High-density lipoproteins (HDLs)**

LDL accounts for approximately 60 to 70 percent of the total blood cholesterol, and VLDL is approximately 10 to 15 percent. HDL comprises 20 to 30 percent. As the percentage ratio of HDL to LDL increases, the less likely the chances of the development of coronary artery disease (CAD). Cholesterol in the diet has been found to increase the risk of coronary heart disease in those individuals with a high circulating blood cholesterol. Blood cholesterol levels should be less than 200 milligrams/deciliter (mg/dl). Any level higher than 240 mg/dl requires close physician follow-up. Although cholesterol is important as a normal component of bile and steroid hormones, it can be synthesized by the liver and does not need to be present in large amounts in our food intake. Saturated fat can be found in meat, lard, bacon grease, and dairy products like butter, cream, and cheese.

The second category of fat is **unsaturated fat**. This category can be further divided into plant fats, which are higher in monounsaturated fats (as in olive, canola, and peanut oil), and polyunsaturated fats, such as corn and soy oil. Recommendations for fat intake suggest that fats should be reduced to 30 percent of total daily intake, and of that 30 percent, no more than 10 percent should be saturated fats.

Proteins are composed of hydrogen, carbon, oxygen, and nitrogen. In addition, some proteins contain sulfur, phosphorus, iron, and iodine. Protein is the "rebuild-and-repair food." It is metabolized at the rate of 4 calories per gram. Since many factors affect tissue needs, there is no set protein requirement for everyone. The recommended formula is 0.4 grams (g) per pound of body weight. However, factors such as age, illness and disease, and quality of protein source affect daily requirements.

When digested, proteins are broken down into **amino acids**. Amino acids are assembled to build proteins and are the end product of protein breakdown or catabolism. There are twenty-two different amino acids, but there are nine that are called *essential*.

TABLE 18-1   Water-Soluble Vitamins: Daily Requirements

Vitamin	Function	Food Source	Daily Requirement (Male and Female)
B$_1$ (thiamine)	Aids in appetite, muscle tone; forms energy from fats and CHO	Yeast, grains, enriched cereals, breads, pork, liver	0.02 milligram (mg)
B$_2$ (riboflavin)	Assists in vision; enhances skin tone	Milk is best source; also eggs, meat, green vegetables	0.02 mg
B$_3$ (niacin)	Provides body energy, growth; promotes healthy skin; assists with nerve and gastrointestinal (GI) function	Meat, poultry, fish, grains, cereals, green vegetables, bran, nuts	0.02 mg
B$_6$	Aids body in use of nutrients	Similar to other B vitamins	0.02 mg
B$_{12}$	Needed for RBC formation; assists with nerve and GI function; aids in use of fats, CHO, and protein	Meats and other animal sources	0.06 microgram (mcg)
C	Aids in absorption and use of iron; strengthens capillary walls; protects against infection	Citrus fruits, melons, strawberries, tomatoes, potatoes, cabbage, green peppers	0.6 mg

Proteins containing all nine essential amino acids are called **complete proteins**. Complete proteins include fish, meat, and dairy products. **Incomplete proteins** contain some of the nine essential amino acids and some of the thirteen others. Incomplete proteins include dried beans and legumes. Partially complete proteins combined with legumes or complex carbohydrates ingested at one meal can be a substitute for complete proteins. For example, combining pasta and beans, rice and beans, or corn and beans as a menu entrée will provide all the necessary amino acids. This is important for vegetarians and those on a fixed income.

Vitamins are organic compounds that assist in the regulation of certain body processes, including the building of tissue. (The word root *vita-* means life.) Vitamins cannot be manufactured by the body but must use the energy from carbohydrates, fats, and proteins. There are two categories of vitamins: water-soluble and fat-soluble. **Water-soluble** vitamins are those that can be dissolved in water and cannot be stored by the body (Table 18-1). Vitamins B and C fall into this category. **Fat-soluble** vitamins cannot be dissolved in water and can be stored by the body (Table 18-2). Vitamins A, D, E, and K fall into this category. In very large quantities, which do

TABLE 18-2   Fat-Soluble Vitamins: Daily Requirements

Vitamin	Function	Food Source	Daily Requirement Male	Daily Requirement Female
A	Promotes normal growth, vision, skin; formation of enamel	Liver, egg yolks, kidneys, whole milk, fortified skim milk, butter, fortified margarine, yellow and dark green vegetables	5,000 international units (IU)	4,000 IU
D	Aids in bone and teeth formation	Fortified milk; also sunshine (Vitamin D is provided by absorbing uv rays from the sun)	200 IU	200 IU

TABLE 18-2   Fat-Soluble Vitamins: Daily Requirements (continued)

| E | Promotes healthy red blood cells | Whole grain cereals, salad oil, shortening, margarine, fruits, vegetables | 15 IU | 12 IU |
| K | Aids in blood clotting | Green leafy vegetables | 0.08 IU | 0.065 IU |

you think can make you toxic (**hypervitaminosis**)? Which do you think require daily intake because of the body's inability to store them? Fat-soluble vitamins can cause diseases related to an overdose because excess intake is stored in the body. Water-soluble vitamins require a daily intake because the body uses the vitamins ingested and excretes the excess through the urine.

Minerals are inorganic (nonliving) elements that regulate fluid and assist in various body functions. There are two categories of minerals: *major* and *trace*. The major minerals include calcium, phosphorus, magnesium, potassium, sodium, iron, and chloride (Table 18-3). The trace minerals include zinc, manganese, boron, copper, iodine, selenium, and chromium.

TABLE 18-3   Major Minerals: Daily Requirements

Mineral	Function	Food Source	Daily Requirement	
			Male	Female
Calcium	Needed for the formation of bones and teeth; aids in clotting of blood; assists in muscle and nerve function	Milk and milk products, dark green leafy vegetables, including mustard greens, kale, broccoli	800 mg	800 mg
Phosphorus	Needed for energy production; needed for nerve and muscle function; aids in bone and teeth structure	Cereals, meats, fish, legumes, eggs, milk, dairy products	800 mg	800 mg
Magnesium	Is a constituent of bone; serves as a catalyst for chemical reactions in the body; builds protein	Brains, sweetbreads, liver, egg yolks, dark green leafy greens, nuts, whole-grain cereals, beans, coffee, tea, cocoa	350 mg	280 mg
Potassium	Aids in energy production; promotes healthy hair, skin, nails	Citrus juices, bananas, protein foods (meats, seafood, fish, poultry, eggs, cheese, legumes)	No U.S. R.D.A. established	
Sodium	Needed for muscle and nerve function	Milk and milk products, meat, deep green leafy vegetables, seafood, salt	1–3 g	1–3 g
Iron	Is needed to carry oxygen to the cells; prevents anemia	Liver and other organ meats, dried fruits, nuts, whole grains, enriched cereals	10 mg	15 mg
Chloride	Needed for muscle and nerve function	Protein foods		

Fiber is all the indigestible carbohydrates and carbohydrates-like components of food. Fiber comes in two forms: *soluble* and *insoluble*. Soluble fiber is a fiber that forms a gel in water. Insoluble fiber is like sawdust and does not dissolve in water. Fiber is important and provides several functions. It acts as a bulk agent to assist with elimination. It acts as a natural appetite suppressant. It acts as a chelating agent, decreasing the absorption of cholesterol and excess minerals from the diet. It also acts as an agent in decreasing the rate of absorption of glucose from meals. Both soluble and insoluble fiber can be found in raw fruits and vegetables, whole grains, seeds, nuts, and legumes. The recommended daily intake of fiber is 25 to 35 grams.

Think of the human body as a house. The framework is your skeletal system. The exterior paint and siding are your skin, muscles, and connective tissue. The appliances are your organs. The electrical wiring is your nervous system. In addition, household functioning requires electricity, a fuel source like oil or gas, reserve fuel such as wood for a fire, and a decent water supply. And years of wear and tear require repairs, remodeling, and maintenance. Quality materials in a house provide quality maintenance. Much like a house, the body requires quality materials for quality maintenance. These are found in our food. Carbohydrates are the main fuel source. Proteins provide the materials for rebuilding and repairing, and fats provide insulation and reserve fuel. Fiber helps to keep our pipes (the digestive system) clean. Vitamins are the caulking and seam tape. Minerals are the nails, screws, and metal fixtures.

The Food Pyramid

You are what you eat. This cliché is true. Malnutrition (*mal-* means "bad" or "poor") doesn't always mean starvation. Let's return to our house. You wouldn't buy a case of paint for a house that needs new flooring. Furthermore, would you think that the purchase of five new stereos in a house with faulty electricity is a wasteful one? What happens when you make purchases that you don't need? Well, generally you store them in the basement until you can't move around in it, or you throw them out or give them away. Our bodies require certain amounts of "food materials" to provide proper body maintenance. How much? The food pyramid is the updated format for calculating basic needs for the average adult. Let's examine the pyramid in Figure 18-2.

There is much flexibility in food selection based on the pyramid. This provides the variety necessary to adhere to healthful eating habits. Notice how the bottom of the pyramid, showing "Grains," represents

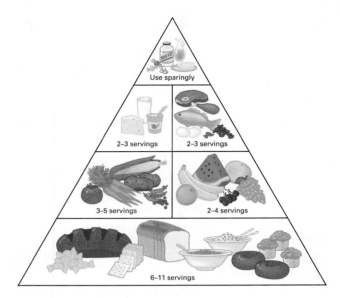

FIGURE 18-2   The food pyramid.

the largest number of servings, and the top, "Fats," represents the smallest number of servings. Wise nutritional planning based on this pyramid can ensure the necessary intake of all the essential nutrients. Examples would be to choose whole-grain bread over white bread. Now hold or limit the butter, margarine, or mayonnaise that you usually slather across it. Choose grain cereals over the sugary ones. How do you know? Read the label for the amount of refined sugar added. Choose brown rice rather than white, and to add some interest, try some of the Eastern grains: couscous, bulgur, and barley. Pizza is a great meal. It can become even better if the sausage and pepperoni (both high in saturated fats) are deleted and vegetables are added.

Cooking methods also affect the vitamin and mineral content of food. When cooking vegetables, steaming is superior to boiling. Of course, raw vegetables are an excellent source of fiber. So why not skip the cooking? Make sure all fruits and vegetables are scrubbed thoroughly before eating. Most produce purchased in the supermarket has been sprayed with chemicals, wax, or coloring agents for increased appeal. In addition, certain microorganisms found on fruit and vegetables can cause digestive disorders. One particular protozoan, cyclaspora, was found on certain berries.

Calories

The number of calories needed per twenty-four-hour period is our daily calorie requirement. One pound of body fat equals 3,500 calories. Therefore, to lose one pound of body fat, 3,500 fewer calories need to be consumed, or energy expenditure through exercise needs to be increased. A general guideline for weight maintenance is 15 calories per pound of body weight. For example, to maintain a weight of 120 pounds, one needs a daily intake of how many calories a day? If you said 1,800 calories, you are correct. Losing weight, a great American obsession, must be accomplished sensibly. A loss of one to two pounds per week is a sane, sensible goal. One should *never* consume fewer than 1,000 calories per day.

The number of calories is not the only important measurement. The number of calories needs to be balanced with the *type* of calories consumed. The U.S. Department of Agriculture has provided recommendations for healthful eating with the food pyramid model.

Some foods are full of nutrients. Others are filled with **"empty calories."** Empty-calorie foods may provide quick energy in the form of refined sugar and saturated fat, but they supply no vitamins or minerals. Foods such as doughnuts, candy bars, potato chips, corn chips, pastries, cakes, cookies, and pies all contain high amounts of saturated fat and refined sugar. Choosing cereal over donuts, fruit over candy, a baked potato over chips, and raw vegetables over desserts can decrease calories while increasing nutrients.

Therapeutic Diets

Therapeutic diets are "prescription diets," modified in some way to improve certain health problems. Modified diets include calorie-controlled, low-sodium, protein, diabetic, low-cholesterol, low-fat, bland, soft, liquid, low-residue, and high-fiber diets (Table 18-4).

Calorie-controlled diets include calorie-restricted and high-calorie diets. Calorie-restricted diets are designed to assist in weight loss. Morbid obesity taxes the heart and blood vessels as well as the musculoskeletal system. Those on calorie-restricted diets should be monitored closely by their physician. Foods to avoid include empty-calorie foods and foods high in fat. High-calorie diets are used in the treatment of anorexia nervosa, cancer, and hyperthyroidism. High-calorie diets increase carbohydrates and protein but do not include empty-calorie foods or foods high in fat.

Low-sodium, or sodium-restricted diets are an adjunct therapy for those suffering from hypertension, cardiovascular disease, congestive heart failure (CHF), and kidney disease. They also assist in controlling edema. Foods to avoid or limit include table salt, smoked meats, pickles, olives, sauerkraut, processed foods, and cheese. Some frozen foods, especially entrées, and some frozen and canned vegetables also contain high amounts of sodium. Reading labels while grocery shopping helps to identify hid-

den sodium in foods. Certain preservatives also contain high levels of sodium, including **monosodium glutamate (MSG)**. Low-sodium diets can be mildly restricting to severely restricting. A mild restriction is 2,000 mg of sodium or a no-added-salt diet; 500 mg of sodium is a severe restriction used in terminal heart and kidney disease.

Protein diets may be high or low in protein. High-protein diets are prescribed to women who are pregnant or lactating, to children with delayed growth, to malnourished patients, and to those suffering from tissue trauma, such as surgery, burns, or infection. High-protein diets may also be used in those with prolonged fever. Foods rich in protein include milk, cheese, eggs, fish, and meat. Low-protein diets are used to reduce the nitrogenous waste buildup in kidney disease. They are also prescribed for certain food allergies. Foods to be avoided are those rich in protein. If you are unsure of protein foods, reread the section "Seven Essential Nutrients."

Diabetic diets are calculated to restrict the number of carbohydrates and calories in the person suffering from diabetes mellitus (DM). Remember that diabetics are unable to metabolize glucose. Therefore, to control hyperglycemia, diabetic diets limit CHO intake and balance fat and protein. Diabetic diets are categorized by the number of calories: for example, 1,200 ADA, 1,500 ADA, 1,800 ADA and so forth.

High cholesterol levels have been associated with cardiovascular heart disease. Studies show that avoiding high-cholesterol foods assists in reducing circulating cholesterol. Foods to be avoided or restricted include egg yolks, organ meats, cream cheese, and milk.

Low-fat, or fat-restricted, diets are used to assist in the treatment of obesity, gallbladder and liver disease, and cardiovascular diseases, such as atherosclerosis. Foods to be avoided are those high in saturated fats or fried in fat. What are the saturated fats? Reread the section "Seven Essential Nutrients" if unsure.

Bland diets are used in certain diseases of the digestive tract. These diets promote foods that are digested easily while avoiding high-fiber and spicy foods, raw vegetables, carbonated beverages, and acid-producing foods, such as chocolate, caffeine, and nuts.

Soft diets are used by those who are edentulous or have teeth and jaw problems. In addition, postsurgical patients may require a soft diet before the return of normal peristalsis. Foods chosen for this diet are easy to digest and easy to chew. Foods to be avoided include tough meats, nuts, raw fruits and vegetables, spicy foods, and rich desserts.

Liquid diets are divided into two categories: clear-liquid and full-liquid. Clear-liquid diets are used post-surgically and before certain x-ray procedures. In addition, certain digestive disorders, such

TABLE 18-4 Therapeutic Diets

Type of Diet	Food to Avoid or Include	Circumstance
Calorie-controlled		
Calorie-restricted	Avoid empty calories, fried foods, foods high in saturated fats	Morbid obesity
High-calorie	Increase carbohydrates and proteins; avoid empty-calorie and high-fat foods; take supplements such as Ensure or Sustacal	Anorexia nervosa, cancer, hyperthyroidism
Low-sodium	Avoid table salt, cured and smoked meats, pickles, olives, certain frozen and canned vegetables	Hypertension, cardiovascular disease, CHF, kidney disease, edema
Protein		
High-protein	Increase meats, fish, poultry, eggs, milk, dairy products, peas, beans, corn, wheat; take supplements such as Ensure or Sustacal	Pregnant and lactating women, children with delayed growth, malnourished patients, tissue trauma, (surgery, burns, infection), prolonged fever
Low-protein	Avoid or limit meats, fish, poultry, eggs, milk, dairy products, peas, beans, corn, wheat	Kidney disease, food allergies
Diabetic	Limit carbohydrates; balance fats and protein; avoid empty-calorie foods and those rich in refined sugar	Insulin- and non-insulin-dependent diabetes mellitus (IDDM and NIDDM)
Low-cholesterol	Avoid or limit egg yolks, organ meats, cream cheese, milk, butter	Cardiovascular heart disease, elevated blood cholesterol levels
Low-fat	Avoid fried foods; limit red meats to 2–3 times/week	Cardiovascular heart disease, hypertension, atherosclerosis
Bland	Eat easily digested foods; avoid high-fiber and spicy foods, raw vegetables, carbonated beverages, and acid-producing foods, such as chocolate, caffeine, nuts	Digestive diseases and disorders
Soft	Choose foods that are easy to digest and easy to chew; avoid tough meats, nuts, raw fruits and vegetables, spicy foods, rich desserts	Toothlessness, teeth and jaw problems, post-surgical patients, transition diet to regular
Liquid		
Clear	Select soup broth, bouillon, clear juice, ginger ale, gelatin, coffee, tea	Post-surgical patients, before certain x-ray procedures, certain digestive disorders, such as partial bowel obstruction, transition diet to full liquid
Full	Choose from all clear liquids, plus cream soups, milk products, custard, pudding, ice cream	Post-surgical patients, GI disorders, elevated temperature, intolerance to solid foods, transition diet to soft
Low-residue	Avoid nuts, vegetables with seeds, seeds, coconut, fried foods, raw fruits and vegetables	Certain digestive and rectal diseases
High-fiber	Increase raw fruits and vegetables	Irritable bowel syndrome

as partial bowel obstruction, may require clear liquids. Clear liquids include clear broth, tea, water, ginger ale, apple juice, gelatin, and ice chips. Full-liquid diets include all liquid foods, including ice cream, custard, frozen yogurt, and cream soups.

A low-residue, or low-fiber, diet is used as a therapeutic approach for those with certain digestive and rectal diseases. Foods to be avoided include nuts, vegetables with seeds, seeds, coconut, fried foods, and raw fruits and vegetables.

A high-fiber diet is prescribed sometimes for chronic constipation and irritable bowel syndrome. **Irritable bowel syndrome** is thought to be a stress-related disorder in which the bowel lumen has areas of constriction. This produces irregular bowel habits with alternating periods of constipation and diarrhea. Bulk-forming foods, such as wheat bran and fresh fruits and vegetables, aid regularity.

Life Span Nutritional Needs

Nutritional needs vary depending on our age, state of health, sex, activity level, and climate. Let's return to the "body as a house" concept. When building a house, many different supplies are required. Until the house is furnished adequately, many purchases are necessary. Similarly, from the time of conception, an abundant supply of nutrients is necessary to build a healthy person. In the growth stages, the body demands a large amount of certain nutrients to build a strong body. Once the nutrients are supplied in the early years of growth and development, the mature body requires fewer "building" supplies, and with the onset of adulthood, demand levels off. Once the house is mature, minor repairs are necessary. If the house has been kept up, even as the house ages, maintenance will be periodic. If the house has been neglected, wear and tear of everyday use will surface, and suddenly everything will seem to require repair or replacement at once. If neglect of the body has occurred, degenerative diseases are apt to surface, and dietary needs must be modified. Of course, disasters can strike along the way, such as storms that carry off the roof, rains that flood the basement, and termites that destroy the foundation. The same is true of our bodies. The assurance of wellness is not absolute, even if an elderly person has practiced nutritionally sound eating habits.

Age-Specific Requirements

An infant begins life with a great need for nutrients because the first year of life is a time of rapid growth. Initially, an infant requires breast milk or prepared formula. Breast milk is the wisest choice, both economically and nutritionally, as it is better tolerated

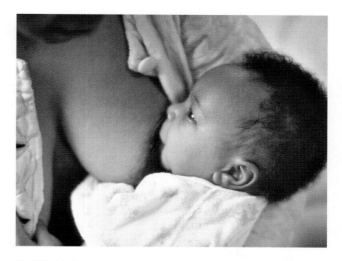

FIGURE 18-3 Breast-feeding provides the infant with natural protection against infection, and it is economical. Suzanne Szasz, Photo Researchers, Inc.

and is more complete than formula. Breast milk is initially expressed as **colostrum**, a thin yellow liquid that provides an immense amount of immune protection for the first six months of an infant's life (Figure 18-3). After the first several months, pureed fruits, vegetables, meats, and cereals may be added to the infant's diet. As the dentition process develops, soft solid foods may be added; later, the infant's digestive system can tolerate most foods.

Toddlers require extra calcium for bone development and protein for tissue growth (Figure 18-4). Preschoolers continue to need protein. Six small meals a day can offer all the necessary nutrients without overwhelming the digestive system.

School-age children are preparing for the growth spurts and reproductive development of puberty. Appetites may vary during these years (Figure 18-5).

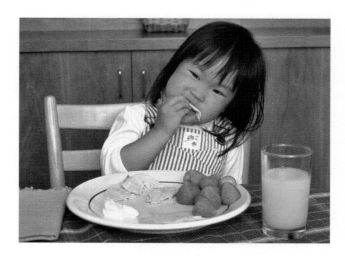

FIGURE 18-4 Toddlers and preschoolers benefit from healthy between-meal snacks. Margaret Miller, Photo Researchers, Inc.

It is important to maintain dietary balances without forcing the child to eat if his or her appetite wanes.

Adolescents require an increase in calories to accommodate the body's development and change. Muscles and bones continue to develop. Therefore, calcium and protein requirements remain high (Figure 18-6). In addition, girls require additional iron after **menarche** (onset of menstruation).

Adult needs vary, depending on exercise level, height and weight, and reproductive activity (Figure 18-7). Pregnant and lactating women require additional protein and calcium to nourish the fetus and infant without strain to the adult body. As the body ages, many body functions are altered. Metabolism slows, along with all digestive processes. Adults can take regular vitamin supplements to make up for changes brought on by aging and to ensure proper nutrition (Figure 18-8).

In older adults, the appetite wanes secondary to a decrease in the sense of taste and smell, a decreased activity level, and possibly a loss of teeth. There is still the need for essential nutrients but a decreased need for calories. Figure 18-9 shows an older adult taking liquid nourishment.

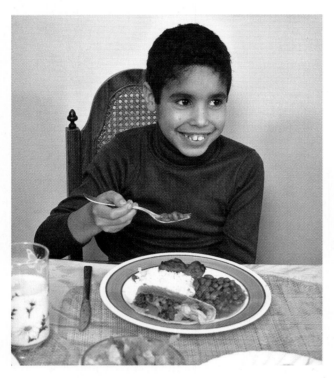

FIGURE 18-5 School-age children experience fluctuations in appetite that should be considered in maintaining good overall nutrition.

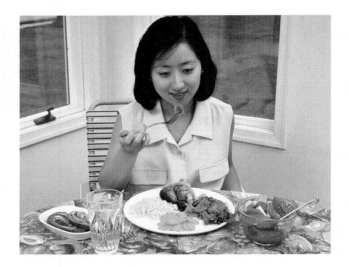

FIGURE 18-7 Young adults require nutritionally balanced meals.

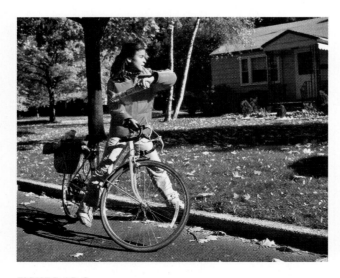

FIGURE 18-6 Adolescent girls and boys require an increased caloric intake.

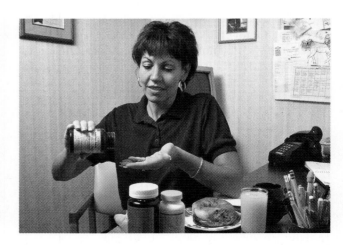

FIGURE 18-8 Middle-aged adults benefit from taking vitamin supplements.

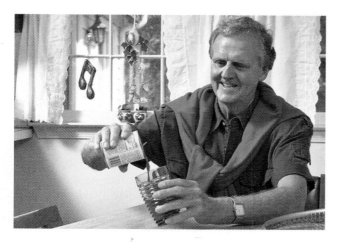

FIGURE 18-9   Older adults sometimes take nutritional liquids to supplement their diet or in place of solid foods.

Alternative Nutritional Support

Alternative nutritional support refers to the administration of water and other liquids through intravenous (IV) and tube feedings. These methods are used to supply fluids and nutrients when there is danger that the patient may become dehydrated or when the patient is not able to eat normally. These nutritional alternatives are usually short-term. Descriptions of the various alternatives follow.

Parenteral Nutrition

Intravenous fluids are administered whenever there is a question of fluid imbalance secondary to dehydration. An IV is a way of maintaining or replacing fluids in an attempt to achieve homeostasis. It does not provide the calories or essential nutrients needed to sustain life. Figure 18-10 shows an IV bag on a pole.

Total parenteral nutrition (TPN), or hyperalimentation, is an intravenous feeding that supplies not only the necessary fluids and electrolytes of an IV, but also the balance of carbohydrates, fats, proteins, vitamins, and minerals to maintain calories and weight. It is used for patients with GI disorders that directly affect the digestion and absorption processes. It may also be prescribed post-surgically for individuals whose intestines require healing. The components may be premixed or may be individualized for each patient.

Peripheral veins are the first choice for IV fluids. Hyperalimentation requires larger veins due to the thick consistency of the fluid. Figure 18-11 shows several types of IV bags.

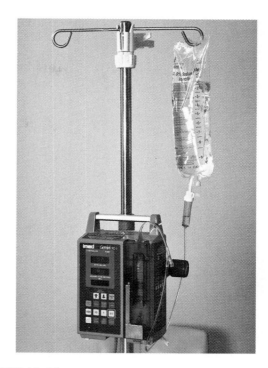

FIGURE 18-10   Intravenous bag on a pole.

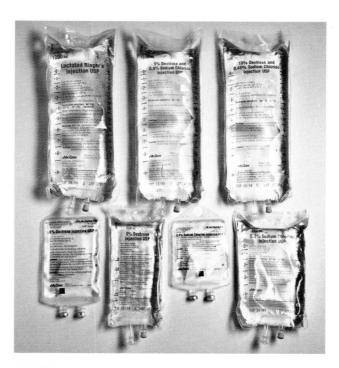

FIGURE 18-11   IV bags may contain additional nutrients to maintain calories and weight.

Tube Feedings

Tube feedings are liquid feedings that are administered through a **nasogastric tube**. This is a tube inserted through the nose, pharynx, and esophagus

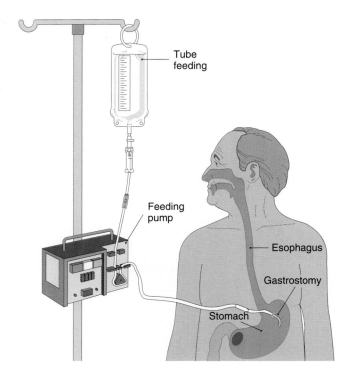

FIGURE 18-12   Gastrostomy tube feeding.

The Cultural and Social Importance of Food

How many times have you associated pasta with Italians? Or fried rice with the Chinese? How about curry with Middle Eastern people? Matzo with Jews? Fasting with Catholics? It is true that culture and religion can influence food choices and food intake and the acceptability of eating certain foods. Cultural and religious practices should be taken into consideration when meals are served, whether they are served in an institution or they are prepared in the home. If a patient refuses to eat a certain food that is served, it is important to question why and to report any cultural or religious preferences so that dietary adjustments can be made.

Table 18-5 lists the major dietary preferences of various cultures and religions.

Many factors contribute to the varying degree of keenness or sensitivity of an individual's palate. Scientific studies indicate that some individuals are born with more taste buds than others. These additional taste cells found on the tongue are what make some palates more discriminating than others. This might account for the people who are sometimes referred to as finicky eaters. Other factors that affect a person's food preferences include finances, lifestyle, and the environment in which the individual was raised.

Poverty frequently contributes to poor nutrition. Federal programs to assist the poor and educational programs designed to teach wise spending and meal preparation can help reduce malnutrition among the poor. Others in our society are malnourished not because they do not have the necessary finances, but because they make very poor food choices.

into the stomach by a nurse or physician. It is a temporary means of administering nourishment to patients who are unable to eat because of stroke, unconsciousness, or coma or who refuse to eat, especially in the elderly. If the disorder becomes long-term, a gastrostomy tube (Figure 18-12) will be inserted by a physician. This tube will enter the stomach directly.

TABLE 18-5   Cultural and Religious Traditions Related to Food

Culture/Religion	Type	Food
Mexican	Cultural	Spicy foods, enchiladas, tamales, tacos, refried beans, rice, tomatoes, chili peppers, stone-ground corn
Native American	Cultural	Beans, corn, squash, chili peppers; varies with each tribe
Chinese, Japanese, Vietnamese, Korean, and Indian	Cultural	Common foods include rice, dumplings, soybean derivatives such as tofu, bean sprouts, bamboo shoots, mushrooms, snow peas. Fish is a very common staple. Food is diced and quickly stir-fried. Chopsticks are used in some cultures.
Middle Eastern, including Greek, Turkish, Iranian, Egyptian, Lebanese, Syrian, Iraqi, Israeli, and Jordanian	Cultural	Lamb and goat, goat products such as goat milk and feta cheese, chickpeas, lentils, eggplant, olives, rice, beans, flat bread such as pita and shepherd's bread, curry seasoning

TABLE 18-5   Cultural and Religious Traditions Related to Food (continued)

Culture/Religion	Type	Food
Caribbean Islands: Puerto Rican, Cuban, Jamaican, Haitian	Cultural	Tropical fruits and vegetables, such as bananas, plantains, mangoes, avocados, citrus. Rice, beans, fish are common staples.
Catholic	Religious	Fasting (one meal per day) during the forty days of Lent; abstinence from meat on Ash Wednesday and Fridays during Lent.
Jewish	Religious	Pork and pork products are prohibited. Other meats are Kosher: drained of blood and soaked in salt before preparation. Meat and dairy products are not eaten at the same meal. Certain holidays require fasting and the use of certain Kosher foods only.

application to practice

Nutrition is essential to life. Meeting the cultural, and religious preferences of patients demonstrates respect for patients' rights. Assisting the patient with diet modifications is part of the clinical assistant's scope of practice. The application of basic nutritional principles, life-span requirements, and therapeutic diets will enhance your ability to meet these needs. Based on what you have learned about nutrition and diet in this chapter, respond to the following situations.

Learning Activities

Situation 1: Nancy Gallagher is a twenty-three-year-old who has come to the emergency room (ER) for possible fecal impaction. She has not had a bowel movement in 10 days. Nancy states that prior to the constipation, she had diarrhea with ribbon-like stools for 3 weeks. She says that this has been her bowel habit for the past 2 years. She is complaining of nausea and belching. Bowel sounds are present in all four quadrants, but her abdomen is distended. The physician orders an enema, which provides relief, and diagnoses her with irritable bowel syndrome. What is your understanding of irritable bowel syndrome?

Author's Explanation: Irritable bowel syndrome is thought to be a stress-related bowel disorder in which the colon spasms, producing alternating periods of diarrhea and constipation.

Situation 2: What diet will probably be ordered for Ms. Gallagher?

Author's Explanation: A high-fiber diet that includes plenty of roughage and a water intake of at least eight 8-ounce glasses will probably be recommended.

Situation 3: What foods does a high-fiber diet include?

Author's Explanation: A high-fiber diet includes whole-grain breads and cereals and fruits and vegetables. Foods to be avoided include empty-calorie foods and those high in refined sugar.

Situation 4: What is refined sugar?

Author's Explanation: Refined sugar is sugar that has been processed from its naturally occurring raw cane form. This includes white and brown sugar. Better forms of sugar are those found in fruits, such as fructose.

Situation 5: Mr. Kilgallan is suffering from malnutrition secondary to metastatic cancer (CA). What kind of diet will probably be prescribed for Mr. Kilgallan?

Author's Explanation: A diet high in protein would be important to a malnourished patient unless the patient has CA of the kidney or kidney disease.

Situation 6: Mr. Kilgallan is edentulous and has difficulty with solid food. How might his diet be modified?

Author's Explanation: He will probably be on a soft diet with foods ground or run through a blender. When he is unable to tolerate a soft diet, he will be moved to full liquids. In addition, he may be given supplements such as Ensure.

Situation 7: Mrs. Smith has been diagnosed with severe hypertension and atherosclerosis. Her cholesterol level is 400. What dietary modifications might the physician prescribe?

Author's Explanation: The physician will probably prescribe a low-fat, low-cholesterol, and low-sodium diet.

Situation 8: What foods should Mrs. Smith avoid?

Author's Explanation: On a low-fat diet, foods to avoid include all fried foods. On a low-cholesterol diet, foods to limit include egg yolks, organ meats, cream cheese, and milk. A low-sodium diet requires the avoidance of table salt. In addition, salt-cured meats, sauerkraut, pickles, olives, and certain frozen and canned foods must be avoided.

Situation 9: Mrs. Fischer is a forty-seven-year-old mother of three who has decided it is time to lose weight. She is being followed by home care after a right total knee replacement. She is 5 foot, 4 inches and 260 pounds. The doctor wants her to lose 100 pounds. How many pounds are safe to lose per week? How many calories must she cut out each week in order to lose two pounds? How many calories should her daily intake be?

Author's Explanation: Mrs. Fischer will be put on a calorie-restricted diet. According to her physician's goal of 160 pounds, her intake should be 2,400 calories per day. One to two pounds per week is a safe weight loss. To decrease her weight by two pounds per week, she will need to decrease her weekly caloric intake by 7,000 calories.

Situation 10: Mrs. Fischer has been given the food pyramid as a guide to developing meal plans. She has developed several sample menus that

the nurse will review. One twenty-four-hour menu is listed below. Here are her menu choices for one twenty-four-hour period:

- Breakfast: three-egg omelette, home fries, two slices of bacon, bagel with cream cheese, and 8 ounces of orange juice.
- Lunch: Swiss cheese and pastrami, a kaiser roll, tossed salad with blue cheese dressing, egg custard, and a can of cola
- Dinner: cheeseburger with bacon on a bun, baked potato, corn and peas medley, and apple cobbler

What do you think about her food choices? Which of the seven essential nutrients is she missing?

Author's Explanation: Mrs. Fischer is including many high-fat products in her diet. In addition, she doesn't have enough servings of fruits and vegetables. She has included refined sugars. Bacon and cream cheese are both considered high in fat, and home fries are fried. Omelettes are generally prepared with butter or margarine.

Better choices would be a two-egg vegetable omelette made with a small amount of cooking spray; two slices of whole wheat, rye, or similar grain bread; boiled potatoes seasoned with herbs, and a fresh fruit cup with citrus fruit. For lunch, the pastrami could be exchanged for fresh turkey breast; the Swiss cheese, for a low-fat variety. The sandwich could include lettuce, tomato, onion, sprouts, green pepper, or another vegetable. The kaiser roll could be replaced by a grain bread. The blue cheese dressing could be exchanged for a small amount of olive oil and some lemon juice, vinegar and olive oil with herbs, or other low-fat salad dressing. Instead of cola, Mrs. Fischer could have a tall glass of water with a lemon or lime slice or a homemade fruit spritzer using half juice and half seltzer. For dinner, the cheeseburger could be replaced with a turkey burger or a lean boneless breast of chicken; the vegetables could be expanded to include carrots or a dark green leafy vegetable. Bread could be added without butter or margarine. The apple cobbler could be replaced with a baked apple. Mrs. Fischer's diet is missing water, one of the seven essential nutrients. These are just some modifications. How many others can you think of?

Examination Review Questions

1. Which is not a type of circulating lipoprotein?
   a. HDL
   b. LDL
   c. VLDL
   d. VDL

2. Which essential nutrient is the most concentrated form of energy?
   a. carbohydrate
   b. protein
   c. fat
   d. cholesterol

3. The essential nutrient responsible for rebuilding and repairing body structures is
   a. carbohydrate
   b. fat
   c. protein
   d. fiber

4. All of the following vitamins are fat-soluble except vitamin
   a. C
   b. A
   c. D
   d. E

5. Which vitamin aids in the formation of bone and teeth?
   a. A
   b. C
   c. D
   d. E

6. Another name for thiamine is Vitamin
   a. B_1
   b. B_2
   c. B_6
   d. B_{12}

7. Which nutrient is an inorganic element necessary in the regulation of fluid and various body functions?
   a. sodium
   b. iron
   c. vitamin D
   d. carbohydrate

8. How many daily servings of vegetables are recommended in the food pyramid?
   a. 4–6
   b. 3–5
   c. 6–11
   d. 1–3

9. Which therapeutic diet is used for the edentulous resident?
   a. bland
   b. soft
   c. liquid
   d. diabetic

10. Which group requires additional protein?
    a. pregnant women
    b. school-age children
    c. adolescent boys
    d. middle-aged adults

The Human Person

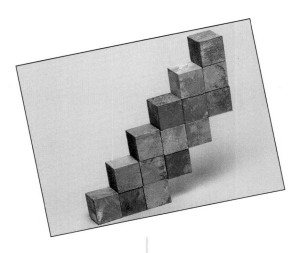

One physician's quest to reverse the process of death and to continue the temporal existence of humans was the theme of one of the most notable Victorian novels, Mary Shelley's *Frankenstein*. Dr. Frankenstein never realized, in his transplanting of various parts to re-create human life, that beyond the human body is the human spirit. Because humans are the highest functioning beings on this planet, their needs are complex and interrelated. Many theories exist about the levels of human needs, the ways in which we meet these needs, and the reasons for our inability to meet these needs. The human spirit drives the need to belong, to be accepted, to feel safe and secure, and, ultimately, to survive when existence is threatened. These elements of the human person—psychosocial, spiritual, cultural, and sexual—are carried through the life journey from the beginning at birth until the final stages of death.

Chapter 19

Care Delivery for the Whole Person

In this chapter, we will explore the human person, complete with needs and stages of development across the life span. We will also explore aspects of the human person that create uniqueness and similarities. The human person is the sum total of physiological, mental, social, sexual, and spiritual components. Each component undergoes stages of growth and development. Each stage presents the human person with spiritual, social, and emotional challenges.

Your work in health care will present you with a range of emotions from joy to grief. Reflect on your experiences with patients and their loved ones and try to gain insight into your life. It is a rich human experience to care for others. Remember that as a human person, the only perfection you will achieve in life is being perfectly human!

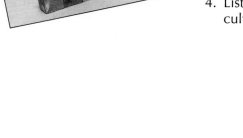

OBJECTIVES

After completing this chapter, you will be able to

1. Describe Maslow's hierarchy of needs
2. List the stages of development and the associated needs across the human life span
3. Define *cultural diversity*
4. List the components of a culture
5. Define *human sexuality*
6. Apply ethical, spiritual, cultural, and psychosocial concepts as they relate to the clinical care associate's scope of practice
7. Define and spell all key terms correctly

The Basic Needs of Humans

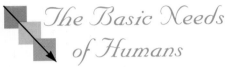

There are many theorists who have examined human growth and development. Through their studies, they developed theories about the growth and development of the human person. **Growth** refers to the physical changes of the human body throughout the life span; **development** is concerned with the psychological, sociological, moral, and intellectual evolvement of the human person.

One theorist, Abraham Maslow, proposed a model of human needs throughout the life cycle. He stated that the primitive needs of humans must be met before higher-level needs can be developed. This model, first proposed in 1902, has become one of the most popular theories of human needs. It is called *Maslow's Hierarchy of Needs,* and it is charted as a pyramid. Let's examine Maslow's model (Figure 19-1).

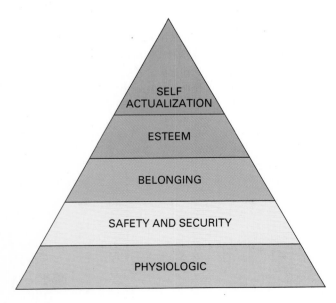

FIGURE 19-1 Maslow's Hierarchy of Needs

Maslow's Hierarchy of Needs

According to Maslow's hierarchy, needs must be met starting at the bottom of the pyramid; these are the primitive, or primary, needs. Needs that are not met at any level of the hierarchy will prevent the person from addressing needs above that level. There are five levels to the hierarchy. These are

- Physiological (water, oxygen, food)
- Safety and security
- Love and belonging
- Self-esteem
- Self-actualization

Let's examine how each of these levels of needs is satisfied.

Physiological needs—the need for oxygen, water, and food—are the most basic. Safety and security needs are satisfied by shelter, clothing, and freedom from harm. To satisfy these needs, we must have money to buy the clothes and to pay for the shelter. So, in modern societies, security needs include a job or a source of money. But even in the wilderness without money, a person will seek shelter and a safe place to live and rest. Love and belonging needs are met through family and friends. Association with others helps us to feel loved and affiliated with a family or a social group.

The esteem needs include self-esteem and the esteem, or value, of others within a social community or group. In infancy and childhood, self-esteem comes from others who make the child feel valued, useful, and worthwhile. We need to feel that there are others with whom we "belong" and who love us. As we develop, we begin to find **self-esteem**—internal value and worth—as well as esteem from others. As an adult, we can praise and reward ourselves when we know that we have done a good job, but as children we need first to learn from others what is "good" or valued.

Self-actualization is the highest-level need, and Maslow tells us that some people may never satisfy it.

Self-actualization is essentially a quest to find out who we are, what our life means, and the purpose for our existence. It can be compared to knowing and achieving our full potential as a human person.

Maslow said that the human person has motivating and demotivating forces that move the individual up and down the levels of this pyramid. If one's most basic need for air is satisfied, then one can meet the need for water. Having satisfied this need, food becomes a priority. No one can live without oxygen. Within minutes without oxygen, life ceases. In just a few days without water, one dies. Let's face it, if you can't breathe, you do not think about getting a drink of water.

An infant is focused on satisfying these most basic needs. In the first seconds of life outside of the womb, the infant begins to "fight for life"; the infant now must gasp for the breath of life and breathe independently. The infant is dependent on the caretaker to provide water and nourishment. Next, the infant needs to feel safe and secure—to be free from harm, sheltered, and clothed. If the need for water and food is not met with consistency, then the infant cannot find the sense of security necessary for development. The infant may fail to thrive. When parents consistently provide for these needs, the infant feels safe and secure. The infant is able to gain a sense of belonging and to experience love.

As this baby grows and develops into a toddler and then a child, life events and nurturing help him or her to build self-esteem. The esteem, or value, provided by others in the social environments of home, school, and friends helps the child to feel a sense of self-worth and the esteem of others. If something happens to threaten the child's self-esteem, he or she is demotivated to the level of love and belonging needs. The child seeks those who provide love to satisfy the child's need for a sense of belonging. If this need is satisfied, then the child is motivated to achieve the esteem needs. If the child's sense of belonging is disrupted by divorce or even changing neighborhoods or schools, the belonging need may not feel fulfilled, and the child is demotivated to find security from home, school, or any safe environment. The need to feel safe and secure becomes more important than love or belonging to a group. Can you remember an argument between your parents that made you feel that you might no longer belong to or be loved by them? You might remember thinking that you would have nowhere to live and no one to love you if your parents separated the family.

Once an individual has achieved the level of esteem needs, he or she can move to fulfilling the next level of need—self-actualization. As an adult, you may be trying to reach for your potential as a human person. You may be striving to achieve goals and to find your purpose in this life. If you no longer have self-esteem or the esteem of others, you may be demotivated and may abandon the quest for self-actualization because you do not have the motivational forces to propel you to the highest level of the pyramid.

How does this model relate to health care delivery? It is important to assess the patient's level of need satisfaction within the hierarchy because this is where the patient is coming from. Table 19-1 presents two cases and relates the circumstances to Maslow's hierarchy of needs.

It is hoped that you can see from these illustrations of the human experience that people are motivated and demotivated by life events and circumstances. Our needs are related to the circumstances of our life events.

Erikson's Eight Stages of Man

Certain needs, such as those in Maslow's hierarchy, are care needs important to humans from birth to death. Other needs, however, are specific to the stages of development across the life span. Maslow's theory deals with the needs of humans within any developmental stage. There are theorists who have described human growth and development within a stage theory. Rather, they are concerned with human development, growth, and needs based on the human person's stage, or period of life. One theorist, Erik Erikson, developed a stage model of growth and development called the *Eight Stages of Man*. This model is based on the biological, psychological, and sociological readiness of the human person to move through the life span. Erikson talks to us about the biological readiness of the human person that propels the person through the psychological and sociological aspects of development within the framework of his or her historical perspective (the period of history experienced by the person).

For example, your grandmother was once thirteen years of age just as you were once thirteen years of age; both of you were biologically ready to perform certain developmental tasks. However, she was thirteen during the time of the Great Depression, and you were thirteen at much later in this century. You both experienced some of the same psychosocial milestones of development for a thirteen-year-old, but each of you experienced this age of life within the historical framework of your time. You and your grandmother had to conquer the psychosocial milestones of a thirteen-year-old, but she saw these through the eyes of a thirteen year old in the 1930s, and you saw them as a thirteen-year-old in the 1960s, 1970s, or 1980s. The world was definitely a

TABLE 19-1 Two Case Studies

Case of Mrs. Wisneski	Level	Response
Mrs. Wisneski lives in a run-down row house in a changing neighborhood. At seventy-nine years old, she is afraid to walk to the corner store to pick up groceries. Many times, she goes without perishable foods because of this fear. In addition, Mrs. Wisneski's plumbing requires major repair, but she doesn't have the finances to fix it. At what level is Mrs. Wisneski in Maslow's hierarchy?	Second level: safety and security	Mrs. Wisneski is at the second level of Maslow's hierarchy.
Her shelter is humble, her food is not always rich in nutrients, and her clothing is worn and dirty. At what level is Mrs. Wisneski? Why is this important?	Second level: safety and security	Mrs. Wisneski's focus is at the second level—the need for safety and security. Mrs. Wisneski will not be so concerned about learning about low-sodium foods and a nutritious diet, for example, if she is too frightened to obtain the foods from the store.

Case of Mr. Thomas	Level	Response
Mr. Thomas is a thirty-eight-year-old married man with two children. He is admitted to the hospital with the diagnosis of ulcerative colitis. He is not eating properly because he is afraid to eat. Each time he eats, he has episodes of diarrhea that are painful and disruptive to his work routine. He is an electrician and works at your hospital. At what level of need is Mr. Thomas focused?	Primary level: water, oxygen, and food	He is focused on the primary level of physiological needs. He probably focuses his conversation with his doctor and nurse on his inability to take adequate fluid and nourishment without discomfort and diarrhea.
Mr. Thomas is put on a low-residue diet and is given medications to help to control his diarrhea and meet his nutritional needs. He is discharged from the hospital. When he returns to work, he is told that his job will be phased out within the month. He needs to find a new job to support his family. What concern will Mr. Thomas now confront on the pyramid of needs?	Second level: safety and security	Mr. Thomas will most probably be focused on the safety and security level of the pyramid. He and his family will still need a home, clothes, and food even if he does not have a job. His family's security and safety are his primary concern.
Mr. Thomas tries to save money by not purchasing his costly prescriptions. He finds a new job in six weeks and is able to purchase his prescriptions again. Now, however, his wife has also found employment as a secretary to the district attorney of the county. She is often busy and works long hours with her boss. She seems to be more interested in her job than in her husband and two children. Mr. Thomas becomes depressed because of this, and he stops caring for his ulcerative colitis. He goes to visit the doctor because he has observed blood in his stool. When the doctor asks him what is happening in his life, he says, "Why bother caring for myself? My wife doesn't love me anymore." What level of need is unfulfilled for Mr. Thomas?	Third level: love and belonging	His love and belonging needs are not fulfilled, and this has demotivated Mr. Thomas.

different place; don't you agree? Grandmother did not know about TV at age thirteen. Your parents saw TV as a new technology, and to you, TV was a common household product. Think of how television influenced your development versus how it influenced your parents or grandparents.

Erik Erikson, a famed psychological theorist, described stages of development in detail. He claimed that all human people, due to their biological growth, are ready to experience social and psychological developmental tasks. It is our biology that propels us to move into social and emotional life events that shape the psychosocial aspects of our development. Let's examine the stages of development as documented by Erikson. Erikson describes the Eight Stages of Man by the biological, psychological, and sociological aspects of life. Table 19-2 outlines these eight stages, including certain concepts, milestones, and age-specific competencies associated with each of the eight stages. Figures 19-2 through 19-9 depict individuals in the various stages of life.

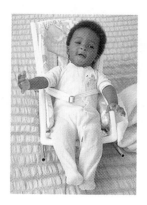

FIGURE 19-2   Infant (age 0–12 months).

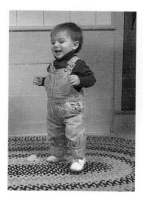

FIGURE 19-3   Toddler (age 1–3 years).

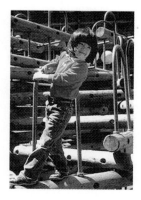

FIGURE 19-4   Preschooler (age 3–6 years).

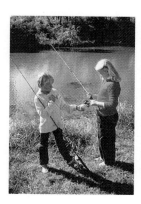

FIGURE 19-5   School-age child (age 6–12 years).

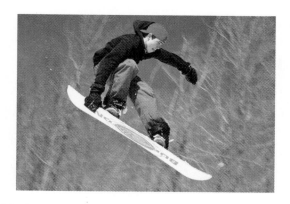

FIGURE 19-6   Adolescent (age 12–20 years). Alan & Linda Detrick, Photo Researchers, Inc.

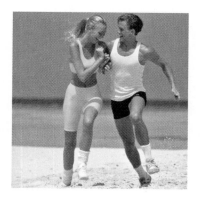

FIGURE 19-7   Young adults (age 20–35 years). Paul Steel, The Stock Market.

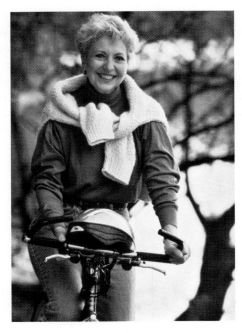

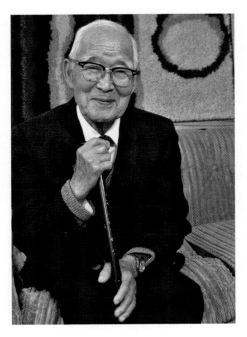

FIGURE 19-8   Middle-aged adult (age 35–65 years). Strauss/Curtis, The Stock Market.

FIGURE 19-9   Older adult (age 65 years and older).

TABLE 19-2   Erikson's Stages of Life

Stage	Age	Psychological Concept	Biological Milestone	Sociological Competency/ Tasks to Be Achieved
Infant	0–12 months	Trust versus mistrust	• Muscles increase in size and precision and control. • Bones harden. • Brain cells grow and specialize. • Weight and height increase. (This growth is faster than in any other stage.) • New brain structures differentiate and specialize.	• Learns to trust mother figure and self. • Starts to feed self, crawl, and stand. • Speaks first words.
Toddler	1–3 years	Autonomy versus shame and doubt	• Nervous system matures. • Walking, eating, and vocabulary skills improve. • Sensory perception and mobility increases.	• Walks, talks, and feeds self. • Begins toileting. • Sees self as separate from mother: *I, me, mine.* • Experiences the "terrible twos." • *No* is a favorite word. • Is self-propelled (crawls, walks, and reaches).
Preschooler	3–6 years	Initiative versus shame and doubt	• Physical growth continues, and vocabulary expands.	• Starts to initiate activities of daily living (ADLs). • Speaks in sentences. *Why* is a frequent word. • Admires opposite-sex parent and wants his or her attention, but wants to be like same-sex parent. • Begins to play with others.

TABLE 19-2   Erikson's Stages of Life *(continued)*

Stage	Age	Psychological Concept	Biological Milestone	Sociological Competency/ Tasks to Be Achieved
School-age child	6–12 years	Industry versus inferiority	• Motor and language skills develop fully. • Puberty begins.	• Begins elementary school. • Teachers are new important adults. • Develops "heroes." • Achieves self-esteem with friends and teachers. • Learns the work of the world. • Motor skills are fully developed by age 12. • Play is organized and cooperative.
Adolescent	12–20 years	Identity versus role confusion	• Growth accelerates, with sexual development and change in body proportion. • Face changes markedly. • Secondary sexual characteristics develop.	• Opposite-sex peers are important. • Achieves with peer groups and school to find self. • Begins to decide on life roles and goals for future. • Wants to be and look like friends to feel accepted by peers.
Young adult	20–35 years	Intimacy versus isolation	• Speed, coordination, strength, endurance, and physical concentration peak. • Reproductive capacity peaks for women.	• Seeks a partner in life. • Establishes life roles. May start a family and career. • Looks for intimacy and fears isolation or being without a partner.
Middle-aged adult	35–65 years	Generativity versus stagnation	• Height decreases slightly between 45 and 50. • Skin elasticity decreases. • Loss of eye accommodation, hearing, and taste begins. • Strength and the ability to perform strenuous physical labor decreases. • Brain weight decreases.	• Is ready to give to the next generation. • Concerns move from self to others and other things (children, society, environment). • May feel stagnate, "stuck in a rut" when children leave home. • Must confront the life issues of menopause and retirement.
Older adult	65 years and older	Integrity versus disgust and despair	• Functional loss occurs. • Cellular regeneration decreases. • Biochemical error of cells increases. • Cardiovascular (CV) and sensory efficiency decreases.	• Looks at the meaning and contributions of his or her life. • May resent retirement and age-related changes of the body. • May enjoy retirement and senior years. • Suffers the loss of spouse, siblings, and friends.

Age-Specific Competencies

Erikson's titles for the psychosocial stages help to describe the **competencies** that people need to achieve during each life stage. These competencies are the accomplishments and learning of the stage. The phrase *trust versus mistrust*, for example, describes the positive and negative learning of the first stage. We learn both the negative and the positive, but the strengths necessary to move us to the next psychosocial stage come from securing the positive. For example, if a baby does not learn to trust others and self, then it will be even harder to secure the sense of autonomy as a toddler. It is difficult to "do for one's self" if trust in oneself and in others is lacking.

Let's examine the meaning of the phrases used to describe the Eight Stages of Man. We'll also review age-specific needs for each stage.

1. *Trust versus mistrust*: This phrase refers to the baby's learning to trust in self and in others. Babies learn to trust that caregivers will care for their needs of food, safety, and love. Erikson says that it is the consistency of "mothering" that allows infants to learn trust. Also, babies learn to trust themselves by testing what can and cannot be done independently. When a six-month-old is learning to sit up without the support of someone else, the baby is learning to trust that he or she can do this alone.

   People need to learn what to mistrust as well as what to trust. A sense of mistrust is necessary for emotional and physical safety. If it is the consistency of the caregiver's behavior that helps a baby learn to trust, then it is inconsistent caregiving that generates a sense of mistrust. If the caregiver is not consistent in loving and caring for the baby, then the baby will be unsure whether his or her needs will be met and learns to mistrust self and others.

   Age-specific needs: The infant needs feeding, changing, touching, comforting, and communicating with eye contact, singing, and talking. Respond consistently to needs and provide for safety at all times. Toys should not be small enough to fit in the baby's mouth; they should be fire-resistant and not have removable parts that the baby can fit into the mouth. Toys should be nonbreakable. If the infant is hospitalized, the parents are encouraged to stay with the baby when they are able. Holding and comforting the baby is important in building trust with the strangers who will care for the infant.

2. *Autonomy versus shame and doubt*: The term **autonomy** means to be self-directed and to do for oneself. The sense of shame and doubt come from the embarrassment and doubt of failing to, or being told that one is unable to, do things that one is ready to do. Toddlers want to and are expected to learn to do things for themselves. Toddlers learn to walk, talk, feed, and toilet themselves. If they are permitted trial and error and are encouraged to be autonomous, they experience less shame and doubt. If they are constantly scolded for their errors, they feel shame, and they doubt their sense of autonomy. The toddler is concerned with "me, my, and mine" and frequently says "no." The phrase *the terrible twos* comes from the toddler's willful need to achieve autonomy.

   Age-specific needs: The freedom to learn to do things independently (with limit setting for safety, security, and development of self-control, of course) is important for the toddler. Praise for accomplishing independence in dressing, talking, feeding, walking, and toileting is also important. Treat regression of learned independent behaviors, such as toileting, in a matter-of-fact manner. **Regression** means returning behaviorally to an early stage of development. Don't scold or embarrass the toddler for performing a task unsuccessfully. Teach the toddler how to perform the task, and be patient with self-centered behavior because toddlers think they are the most important person in their world. Toys should be nonbreakable and a safe size because toddlers still like to test things with their mouths. They can choke or injure themselves easily with toys that are breakable or have removable parts. Toys that support the learning of motor control, sizes, colors, names, and shapes are best for toddlers. If hospitalized, the toddler needs to have parents stay if possible. Encourage independence in activities that the toddler has been doing at home. Keep the safety of the toddler foremost in all aspects of care. Allow time for play, and be patient with fearfulness of strangers, procedures, and the hospital environment.

3. *Initiative versus guilt*: Preschoolers want to and are biologically ready to **initiate** (start) certain activities. Once they gain a sense of autonomy, they are more certain of themselves. They begin to play with other children, ask many questions, and try to accomplish things on their own. "I do it myself" is a frequent phrase of preschoolers because it is important to them to initiate and accomplish tasks independently. Preschoolers may imitate the actions and roles of their parents. They learn guilt by initiating tasks that they are not permitted to do. They begin to recognize the consequences of their actions. Preschoolers also learn this sense of guilt when parents set unreasonable expectations and demonstrate extreme

disappointment in the child. Preschoolers try to disguise their wrongdoing by hiding something they have broken or lying about who broke it to escape parental dissatisfaction or punishment. Some children gain a strong sense of guilt because of the criticisms and the nature of the consequences that the caregiver imposes on them.

Age-specific needs: Preschoolers need to initiate tasks and should be permitted to take the lead in activities of daily living. Although children may choose clothes that do not match, they should be praised for trying. Their curiosity about the world and eagerness to learn is demonstrated by frequent questions about how, who, and why things and people are certain ways. Play with other children is important, and preschoolers need to learn cooperativeness in play. Toys that encourage verbal skills and motor dexterity are needed. Preschoolers need to learn about safe and unsafe places, people, and things. Answers to questions should be honest and aimed at the child's level of understanding. When the preschooler is in the hospital, it is important to explain all activities to him or her. This will encourage cooperation. Parents are encouraged to stay with the child. Maintain independence in ADLs, and honestly answer questions in simple language that the child can understand.

4. *Industry versus inferiority*: School-age children gain a sense of **industry** from their work: school and play. Before formal schools were established, children learned this sense of industry by working beside their parents. Usually, the parent taught the child a trade or profession. Today, children also learn to be industrious in the home by doing chores and errands. School is a major source for gaining this sense of industry. Achievement and hard work at play, chores, and studies help the school-age child to have this sense of industry. However, children also gain a sense of **inferiority** as they recognize their failures and weaknesses. They may develop a stronger sense of inferiority if they are put down, or criticized, for trying and failing to meet the expectations of parents, teachers, and friends. We all learn that we are not the best at everything we try to do. When others accept our weaknesses and praise our strengths, we learn to strive for success, set goals, and gain self-esteem.

Age-specific needs: School-age children need time to play and interact with their peers. They need opportunities to play at activities that further develop motor skills, for example bike riding, skating, and organized sports. Playacting adult roles—teacher, mom, dad, pilot—is important for social and emotional development.

Achievement in school is important in building self-esteem. The need exists for structured time for study, including supervision and assistance with study and school projects. School-age children benefit from participating in organizations, such as soccer and softball leagues, school sports, and other activities like Boy Scouts of America and Girl Scouts of America. These activities help children at this age to learn the value and the importance of cooperation and contribution in group activities. If the school-age child is hospitalized, parents may be encouraged to stay with the child. Explain and be honest about all tests, procedures, and care given. School work can be continued if needed. Allow time for telephoning friends, and provide activities and games that are age-appropriate. Remember that privacy will be important for the child who is going through puberty.

5. *Identity versus role confusion*: Adolescents are trying to gain a sense of identity but are often confused about who and what they want to be. During adolescence, the teenager is expected to prepare for the roles of adulthood. During high school, choices of college, job training, or fields of work are considered. Teens try to define their **identity** (who they are) by the groups with whom they associate and the friends that they choose. They rebel against parents and the norms of society to demonstrate this identity. They are no longer children and not yet adults, but their bodies are changing into adult bodies. Adolescents often want to participate in activities that are considered adult activities (e.g. sexual relationships). Acceptance among peer groups is very important, and sometimes teens participate in activities with peers that their parents do not approve of. They want to do what the other teenagers are doing because they want to be like them. It is in trying to be like others, and at the same time trying to be unique, that teenagers establish their identity. They face much confusion in finding this identity.

Age-specific needs: Peers of both sexes play an important part in the adolescent's development. Talking on the telephone and listening to music are favorite activities for many teenagers. The physical changes associated with growth in height, weight, and sexual development make teenagers acutely aware of and sensitive to their body and appearance. In puberty, some teens are awkward about their physical development, so privacy is important. Teenagers need support in developing adultlike behavior and in making career choices. They need independence, but limit setting is also important. Honest discussions about their recreational activities, sexuality, and lifestyle choices are essential to the guidance that adolescents need in preparing for young adulthood. Adolescents need support to affiliate with different groups of friends and organized groups, such as school clubs, sports, band, and competitive activities. These help to build their identity. If hospitalized, adolescents need to be able to visit with their friends and to use the phone to communicate with their peers. They need the same privacy and respect as adults. They may not ask questions about procedures and diagnoses, but they should be encouraged to ask questions and should be given honest answers. Encourage adultlike behavior, but recognize and be patient with their childlike frustrations.

6. *Intimacy versus isolation*: In young adulthood, people are searching for intimacy with another person. Sexual intimacy is often confused with true intimacy because young adults have not yet gained a true sense of identity and intimacy with themselves. To be truly intimate with another, we must first be intimate with ourself, have a real sense of personal identity, and love who we are. Failure to find a partner with whom we can give of ourself may heighten our sense of fear and isolation. Society expects young adults to look for and to find a mate. This societal pressure imposes a sense of aloneness and isolation for those who remain unattached. When a person has established a relationship that is without intimacy, both partners experience a sense of isolation. Divorce, separation, and the isolation of marriage partners are the by-products of disrupted intimacy in a relationship. During this time of life, young adults choose careers and establish homes for themselves and their families.

Age-specific needs: Young adults need to form bonds with people of both sexes. Most are searching for a mate and are exploring new relationships in an attempt to find someone with whom they can be intimate. Young adults need to learn the responsibilities and roles of adulthood. Attending college or postsecondary training programs and working are necessary to prepare young adults for careers and for independent living. Young adults need to learn to budget money and to arrange for independent living. If they are sick or hospitalized, they are concerned about the safety and care of their children, their home, and job security.

7. *Generativity versus stagnation*: In the years of middle adulthood, life undergoes many events and changes. People establish and change careers and lifestyles, raise children, go through meno-

pause, and plan for life after retirement. There is a readiness to be **generative** (to demonstrate concern for the next generation). Whether they have married or have had children, middle-aged adults embark on or are thrust into the caring of others, society, and the world. Most people find the sense of generativity through caring for their children and home. But those who have no children of their own can find this sense of generativity by an interest and concern for others through careers and life activities. The inability to move beyond oneself and one's interests and concerns is referred to as **stagnation**. Sometimes, when children move on to establish their own lives with home and family, parents may feel this stagnation. The expression *empty-nest syndrome* comes from this experience of stagnation. Generativity is gained when people see the contributions they have made to family and society.

Age-specific needs: Adults in this age group need to be productive in family, work, and community. Some adults at this age are not only caring for their children, but are also caring for their parents. If they become ill or hospitalized, they worry about their responsibilities to home, job, and family. Finances are often a major concern because of mortgages or rent, children's college tuition, insurance, and other responsibilities that require them to work. Midlife physical changes (menopause) and the loss of the physical appearance of youth (hair loss, graying, wrinkles, and so on) may not be accepted easily. Middle-aged adults need emotional support and reassurance about their desirability and value to others. Planning for retirement and the fact that the children are leaving home to start their own families are significant issues during this stage of life.

8. *Integrity versus disgust and despair*: In late adulthood, the accomplishments of the other seven life stages are realized in the sense of integrity. **Integrity**, the last of the psychosocial competencies, is linked to the trust of the first stage of life, for trust is belief in the integrity of others. Integrity is felt in the sense of the wholeness or completeness of one's life; the belief that one's life has had meaning and purpose. It is the belief that you have done the best that you could with your life, based on the circumstances of your life history. The sense of **despair** and **disgust** often comes from the feeling that one's life has not been meaningful and that there is not enough time left to accomplish tasks that would give life purpose and meaning. Many elders are confronted with situations that lead them to feel disgust and despair.

Failing health, loss of independence, limited finances, and the death of loved ones present elders with stress and frustration. And for some, these stressors lead to feelings of disgust and despair about growing old. Reminiscence about life events and preparation for life's ending or death are important tasks of this stage. Different cultures regard elders and care for elders in different ways. In some cultures, the elder's wisdom and life experience are valued and treated with great respect. In the United States, many elders feel that youth is what is valued and desired and that, because of their age, they are no longer valued and needed.

Age-specific needs: Elders' needs vary greatly, based on physical and financial status. Some elders remain independent in all aspects of life, and others need partial or total assistance. Elders may be retired or widowed, and social activities with family and friends are important to their emotional well-being. Older adults need to maintain as much independence as possible. They need to know that they are useful and valued regardless of their level of independence. The need to reminisce and tell stories about the past is important for elders' self-esteem. Reminisence is an evaluation of what their lives have meant to them and to others. Older adults who are in long-term care or hospital care need to be treated with dignity and respect and should not be called "Granny," "Sweetie," or other "pet" names. They are not children, and even those who have cognitive impairments should not be treated or encouraged in a childlike fashion.

Human Sexual Behavior

Throughout the history of humankind and the life history of any person, sexuality and sexual behavior cannot be ignored. It is sexual behavior that leads to reproduction and the continuation of a species. In all animals other than single-cell animals, reproduction involves the coupling of **gender** (opposite-sex) partners. Artists, writers, and theologians, as well as scientists of biology, sociology, psychology, and anthropology, have studied and described animal sexual behavior, most especially human sexuality.

Sexual Behavior Research

In 1897, an English psychologist, Havelock Ellis, shocked Victorian English society with his *Studies in the Psychology of Sex.* His work openly refuted the idea that homosexuality is a sickness because he be-

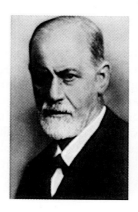

FIGURE 19-10   Sigmund Freud.

lieved that it is inborn. He declared that the legal system should have no part in the private sexual relationship of two consenting adults.

Sigmund Freud also studied human sexuality in the late nineteenth and early twentieth centuries (Figure 19-10). He believed that one's sexuality is rooted in the unconscious mind and is influenced by childhood episodes that led to what and whom individuals search for in adult love. Freud's study of human sexuality was based on his psychoanalytic treatment of patients. His study was conducted during the Victorian era—a period of history that emphasized morality and frowned on the discussion of sex. Sexual behavior was necessary for reproduction, but it was considered vulgar to discuss sexuality in polite society. Freud and Ellis did much for the initial and formal study of human sexual behavior. They opened the door for the discussion and study of the topic.

In the 1950s, two more daring scientists, William Masters and Virginia Johnson, conducted research of hundreds of men and women. Their laboratory studies monitored the male and female responses during sexual intercourse. For the first time, the physiological response of sexual stimulation was researched. They found that the human sexual response consisted of four phases: *excitement, plateau, orgasm,* and *recovery.* They found that men and women had very similar sexual responses, both psychologically and physiologically. These two scientists continued to open the "closet" door and the frontier to the study of sexuality. Now, all medical and nursing schools include a human sexuality course in their curricula.

Sexual Behavior and Patient Care

It is important for the clinical care associate to have an understanding of the importance of human sexuality in the holistic care of patients. One's sexuality is not something that can be separated from the person, any more than one's spirituality can. A patient or client does not leave this aspect of self at home when entering the doors of a health care facility. **Sexuality** is the awareness of one's sexual qualities as a man or a woman. It is influenced by many factors and is expressed in one's attitudes and behaviors. Gender, culture, religion, age, health, environment, and physical appearance all influence sexuality and sexual behavior. Sexuality is psychologically and physiologically developed and is influenced throughout one's life.

Growth and Development and Sexuality

In infancy, the baby learns about love and physical closeness from caregivers in the baby's environment. Research has shown that parents tend to cuddle baby girls more and dress them in clothes to identify femininity. Baby boys are typically cuddled less than girls, and their sexuality is identified by clothes with designs of cars or sports.

Toddlers are usually given toys that are descriptive of traditional male and female roles. Girls are given soft, cuddly toys, while boys are given trucks and cars. Toddlers begin to recognize the physical differences of boys and girls, and they are interested in learning about the names of their sexual organs.

Preschoolers are more aware of the physical differences of the sexes and are curious about the differences in adult and child sexual organs. They begin to ask questions about these differences. They often are most interested in the attention of the opposite-sex parent; preschool girls may want to behave like Mommy to get Daddy's attention, for example.

School-age children are most interested in the sameness of their gender. They play typically with children of the same sex and easily become embarrassed by demonstrations of interest or attraction from the opposite sex. By the end of the school-age period, children start to experience the physical changes of puberty. Some children seem comfortable with these changes, and others seem ashamed and try to conceal them.

By adolescence, the secondary sex characteristics are apparent. Sexual curiosity and interest peak, and for many adolescents, sexual experimentation begins. At this age, boys are capable of impregnating a girl, and girls are able to become pregnant and bear children. Out-of-wedlock teenage pregnancy is not uncommon in today's society, and it is a topic of medical and political concern. In the early part of this century and in centuries past, marriages began

in adolescence. The life expectancy was shorter, and people compensated for this by having children in adolescence. Today, many people in Western societies find it preferable to establish careers and wait until they are in their late twenties, thirties or forties to start families.

In young adulthood, the body matures, and sexuality continues to be defined. People look for intimacy in a relationship, and they choose a spouse or a life partner. Whether heterosexual (sexually attracted to members of the opposite sex) or homosexual (sexually attracted to members of the same sex), people want to share themselves intimately with another. Young adults establish a level of comfort and acceptance with their sexual identity.

In the middle adult years, sexual activity may be less frequent than in young adulthood. The pressures of work, home, and raising children may decrease the availability or opportunity for sexual activity. As women undergo menopause, hormonal changes affect them physically and psychologically, but this does not make a woman less attractive or less interested in a sexual relationship. It is the person's sense of self-esteem and self-image, along with the closeness of the relationship with her partner that have a greater impact on the sexual relationship than the changes of menopause. For some women, the decline of feminine hormones causes dryness of the vagina and may make intercourse painful. Impotence may affect some men at this age because of vascular disease, or medications (such as antihypertensives) may cause impotence or decreased sexual desire. A woman's libido (sex drive) can also be affected by menopause or medications. At any age, illness and medications can impact one's sexual interest and response. As people age, arthritis and other conditions decrease physical agility and mobility. This makes it necessary to adapt former sexual positions and activities to accommodate physical needs in order to continue to be sexually active. Some individuals find the period of middle adulthood to be one of sexual freedom. After menopause, the fear of unwanted pregnancy is no longer an issue, and the children are grown and are less demanding of their parents' time and energy.

In spite of many myths about old age, senior citizens are still sexual beings. Some seniors are limited only by the absence of a partner. More women than men are widowed and have no available partner for sex. Those who are fortunate enough to have a partner and who are in reasonably good health are able to remain sexually active. Even those who are no longer engaging in sexual intercourse find that the closeness and comfort of a sexual partner is desirable, and intimacy is wanted. Figure 19-11 shows an elderly couple who benefit from a shared relationship.

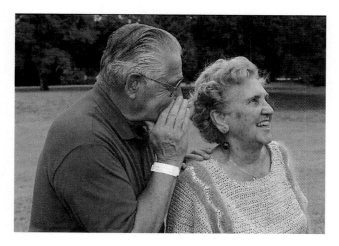

FIGURE 19-11 Elderly couple.

Care Delivery and Patients' Sexuality

You may be wondering how you, as a clinical care associate, will be involved in the sexuality of your patients. It is most important for health care workers to be supportive and nonjudgmental of the sexual preferences and lifestyles of their clients. Respect for the individual as a human being must be foremost in your care. Patients from varying sexual backgrounds and preferences will be in your care. You should be attentive to their expressions of sexuality. When people are ill or in an institution for acute or long-term care, their sexuality is affected. Disease, surgery, medication, and rehabilitation affect the patient's self-image, physical stamina, social and emotional well-being, and libido.

Conditions such as paralysis; cancer of the reproductive organs; neuromuscular, skeletal, and cardiovascular diseases; medications; radiation therapy; surgeries that cause any real or imagined disfigurement; mental illness; and depression all affect sexual image. Be attuned to any behavior, mood, questions, or comments that express patients' need to validate their sexuality, desirability, or ability to engage in sexual activity. Often people are embarrassed to ask questions about sexual activity and seek permission to talk about their fears and worries. They should be encouraged to discuss any such fears or worries with the physician and the nurse. If sexual counseling is necessary, the physician can refer the patient to the appropriate specialist.

Role of the Clinical Care Associate

You should also be aware of your own sexuality and patients' responses to you as a sexual being. Obviously, you should not have sexual relationships with your patients, but you should not deny that patients are people, too, and that they may be attracted to you. You should respond professionally and directly if a patient makes sexually suggestive comments or gestures toward you. You should calmly let the person know that you are uncomfortable with the behavior and that it is not appropriate for your relationship with them. Sometimes a male patient may get an erection while you are providing care, and you should not respond in a fearful, rejecting, or childish manner. You should simply state that you think he needs some time alone and that you will return in a little while. Couples will need time alone and may request that you shut the door to give them privacy. You should respect their wishes and let the nurse in charge of the patient's care know about the request.

Privacy for Residents of Long-Term Care Facilities

Married couples in nursing homes are usually in a private room, and they should be permitted privacy. Sometimes residents in nursing homes form relationships that are sexual in nature. They are adults and have this choice as adults. Nonetheless, if a resident is unable to consent to this type of relationship, the nursing staff will have to advocate for him or her. People who have cognitive impairments, such as Alzheimer's disease, or any disability that interferes with their judgment or reasoning ability must be protected.

Counseling for Clients

You will have patients who have sexually transmitted diseases who need counseling and education. A professional nurse, physician, or counselor will provide this education and counseling.

Couples who are experiencing infertility will need counseling and guidance from physicians and counselors. Infertility, or the inability to become pregnant, may pose a threat to the relationship. Both partners may feel inadequate because each feels responsible for the infertility. One's sexuality may be threatened because the individual feels that he is not man enough or that she is not woman enough to achieve the desired pregnancy.

Children and adolescents will ask questions about sex, and they may exhibit sexual behavior, such as masturbation, while in a health care facility. You should not respond with judgment and should recognize that this is not abnormal behavior. Provide privacy, and let the patient's nurse know about the behavior and any questions the patient has asked. With small children, you may want to direct the questions to the parents or guardians if appropriate.

Sexual Abuse and Rape Victims

If children or patients of any age report what sounds like sexual abuse, you should immediately report this to the nurse so that the appropriate interventions can take place. If you notice bruises of the breasts, genitals, or anal area, you should report this to the patient's nurse.

If you have a patient who has been raped or sexually molested or abused, your gentle emotional support is needed. **Rape** is defined as a criminal act of sexual assault without the consent of the victim. Men as well as women can be raped. Penetration of the anus or vagina against the will of the victim is rape; this results in physical and emotional trauma. Victims of sexual assault should be counseled by a trained professional. If you become involved in the care of a rape victim, you should stay with the patient. Rape victims may be frightened and may feel shame over being raped. Your quiet reassurance, comfort, and listening will be valued. Do not throw away or clean any evidence. Do not allow the patient to wash or bathe until examined and until specimens are collected. With the patient's permission, the physician or nurse will take pictures of any injuries as evidence. Clothes will also be kept as evidence. This patient needs reassurance that the sexual assault was not provoked. No one wants to be raped. Help this patient to feel safe and accepted.

The Spiritual Needs of Patients

The care of another person involves caring for the whole person, and that includes the person's spirituality—what the person believes. Many people believe that there is a world beyond the physical world and that the human spirit longs to be filled with much more than this earthly world has to offer. And though some people pursue worldly treasures with a vengeance, they indicate from time to time that they feel there is something more to life. Some call this a thirst for the Almighty. Whether the Almighty is called Yahweh, Jehovah, Lord, or Higher Power, those with faith know that the title is not the belief. Faith is the belief that there is more to the human person than what is known and seen in our current state of existence. This thirst creates spiritual needs.

Among those who believe, the need for spirituality is manifested in different ways. Some contemplate or meditate on the mysteries of their faith; others pray audibly, repeating words long since committed to memory; still others find comfort in listening to or reading passages from the Bible, the Koran, or other Scripture. The human person is truly a composite of body and spirit. Some claim to see the human spirit through an aura, a word used to describe the glow of color emanating from a person's energy field. Whether seen or not, its existence is not disputable to those with faith. Since this hunger exists, meeting the patient's spiritual needs is important for a holistic approach to care. Remember that as a health care team member, you are there to care for the patient's needs, and for many patients' spiritual needs are often overlooked.

There are people who do not believe in a higher power or God; the term used to describe this type of person is **agnostic**. (*Agnostic* literally means "without knowing.") It is important not to try to impose your beliefs on others. The individual's right to choose to believe or not to believe in God must be respected.

Erik Erikson says that people may not experience this spiritual need or longing until they face death. Some people look for spirituality in late adulthood to give life meaning as they approach inevitable death. As a person who provides care to others, you need to attend to what the patient needs for spiritual support and holistic health.

An important part of the nurse's assessment of a patient includes an interview about the person's health and social history. One question in the assessment profile is religious affiliation. It is important for the team to know if the client would like to talk with a priest, a minister, or a rabbi. Even people who do not belong to a particular religious group may have faith in God and find the need for spiritual guidance. Many hospitals have pastoral care departments to meet the spiritual needs of the patient and the family. The employees of the pastoral care department can be clergy or religious leaders from any organized faith. They are members of the multidisciplinary health care team, and they participate in care conferences and patient treatment.

Visiting clergy from all denominations of faith also see patients and families to provide the blessings and guidance of the patient's specific religious group. Priests or lay religious come to hospital rooms to deliver Communion to patients. Patients should be offered the opportunity to visit with someone from pastoral care. They need to know that spiritual guidance and life counseling are accessible twenty-four hours a day. When hospitals do not have a pastoral care department, they have clergy on call from the community to meet patient and family needs. Health care team members must respect patients' spiritual rituals and allow them the opportunity to express their spiritual needs. Even though you may not understand these rituals, you must respect them.

Illness presents the patient, family, and friends with decisions and dilemmas that may be easier to bear with guidance or counsel from a religious leader. If you are caring for a client in a community setting or in home care, you, the nurse, or a professional team member should ask about the client's interest or need to attend services or to visit with a religious leader. Clients in community care should not be denied their spiritual needs. Efforts should be made to assist the individual in meeting these needs.

We must be respectful of religious practices that affect the patient's health care decisions. Jehovah's Witnesses and Seventh-Day Adventists will not accept blood or organ transplants. This causes conflict for health care teams when the patient is medically in need of blood and the patient refuses because of religious beliefs. Hospitals sometimes get court orders to impose the life-saving treatment against the wishes of the family when the patient is a minor or an incapacitated adult. Certainly, this creates an ethical dilemma for family and team members.

Cultural Diversity

Traditions are certain practices that are customary and special and are carried on generation after generation. A tradition such as eating special food on a holiday, saying grace before meals, or holding a yearly family reunion picnic creates an environment of stability and security. Traditions can cross a large segment of people (like a Christmas tree at Christmas), or they may be unique to one family. Dietary practices are part of one's culture. Some are based on religion, such as the Jewish celebration of Passover, and some are part of immigrants' attachment to their native land and their desire to eat familiar ethnic dishes. Values are codes by which to live. Values begin in the home, based on culture and religion. Religion and the belief in a higher authority provide comfort to individuals and support to each believer. Religion provides a sense of belonging and strength to cope with adversities, such as illness and death.

Ethnicity influences culture because certain ethnic groups hold strong to beliefs and customs unique to them. **Ethnicity** (ethnic affiliation) is identified by the heritage of one's native land. Some classifications of ethnic groups are African-American, Latino, Asian, Pacific Islander, and so on. In the United States, there are numerous ethnic groups that form the American culture. **Culture** shapes an individual's beliefs and social expectations. It also influences interactions with others. Cultural traditions—diet, language, values, religion, and customs—are passed from generation to generation. Our quest for global unity requires an acceptance of the diversity of the cultures existing in our world today. Stereotyping must be replaced with genuine understanding and respect for cultural differences (Figure 19-12).

Our perceptions are influenced by our culture; we may see things differently based on the culture and traditions of our lives. Remember, as you work with and care for others, that their behavior and values are a part of their culture. Everyone does not see the world as you see it. What a person from one culture considers beauty may not be apparent to a person from another culture. Taste, beauty, value, customs, and social norms are as diverse as the many cultures that exist in this world. What may seem abnormal or unusual behavior to you should be seen within the context and perspective of another's experience and culture.

Different cultures and religions view life and death based on their beliefs and traditions. This aspect of the human person is discussed in Chapter 20.

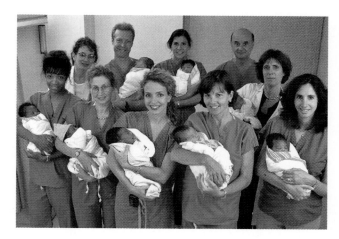

FIGURE 19-12 Cultural diversity.

![application to practice]

Understanding the stages of human growth and development, the human spirit, the need for spirituality, and the range of human sexual experiences is essential to caring for people in a holistic manner. Based on your learning from this chapter, respond to the following situations.

Learning Activities

Situation 1: Mrs. Jones is a forty-year-old woman who had a total hysterectomy for ovarian cancer. She is married and has three children. Two days post-op she tells you that she is "no longer a woman." What will you say?

Author's Explanation: You should ask Mrs. Jones what she means by this comment. She should have your undivided attention so you can hear the feelings underlying this statement. You might assume that she is concerned about her inability to bear more children, but it could be a concern for her life and the cancer that was found in her ovaries that is her pressing fear. Listen to her concerns, and report her concerns to the nurse.

Situation 2: Tim Morgan is a seventeen-year-old who is a resident in a rehabilitation center. He was admitted for injuries resulting from an automobile accident. He has paraplegia as a result of the accident. He is visited often by friends. One night you find him and his girlfriend in bed together. You do not know what they have been doing, but you are upset by this. You tell her to leave immediately, and you tell Tim that you are going to tell his mother what you saw. If you could replay this scenario, how would you replay it, and why?

Author's Explanation: Consider Tim's age and his disability. Remember that you did not see them engaged in any sexual activity. You overreacted and jumped to conclusions. You also passed judgment and treated Tim like a child. He probably felt embarrassed and ashamed in front of his girlfriend. He was also helpless to respond to your anger. He couldn't get up and run after his friend to apologize for your behavior. You needed to respond to Tim as an adult without judging him and involving his mother. You should have talked with the nurse about how to proceed. You and the nurse could have approached Tim, asked him what he was doing, and told him of your concerns. Tim is an adolescent in search of his personal and sexual identity. He probably was not having intercourse, although sometimes males with paraplegia can get an erection.

Situation 3: Mr. and Mrs. Snow are residents in the long-term care (LTC) facility where you work. They share a private room and are happy and enjoy time alone together. One night, you forget to knock on the door before you enter, and you see them naked in bed together. What should you do?

Author's Explanation: Close the door quietly, and leave them alone. If there was an urgent reason why you entered, you should close the door, knock, and announce that you have an urgent reason to see them. Let them tell you when it is acceptable to reenter the room. When you do enter the room, apologize for the rude interruption.

Situation 4: Jane Ruccocas is a three-year-old patient in the pediatric unit. She is playing with a doll, and she is talking to it about touching her "privates." She starts to get angry with the doll and throws it on the floor, saying, "Jane's a bad girl and needs to be punished." What do you do?

Author's Explanation: Ask Jane why she threw the doll on the floor and what she means by saying that "Jane's a bad girl and needs to be punished." Let Jane tell you in her own words; don't lead her in any direction. Tell the nurse what you saw and heard, reporting Jane's responses to your questions.

Situation 5: Harvey Sherr is a fifty-six-year-old patient who is being discharged from the inpatient psychiatric unit. He has been treated for depression and seems ready for discharge. While you are helping him pack his bags, he says, "You are such a kind person, and you helped me so much." He tells you he finds you attractive and that he would like to see you after he has returned home. What will you say?

Author's Explanation: You should let Mr. Sherr know that you like him as a person and that you are glad to see him taking an interest in others. Let him know that you and he have had a therapeutic relationship and that often people feel comfort from this relationship. Tell him that you will not be able to see him when he returns home and that your relationship with him will remain one of caring, but of a professional nature. Avoid using the easy way out: "I'm married" or "Policy says we can't date patients." While these may be true, they do not adequately address the patient's intentions and the purpose of maintaining a therapeutic relationship.

Situation 6: Susie Mantra is a four-year-old girl whose parents are devout Jehovah's Witnesses. One night she is sick with fever, and her father takes her to the emergency room (ER) of a children's hospital for treatment. The doctor finds that Susie has a heart murmur and a temperature of 104°F. He admits her for treatment of acute infection of the heart. The child is severely anemic and is in need of blood. Her parents will not give permission for a transfusion. Upon further examination of the heart murmur, the doctor determines that she will not survive without a heart transplant. The team decides that they must seek legal permission to give blood transfusions. The court overrules the parents' decision, and the hospital is permitted to give the child blood. The doctors and nurses explain once again to Susie's parents that she will die very soon if she does not receive a heart transplant. The parents refuse, knowing that blood will be given to Susie against their will. The transfusions are given while the distressed parents pray for guidance. The child dies two days later. At the memorial service for Susie, the parents and congregation are calm and without tears or remorse about the decisions they made.

Respond to the circumstances of this case by discussing your thoughts and feelings with a small group of classmates. Consider the intervention of the court order and the importance of faith and adherence to a religious doctrine versus the use of available life-saving measures. Should the age of this patient be a consideration? Would your response as a health care provider be affected by the age of the person?

Author's Explanation: No answer is given here because there is no "right" answer. The answer lies within you and is tied to the value you place on human life, the measures used to prolong life, and your spiritual and religious beliefs.

Situation 7: What would you do if a physician asked you to assist with a therapeutic abortion and you were opposed because of religious convictions?

Author's Explanation: There are times when health care workers may face conflict in participating in treatment or procedures that are against their religious beliefs. One example is abortion. In this situation, you should speak with the physician and explain your feelings and beliefs. Ask to be relieved of this task and offer to do the tasks of another assistant who is not in conflict over the procedure. Logically, you would also not seek employment in a clinic that performed abortions because you would not be able to do your job.

Situation 8: Reflect on a stage of your development. Consider Erikson's phrase for the competency of that stage. Discuss with a classmate your acquiring a sense of "trust versus mistrust" or another competency. Discuss the events of your family life, friends, health, or illness at this time. Consider the historical events that took place at this time in life as you reflect and discuss.

Author's Explanation: Responses will vary according to each participant's personal situation and personal background.

Situation 9: Mrs. Mark is an eighty-eight-year-old woman with congestive heart failure (CHF) and chronic obstructive pulmonary disease (COPD). She has been depressed since the death of her daughter at age 47, which occurred 11 years ago. Since her daughter's death, she has been disinterested in food, and she eats just enough for survival. Her husband died 20 years ago, and her youngest son has been overseeing her care. Mrs. Mark's condition of COPD worsens, and she becomes full of despair and seems very self-focused and even less interested in eating. Based on Maslow's Hierarchy of Needs, discuss the possible cause of her demotivation.

Author's Explanation: Because her COPD has become more severe, she is probably focused on her most basic need of life—oxygen!

Situation 10: Why would Mrs. Mark develop a sense of despair when she has lived such a long life?

Author's Explanation: Mrs. Mark is in a stage of human development in which she is reflecting on her life and her accomplishments. At eighty-eight years, she is now dependent on her son, she has lost her husband, and she has had to bury a child. She is no longer fully independent and suffers from a disease that affects her most primitive need—oxygen.

Examination Review Questions

1. Defining *who we are* falls into which of Erikson's stages?
   a. autonomy versus shame and doubt
   b. initiative versus guilt
   c. identity versus role confusion
   d. industry versus inferiority
2. Reaching your potential as a human person defines which need, according to Maslow?
   a. self-esteem
   b. self-actualization
   c. physiological
   d. safety and security
3. When a person becomes acutely ill, at what level of Maslow's hierarchy will they be functioning?
   a. safety and security
   b. love and belonging
   c. physiological
   d. self-esteem
4. *Autonomy versus shame and doubt* is addressed by what age group?
   a. 0–12 months
   b. 1–3 years
   c. 3–6 years
   d. 6–12 years

5. During which stage does the biological milestone cited by Erikson for full development of motor and language skills occur?
   a. toddler
   b. preschooler
   c. school-age child
   d. adolescent

6. Generativity is a concern of which stage in Erikson's *Eight Stages of Man?*
   a. young adult
   b. middle-aged adult
   c. older adult
   d. adolescent

7. Which famous theorist equated sexuality with childhood experience?
   a. Ellis
   b. Maslow
   c. Erikson
   d. Freud

8. Our perceptions are influenced by all of the following *except*
   a. religion
   b. customs
   c. values
   d. knowledge

9. Meeting the spiritual needs of patients is appropriate in all of the following *exept*
   a. calling their minister
   b. transporting them to services
   c. reading their Bible
   d. encouraging their making peace

10. The most important reason for meeting a patient's spiritual needs is to
    a. respect the patient's rights
    b. provide holistic care
    c. prevent legal ramifications
    d. promote quality health

Care Delivery for the Dying Patient

In the United States in the early 1950s, death was moved from home to the hospital. The advent of advanced technologies and capabilities to offer support and care for the dying in hospitals affected the way society viewed death. Today's increased number of aging individuals whom will die from "old age," is changing the trend. Individuals are choosing a more natural dying process at home rather than in the hospital surrounded by "fancy technical stuff." Today's youth-oriented culture doesn't easily discuss or face dying, but no one escapes death. Eventually, everyone faces his or her mortality. It is part of the human experience. This chapter explores current trends in caring for the dying patient.

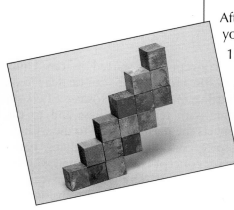

OBJECTIVES

After completing this chapter, you will be able to

1. Describe the stages of dying
2. Define *hospice*
3. Describe hospice care
4. Identify your stance on ethical decisions at the end of life
5. Apply ethical, spiritual, cultural, and psychosocial concepts as they relate to the clinical care associate's scope of practice
6. Define and spell all key terms correctly

k e y   t e r m s

acceptance	death with dignity	incompetent
advanced directive	denial	living will
anger	depression	overt
attorney-in-fact	durable power of attorney	Patient Self-determination Act
bargaining	ethical dilemma	surrogate decision maker
competent	hospice	
covert	incapacitated	

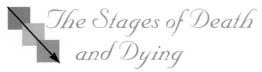

The Stages of Death and Dying

Elisabeth Kübler-Ross has devoted her life's work to exploring the dying process and ministering to those facing death. In the process, she has observed and noted the feelings that accompany what she calls the *five stages of death and dying.* She has also noted that these stages accompany the bereavement process and are universal in all cultures. These five stages are *denial, anger, bargaining, depression,* and *acceptance.* Not all people experience all five stages, nor do they run in any sequential pattern. But in most cases, all five stages are experienced by the dying person, the family, and their friends. Let's explore each stage in turn.

- **Denial** is a coping mechanism in which the person does not believe reality. Denial is not lying. It is unconscious; the person's mind refuses to believe the reality of the situation.
- **Anger** can be **covert** (hidden) or **overt** (blatant). Anger can be manifested physically through aggressive behavior or verbally through caustic remarks.
- **Bargaining** is a response of promises with God or the, "Let's make a deal, God. If you cure me, I will . . ." The "I will . . ." part depends on the individual. It could be, "I will attend church faithfully" or "I will be a better or changed person." Just as Ebenezer Scrooge in Charles Dickens's *A Christmas Carol* bargained with death to change his behavior and to share his riches with others, people bargain for life.
- **Depression** is withdrawal and an expression of sadness (see Unit 8 "Mental Health Needs").
- **Acceptance** is coming to grips with the diagnosis, the treatment, the pain, and the truth—the living of each moment for all that it holds.

Individuals can move in and out of these stages during their illnesses, or they can progress along the first four stages until acceptance is reached. It is important to comprehend these stages and to work with the patient and family to support them through these difficult moments. It is imperative not to try to force the patient and family out of any stage. All that you can do is recognize the stage with its manifesting signs and support the client in that stage. Coping with defense mechanisms is not always easy. You may see the depression or anger and want to move the patient or family toward acceptance. People cannot be coached through this natural process. The family might be in the anger stage and the patient in the denial stage. Family members will move through these stages before and after the patient dies. Sigmund Freud claimed that there are two basic drives in all humans. These are the drive to live, Eros, and the drive to die, Thanatos. We confront and battle the drive to live and to die throughout our time on earth. When confronted with the knowledge of imminent death, we struggle to fight for life.

You will face life and death issues in your work and in your personal life. You will need the guidance of professionals in hospice services to assist you in caring for people who know that their lives will soon end.

Hospice

Hospice is a concept that started in the United States in the 1970s. Hospice care can be delivered in a residential setting or at home. Hospice offers support to patients with terminal illness and to their families; it respects the person's need to die with dignity. The hospice concept is to the dying patient what the Lamaze concept is to the woman who is in the process of childbirth. The goal is for a natural process, one that provides a smooth transition of a life change without artificial intervention. All hospice personnel are specially trained to care for the physical and psychological needs of the dying patient and the family. Hospitals and home care agencies use professionals, support staff, and volunteers to care for the needs and wishes of the patient and the family. Hospice services provide physical, emotional, social, and spiritual support to the dying person and his or her family. They help the individual with pain relief and comfort needs, provide grief counseling, and assist the patient and the family in addressing issues of death and dying (Figure 20-1).

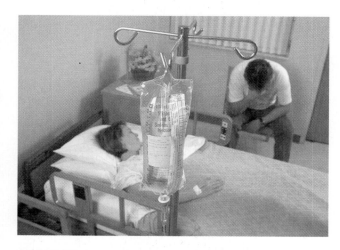

FIGURE 20-1 Grief can be a lonely, isolating personal experience.

Decisions at the End of Life

We all must face the inevitable end of our life—death. This is not an easy topic for most people to discuss when they are well or when they are gravely ill. Nonetheless, we must address this issue and recognize that there are decisions that we can make about end-of-life choices (Figure 20-2).

Some people imagine that it would be easiest to die in their sleep, others want to have the time to say good-bye, and some cannot bear to think about end-of-life decisions. Have you ever considered your own dying and death? The following list of questions is provided here for your consideration. The questions cover various aspects of death and dying that every person should address while he or she has the opportunity and the mental and physical capacity to do so.

1. Have you imagined how you would want to see your last wishes honored?
2. What can you do to let others know what you would want if you were in a coma, needed to be

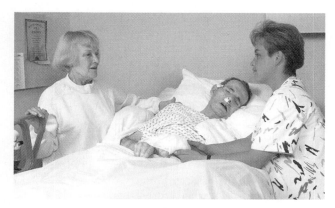

FIGURE 20-2 Decisions at the end of life.

on a respirator, or had no hope for regaining consciousness? Do you want to be alive in that state?
3. If you were terminally ill with cancer or acquired immunodeficiency syndrome (AIDS) and you ceased breathing, would you want to be resuscitated? Would you want, cardiopulmonary resuscitation (CPR)?
4. If you have already decided what efforts you want used to save your life (in life-or-death emergencies), have you let anyone know your thoughts about these situations? Have you expressed your wishes in writing?

Without written directives detailing your wishes, emergency services personnel and hospital intensive care units (ICUs) will pull out all the stops and make every effort to revive the patient—you or someone you love. Advanced directives are discussed in the next section. Whether or not you have had personal experience caring for a seriously ill or dying relative, it is important that you understand advanced directives.

Types of Written, Advanced Directives

There are three different written documents regarding advanced directives: advanced directives, living wills, and durable power of attorney for health care. These documents were sanctioned in the **Patient Self-Determination Act** of 1990. This act ensures that people who are admitted to hospitals, long-term care facilities, and home care are asked about advanced directives.

Advanced Directives

An **advanced directive** is a legally valid written or oral statement that states an individual's treatment decisions and designates a surrogate decision maker. A **surrogate decision maker** is a person who acts on behalf of the patient when he or she is unable to make decisions because of permanent unconsciousness or incapacitation. In an advanced directive, an individual can indicate decisions about life-saving measures—CPR, blood transfusions, tube feedings—to be initiated if death is inevitable or if the person would remain in a permanent unconscious ("vegetative") state of existence.

Living Wills

You can have your wishes written and predetermined in a living will. A **living will** is a type of advanced directive in which an individual states specifically the exact life-sustaining or life-prolonging treatments that the person would want if terminally ill or unable to make decisions on his or her own behalf. A living will does not have to indicate a surrogate decision maker. Figure 20-3 illustrates a living will.

Durable Power of Attorney for Health Care

The **durable power of attorney** is a document that appoints a specific person as the **attorney-in-fact**. This person is also a surrogate decision maker who makes treatment decisions for the individual when the patient is unable to make those decisions personally. The attorney-in-fact can authorize admission to a health care facility and can authorize medical or surgical treatment for the patient if he or she is incapacitated or unable to make a decision because of unconsciousness. If an advanced directive does not indicate specific refusal or permission for certain types of treatments, then the attorney-in-fact is authorized to make decisions based on knowledge of the patient's values and choices in life. The attorney-in-fact is guided purely by his or her belief of what the patient would want. The attorney-in-fact may not have the authority to refuse treatment for the patient, especially if the treatment would be beneficial.

These documents can only be created by a person who is competent to make decisions. Evidence of competence must be documented. Any form of advanced directive should be kept in the patient's chart when admitted to a hospital and should be made known to the personal physician, nursing home administrator, or home care agency. Whenever patients are admitted to a hospital, home care, or long-term care agency, they must be asked by a health care professional if they have any form of an advanced directive. If they do not, they are asked if they want information about these documents. If they do have any type of advanced directive, they are asked to provide a copy of the document for the medical record.

Competent versus Incompetent

There are some important terms that need to be defined to understand the full meaning of the directives and the surrogate decisions. These are *competent* and *incompetent* or *incapacitated*. **Competent** means that the person is able to recognize, comprehend, and weigh the risks of alternative treatment options. The person's general orientation and mental functioning are considered. Another factor considered is the person's ability to understand the nature of the illness and proposed treatments. A person may have a mental illness yet be competent to make decisions about treatments and to understand the nature of the illness.

The famous case of Mary Northern on this page brings home the issue of competence.

Incompetent and **incapacitated** are the terms used to describe a person who is unable to recognize, understand, or weigh the risks, benefits, and alternatives of a proposed treatment. The word *incompetent* was formerly used to describe a person who is unable to make decisions. Now the term *incapacitated* is used more regularly. A legal hearing or a court decision determines incapacity. A person cannot be considered incapacitated without sitting before a judge or mental health magistrate who makes the determination of competence for this person in the particular situation. Described on page 266 is the case of a woman who had severe coronary artery disease that her physicians believed could be treated successfully with a coronary artery bypass graft (CABG). Not only would this surgical procedure have saved her life, but it would also have improved the quality of her life.

Advanced Directives Take Effect

Any type of advanced directive can take effect only in specific situations. The following conditions must exist for an advanced directive to take effect: The patient must be incompetent *and* in a terminal condition or permanently unconscious. The treatment must serve only to prolong the process of dying or to maintain the patient in a state of permanent unconsciousness. If the care or treatment is medically beneficial, not futile, it cannot be refused on the basis of a living will.

Honoring Advanced Directives

Advanced directives may not be honored by the health care provider when he or she is of the belief

The Case of Mary Northern

Mary Northern was a senior citizen receiving home care services for foot ulcers. She developed gangrene of the foot. She told her doctor that it was soot on her foot, and this was causing the blackened skin color. She knew what the doctors meant when they talked about surgical amputation of the foot as a life-saving measure, and she refused the surgery. She was delusional about the foot condition, but she understood that the risk of refusing surgery meant death. The doctors thought that her delusional thinking was reason to petition the court for a competence hearing. The court declared her incompetent. She was admitted to the hospital against her will for amputation of her foot, but the surgery was never performed. She died shortly before the scheduled surgery. Mary Northern's case established a legal precedent.

PENNSYLVANIA LIVING WILL DECLARATION

I, _____, being of sound mind, willfully and voluntarily make this declaration to be followed if I become incompetent. This declaration reflects my firm and settled commitment to refuse life-sustaining treatment under the circumstances indicated below.

I direct my attending physician to withhold or withdraw life-sustaining treatment that serves only to prolong the process of dying, if I should be in a terminal condition or in a state of permanent unconsciousness.

I direct that treatment be limited to measures to keep me comfortable and to relieve pain, including any pain that might occur by withholding or withdrawing life-sustaining treatment.

In addition, if I am in the condition described above, I feel especially strong about the following forms of treatment:

I ( ) do ( ) do not want cardiac resuscitation.
I ( ) do ( ) do not want mechanical respiration.
I ( ) do ( ) do not want tube feeding or any other artificial or invasive form of nutrition (food) or hydration (water).
I ( ) do ( ) do not want blood or blood products.
I ( ) do ( ) do not want any form of surgery or invasive diagnostic tests.
I ( ) do ( ) do not want kidney dialysis.
I ( ) do ( ) do not want antibiotics.

I realize that if I do not specifically indicate my preference regarding any of the forms of treatment listed above, I may receive that form of treatment.

Other instructions: _____
_____

SURROGATE DESIGNATION

I ( ) do ( ) do not want to designate another person as my surrogate to make medical treatment decisions for me if I should be incompetent and be in a terminal condition or in a state of permanent unconsciousness.

Name and address of surrogate (if applicable): _____
_____

Name and address of substitute surrogate (if surrogate designated above is unable to serve): _____
_____

ANATOMICAL GIFT DONATION

I ( ) do ( ) do not want to make an anatomical gift of all or part of my body, subject to the following limitations, if any: _____

DECLARANT SIGNATURE

I made this declaration on the _____ day of _____ (month, year).

Declarant's signature: _____

Declarant's address: _____

WITNESS SIGNATURES

The declaration of the person on behalf of and at the direction of the declarant knowingly and voluntarily signed this writing by signature or mark in my presence.

Witness signature: _____

Witness address: _____

Witness signature: _____

Witness address: _____

FIGURE 20-3 An example of a living will.

The Case of the Coronary Artery Bypass Graft

The woman was disoriented and at times forgetful and confused about money matters. The physicians requested a competence hearing to determine if she was competent to decide to refuse surgery. When the judge asked her about her understanding of coronary artery disease, she was able to define it appropriately, and when asked about the nature of the CABG, she was able to describe that a new "tube" would replace the sick arteries in her heart. She was not able to correctly identify the day or date and was not able to recall the president's name. The judge did not deem her incapacitated because she was able to comprehend the risk of refusing surgery and she understood the nature of the illness and the surgery.

that adherence to the patient's wishes under the advanced directive cannot be executed in good conscience. Essentially, the decision to honor or not to honor a patient's advanced directive creates an ethical dilemma for the people involved in the situation. The surrogate decision maker or attorney-in-fact has the right to appeal the health care provider's decision and may file a grievance with the state certification agency against him or her. The surrogate may feel that it is an ethical duty to honor the patient's wishes or directives. A health care provider who believes it is wrong to honor the advanced directive should direct the family or surrogates to a health care provider who will honor these wishes. This should be discussed with the surrogate and significant others so that they can proceed in the patient's best interest. When a situation arises about honoring an advanced directive, the ethics committee of the health care facility is used to help resolve or shed light on the choices to be made regarding this ethical dilemma.

Death with Dignity

The phrase **death with dignity** describes the idea that every person should have the right to decide during the course of a terminal illness when death is near, to refuse treatment, and to die without pain and in a peaceful manner. Death with dignity encourages realistic treatment, pain reduction, home care or hospice care, and the involvement of significant others in the care of the dying person. Without a doubt, there are obstacles to death with dignity. These issues arise when pain relief cannot realistically be achieved, when tube feedings are forced, and when home care or hospice care is not available for

the patient. Much consideration must be taken in the care of a dying person. The patient's wishes and decisions, as well as those of the significant others, must be considered in the treatment decisions. It is often hard for significant others (family and friends) to watch the patient suffer and die. When choices are discussed, the patient and significant others must be presented with the choices, risks, benefits, and prognosis. They must know that no treatment is an option. They must have time to make decisions and must consider the values and beliefs of the dying person.

It is hard to imagine not providing nutrients to a person because food is nurturing. Food is loving. But there are times when nutrients are not enough to prevent the disease process from proceeding. Food alone will not nurture a terminally ill person back to health or even sustain life. Pain management is also an issue for the patient, the family, physicians, and nurses. Today, physicians and nurses are less fearful of addiction to narcotics with patients in severe and terminal pain. It is important to evaluate the patient's pain tolerance and vital functions when providing pain relief. It is also essential to consider the patient's wishes for pain-relieving drugs. Sometimes patients will want to withhold pain-relieving medications because they would rather feel the pain than be less aware of their surroundings because of the effects of the narcotics. Some patients might say that the pain is the only thing that makes them still feel alive, and they resist pain-relieving drugs. The nurse must act as the patient's advocate and assist in providing the prescribed medications within the patient's tolerance.

The risk of addiction should not be a factor in providing adequate pain relief to a person with a terminal illness. Comfort measures are essential. The clinical care associate is key in providing emotional and physical comfort to the dying patient. Sometimes it is the gentle touch, cool washcloth, sips of water, and quiet presence of the care associate that help to relieve the loneliness of pain. Alerting the nurse to the patient's discomfort and reminding the patient to use the patient-controlled analgesia pump are vital to comfort for the patient in grave pain. Turning, changing, feeding, and gently rubbing a sore back or foot can help the patient to rest and find temporary relief.

Remember that death with dignity should not be a privilege, but a right, for those who are facing death.

Ethical Dilemmas

In Unit 5, ethical principles were discussed. These principles are the fundamentals that the clinical care associate should apply in providing care for clients.

These ethical principles were beneficence, nonmaleficence, justice, and autonomy. Remember, they serve as a guide and a foundation for the behavior, actions, and decisions of all members of the health care team. Here we will list and describe the characteristics of ethical principles and ethical dilemmas.

An **ethical dilemma** sometimes arises when decisions and choices must be made about the welfare of a patient. This creates conflict and debate about which alternative should be chosen in a particular case. In essence, an ethical dilemma presents itself when there is difficulty in decision making because there is no "right" choice or "absolute" decision to be made. It is the weighing of what to do; it is the balancing of what would benefit the patient, the family, and perhaps the greater good of a system or a community. Sometimes ethical dilemmas involve more than what is good or best for one person; they include the collective good of many people.

A Case in Point

Let's imagine that a family has $5 million of health care insurance that could be spent for the lifetime health care of the family. There are four people in the family. Does it sound "fair," based on the ethical principle of distributive justice, to say that each family member would have $1.25 million to spend on health care? Each would have an equal amount of money to be used for a lifetime of health care. Suppose that the father is sixty-four years of age, needs open-heart surgery, and has multiple complications following the surgery that require extensive days of hospital care. Within a month's time, the father has used his $1.25 million. Now the doctors say that he will need expensive medications, tests, and treatments to maintain his health needs. He could live another 20 years if he is well cared for. The other members of the family are twelve, twenty-two, and

fifty-eight years old. No one knows what their health care needs will be during their lives.

What should the family do? Should the family redistribute the remaining $3.75 million equally among the four members? Should they each give a portion of their share to the father? Or should they adhere to the "fair" distribution that was established? Seriously consider and discuss the nature of this situation with your friends, family, or classmates.

The nature of an ethical dilemma is that there doesn't seem to be one "right" or "absolute" answer. Table 20-1 highlights the major points or characteristics common to all ethical dilemmas. The situation described above is used to explain each of the characteristics listed in the table.

The principle of equal distribution of resources may have justified the actions of this family if they had decided that they would each have $1.25 million of health care insurance and that, no matter what happened, they would adhere to this principle. The father would have taken his chances and spent whatever cash the family could afford to buy medications and pay for medical care. Then each would have had an equal pool of insurance money to use. But who knows? Maybe the twelve-year-old would not have developed leukemia and the twenty-two-year-old would never have been in an automobile accident. The father may have died at sixty-five. This family might have looked back thirty years later and felt that they were not just in their actions and that they failed to fulfill their duty to the father.

The principles of ethics are used to suggest direction and the actions to be taken. They are not absolute; there are always exceptions to the rules. The principles of ethics are used to resolve conflicts and to help weigh the consequences of actions. They are the reasons that justify moral actions. They are not rules or values. They are guides to organizing and understanding information in an ethical dilemma.

TABLE 20-1 Characteristics of Ethical Dilemmas	
Characteristic	Description
The choice is between equally undesirable alternatives.	Any alternative this family chooses could have an undesirable outcome for the entire family or for individual members of the family.
Real choice exists between the possible courses of action to be taken in the situation.	There are definitely real choices between all the possible courses of action. These are choices that are not easy to make because the future needs of the other family members or even the sixty-four-year-old father cannot be predicted.

TABLE 20-1   Characteristics of Ethical Dilemmas (continued)

Characteristic	Description
The people involved place a significantly different value judgment on the possible actions or on the consequences of those actions.	Each member of this family would probably have a different perspective about the decisions to be made. Suppose you are the twenty-two-year-old, have asthma, and know that you will need continued medical care for this. You may wonder what will happen if you get into an accident and need surgery or rehabilitation and there is not enough money left when you need it. What about the fifty-eight-year-old mother, who has a family history of cancer and heart disease? She may be healthy now, but what if the family history of cancer affects her? Will there be enough insurance money left to save her life?
Data alone will not help resolve the dilemma.	The doctors predict another 20 years of life for the father if given the needed medication, tests, and treatments. This prognosis is based on data from studies of people who survived heart disease after open-heart surgery and followed a prescribed course of diet, exercise, and medications. But will these data help the family to make a decision? What if we could predict the odds as 1 in 20 that you would have an automobile accident that resulted in serious injuries? Would you be willing to give up some of your share of the pool of insurance dollars?
"Answers" to an ethical dilemma are influenced by several disciplines—psychology, sociology, theology, and medicine.	The family must make this decision by considering its religious beliefs and its individual and collective emotional and social well-being. They would want to know all the possible information that the doctors could give them. What decision could you live with as an individual member of this family? Would a decision to redistribute the pool of insurance money cause distrust or disharmony in the family?
Actions taken to respond to a dilemma will result in unfavorable outcomes or breach one's sense of duty to another person or group of people.	Suppose the family decides to provide the father with all necessary medications and treatments, regardless of the future needs of other family members. They all feel that it is their duty to provide what is needed because they love the father. Four years later, he dies. The twelve-year-old son is now sixteen and is diagnosed with leukemia. There is $3 million of health care insurance money remaining for the family. The only hope for his surviving the leukemia is a bone marrow transplant. This will be costly and will require a lengthy course of treatment and follow-up care. The expected cost is $1.8 million. Imagine that you are now twenty-six and need lifetime care because of paralysis resulting from an automobile accident. The remaining $1.2 million of insurance money will not last very long. Who will benefit from the remaining insurance money? The outcome will be unfavorable for some member or members of this family. Is the duty to one member greater than the duty to the others?
The choices made in an ethical dilemma have effects that are far-reaching. They affect our perception and definition of the value of human beings, relationships, and society as a whole.	The choice made to extend the life of the sixty-four-year-old has far-reaching effects. It has made this family examine the value of each human life in the family. The principle of distributing the resources equally now creates even greater dilemma and confusion about the meaning of fairness and equality.

TABLE 20-1   Characteristics of Ethical Dilemmas (continued)

Characteristic	Description
Any ethical decision involves using financial, material, or human resources that are finite or limited in nature.	While $5 million seemed like a significant pool of insurance money at the start of this dilemma, it now seems very finite. The extent of human resources, or the amount of emotional and social support for one another, is also finite. Members of this family may be feeling that they have given and have suffered as much as they can bear.
Ethical dilemmas are not solvable, but they are resolvable.	A decision had to be made, but it did not truly solve the problem. It resolved the original dilemma of prolonging the father's life, yet it created future dilemmas that can also be resolved, but never solved.
There is no "right" or "wrong" when dealing with two equally unfavorable actions.	As you can see, there was no right or wrong solution to the original dilemma or to the future dilemmas of this family. The choices they had to make had no favorable action or consequence for all. The decisions had to be based on what they could live with based on their beliefs, values, and knowledge at a given point in the history of the family's lifetime.

application to practice

Use what you have learned in this chapter about care delivery and supporting the dying person to consider the situations presented here.

Learning Activities

Situation 1: Mr. Fiore was just diagnosed with cancer of the pancreas. He feels well and doesn't believe the physician, who says he may have as little as six weeks to live. He refuses home care. What stage of death and dying is Mr. Fiore exhibiting?

Author's Explanation: Mr. Fiore is in denial. Because he is not manifesting any physical problems related to the cancer, he does not believe the physician's diagnosis.

Situation 2: Mr. Fiore's skin and sclera turn yellow two weeks after his diagnosis. He tells his wife that the doctor poisoned him with that biopsy test he was given. What stage is Mr. Fiore in now?

Author's Explanation: Mr. Fiore is angry and using displacement, a defense mechanism that focuses the anger outside of himself onto someone or something unrelated to the source of emotional pain.

Situation 3: His wife calls your home care agency and asks for activation. She is frightened by her husband's change of status. She says she hasn't slept since the diagnosis was pronounced, and she has done nothing but cry. She begs for help. What stage is Mrs. Fiore exhibiting?

Author's Explanation: Although Mr. Fiore is in the anger stage, Mrs. Fiore is in the depressed stage.

Situation 4: Mr. Fiore has a home evaluation, and as a result, home care is activated. When you arrive for personal care assistance, Mr. Fiore asks, "What is cancer of the pancreas?" What do you say?

Author's Explanation: Reflect the question back to Mr. Fiore. For example, "Mr. Fiore, what do you know about cancer of the pancreas?" He probably is questioning the reality of the diagnosis and needs to express his concerns. Reflecting the statement back to him affords him the opportunity to discuss what is really on his mind.

Situation 5: You assist Mr. Fiore into the shower and tell him you'll be right outside the door, changing his bed linens. You overhear Mr. Fiore crying and saying, "Please, God, I promise to be a better husband to Mary if you'll just let me live." What stage is Mr. Fiore in now?

Author's Explanation: Mr. Fiore is in the bargaining stage. He is bargaining with God to change reality and promising to change if he is given more time.

Situation 6: When he gets out of the shower, he is crying and asks you to pray for him. He tells you he is too young to die. How will you respond?

Author's Explanation: Console Mr. Fiore. Tell him you are going to be a support to him and to Mrs. Fiore. Ask him if he has a priest or minister who could be called to visit with him. If he says yes, report this to the agency's nurse.

Situation 7: You have finished with Mr. Fiore's personal care. As you are leaving, Mrs. Fiore corners you at the door. She grabs your arm and begs you not to leave. She is holding you very tightly, and tears are in her eyes. What will you do?

Author's Explanation: Ask Mrs. Fiore what she needs at this time. Perhaps she is frightened. She may be frightened that her husband will die at home, and she will be alone. Permit her to express her fears, and assure her that the agency team will be available to assist her in this very difficult time. When you return to the agency, talk with the registered nurse in charge of Mr. Fiore's case about hospice intervention.

Situation 8: You finally leave the Fiores. You have spent two hours there, but it felt like two days. You have three more clients to visit. What can you do to replenish your drained energy? Right now you feel as though you've worked 12 hours.

Author's Explanation: Acknowledge to yourself what you are feeling. You are allowed to feel sad and frustrated. Recognize that you cannot cure the patient or solve all his issues. Remember the resources that can be made available to this couple. Appreciate the fact that you have provided needed support for them. Tap into your favorite portable activity. Listen to your favorite music, sing a song, take a short walk, say a prayer, breathe deeply. When you have finished work for the day, be sure to make time for yourself, even if it is only 10 minutes. A hot shower or bath, a few minutes with a good book, or a short phone conversation with a trusted friend can help you to cope with the stress of working with a patient with a terminal illness.

Situation 9: Becky Brownley is a four-year-old who was diagnosed with a rare type of blood

dyscrasia. You are the clinical care associate (CCA) on the pediatric floor. Lately, it seems all the clients have had a terminal illness. How will you cope with all the emotions that you are feeling?

Author's Explanation: Be sure that this issue is discussed in team report. If you are feeling this way, it is probable that others are experiencing similar emotions. Team members help each other to cope with these painful and confusing feelings. Don't go it alone; seek the support of others who know this experience.

Situation 10: You have seen this scenario before. The parents are filled with guilt and are blaming everyone—themselves, the doctors, even God. In what stage are the Brownleys?

Author's Explanation: The Brownleys are in the anger stage of dealing with illness. Their helplessness to heal their daughter makes them feel this anger.

Situation 11: Becky knows something is wrong. She doesn't feel well and has been throwing her toys all over the room. What are some techniques to help Becky deal with her anger?

Author's Explanation: Have Becky draw some pictures and then describe what the pictures represent. Also have Becky role-play using the stuffed animals. Talk with the team leader about Becky's behavior. There are play therapists—specialists who help children deal with difficult situations through play. Be tolerant, and ask Becky to tell you about why she is throwing her toys.

Situation 12: The Brownleys have been participating in the group counseling available at the hospital. Every day they come in to see Becky, and they find something to criticize. Today, it's the way you made Becky's bed. How will you respond?

Author's Explanation: Recognize that the Brownleys are still in the anger stage of dealing with Becky's illness. Ask the Brownleys how they are doing. Do not even comment on their critical remarks. Recognize that these remarks are manifestations of displaced anger.

Situation 13: Becky takes a sudden turn for the worse. When you arrive on shift today, she is unconscious and hooked up to a ventilator. The shift report reveals a chain of events including a hemolytic reaction secondary to blood transfusion. As you enter Becky's room, the parents greet you with, "If she doesn't pull out of this, we're going to sue this hospital and everyone who has even touched Becky. That includes you." How will you respond?

Author's Explanation: Once again, do not take the comment personally. The Brownleys are stuck in the anger stage of dealing with this illness. They are continuing to displace their anger. They are unable to save the life of their four-year-old daughter. In response to this helpless feeling, they misdirect their anger onto you.

Situation 14: Mrs. Valisha is from India, and she is visiting her brother in America. She was admitted to your unit with severe chest pain to rule out myocardial infarction. Her diagnostic workup gives a poor prognosis, severe cardiomyopathy. Heart transplant is not a realistic option; she is eighty-four years old. You see her brother grieving and frightened. Mrs. Valisha is gasping for each breath. You want to communicate with the patient and to comfort her and her brother. Mrs. Valisha speaks little English. You are told she is Hindu. What does this mean to you? How will this affect your care delivery?

Author's Explanation: According to the Hindu religion, the head is the seat of the soul; therefore, never touch a Hindu's head. Know that only westernized Hindus will shake hands with the opposite sex. Do not hug or touch in greeting. Pointing with a finger is considered rude. Ears are considered sacred appendages. Hindus do not eat beef or use beef products (for example, leather). Women must keep their upper arms, chest, legs, and back covered at all times. The head, when tossed up and down, means no. Side-to-side head movement indicates agreement. This is the opposite of Western tradition.

Situation 15: What can you do to comfort Mrs. Valisha and her brother?

Author's Explanation: Respect their culture, and recognize that your western style of comfort may seem disrespectful. Assist Mrs. Valisha and her brother in the grief process by identifying their behavioral indications for solace and comfort. Listen to what the brother communicates about his sister's needs. Make certain that her dietary restrictions are followed. Ask her brother how you can help them. Let them know that you are available to meet their needs.

Situation 16: Mr. Kashmir has been in and out of a coma for the past three days. His family doesn't understand why he is "hanging on." What are some possible reasons? How can you find out?

Author's Explanation: Sometimes a patient will hang on because of something that is unresolved. It could be wanting to see a particular person or to give a message to a family member or because the patient senses the family has not resolved to let go. The person may have unfinished business. Some may say it is God's will and it isn't their time yet. Often, however, it is because of an unmet spiritual need. Check the chart for the client's religion. Report your observations and the family's to the nurse. Ask if a short team meeting can be held or if it can be brought up during report.

Situation 17: You check Mr. Kashmir's chart and see the client's religion listed as Presbyterian. The staff meeting reveals no contact by a minister. The nurse asks the family if the minister was contacted and explains that often the patient needs this support. The family states that the client hasn't been to church in years. Why do you think this argument may be invalid?

Author's Explanation: Values hold firm. Even if the client hasn't been to church in years, his values are still a part of him. He still considered himself a Presbyterian even though he didn't go to church. He may still have faith, and he may still believe in God and pray.

Situation 18: Mrs. Swietzer, a recent nursing home resident, has been diagnosed with stage 3 Alzheimer's disease. She has a very caring family that has been very anxious and somewhat guilty about her placement in the facility. She receives daily visits from family members, who always have many questions about her status. Her husband spends most of his day sitting by her side holding her hand and talking to her, even though she doesn't respond. She is a total care patient who requires close supervision. The physician has written an order for "DNR." This morning at her bedside while you are feeding Mrs. Swietzer, she chokes and begins to turn blue. According to the cardinal signs, she must have a complete airway obstruction. You call for the nurse and begin emergency procedures. If Mrs. Swietzer codes, should you begin resuscitation?

Author's Explanation: *DNR* does not mean "do not provide care." An airway obstruction from aspiration of food is not a usual event in the process of natural death. *DNR* means "do not resuscitate"; it does not mean do not perform the Heimlich maneuver if the person is choking on food. It means if you find the person without respiration or pulse that you should not resuscitate or start CPR. Airway obstruction of a conscious victim should be relieved. If you do not resuscitate you could be considered negligent of care.

Examination Review Questions

1. Which of the following was *not* part of the Patient Self-Determination Act of 1990?
   a. advanced directive
   b. ethics committee
   c. durable power of attorney
   d. living will

2. Who makes the determination of incompetence for the enforcement of surrogate decision makers?
   a. physician   c. family
   b. judge   d. nurse

3. The term used to describe the coping mechanism used to unconsciously refuse to believe one has a terminal illness is
   a. denial   c. bargaining
   b. anger   d. depression

4. Which statement about the stages of death and dying is *not* true?
   a. A person might move in and out of the various stages.
   b. A person might progress along the first four stages before reaching acceptance.
   c. Everyone always follows the stages in order.
   d. A person might remain in one stage until death.

5. What stage of death and dying is exhibited through caustic remarks?
   a. covert anger   c. covert depression
   b. overt denial   d. overt bargaining

6. The purpose of the durable power of attorney document is to
   a. appoint an attorney-in-fact
   b. interpret the living will
   c. authorize one's death
   d. open the patient's record

7. Which of the following will *not* affect an advanced directive?
   a. terminal illness
   b. permanent unconsciousness
   c. mental incapacitation
   d. controversial treatment

8. Complex decisions regarding terminal treatment create
   a. ethics committees   c. ethical dilemmas
   b. surrogate decisions d. attorneys-in-fact

9. The Lamaze concept is to childbirth what the hospice is to
   a. growth   c. dignity
   b. development   d. dying

10. The term used to describe a person's inability to recognize, understand, or weigh the risks, benefits, or alternatives of proposed treatment is
   a. competent   c. incapacitated
   b. capacitated   d. dilemma

Mental Health Needs

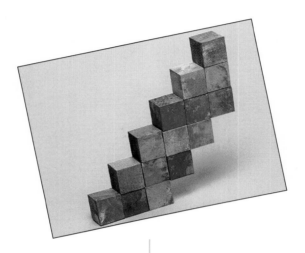

In 1978, the Commission on Mental Health concluded that mental disorders or emotional disturbances would strike one in seven Americans. Many people live part or all of their lives with psychological pain and suffer quietly without professional help.

Genetic or environmental factors (or both) can create a mental environment ripe for instability. Scientists are just beginning to understand the human mind and the internal environment, which is rich in neurochemicals that affect our sense of well-being and mental stability. For example, the neurochemical serotonin and its link to clinical depression have spurred changes in the treatment of depression. Now, medications are able to balance this neurochemical imbalance. Diet and its proven effect on mood has opened up new schools of thought on nutrition and mental well-being. Researchers are searching constantly for the genetic and biological causes of various mental disorders.

Chapter 21

Understanding Mental Illness

In this chapter, you will explore the mind and the signs and symptoms of mental illness. Abnormal psychology—the study of emotions, thoughts, and behaviors that deviate from a society's norms or the expectations of normal—is in a constant search for knowledge about abnormal conditions of the mind. The stressors and unique pressures of this fast-paced, technological society require strong coping strategies to enable people to function optimally. Cracks in mental coping can cause "crack-ups." Unfortunately, some individuals do not have the mental capability to maintain mental health because of environmental factors or a genetic predisposition to mental illness.

OBJECTIVES

After completing this chapter, you will be able to

1. List and describe the psychotic disorders
2. List and describe the common defense mechanisms
3. Compare and contrast the thought, personality, mood, anxiety, addictive, and cognitive disorders
4. List the cognitive brain disorders and describe their features
5. Differentiate between delirium, depression, and dementia
6. List the categories of mental retardation
7. Define and spell all key terms correctly

key terms

Alzheimer's disease
antisocial personality disorder
anxiety disorders
avoidant personality disorder
bipolar mood disorder
borderline personality disorder
catatonia
catatonic schizophrenia
cognitive disorder
cyclothymic disorder
defense mechanisms
delirium
delirium tremens (DTs)
delusional disorder
delusions
dementia
dependence
dependent personality disorder
depressive episodes
disorganized schizophrenia
dissociative disorder
distorted thinking patterns

Down's syndrome
dysthymic disorder
euphoria
flat affect
general anxiety disorder
grandiose delusion
hallucinations
histrionic personality disorder
hypersomnia
insomnia
intelligence quotient (IQ)
least restrictive alternative
mania
mental retardation
mood disorders
narcissistic personality disorder
neurosis
nihilistic delusion
obsessive-compulsive personality
  disorder
panic disorders
paranoid schizophrenia

passive-aggressive personality
  disorder
persecutory delusion
personality disorder
phobia
psychoactive substances
psychosis
reactive psychosis
residual schizophrenia
sadistic personality disorder
schizoaffective disorders
schizoid personality disorder
schizophrenia
schizotypal personality disorder
substance abuse
substance dependence
tolerance
undifferentiated schizophrenia
waxy flexibility
withdrawal

Mental Health

Most of us fall into the categories of sane and well. In other words, according to society's norms, most of us are normal. The definition of *normal* is not simply stated. It is defined by the functioning of an individual within the structure of a given society. *Normal* is also defined by the conclusions of a society about what is abnormal. It is difficult to ascertain the normal or abnormal behavior of an individual unless you know the historical and societal expectations of "normal" in a given culture.

Most individuals appreciate and nourish the richness of the human mind, with its magnificent capability for thought and emotion. Each person learns (sometimes unknowingly) how to develop the mental strategies necessary to promote and maintain good mental health (Figure 21-1). However, at some time in their lives, even the most well balanced individuals experience confusion, temptation, abuse of addictive substances, depression, desperation, or fear. They learn to work through the difficult times with the support of friends, or they seek the counsel of professionals who can help them recover from their mental traumas. Unfortunately, there are individuals who struggle throughout their life with the burden of mental disorders. These disorders paralyze, disarm, and disable thoughts, emotions, behavior, intellect, judgment, or personality. Let's examine the classifications of mental disorders.

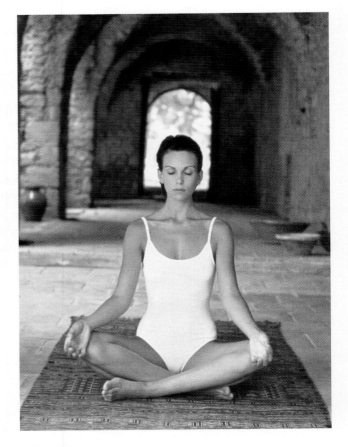

FIGURE 21-1   Yoga is practiced by many who strive to improve their mental and physical well-being. Rex Rauchon, Explorer, Photo Researchers, Inc.

Diagnostic Categories of Mental Health

It is not possible to discuss all of the mental health disorders in this text. The mind is complex, and the study of mental illness is an extensive topic. This chapter introduces you to the most common disorders to assist you in understanding the nature of mental illness. The diagnostic categories discussed within this unit are disorders classified in the *DSM IV*. The *DSM IV* is the fourth edition of the *Diagnostic and Statistical Manual of Mental Disorders*. This edition of the manual was published by the American Psychiatric Association in May 1994. The mental disorders discussed here do not include all of the classified psychiatric/mental health disorders. Disorders of childhood, adjustment disorders, eating and sleeping disorders, impulse disorders, sexual and gender-identity disorders, some of the addictive disorders, and disorders of conduct are not included. The possible physiological, environmental, and psychosocial causes and treatments for these disorders cannot be discussed in one chapter of a text.

Psychotic Disorders

A **psychosis** can be the most severe and disabling of the mental illnesses. The psychotic disorders involve disturbances of thought, mood, social behavior, and judgment. They disable the individual's ability to recognize and respond to reality. The psychotic disorders discussed in this section include *schizophrenia, reactive psychosis, schizoaffective disorder,* and *delusional disorder.*

Thought Disorders

Psychotic disorders are thought disorders that create gross distortions of reality (Figure 21-2). The individual's perceptions, thinking, and emotions are so distorted that they are severely disabling. The most common disorder of thought is schizophrenia.

Schizophrenia

Schizophrenia literally means "split or fragmented mind" (*schizo-* means "split," and *-phrenia* means "mind"). Actually, there is gross fragmentation of thought and great disorganization of behavior and judgment. Hence, the term *splitting* actually means "splitting from reality." There is an intellectual split between thoughts and emotions. There are several types of schizophrenia. Each is named by the predominant features of the particular type, but all involve distortions in thinking. Schizophrenia can

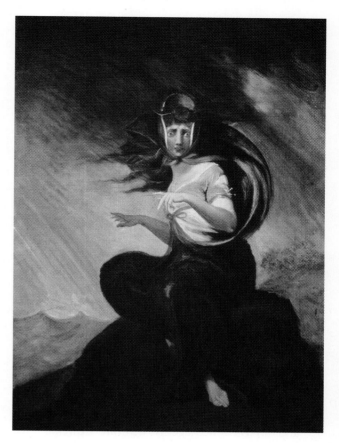

FIGURE 21-2 Example of someone suffering from a thought disorder. Mad Kate, 1806–07 (oil on canvas) by Henry Fuseli (1741–1825). Goethe Museum, Frankfurt/Bridgeman Art Library, London/New York.

occur in childhood and older adulthood, but it is found most commonly in people between fifteen and forty-five years. A list of diagnostic criteria for schizophrenia follows.

Diagnostic Criteria for Schizophrenia

1. **Delusions**—beliefs that something is true when it isn't; false beliefs that cannot be altered by relating the truth. The most common types of delusions are persecutory, grandiose, and nihilistic.

   - **Persecutory delusion** is the delusion that someone or something is out to harm the person. (Example: "The people in this hospital want to kill me, and they are poisoning the food.")
   - **Grandiose delusion** is the delusion of ideas of grandeur. The person falsely believes the exaggeration of personal status, power, or beauty. (Example: "I am Queen Victoria.")
   - **Nihilistic delusion** is the delusion of denying the existence of some part of the self. (Example: "I can't eat because I have no stomach.")

2. **Hallucinations**—false sensory perceptions or distortions of the senses in which the person hears (auditory hallucination), sees (visual), feels (tactile), tastes (gustatory), or smells (olfactory) objects or people that are not real. Generally, the hallucinations with schizophrenia are auditory or visual. The person with schizophrenia actually believes the voices are real. Often, these voices are threatening to the individual. The visual hallucinations are equally as frightening.

3. Meaningless speech—a pattern of speech that is confusing to the listener.

4. Unusual or absent body movements (**catatonia**)—posturing or repetitive, useless movements or rituals of movement. For example, the person who exhibits catatonia does not move, and pulse, respirations, and blood pressure are barely audible or palpable. When someone is in a catatonic state, he or she has **waxy flexibility**, which means that if you raise the person's arm, it will remain in that position until you move it again.

5. Flat or absent emotional tone (**flat affect**)—a condition in which the person has no emotional expression; the person does not look happy, sad, and so on; the face is without expression of mood.

6. Incongruent affect—a display of emotion that is not consistent with the thoughts the person is expressing. For example, a person may be laughing when she tells you that her mother just had a heart attack.

7. Gross decrease in social and occupational functioning.

8. Decrease in personal hygiene and grooming.

9. Magical thinking—a condition that equates thinking with doing. (Example: "Step on a crack and you break your mother's back.")

10. Unusual perceptual experiences, such as illusions or misinterpretations of real sensory experiences. (Example: The person hears the sound of the wind and thinks someone is calling his name.)

11. Decline in motivation, focus, and energy.

12. Ideas of reference—relating something that is coincidental as being related directly to oneself. (Example: The person hears something in a news report and interprets it as if it related to her.)

Medications that help to improve thinking and reduce agitation are used to control the symptoms of schizophrenia. There is no known cure. The cause at this time remains unknown, but it is believed to be neuroanatomical, or neurochemical, or genetic. Some of the types of schizophrenia are **paranoid**, **catatonic**, **disorganized**, **residual**, and **undifferentiated**. These types of schizophrenia are categorized according to the prevailing features of the disorder.

Reactive Psychosis

Reactive psychosis is a short-term psychotic episode that evolves from an emotional turmoil and produces a brief period of schizophrenic manifestations with a return to the preillness state after days, weeks, or months. This disorder may appear after a severely stressful situation takes place and the individual does not rest or eat adequately during the period of extreme stress. Normal coping patterns are disrupted; the person may drink alcohol or use illicit drugs to reduce the anxiety during the stressful period. The combination of all or some of these factors may be sufficient to produce a reactive psychosis.

Schizoaffective Disorders

Schizoaffective disorders involve schizophrenic features along with coexisting manic or depressive symptoms. The mood is disturbed as well as the thoughts. (See "Mood Disorders.")

Delusional Disorder

People with a **delusional disorder** appear to function within normal limits in most life situations except for one irrational belief. This belief cannot be shaken, even when logical evidence supports its fallacy. There are five main areas for delusional disorders. These are

1. Erotomania—the irrational belief that someone is in love with you.
2. Grandiose—the irrational, overinflated belief of self-worth, power, or importance.
3. Jealous—the irrational belief that a partner is unfaithful.
4. Persecutory—the irrational belief that someone is out to get the person.
5. Somatic—the irrational belief of suffering from a physical disease, ailment, or defect.

The delusion is very real to the individual, and it is organized and not bizarre, unlike the delusions of people with schizophrenia. The presence of logical, well-structured delusions is a distinguishing feature of this disorder. Let's look into the delusion of Mr. Ordotti on page 279.

What is striking about delusional disorder is that the delusion has threads of reality that seem plausible or believable in part. The person with this disorder builds an airtight delusional system that is difficult to

Mr. Ordotti's Delusion

Mr. Ordotti is suffering from a delusional disorder. He believes that he is being sought by the Mafia. Mr. Ordotti's next-door neighbor was shot by the Mafia. Now, Mr. Ordotti believes that he will be shot also because they were neighbors. Mr. Ordotti begins to look for clues to substantiate this false belief. He believes that he is being followed by someone who worked with his neighbor. When this coworker comes to pay his respects to the neighbor's wife, he accidentally knocks on Mr. Ordotti's door. Each time Mr. Ordotti sees this man in the neighborhood, he imagines that he is spying on him. The neighbor's coworker looks at him and says "Hello" each time he sees him, and this makes Mr. Ordotti feel suspicious and frightened. Soon, Mr. Ordotti refuses to leave his home. He hides behind the curtains, looking for this man.

What is a striking feature of delusional disorder?

penetrate with the facts of reality. The person may continue to work and function in other areas of life. The behavior, mood, and thoughts that are not connected with the delusional system are organized and based in reality.

Sometimes, psychotic reactions are directly related to a medical condition. When there is a disturbance of electrolyte balance, such as high blood calcium, the person will experience delusions, hallucinations, and illusions. The appearance of these symptoms is abrupt, and the nature of the hallucinations may be tactile or olfactory as well as visual or auditory. It is essential for the physician to look for underlying medical conditions to diagnose any mental disorder correctly. Liver, endocrine, and kidney disorders can lead to extreme confusion, disorientation, hallucinations, and disturbances in thought or mood.

Personality Disorders

Attitudes shape our personality. Attitudes direct our definition of ourselves and the world around us. How we perceive reality may be distorted by our attitudes, distorted patterns of thinking, and use of defense mechanisms. When these **distorted thinking patterns** interfere with our relationships, work, and social life, a **personality disorder** results. The most striking feature of personality disorders is that the person with the actual disorder does not recognize the problem; it is usually brought to the attention of professionals by someone who is close to the individual. The significant other experiences the anxiety from this person's behavior. The person with a true personality disorder may not experience anxiety or perceive any accountability for generating the problems that he or she faces. It is the experience of "She

made me do it" or "I didn't do anything. He led me to . . ." We all have personality tendencies. In fact, when reading about the types of disorders, you may find some elements that resemble your behavior. The following is a brief list of personality disorders. Remember, only a trained mental health professional can diagnose and treat mental disorders.

Types of Personality Disorders

Types of personality disorders include *antisocial, avoidant, borderline, dependent, histrionic, narcissistic, passive-aggressive, sadistic, schizoid, schizotypal,* and *obsessive-compulsive.* Let's examine each briefly.

Antisocial personality disorder is manifested by irresponsible behavior and the inability to conform to social norms. This disorder was formerly called *psychopathic* or *sociopathic disorder.* The individual can be very convincing and appealing in nature. Con men and "shysters," or unethical lawyers, doctors, and businesspeople, are best described as antisocial. They have no remorse for their actions and feel justified in their antisocial or manipulative behavior. They can take advantage of people and believe they are not doing any harm. They fail to feel any shame for their behavior.

Avoidant personality disorder manifests as general fear, fear of negative evaluation, and great social discomfort. People with this disorder avoid any situation that will show them in a negative light. By avoiding work and responsibility, they seem passive and perhaps, neurotic. Their avoidance inflicts harm on their relationships and causes distress for others. They cannot see how they contribute to their problems. They are extremely hurt by even the slightest sign of disapproval. They avoid making friends because they will not risk being disliked by someone. In addition to these, they are prone to exaggerate the potential dangers of ordinary situations.

Borderline personality disorder is characterized by unstable moods, self-image, and inconsistent interpersonal relationships. The person may at times seem psychotic and, at other times, seem neurotic. They are usually very narcissistic (self-absorbed) and create conflict in relationships because of their reactive nature to any insult to their self-esteem. Their relationships are intense and unstable, and they fear abandonment. Often, they quickly become intimate and intense in their relationships with others and rarely feel that the other person loves or gives enough to them. They are prone to acting out their problems on themselves and others. They may also appear very depressed and may make attempts at self-mutilation or suicide because they do not have healthy coping skills. They impose the "fault" of their self-harm as the responsibility of others. Typically, a person with borderline personality disorder will engage in "splitting" behaviors. Splitting is a mechanism whereby the individual divides the perception, loyalty, and trust of others in the social environment for the purpose of self-gain. Some people will believe this person and see him or her as helpless. Others will see this individual as manipulative and untrustworthy.

Dependent personality disorder is characterized by submissive behavior, helplessness when alone, fear of abandonment, and inability to make decisions. While this individual seems to be the caretaker of others, the caretaking is in the interest of keeping others in the relationship dependent on them. They have difficulty expressing disagreement, especially with the person on whom they are dependent. The fear of separation or rejection by the person on whom they depend is intense, and they will become involved in activities they feel are wrong just to keep the other person involved in the relationship.

Histrionic personality disorder is characterized by displays of melodramatic and attention-seeking behavior. People with this disorder seem to have their egos bruised easily and act out these injuries to the self in methods that are dramatic beyond the actual situation. Often, they find themselves going from one relationship to another, seeking validation of their worth and attractiveness. The other person in the relationship often feels that they will "blow off" at the slightest infraction against this person's self-esteem. Individuals with this disorder feel uncomfortable and unappreciated when they are not the center of attention. They are initially charming, flirtatious, and engaging, but this soon wears thin as they continue to need to be the center of attention. These individuals are dramatic in their emotional expressions and often embarrass friends and family with an excessive display of emotion in public situations. They express strong opinions but have no valid reasons for these strong opinions. For example, the person may say that someone is a beautiful and wonderful individual but cannot give you any reasons or descriptions of the individual to explain why the other person is so wonderful.

Narcissistic personality disorder is characterized by a grand sense of self-importance and lack of empathy for others. This includes being overly sensitive to the evaluation of others. Emotionally, this individual is wounded easily and does not realize the emotional scars inflicted on others. At all costs, this person tries to preserve self-esteem and self-worth. These individuals are often preoccupied with fantasies of unlimited success, power, brilliance, or beauty. They never feel admired enough by others. They feel entitled to great respect and admiration. They are puzzled or angry when they do not get the attention they feel they deserve from others. Because they lack empathy (concern for others), they do not praise or show concern for another person's success or problem. Criticism may haunt these individuals and lead to rage or social withdrawal.

Passive-aggressive personality disorder is characterized by a very submissive appearance, but the unexpressed anger these people internalize causes them to be aggressive in situations unrelated to the anger. Often, these individuals are unable to explain why they acted against another person. They do not see how they acted aggressively, and they feel attacked by others who point out their aggressiveness.

Sadistic personality disorder is manifested by cruel and very aggressive behavior without concern for others. People who are sadistic may feel powerful or gain self-esteem when they are able to hurt others emotionally or physically. They are gratified by the act of inflicting hurt or pain on others.

Schizoid personality disorder is seen in people who demonstrate indifference to the social arena and those who have restricted affect or expression of mood. They lack the ability to experience emotion. People with schizoid disorder neither desire nor enjoy social relationships, including family. They lack close friends and confidants, and they are indifferent to the praise or criticism of others. Typically, these people work best in solitary jobs that do not require much interaction with others. They are often described as "loners."

Schizotypal personality disorder is displayed by defects in interpersonal relationships and oddities in appearance, thinking, and behavior. Typically, these people have odd beliefs or magical thinking. They may also experience strange perceptual experiences, including bodily illusions. They lack close friends and are extremely uncomfortable in social situations. They may have strange rituals that are noticed by others and may seem schizophrenic, but they do not have a true thought disorder.

Obsessive-compulsive personality disorder is characterized by excessive orderliness, preoccupation with perfectionism, and mental and interpersonal self-control. People with obsessive-compulsive disorder attempt to maintain order and control through painstaking attention to rules, details, procedures, lists, and schedules. They check repeatedly for mistakes and are preoccupied with doing activities in precisely the same way all the time. Deviation from a task's precise order of steps leads to anxiety and irrational fears. People with this disorder are scrupulous, inflexible, and overconscientious about matters of morality or values. These individuals are rigid and stubborn and hoard and save objects that are not needed and have no sentimental value. They are miserly in spending money on themselves and others. Usually, they cannot delegate a task unless the other person agrees to perform it in precisely the same manner that the individual would perform it. They spend excessive amounts of time performing rituals that interfere with their daily activities. These individuals may spend the entire day handwashing or checking the locks or electrical outlets hundreds of times. This is done to reduce anxiety and to control the environment. The person may be unable to have social relationships that are pleasurable because of the time "wasted" in organizing tasks or performing rituals.

Mood Disorders

Mood disorders are sometimes called *affective disorders*. Our mood involves our feelings. *Mood* is what you feel, and *affect* is the outward expression of mood. Our feelings are affected by our thoughts and are a reaction to mental stimuli. Feelings motivate our life decisions. Feelings are powerful. Dealing with feelings in a healthy way is important to our mental wellness. Mood disorders may appear "out of the blue" or may result from prolonged grief. Research has proven that mood disturbances are linked to neurochemical imbalance (Figure 21-3). What creates the imbalance of neurochemicals like serotonin or epinephrine is not clear. Mood disorders include *bipolar mood disorder*, formerly called *manic depression*, *major depression*, *dysthymic disorder*, and *cyclothymic disorder*.

Bipolar Mood Disorder

Bipolar mood disorder is characterized by episodes of mania and depression. At least one episode of mania must have occurred to result in this diagnosis. **Mania** is an expansive, persistent, elevated, or irritable mood that lasts for at least one week. During a manic episode, the person experiences inflated self-esteem or grandiosity and a decreased need for sleep and is distracted easily by unimportant stimuli in the environment. Delusions of grandeur and persecution are commonly experienced. The individual may be excessively talkative and have pressured speech. *Pressured speech* is speech in which the person seems pressed to keep talking. There may be *flight of ideas*, in which the person may jump from one topic to another in a conversation. The individual jumps from one loosely related topic to another, and it is difficult for the listener to understand what stimulated the sudden change in topic.

In the initial manic phase (hypomania), this person may seem highly effective and goal directed. Eventually, the schemes and great ideas lead to financial, occupational, and interpersonal losses. The individual is involved excessively in pleasurable activ-

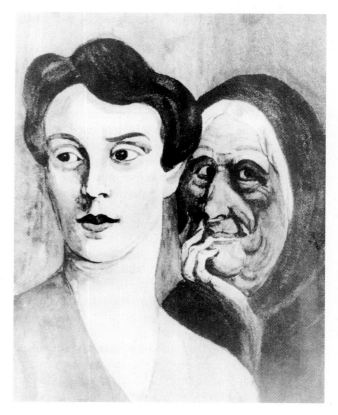

FIGURE 21-3 Mood disorders are linked to neurochemical imbalance. Reprinted by permission of the publisher from *Thematic Apperception Test* by Henry A. Murray, Cambridge, Mass.: Harvard University Press, Copyright © 1943 by the President and Fellows of Harvard College, © 1971 by Henry A. Murray.

ities that have a high degree of risk. The person may go on unrestrained shopping sprees, engage in risky sexual liaisons, or make foolish business decisions. This manic mood may range from a mild manic disturbance to a delirious mania in which the person cannot sleep or cannot stop talking. The person becomes extremely irritable and aggressive.

The **depressive episodes** are characterized by the same features as a major depressive disorder. Lithium and antidepressant medications are used to treat these disorders. Lithium is a naturally occurring chemical salt. It is used as a medication to help balance the mood disturbances of someone with a bipolar disorder. Antidepressants are used to treat depression.

Major Depression

The symptoms of a depressive episode include at least five or more of the following symptoms. The person feels sad or depressed most of the day every day and lacks interest in pleasurable activities. The individual may lose or gain weight when not trying to lose or gain. **Insomnia**, the inability to fall asleep or stay asleep, or **hypersomnia**, excessive sleep, may be present. Also, the motor activity can be extremely slow or agitated. Feelings of worthlessness, uselessness, helplessness, and hopelessness are present. There may be preoccupation with feelings of guilt, and there is an inability to concentrate or to think. Recurrent thoughts of death or suicidal thoughts may be present. Suicide attempts are most likely to occur when the person seems less depressed and able to make decisions. During deep depression, the individual may not be able to concentrate long enough to plan and organize. These symptoms cause significant distress that impairs occupational and interpersonal functioning.

Dysthymic Disorder

Dysthymic disorder is characterized by depressed mood most of the day for a period of at least two years. Two or more of the following symptoms must be present: poor appetite or overeating, insomnia or hypersomnia, low energy or fatigue, low self-esteem, poor concentration or difficulty making decisions, and feelings of hopelessness. These symptoms are not as pervasive or intense as in a major depression or a depressive episode in bipolar disorder.

Cyclothymic Disorder

Cyclothymic disorder is a disorder in which the symptoms are present for a period of at least two years. The symptoms include features of a bipolar disorder, but the symptoms are less severe and disabling for the individual. The symptoms of hypomania and dysthymia are present and alternating in occurrence.

There are other mood disorders that are associated with medical conditions. Some are related to substance abuse, and others may be related to a dementia, such as Alzheimer's disease.

Neurotic Disorders

Neurosis literally means "condition of the nerves." A **neurosis**, or anxiety-based disorder, is not a neurological condition that results from specific impairment of the nervous system, like multiple sclerosis or amyotrophic lateral sclerosis. Nonetheless, those who have been diagnosed with a neurosis often feel "nervous." There is a persistent feeling of anxiety, threat, and fear in facing everyday life situations. In these disorders, the maladaptive reactions to life events usually can be traced to coping patterns developed in childhood (*mal-* means "poor" or "bad"; *adaptive* refers to the ability to adjust and cope). The person's usual or normal coping methods are not successful in relieving the fear or anxiety.

Defense Mechanisms

Those who have no mental health diagnosis and those with all categories of mental disorders use what are called *ego-defense mechanisms* to protect their egos. The major **defense mechanisms**, or coping strategies, include *denial, compensation, suppression, repression, regression, projection,* and *displacement*. Defense mechanisms are used by all people to help "save face," to disguise or to deny any apparent flaw or personal weakness. They usually help us to cope with the anxiety or threat of the moment. Defense mechanisms are normal, useful, and healthy when they aid an individual to resolve and redirect fears and anxiety successfully. They become unhealthy when they are overused or are the sole source of the person's coping with problems of everyday life.

People with neuroses use these defense mechanisms in an unhealthy way. When the defense used to cope with the source of anxiety becomes the reason for the anxiety, it is called the *neurotic paradox*. A paradox is something that is in direct contrast to what is expected. An example of a paradox is hot ice or nonhurtful pain. Essentially, what happens is the person relies extensively on the use of defense mechanisms to protect against emotional harm, and eventually, the defense becomes the source of the person's anxiety. Defense mechanisms are not only used in excess by those who suffer from neuroses, but also by people with other mental health disorders. Let's examine these defense mechanisms.

- *Denial* is the refusal of the mind to accept the truth about a situation. If you are told by your physician that you have a terminal illness, you might not want to accept this fact readily. Your mind might deny the impact of this reality in an attempt to help you survive. When you are asked, "What is the physician's diagnosis?" you might not say, "I was told that I have cancer." Instead, you might say, "The doctor said I have a growth. It's nothing life-threatening."

- *Compensation* is making up for a lack or weakness in one aspect of life by excelling or overperforming in another area of life. For example, if you are a student who is not a good athlete, you might become a terrific student or excel in art or music. We compensate for weaknesses so that we can feel okay about ourselves. Compensation is unhealthy when we overcompensate in something and fail to feel better about ourselves or to work on our weaknesses.

- *Suppression* is pushing something out of our conscious thoughts that we find too uncomfortable or unbearable to deal with at the moment. We know that the issue is there, but we try not to remember it. If you hate to go to the dentist and you have an appointment at 3:00 P.M., you may find that you forget the appointment. When someone reminds you that you are late for the appointment, you suddenly remember you forgot. When you were in elementary school, if you ever failed a test that your parents needed to sign, you may have forgotten to show it to them because you couldn't face the consequences. You wanted to avoid thinking about the failure. The next day, when the teacher asked for the test, you suddenly remembered that you forgot to get it signed. This is not lying, nor is it denial. Lying is a conscious decision not to do something. This defense mechanism, like most defense mechanisms, is used without decision and without an awareness of using it.

Repression is the act of pushing thoughts, events, or feelings deep into the unconscious so that they are not remembered even when someone reminds you of them. If you were abused as a child, you may have repressed these memories because they were too painful to think about. To protect yourself, your mind pushed these memories away from conscious recall. Hypnosis is often used to help people remember repressed memories. Sometimes, the expression *Freudian slip* is used to describe the unconscious slip of repressed memories. When people are under the influence of drugs, sedatives, or alcohol, the memory or thought may unconsciously "slip out."

Regression is the defense mechanism in which a person reverts to an earlier stage of behavior or to a previously used coping strategy to manage the anxiety-producing events in the present. Children regress to earlier stages of behavior when they feel threatened by something with which they can't cope. You may know a small child whose family just brought home a newborn infant. The child who was "potty-trained" begins soiling again. Unconsciously, the child is trying to return to a stage of life like the infant's when this function was cared for by the parents. People who quit smoking cigarettes may find themselves regressing and smoking again when they are under stress.

Projection is placing unacceptable or uncomfortable emotions onto someone else. If you did something that you find unacceptable to your self-image, you may not be able to accept this feeling readily. Unconsciously, you may place the blame for this on someone else. You probably know people who drink too much alcohol, and when they are confronted about this behavior, they say they wouldn't drink so much if their spouse treated them better. They unconsciously put the blame for their behavior on someone else: "She makes me do it."

Displacement is taking a feeling about a person or situation and directing it at someone or something other than the source of the negative feeling. Usually, the person who generates this negative feeling is somebody that we do not feel safe in confronting. Imagine that your boss tells you that you are performing your job inadequately. You feel that you are doing everything you can to meet her expectations. You can't tell your boss that you dislike her and that you are angry with her. You hold this feeling inside. When you get home, your husband asks you how you feel, and you scream at him for not folding the laundry. He's confused about why you are so angry. You can't remember why you are feeling so frustrated. Your husband decides he can't tell you to be quiet and leave him alone because he needs you to cook dinner, so he displaces his anger on your son, who can't yell back at dad. Later, your son kicks the cat, and when you ask him why he did that, he says, "I don't know."

There are many defense mechanisms that we use to cope with daily life; these are examples of the most commonly used defense mechanisms. Remember that defense mechanisms can be useful or hurtful, healthy or unhealthy. They are no longer healthy when we use them to excess. When they become our main means of coping with the stressors of life, they fail to control our anxiety.

Anxiety Disorders

Anxiety disorders stem from a distorted perception of events. Anxiety disorders fall into four categories:

- General anxiety disorder
- Panic disorder
- Phobia
- Dissociative disorder

General anxiety disorder is associated with an unrealistic or excessive worry about life circumstances for at least six months. Symptoms may be physiological or emotional. Physiological symptoms include trembling, tension, fatigue, facial straining or brow furrowing, sweating, clammy hands, dizziness, tingling of the extremities, urinary frequency, diarrhea, apprehension, worry, anticipation of mishappenings, hyperattentiveness, difficulty focusing, irritability, and impatience. The anxiety felt is not related to a specific "something." It is vague and generalized. Depression is often associated with anxiety. The person experiences difficulty making decisions, fear of making errors, rumination over consequences of prior actions, and excessive worry about everything.

Panic disorder is characterized by an attack of acute anxiety and fight-or-flight physiology. The onset of symptoms occurs without an apparent trigger. The symptoms of fight-or-flight include heart palpitation, dizziness, sweating, trembling or shaking, difficulty breathing, or tingling of the hands and feet. In addition, the person has a fear of going "crazy," dying, or losing control. These panic attacks can incapacitate the individual and lead to other neurotic disorders, such as phobias.

A **phobia** is an intense, irrational fear of a person, place, object, activity, or situation. It is irrational because the perceived fear is far greater than the real danger. People with phobias often admit that the fear is not logical, but they do not change the emotional response to the fear. If the phobia prevents normal activities of daily living (ADLs), the person suffers from a phobic disorder. There are three types of phobic disorders: *simple* or *specific*, *social*, and *agoraphobic*.

- *Simple phobic disorders* include fear of heights, germs, spiders, bridges, water, and so on.
- *Social phobias* include fear of delivering public speeches or communicating in public.
- *Agoraphobia* is a complex anxiety disorder in which the person fears a variety of ADL situations, such as driving, standing in line, and crossing the street (*agora-* means "marketplace," and *-phobia* means "fear"). Doing these things produces severe anxiety and panic attacks. People with agoraphobia become so disabled that they never leave home because to do so produces severe anxiety, panic, and an impending sense of doom.

Dissociative disorder, or multiple-personality disorder, evolves as a response to deep emotional and physical abuse and results in a lack of personality integration. Children who have been abused often try to resist the internal agony of the abuse by developing an alternate personality that will handle the abusive situation. The child escapes from the abuse by allowing an alternate personality to appear—one that can manage the trauma. Alternate personalities may be any age, any ethnic group, and either sex. An adult female may have alternate personalities of a male child, a woman who is very different in behavior from the core person, a mute individual, and so on. The core personality does not usually recognize the presence of the alternates. The alternates may identify the core personality. The person often cannot explain or account for periods of time when an alternate appears to help the core person manage an anxiety-producing situation. This disorder is very disabling, and many years of therapy may be needed to try to reconstruct and integrate the personalities. Dissociative disorder is now a separate classification in the *DSM IV*. It was formerly included in the neurotic or anxiety disorders.

In addition, there are other dissociative disorders such as amnesia, fugue states, depersonalization disorder, and conversion reactions. The essential features are disruption of memory and identity.

Addictive Disorders

One can be addicted to almost anything, but the major recognized addictions are drugs, alcohol, sex, gambling, work, caffeine, tobacco, and food. Why do people become addicted? There are several theories. One is that addiction is the outward expression of underlying emotional problems. Another is that the person is a dependent personality who has transferred his or her dependence onto a substance or activity. Social theorists believe that a person learns to be an addict. Biological theorists hold that the person has an inborn trait or physiological craving for a substance that is lacking or is not sufficient to meet biological needs once the person has introduced the body to the substance. The **euphoria** (sense of well-being) that the initial indulgence produces sparks a positive reinforcement for continued use of the substance. The person with an addiction expects enhancement of self-image or abilities and thinks the addiction will be transforming. Self-image and normal social barriers are distorted by the presence of an addictive substance. The person's usual social behavior or performance is altered.

Can you remember your first alcoholic beverage, cigarette, binge on chocolate, or cup of coffee? Did it make you feel different, pleased, happy, or confused? Probably, addiction is both physiological and psychosocial in nature. Why do some people become addicted to alcohol and others to heroin? Why do some people crave coffee and others crave cigarettes?

Consider the fact that you have been introduced to many possible addictive substances. If you have an addiction, why did your mind and body choose to seek one particular substance over another addictive substance? Why doesn't a person who is addicted to cocaine choose a narcotic? Did he or she learn to like this drug and its effects because of environmental or social factors, or did he or she have an inborn attraction to this particular substance? Whatever addictive substance is pursued, those who do not control or reject the urge to pursue it have a problem. Theorists have been searching for an answer, a cause, and a cure for addiction for many years.

Substance-Related Addictive Disorders

The diagnosis of **substance dependence**, or **substance abuse**, is a maladaptive pattern of substance use that leads to a clinically significant problem or impairment based on at least three or more of the following conditions occurring at the same time for a period of at least 1 year. The conditions include these:

1. Tolerance of the substance is established. **Tolerance** is defined as a need for increased amounts of the substance to achieve intoxication or the desired effect. Tolerance is also the use of the same amount of the substance with a diminished or lessened effect. (For example: If you started drinking alcohol at age eighteen and you continued to drink one glass of beer every day for several years, you would no longer feel the intoxication of the alcohol. If you started drinking at age eighteen, by the time you were twenty-one you might have needed to drink three to four glasses of beer to achieve a high, or intoxication.)

2. Withdrawal symptoms occur when the substance is not taken into the body or, another similar substance is used as a substitute, producing effects similar to the original substance. The symptoms of withdrawal are based on the nature of the substance. (For example: You might feel agitated and nervous if you are addicted to alcohol and you have no alcohol. You might substitute by taking a Valium to "calm you down." If you used to drink three shots of whiskey daily and you have no whiskey to drink now, you may feel the symptoms of withdrawal.)

3. A substance is taken in larger amounts or over a longer period of time than it was intended to be taken or prescribed.

4. There is a persistent desire for the substance, or there are unsuccessful attempts to cut down or to stop the use of the substance.

5. A great deal of time is spent in trying to obtain the substance, use the substance, or recover from the effects of the substance. (For example: An addicted person might spend much time trying to purchase the substance by going to several doctors or making numerous calls and visits to drug dealers, might spend a lot of time chain-smoking cigarettes or preparing to smoke crack, or might drink too much alcohol or ingest too much Valium and need extra hours of sleep to recover from the intoxication.)

6. Important occupational, recreational, and social events are missed because of the use or lack of availability of the substance.

7. In spite of knowledge of a psychological or physical problem caused by the substance, the use of the substance is persistent. (For example: The person recognizes the source of the problem and feels depressed and exhausted after using cocaine but continues to use it, or a person has a stomach ulcer and continues to drink alcohol, despite the knowledge that alcohol is a contributing factor.)

Dependence on **psychoactive substances** implies that there is a physiological or psychological addiction. **Dependence** is the need to use a substance. Physiological dependence is featured by items 1 and 2. Substances like alcohol, barbiturates, narcotics, nicotine, and alcohol create a physical dependence. Tolerance and withdrawal are experienced with these substances. Psychological dependence is usually associated with physical dependence. However, some substances do not create a physical dependence. Substances like marijuana, hallucinogens, and amphetamines create a psychological dependence. Although the individual may feel negative effects physically because he or she has not taken the substance, these substances do not have a physical basis for dependence.

An individual can be physically dependent and experience tolerance and withdrawal symptoms but not be psychologically dependent. If you were in severe pain for a period of time and required a narcotic (codeine or morphine) to manage the pain, you may not seek this drug when the pain subsides. Nonetheless, you will feel the negative physical symptoms when the drug is stopped.

Some substances can have severe and life-threatening withdrawal effects. Barbiturates, anti-anxiety agents, and alcohol can have life-threatening withdrawal symptoms. A physician should always be consulted when an individual will undergo **withdrawal** (complete and immediate removal of a drug on which the person is dependent). A person who wants to withdraw from some substances, such as Valium, which can cause life-threatening effects if withdrawn abruptly, needs to be monitored for seizures and severe agitation. The substance should be slowly reduced in frequency and dosage.

Withdrawal from alcohol can lead to seizures, severe agitation, confusion, and hallucinations. The condition is called **delirium tremens (DTs)**. Substance abuse can lead to or can be the source of other mental health disorders. Some drugs may create extreme anxiety, paranoia, depression, and psychosis. Prolonged use of some substances can cause organic brain disorders that are permanently disabling.

Dependence, tolerance, and withdrawal are not to be taken lightly. Treatment should not be managed by an unskilled individual. Treatments for managing withdrawal and maintaining abstinence include medical care and, if needed, detoxification in an inpatient setting, individual counseling, supportive group therapy, vocational counseling, or membership in a twelve-step program like Alcoholics Anonymous (AA) or Narcotics Anonymous (NA).

Table 21-1 lists and describes the substances that are commonly abused.

Cognitive Disorders

Cognitive disorders are in contrast to the previously described mental disorders because the abnormalities of thinking, mood, and behavior are caused directly by a physical defect in the brain that impairs normal brain functions. Usually, when there are defects in

TABLE 21-1   Substances That Are Commonly Abused

Classification	Substance	Use	Medical Use	Tolerance	Physical Dependence	Psychological Dependence
Sedatives	Alcohol	Reduce tension	No	Yes	Yes	Yes
	Barbiturates	Relax in social situations, cause relaxation and sleep	Yes	Yes	Yes	Yes
Stimulants	Amphetamines • Speed • Crank • Dexedrine • Methamphetamine	Increase feelings of confidence and alertness, decrease fatigue, stay awake, increase endurance, stimulate sex drive	Yes	Yes	No	Yes
	Cocaine		No	Minimal	No	Yes
	Crack cocaine		Yes	Yes	Yes	Yes
Narcotics	Opium, heroin, morphine, Demerol, Dilaudid, Hydrochloride, Percodan, codeine	Reduce physical pain, reduce anxiety and tension, aid sleep	Yes (except heroin)	Yes	Yes	Yes
	Methadone	Treatment for heroin addiction	Yes	Yes	Yes	Yes
Hallucinogens	Marijuana, hashish, peyote, LSD, PCP	Relax; change mood, thoughts, and behavior; "mind expansion," "tripping"	No (THC, the active ingredient in marijuana, is used to reduce nausea associated w/terminally ill patients)	No	No	Yes
Tranquilizers (antianxiety drugs)	Librium, Valium, Ativan, Serax, Zanax	Reduce anxiety, induce sleep	Yes	Yes	Yes	Yes

the brain before birth or at an early age, mental retardation results. The severity of the defect in the brain is related directly to the severity of the retardation or dysfunction of mental and brain functions. People who sustain structural or chemical damage to the brain after the brain has fully developed, have a **cognitive disorder**. The term *cognitive disorder* is the current term used to describe what was formerly classified as an *organic mental disorder*. The cognitive disorders that will be discussed in this section are delirium and dementia. In the next section, we will review the classifications of mental retardation.

Delirium

The term **delirium** is used to describe the grossly abnormal impairments of mental functioning that result from a medical condition or a chemical or substance-induced cognitive dysfunction. Cognition is thinking. Thinking involves the ability to interpret incoming information from the environment, to process the information, and to form a response. Usually, disturbances in cognition include symptoms and signs of confusion, disorientation, lack of reasoning ability, lack of judgment, and distortions of thought, speech, mood, and perception. In delirium and dementia, cognition is impaired. Definitions and descriptions of these terms follow.

- *Confusion* is the inability to understand and make sense of a situation.
- *Disorientation* is the lack of orientation to person, place, or time. *Orientation* refers to knowing and identifying people, places, and time (day, date, year, season). Orientation is assessed in these three spheres and is documented as oriented × 1, oriented × 2, or oriented × 3. If you are oriented × 3, then you know who you and others are by name or association. You know and can state where you are (the location or type of environment). You can identify the date, day, year, season, or the approximate time of year. Most frequently, disorientation involves not knowing the time, day, and date. If this were the case, you would say that a person is oriented × 2 and note that the person is disoriented to time. Disorientation to time is the first sphere or area of orientation to be impaired when someone has dementia or delirium. The more severe the impairment of cognition, the more disoriented the person is. A delirious person may be disoriented × 3.
- *Judgment* is the ability to evaluate by comparing and using reasoning to form an opinion about someone or something. When judgment is impaired, a person will not be able to process the situation at hand and will respond in a manner that is unsafe, unreasonable, or inappropriate.

The disturbances of delirium develop over a period of days or hours. The person who is delirious is unable to focus attention, is distracted easily, and has wandering attention. Because of this, it may be impossible to engage in logical communication with the individual. Recent memory is impaired, and the person may not be able to remember anything from one minute to the next. The disorientation is noted because the individual is unable to correctly identify time, place, or person. Speech may be rambling and incoherent. *Incoherent speech* is speech that does not make sense and is related to confusion of thought. As the person speaks one thought, it does not connect with the next.

The person with delirium usually experiences illusions and hallucinations. The illusions and hallucinations can be auditory, visual, tactile, olfactory, or gustatory. Hallucinations other than auditory ones should always trigger the nurse and physician to assess for possible delirium and to look for the medical or substance-induced cause of such hallucinations or illusions. These false sensory perceptions create fear and may cause the person to have unpredictable behavior and rapid changes in mood. Delirium is generally more evident in the nighttime hours. The patient may seem alert and oriented in the morning and, as the day progresses to nighttime, become grossly confused and disoriented. This is called *sundowning*. During the late night hours, you might find this person completely disoriented, confused, uncooperative, and agitated. Movements can be hyperactive or hypoactive or can rapidly alternate from sluggishness to rapid, sudden, and unsafe or untimely movements. The person may pick at clothes or grope at real or imagined people or things. The individual may pull out IV lines or tubes because they do not know what they are doing, and it may be impossible to get the person to consent to necessary medical care because of their mental state.

Delirium can be caused by head injury, disrupted blood flow to the brain, electrolyte imbalances (high blood calcium), kidney failure causing uremia, or liver failure causing toxins to build up in the blood. Substance-induced delirium results from intoxication by hallucinogens, cocaine, alcohol, barbiturates, or PCP and from high doses of prescribed medications. Combinations of two incompatible medications can cause delirium. Withdrawal from alcohol, Demerol, and barbiturates can cause delirium. Toxic substances such as insecticides and fumes from gasoline, paint, glue, and carbon monoxide can produce delirious states. High fevers can cause delirium. Sometimes, patients who have a dementia can become delirious when they are admitted to a hospital or nursing home. The change in the environment may be sufficient to cause confusion and disturbances in the sleep-wake cycle. About 10 percent of older patients, become delirious when they are admitted to a hospital. Prolonged length of stay in an intensive care unit (ICU) can cause delirium; the environment of an ICU can be very confusing and can alter sleep patterns. Patients who have had extensive and prolonged surgical procedures or who were under anesthesia for long periods of time may exhibit delirium post-operatively. Infections of the brain, tumors of the brain, cerebral vascular accidents (CVAs), and late stages of acquired immunodeficiency syndrome (AIDS) may cause delirious states. AIDS can also lead to dementia.

Dementia

Dementia was once referred to as *senility*, and the individual was described as being *senile*. Dementia results from a degeneration of brain tissue. Unlike delirium, dementia is chronic in nature and has a slow onset. Most often, it is associated with deterioration of the brain from aging. However, the majority of elders do not suffer dementia. There are dementias that occur before old age, and these are related generally to cerebrovascular diseases, the late stages of untreated syphilis, AIDS, Huntington's disease (a genetic disorder of the nervous system), Pick's disease (a rare neurological disorder that causes slow deterioration of the brain between forty-five and fifty), and Alzheimer's disease. The abuse of substances such as alcohol can lead to dementia in some people, and it may appear before old age. Head injuries can lead to forms of dementia. If a head injury causes cognitive impairment before the age of fifteen to eighteen years, it is classified as mental retardation.

The clinical picture of dementia includes intellectual impairments in adults who are otherwise alert and attuned to events in the environment. Memory is virtually always impaired, as is the ability to learn new information or skills. Memory is evaluated as short-term memory, recent memory, and long-term memory.

Short-term memory involves the processing and storing of information that occurred within the past minute. *Recent memory* relates to remembering information that occurred within the past hours and days. *Long-term memory* involves retaining information that occurred days or years ago. In dementia, short-term and recent memory are impaired most frequently. Long-term memory, especially memories stored years before, may remain intact in certain dementias. Sufferers may not recall what you just said to them or what they wore yesterday, but they might be able to recall what they did on the day they were married.

Judgment and problem solving are impaired. Disorientation to time is noted initially, and eventually, places and people are also not recognized.

Alzheimer's disease accounts for approximately 50 percent of the cases of dementia, and it is the dementia seen most frequently in long-term care and home care.

Alzheimer's Disease At whatever age it strikes, **Alzheimer's disease** is the degeneration of neurons and the accumulation of tangles and plaques of the neurons in the forebrain. There is a gross loss of neurons—up to 75 percent of the nerve cells in the forebrain. The cause of this disease is still unknown and under investigation. The disease proceeds slowly, with initial changes noticed in memory and gradual withdrawal from life activities, especially work and social events. Changes in routine and new events or expectations cause confusion and frustration. In the early stages, Alzheimer victims may seem forgetful. Judgment in social situations is also affected. They may choose inappropriate attire for the temperature or event and may behave in ways that are atypical. They may say things that are out of the ordinary or use language that is not appropriate. The course or pattern of this disease is not predictable or the same in all people. The cognitive losses become more pronounced and involved as the disease progresses. Some people may demonstrate agitated behavior, paranoid thinking, depression, or euphoria (an extraordinary sense of well-being). Those who live long enough with this disease will become unable to recognize family or home. They will not be able to perform simple activities of daily living and will need total assistance with all feeding, toileting, dressing, and walking. In the final stage of this illness, the victims are in a vegetative state and may not respond to stimuli in the environment. The tragedy of this illness is as much a tragedy for the loved ones as it is for the individual. Even though the person is alive, the spouse or children lose "the person they knew." The family is helpless in controlling the "slipping away" of the person they love.

Mental Retardation

Mental retardation is characterized by a significantly less-than-average **intelligence quotient (IQ)** that is present before the age of eighteen years. IQ is determined by standardized tests that are designed to measure an individual's performance of typical academic—math, reading, science—content on paper-and-pencil tests. Such tests were used originally to predict how well schoolchildren would perform "everyday" academic tasks.

IQ and the ability of the individual to perform ADLs, to perform personal and occupational tasks independently, and to adapt to the social environment are used to classify the levels of mental retardation. There is a formula used to approximate IQ:

$$\text{mental age} \div \text{chronological age} \times 100 = \text{IQ}$$

For example, if a child is 10 years old and functions at the age of a five-year-old, the child's IQ would be 50.

$$5 \div 10 = 0.5 \times 100 = 50$$

If a child is ten years of age and functions at the age of a six-year-old, what would the IQ be?

This child's IQ would be 60.

$$6 \div 10 = 0.6 \times 100 = 60$$

While IQs are used to classify the severity of mental retardation, it is the person's ability to adapt to the demands of the environment, along with less-than-average IQ, that provides a definitive diagnosis of mental retardation. People with normal or average IQ may have difficulty adapting to the demands of the environment, but they are not diagnosed with mental retardation. Let's examine the levels of mental retardation.

Mild mental retardation is an IQ of 50 to 70. The majority of individuals diagnosed with mental retardation fall into this group (Figure 21-4). As adults, their intellectual level of functioning is that of an eight- to eleven-year-old. These people can learn to read and write and do simple math calculations. Socially, they may adapt to the level of an adolescent, although it is not fair to indicate that all people with mild retardation function socially as teenagers. Some are more adept socially; however, their judgment and impulse control only develop to that of an adolescent. The person can obtain employment in jobs that do not demand high levels of problem-solving and reading ability. They can learn to perform ADLs independently and form social and vocational relationships. Judgment may be limited because they may not be able to foresee the consequences of their actions. This makes those with mild retardation vulnerable to people who take advantage of their limited judgment.

Moderate mental retardation is the term used for people with an IQ of 36 to 50. They can be trained to perform the tasks that a four to seven-year-old can learn. Dressing, feeding, and household tasks can be learned. Some people with moderate mental retardation learn to read and write at the level of a child of four to seven years of age. They may work in shel-

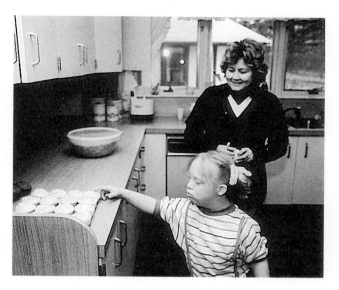

FIGURE 21-4   Down's syndrome is a cause of mental retardation.

tered workshops and earn money for their work. Vocational training in jobs that require simple repetitive tasks, such as assembling, stacking, packaging, stocking, and boxing items are usually the nature of vocational work.

Severe mental retardation is an IQ of 20 to 35. The level of motor and intellectual functioning is that of a preschooler. The person may learn to speak, feed, dress, and walk. Supervision is required for safety and protection. This person will not travel independently. Communication will be limited to short, concise directions and interactions. The individual will have limited language skills and may have difficulty with any complex motor skill (for example, cooking and cleaning). Most often, vocational training is provided, and the person is supervised continually in the performance of any vocational tasks. Sheltered vocational workshops have direct vocational trainers who work with small groups of people who need much supervision to stay focused and to complete repetitive tasks. Generally, people with this level of retardation require assistance with all activities of daily living.

Profound mental retardation is classified by IQs under 20. These individuals are totally dependent on others for personal care and protection. They may learn to feed themselves and may learn to speak simple words. Generally, they have profound motor disability and behavioral abnormalities.

People with mental retardation are as unique and diverse as those with average intelligence. It is important to treat the people who have mental retardation as you would treat any person in your care. These individuals may have subnormal intelligence, but they are not stupid. When they are adults, they should not be treated as children. They have feelings, needs, and desires as everyone else does. When people with mental retardation are treated without consideration for age and without respect for their freedom of choice, it is not only disrespectful, but it could be abusive. People with retardation should not be limited by their IQ; they should be educated and trained to perform to their highest potential. Schools mainstream children with mental retardation into regular academic and vocational classrooms. Vocational training opportunities are available, and those individuals who can work in industry are encouraged and supported to work and to earn a living. People with mental retardation may fall in love, marry, work, and have children. This is limited only by the person's social and adaptive abilities.

The institutionalization of people with mental retardation is no longer permissible simply because the person has mental retardation. In schools and in living arrangements, the focus and goal is to provide the **least restrictive alternative** possible. The least restrictive alternative is a concept that is employed to make decisions about living arrangements, classroom settings, vocational or job settings, and treatment measures. In essence, whenever possible, independent living in an apartment should be opted for over a group home. If the person's behavior is inappropriate or uncooperative, locking the person in a room is illegal. The staff in a treatment facility should attempt to help the person gain control over this behavior first by talking to the individual. If that is not successful, the staff should remove the person from the situation for a time-out. Whenever any restrictions are placed on an individual in your care in any environment, you should employ the concept of least restrictive alternative.

Sometimes, it is the label of "disability" that is as disabling as the disability itself. You should be cautious about referring to any person with a disability by the nature of the disability. In other words, you should avoid saying "that mentally retarded person"; instead, say "the person who has mental retardation." If you had blindness, you wouldn't want to be called a "blind person," because first you are a person and then you are blind. Being blind does not define a person. The same holds true for people with physical or mental illness.

Causes of Mental Retardation

The causes of mental retardation are numerous. Some causes begin before birth, some during the birth process, and some after birth. The causes include the following:

- Genetics
- Infections and toxins
- Prematurity and trauma
- Radiation
- Malnutrition
- Metabolic disorders
- Cranial abnormalities
- Environmental deprivation

The largest number of people with mental retardation have suffered from environmental deprivation. This means that the individual was deprived of usual stimulation or lived in adverse or harsh environments that failed to promote intellectual and social interaction and stimulation. Three-fourths of the individuals diagnosed with mental retardation suffered extreme isolation and received no sensory stimulation from those in the home during the developmental years. In addition, they had no play or social interactions.

One of the genetic causes of mental retardation is **Down's syndrome**. This syndrome results from trisomy of chromosome 21. This is not an inherited chromosomal defect. During embryonic development, chromosome 21 develops a third attachment instead of having the normal two. Why this chromosome develops this defect is unknown. A woman may have other children who are born without this abnormal chromosome because it is not passed along as an inherited trait.

The baby born with Down's syndrome has an appearance that characterizes the syndrome. Typically, children with Down's syndrome have almond-shaped eyes, short thick necks, flat noses, and hands that are thick with creases across the palm. The iris of the eye is speckled, and the tongue is usually thick, with deep fissures. Although people who have Down's may look alike, they are not all the same in behavior or intellectual capacity. Similarly, these children and adults should be treated as unique individuals.

application to practice

At the end of Chapter 22 is a "Learning Activity" section that uses information you have learned in this chapter about mental health and mental illness.

Examination Review Questions

1. Which of the following is *not* a thought disorder?
   a. bipolar disorder
   b. schizophrenia
   c. delusional disorder
   d. schizoaffective disorder

2. Which is *not* a marked feature of dementia?
   a. is chronic in nature
   b. has a slow onset
   c. occurs with old age
   d. is associated with degeneration of the brain

3. Which disorder is characterized by episodes of mania and depression
   a. schizophrenia
   b. bipolar disorder
   c. major depression
   d. dysthmic personality disorder

4. The cause of most mental retardation is
   a. environmental deprivation or lack of healthy stimulation during early development
   b. cranial abnormality
   c. infections and toxins
   d. prematurity and trauma

5. Down's syndrome results from a defect on chromosome
   a. 15
   b. 17
   c. 21
   d. 23

6. A display of emotion that is inconsistent with the thoughts a person is expressing is said to be
   a. flat
   b. absent
   c. incongruent
   d. waxy

7. Which personality disorder is characterized by displays of melodramatic and attention-seeking behavior?
   a. dependent
   b. avoidant
   c. sadistic
   d. histrionic

8. Kicking the dog after a bad day at work is an example of which defense mechanism?
   a. regression
   b. displacement
   c. projection
   d. compensation

9. Which of the following is *not* a symptom of delirium tremens (DTs)?
   a. confusion
   b. hallucinations
   c. seizures
   d. euphoria

10. The inability to understand and make sense of a situation defines which symptom of cognitive impairment?
    a. disorganization
    b. confusion
    c. Alzheimer's
    d. dementia

Chapter 22

Treating Mental Illness

Chapter 21, "Understanding Mental Illness," introduced the major diagnostic descriptions of adult mental illness. In this chapter, an overview of therapeutic interventions will be discussed to help you to understand the fundamental principles of assisting in the care of people who have been diagnosed with a mental illness or mental retardation. If you choose to use your health care skills to assist people with mental illness or mental retardation, you will need to pursue further course work in this field. With further study, you will gain a richer understanding of the range of disorders, available treatment options, and therapeutic techniques used currently in the treatment of mental illnesses.

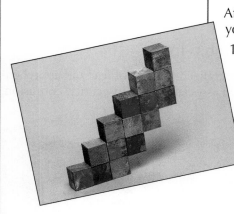

OBJECTIVES

After completing this chapter, you will be able to

1. List and describe the general guidelines
2. Explain the therapeutic techniques for managing specific behaviors
3. Describe the behavior-modification strategies
4. Describe the elements of the mini mental-state examination
5. Apply mental health concepts as they relate to the clinical care associate's scope of practice
6. Correctly define and spell all key terms

key terms

ambivalence	depression	ritual
anxiety	end-result reinforcement	shaping
baselining	immediate reinforcement	stimulus
behavior	intermittent reinforcement	suicidal ideation
behavior modification	negative reinforcement	task analysis
chaining	obsession	
compulsion	positive reinforcement	

General Guidelines

Assisting in the restoration of mental health and caring for people who have mental illness or mental retardation are different from caring for people with physical illness. Although you communicate in a therapeutic manner with all patients, there is an even greater need to possess a sense of personal awareness and to know personal expectations and prejudices when you care for people with mental disabilities (Figure 22-1). When someone has a fever, the treatment team can usually isolate the cause of the fever, treat the cause, and relieve the patient's discomfort. However, when someone has depression, psychosis, and so on, it is not easy to identify the cause. Treatments may not relieve the problem or discomfort of the client. Many forms of mental illness are not curable. One example is schizophrenia. However, mental illness is treatable, and symptoms are manageable. In medical environments, the physical care that you will provide will produce a feeling of accomplishment and comfort.

In a mental health treatment setting, the care is not visible. You listen, support, counsel, guide, and redirect. Communication skills are of the utmost importance. The therapeutic tools used in mental health settings are the communication skills of the treatment staff. These are a few general points to remember about caring for the mental health of another person. Examine Table 22-1 for a comprehensive list.

Managing Behavior: Guidelines and Therapeutic Approaches

In this section, we will discuss some guidelines and approaches that can be useful in managing the behavior of clients who are experiencing anxiety, hostility, depression, and hallucinations or delusions. It is more appropriate for the clinical associate to learn how to manage behavior (Figure 22-2) than to learn the standards of care for the mental health diagnoses. You may not know the patient's diagnosis, but you will recognize the behavior.

Anxious Behavior

Anxiety is generalized feelings of fear and apprehension. It is often associated with insecurity, confusion,

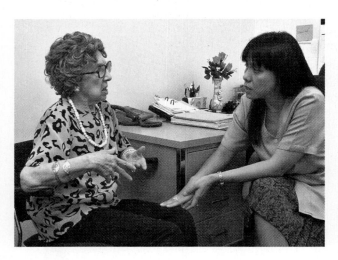

FIGURE 22-1 Therapeutic session with an outpatient.

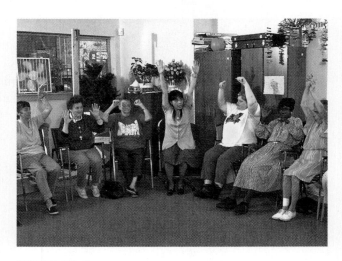

FIGURE 22-2 Group activities like exercising can be therapeutic.

TABLE 22-1   General Guidelines for Mental Health Care Providers

General Guidelines

1. Remember that expectations and prejudices complicate communication with the client.
2. You are the *only* person that you can control.
3. Know yourself. This is the most critical aspect of communication with any person.
4. Subtle things about a person's behavior, physical characteristics, and communication style affect our responses to others. Sometimes, we are influenced by things of which we are not aware. What you hear, see, smell, and feel on your first encounter with someone sets up your impression and response to that person.
5. Know which behaviors or traits in others trigger automatic feelings of like and dislike in you.
6. Learn about your biases in communication styles or behavioral patterns. You will probably always have these biases, but you can learn to manage your behavior toward another person's style or behavior.
7. Develop a skill for recognizing your immediate feelings toward others, and develop a set of responses that work in dealing with the situation or person without judgment.
8. Do not judge your clients. You do not have to like your clients, and they do not have to like you. Your goal is to help your clients and to do so fairly. Remember patients' rights.
9. All clients deserve respect and fair treatment.
10. You work in a mental health treatment setting to meet the needs of the client—*not your needs.*
11. Deal with your feelings with someone you trust, *not* with the client. Clients should not help you manage your feelings.
12. Examine your feelings *before* you react.
13. Learn to accept the fact that you do not have to be right; you can "win" even when you appear defeated. Winning an argument with a client is not important, nor is it therapeutic or permissible to argue with clients.
14. You can agree to disagree with others.
15. Remember that the client has to be in agreement with a goal to work on that goal.
16. Feelings are feelings. They are neither right nor wrong, good nor bad. Clients should feel free to tell you their true feelings.
17. People are entitled to feel what they feel. Your job is to help them manage the behavior that results from those feelings.
18. Remember that clients are reacting to illness, hospitalization, loss of control, and fear.
19. Know that people respond to situations with a set of behavioral responses that they have learned throughout life. These may not be healthy responses. The goal is to help the patient to develop healthy coping behaviors.

agitation, cognitive distortions, and inner conflict. Remember, it is the prevailing symptom of an anxiety-based disorder. Table 22-2 provides a list of guidelines and therapeutic approaches to use when caring for clients with anxious behavior.

Anxiety can be manifested in many ways. Sometimes, it is in the form of numerous and frequent physical complaints, hand-wringing, pacing, talking excessively, frequent questions, chain-smoking, rituals, and obsessive-compulsive behavior. Some anxiety is internal and not displayed to others. People who have panic attacks may feel the racing of the heart, tingling sensations, shortness of breath, and dizziness. They feel out of control and may feel that they are going to die.

A **ritual** is a repetition of an act or acts. Rituals are not necessarily the result of an obsessive thought, but usually they are used to reduce a nervous, tense, or anxious feeling. An **obsession** is a persistent and often unreasonable thought that preoccupies one's thought processes. Germs, safety, fairness, and morality are common obsessions. A **compulsion** is the action that is used to relieve the anxiety produced by an obsessive thought. Washing hands, checking door locks and alarms, repeating words or phrases, and smelling food are all compulsions when performed to excess and when performed in an effort to reduce the anxiety of an obsessive thought.

Angry, Demanding, and Verbally Abusive Behavior

You may see this behavior manifested in clients with any mental health or mental retardation diagnosis. Frequently, the individual is unable to control feelings of frustration and hostility. At times, the behavior may be a sign that the patient is frightened or fears rejection and is unable or afraid to show the fear.

In contrast to this, some clients attempt to control others. These individuals attempt to control those around them, regardless of the consequences. There may be some unfulfilled desire or need that the client is unable to identify or explain. Anger and frustration may be voiced by abusive or foul language, threats, or actual physical abuse. Table 22-3 offers

TABLE 22-2	Therapeutic Approaches to Reduce Anxiety

Therapeutic Approaches

1. Remember that the person's behavior is aimed at reducing his or her anxiety.
2. The behavior that is displayed is telling others that something needs to be done. The person may be too anxious to make a decision about what to do with this feeling.
3. Unfamiliar and new surroundings and situations can produce anxious behavior. Anxiety increases when the person doesn't know what is expected.
4. Provide concise, clear, and simple directions.
5. Tell the person what is expected and what to expect from a situation or procedure. Tell the individual what is going to happen with each step or what will happen next.
6. Sometimes, what you are asking the person to do is causing anxiety.
7. The person may feel uncertain of what you are asking. Ask the individual what information he or she needs to proceed.
8. When you perceive that a patient is anxious, make a process statement about your perception: "You seem anxious or uncertain about what is happening." A process statement is stating what may be the underlying emotion rather than focusing on the obvious or observed behavior.
9. Allow the individual time to respond. Do not try to rush responses or actions when someone is anxious because this will only increase the anxiety.
10. It may be helpful to give directions about what to do rather than to ask the individual.
11. If you are involved in a discussion with someone who becomes nervous about a topic, it may be helpful to move the discussion off the "hot" topic. You might say, "We don't have to talk about this now. We can talk about this when you feel ready."
12. If there are time constraints, gently let the person know the expected time frame. Sometimes, compulsive actions and rituals cause delay. The client may need to handwash after every step of getting dressed or may need to check the locks and lights numerous times before leaving the room or building.
13. Try not to interrupt a compulsion or ritual because this is what the person feels he or she must do to manage anxiety. When you take away the opportunity to act out the ritual or compulsive behavior, you increase the anxiety.
14. Rituals and compulsions need to be controlled when they are harmful to the patient. If a client handwashes one hundred times a day, the healthy state of the skin might be in jeopardy.
15. Compulsive behavior must be withdrawn gradually. A plan to manage the compulsive behavior is provided by the patient's therapist and doctor.
16. Don't check your watch too often when you are helping an anxious person to communicate feelings or to prepare for an event.
17. Be aware of your frustration with these compulsions and rituals. Do not demonstrate your frustration to the client. This increases the anxiety and the need for the ritual.
18. Get the client started ahead of time so that neither of you becomes frustrated.
19. Do not tell this person about events too far in advance, as this will give him or her more to worry about. Tell the patient in enough time to give direction, to answer questions, and to prepare for the event or procedure.
20. Use a matter-of-fact or businesslike tone of voice when you are assisting someone who is anxious. A cheerful, overly friendly tone or a demanding or bossy attitude can overwhelm the person and will increase anxiety. The individual will wonder what is expected and what must be done in return for your friendliness. If you are demanding, the patient will feel that you cannot manage this display of anxious behavior.
21. It will take time for the anxious person to trust you and to recognize that your only interest is his or her well-being.
22. Your patience, calmness, and assurance of safety will build trust.
23. Do not expect anything in return for your efforts. The person's anxiety will prevent recognition of your efforts to help.

numerous constructive approaches to employ when caring for individuals who exhibit angry, demanding, and verbally abusive behavior.

Depressed Behavior

Depression is an emotional state characterized by extreme feelings of dejection, worthlessness, hope-

lessness, and sadness. Depression is associated with a real or perceived loss. The depression that you will see in clients who require inpatient and extended outpatient treatment is different from the normal process of grieving and feeling "blue" (Figure 22-3). The behavior, thoughts, and feelings of a person with major depression are causing the individual great distress that will not resolve spontaneously. It

TABLE 22-3   Constructive Approaches to Patients Exhibiting Angry Behavior

Constructive Approaches

1. Remember that the person may be reacting to frustration that is beyond his or her impulse control. The anger may be misplaced and may have nothing to do with you.
2. Sometimes, the patient displays this anger because of the belief that you can and will handle it to help him regain control.
3. *Always pay attention to your feelings and intuition when you feel threatened by a hostile or physically threatening person.* If you feel physically threatened, get help before attempting to control the outburst.
4. If you sense that the person is acting out because he or she is threatened by hallucinations or delusional thinking, try to reassure the client that he or she is safe. Assure the client that you do not want to cause him or her harm.
5. Set limits on behavior, not feelings. Let the person know that you recognize the anger or frustration but that you cannot allow this person to hurt others.
6. Be willing to accept the person and the feelings, not the behavior.
7. Do not get drawn into an argument. If you do, the patient has "one up on you." The client has caused you to lose your temper and self-control. Anytime you argue or lose your temper with a patient, the patient wins. You are there to teach appropriate and healthy coping skills. You are perceived in a negative and unprofessional way when you forget this fact. You can expect that patients will not be able to act rationally, but *you* are expected to be rational.
8. Remain in control. Be aware of your body language, voice tone, and volume. The louder you get, the louder the client needs to be to dominate the situation.
9. Try to reduce the possibility of an audience. Try to remove the client to an area where others cannot see his or her loss of control. When the situation is over, the person will be embarrassed. The client may be angry with you because you let other clients see the display of hostility.
10. Do not attempt to do this alone. Have other staff help you to remove the person to a more private area.
11. If the client is physically violent, you or other clients could be injured.
12. When the available staff assemble to manage the violent or potentially violent client, you *must* plan your actions. Determine who will verbally direct the situation. Plan for the real possibility that the client will not cooperate with directions. Determine the number of staff needed, and decide how each staff member will respond to control the client's violent behavior.
13. Remember that other clients will be frightened by the hostile outburst. They want to see that the staff is in control of the person and situation.
14. Try to determine the reason for the outburst. Ask questions in a matter-of-fact but controlled tone of voice.
15. Do not engage the person in explaining this behavior in the heat of the moment.
16. If the patient identifies that you are frightened and uncomfortable, don't say, "I am not afraid," if you are. Simply state that his or her language or behavior is threatening and that you want to help him or her regain control.
17. Examine your attitude. Patients are very perceptive of rejection and hostility. Talk about your feelings with a neutral person to cool down before you face the patient again.
18. Be safe, and believe threats.
19. Get help from other staff. Follow the guidelines and procedures of the facility for controlling physical threats or actual acts of violence.
20. Keep a safe distance from a patient who is verbally threatening. Do not stand too close.
21. Make process statements rather than judgments. Say, "You are angry because you didn't get _____," rather than, "You didn't get _____, so now you are acting out to get _____."
22. First, try to deal with the fact that the person is angry. Then move on to find out why.
23. Sometimes, demanding behavior is in the form of passive, whining behavior that demands your reassurance and support. You may begin to feel that nothing you do for this client is satisfactory.
24. The client may try to control the amount of time that you spend with him or her. This person views the amount of time spent as an indication of personal worth.
25. Let the person know that you are interested and concerned by providing frequent and short interactions.
26. Whining is a style of passively demanding attention. When this is the case, give praise and spend more time with the individual when he or she is not whining. Assess the situation, and find out what the need is. Attend to the need, not the whining behavior.
27. Be kind and courteous, but set limits. Be specific about the amount of time you are prepared to provide.
28. If the person wants something *now* and you cannot do it now or the need is not immediate, tell the person when you will have time to meet the request. Do not say, "I will do this later." Explain when later is: "I will be able to help you with this at 1:00 P.M."
29. Process behavior that doesn't make sense to you with other staff so that, as a team, you will understand the possible underlying reasons for the behavior. *All behavior has a purpose.*

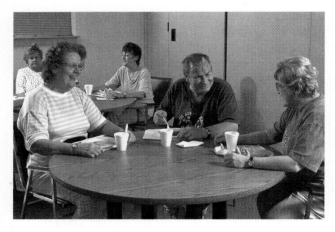

FIGURE 22-3   Mealtimes frequently provide opportunities to increase social interactions among clients and to help clients overcome grieving and feeling "blue."

requires medical and psychological interventions. Depressed people may have thoughts of suicide and may attempt suicide. When clients talk about suicidal thoughts or make attempts, they must always be taken seriously. Table 22-4 gives a list of constructive approaches in caring for depressed patients.

Hallucinations or Delusions

The person who has false perceptions of sensation (hallucinations) or delusions is unable to differentiate real from unreal. Often, these patients are frightened themselves, but their behavior is frightening to us because it is unusual and unpredictable. At times, it is difficult to determine if what the person is reacting to is something that is actually occurring in the environment or if it is a faulty perception. Table 22-5 provides strategies for intervention to be used when caring for individuals experiencing hallucinations or delusions.

Behavior Modification

Behavior modification is a treatment technique that helps to reduce the occurrence of undesirable or unwanted behavior. This may sound like a fancy term for actions that you use as a parent or as a teacher. You may have even used these techniques on yourself to help to control smoking, overeating, or other behaviors that you wanted to modify (Figure 22-4).

Behavior refers to the actions or responses that one produces in reaction to a given stimulus. A **stimulus** is something that triggers a behavior. A behavior is reinforced or rewarded by your response or the response of others to the behavior. For example, if a dog rolls over (the behavior) when it sees a bone

(the stimulus) and then it receives the bone (the reward), the behavior has been reinforced. The next time the dog sees the bone, it will roll over.

Modification refers to the conditions or actions that are formed to change, modify, eliminate, increase, or decrease a behavior. Let's examine a situation to explain behavior modification. Let's imagine that you like chocolate cake! The behavior is eating the chocolate cake. The stimulus to eat it may be that you are walking through the cafeteria food line and you see a delicious-looking piece of chocolate cake. You hadn't thought about buying a piece of cake, but then you saw this luscious piece and thought, "That would taste so good." You resist putting it on your tray because you're on a diet, and after you finish your salad with low-fat dressing, you think, "I would really like that cake," so you go back into the line, and you get it.

Forget the diet; you were stimulated to eat the cake. The reinforcement for eating the chocolate cake was the pleasure of the smell and taste of the cake. You would have modified this response if you hadn't eaten the cake, had selected instead low-fat frozen yogurt, or had gone for a brisk five-minute walk. You would have been rewarded by the lower weight that resulted on the scale if you had stuck to your diet plan.

In theory, behavior modification is just that simple. However, in reality, modifying behavior is *not* that simple. It's hard to resist a stimulus. It is not always easy to find a new reward or reinforcement to replace the original reinforcers. We use and "abuse" the principles of behavior modification all the time.

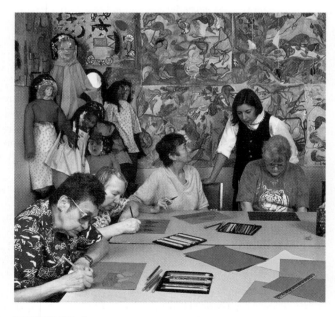

FIGURE 22-4   Art therapy is used as a therapeutic approach.

TABLE 22-4   Constructive Approaches to Caring for Patients who are Depressed

Constructive Approaches

1. Provide interactions and attention that are not associated with compliance or pleasing others' wishes or rules. Often, depressed people do not share their feelings because of the distorted perception that they have nothing to give in return for the "favor" of listening to them.
2. Know that you will identify with the person's depression. When you are emotionally engaged by the client's sadness, you may begin to feel sad yourself. Guard against internalizing the sadness because you will be less therapeutic if you internalize the client's sadness.
3. You will not be helpful if you are also overwhelmed by the person's pain. You may feel sad and empathize with these feelings, especially after the individual has shared his or her emotional pain.
4. Avoid making statements like "I know just how you feel" or "Everything will be all right" or "Just trust in the Lord. He will heal your pain." While these statements express sympathy for the person's sadness, they do not help to make anyone feel better. They also make the person feel that you view the problem as trivial. They may convey that the problems in this client's life are not important enough to warrant what the person is feeling.
5. You do not know just how the client feels. You are not in the Client's life situation.
6. Do not try to minimize the depressed patient's problems, even though the complaints may seem simple to solve. To this person, the problems are very real and may feel insurmountable. When you minimize the problem or the reason for the depression, it does not make the person feel better. It makes the feelings worse. "I must really be inadequate if I can't solve this little problem."
7. Tolerate silences. When you are trying to communicate with people who feel very depressed, there will be many periods of silence. The person may not have enough energy to speak. Thoughts and ideas may come slowly.
8. Your ability to tolerate silences tells the depressed person that you care and that you are willing to accept the person "as is."
9. If the client says to you, "Don't bother to talk to me. I don't have anything to say," or asks, "Why bother with me? I'm hopeless," let the person know it's okay not to talk and that you want to sit with him or her quietly for a while. If the client wants to talk, he or she can, and if not, it's okay.
10. Often, people who are depressed feel devalued and have low self-esteem. Sit with the person in silence to demonstrate that this is time well spent. Quiet time assures the client that you are interested and that you care.
11. Tell the client that you will set aside 10 minutes to spend with him. "We can sit quietly or have a conversation; I will respect your need for silence." When the 10 minutes are almost up, remind the person that you have just a few minutes left. If nothing is said throughout the entire period of time, simply thank the client for sitting with you. Tell the patient that at a specific hour you will come back and spend another 10 minutes. Be specific about where you will meet.
12. Be sure to return at the stated time. This builds trust. If something prevents you from keeping the appointment, let the patient know you didn't forget your appointment, and explain what kept you away.
13. Do not probe the client for information about the depression. Many questions will make the person feel anxious and unable to answer. This reinforces the client's feelings of inadequacy.
14. When you ask questions the client cannot answer, let the client know it's acceptable not to have an answer: "You can answer that question when you've had more time to think about it."
15. If the client has a tendency to magnify negative aspects of a situation or a task he or she is asked to perform, try to shift the focus to a positive outcome. Shift the focus by emphasizing strategies for solving the problem rather than dwelling on the problem itself. "I know that _____ is a problem—this is one way of resolving this type of problem."
16. Look for and try to help the person find the positive aspects of his or her life. Do not exaggerate strengths. Look for real strengths. "You lost your job, and this was a job you held for _ years. That is a significant amount of time in one position. You must have been a productive employee for those years."
17. Give genuine praise for efforts made to accomplish activities of daily living (ADLs) or tasks. Do not give false praise. The person will know it is not real.
18. If the patient has not gotten out of bed for several days, offer praise when this behavior occurs. Say something like, "It's good to see you out of bed."
19. When patients cannot accept praise directly, offer it indirectly. Instead of telling the patient, tell another person so that the patient can hear your statement but does not have to directly accept your compliment.
20. When the patient tends to overdramatize everything, use this equation:

$$\text{action} = \text{benefits obtained} \div \text{risks to be taken}$$

In other words, if you ask Mr. Jenkins to get out of bed and he says, "I can't do it," try this: "How badly would you say you feel staying in bed? Rate it on a scale of 0 to 10, with 10 being the worst feeling you have ever experienced." If Mr. Jenkins says any number, there is nothing to lose. If he says 10, say something like, "If staying in bed feels like a 10, try getting out of bed, and we will evaluate how that feels. It can't be worse than a 10."

TABLE 22-4	Constructive Approaches to Caring for Patients who are Depressed (continued)

Constructive Approaches

21. Help the person to realistically look at the action or task you want the person to perform. Evaluate the task in terms of the client's worst fear or what could happen. Help the patient to separate realistic consequences from self-imposed suffering. Present the positive and negative aspects of accomplishing the task. "If you get out of bed and feel worse, you will at least know that you have tried. You may find that it doesn't feel any worse. You will have accomplished something you haven't tried to do in several days, and that's a start. If it feels worse, then we can discuss going back to bed."

22. With depression, the person often avoids activity because he or she feels incapable of completing the task or fears failure. Help the person to look at the extremes on a scale of 0 to 10.

23. Be alert to clues of **suicidal ideation**, and examine these with the nurse. Suicidal ideation refers to thoughts or ideas of suicide or of killing oneself. An individual may be thinking of suicide as a means of ending his or her emotional pain.

24. Clues may include saying good-bye to significant others, making peace for wrong doings, talking about death as an option, giving away possessions, writing lists of things to do, suddenly appearing happy or "fleeting to health," and asking to be discharged. Fleeting to health refers to a sudden appearance of improvement from the depressed state. The person is said to "flee" to a healthy state when nothing has changed or improved in the person's life or mental condition. It is often used in association with the depressed client who has a sudden change in mood and behavior.

25. People who have made a plan for suicide usually feel a sense of accomplishment, and this may improve their mood and energize their behavior. Be alert to sudden improvements in the mood and energy level of depressed patients. This may be a danger signal. When people are extremely depressed, they usually do not have the organization of thought or the energy level to form a plan for suicide or to act on it.

26. When the energy level and thought organization of the depressed patient improves, he or she is more likely to attempt suicide.

27. If a patient discusses suicide, do not be afraid to ask about these thoughts. Asking about suicide does not give the person the idea to commit the act. Chances are the option of suicide has already been considered.

28. It is more important to find out if the patient is thinking about suicide than to avoid the topic.

29. If a patient expresses suicidal ideas, ask about a plan: "Have you thought of a plan for suicide?" If the person says yes, ask, "What are you considering as a plan?"

30. A patient who has a plan is serious. Even if the person has not thought of a plan but mentions the idea of suicide, *tell the nurse or supervisor stat.*

31. If you ask a question about suicide or a suicidal plan, you *cannot* promise to keep the response a secret, no matter how important you think it is for the patient to share suicidal thoughts. This is worth repeating: You must inform the nurse stat.

32. Whenever any client says, "Promise that you will keep this a secret," you must tell the patient that you *cannot* keep any secrets because the secret could be vital to their health and well-being. Say something like this, "I really want you to tell me your thoughts, but I cannot promise that I won't tell anyone involved in your treatment," or "If it is important to your safety or health, I cannot keep the secret; it is up to you to tell me."

33. If you promise to keep a secret and then find out that the person has ideas of suicide or homicide or that the person has been a victim of abuse or has abused others or that the person has committed a crime, you must tell the person in charge. Now, you are caught in the bind of having to break a promise to a patient. You must tell the patient that someone in authority on the treatment team must know about this "secret." You risk losing the patient's trust when this happens. It is better to tell the patient up front that you cannot promise to keep a secret; this is for the patient's benefit.

34. People who express suicidal thoughts are often ambivalent about the wish to die and the wish to live. **Ambivalence** means having two opposite thoughts and feelings at the same time. It is like sitting on the fence and thinking, "Should I jump, or should I just sit here?"

35. It is important to allow the person time to discuss this ambivalence: "You say you want to die, and you are questioning this; tell me about wanting to live."

36. Patients who express suicidal thoughts and patients who have made suicide attempts are placed on special precautions. You must follow your agency's policy and procedures for "suicide watch" or "suicide precautions."

37. These special precautions could mean keeping the patient in eyesight at all times, making rounds on the patient every 15 minutes, documenting the patient's whereabouts and condition every 15 minutes on the rounds sheet, or a one-to-one observation.

38. The treatment team will determine the level of the precautions. If you are assigned, you must adhere closely to these policies.

39. A one-to-one observation means that one staff member is assigned to stay with the patient at all times. This means that you never leave the patient alone, that you stay within an arm's length of the patient, even when he or she is sleeping or in the bathroom or shower. Always follow your agency's procedure, and take this one-on-one observation very seriously.

40. Safety is the primary issue with all patients and especially patients who are thinking about suicide.

41. Every suicide attempt is a cry for help.

TABLE 22-5	Intervention Strategies for Patients who are Hallucinating or Delusional

Intervention Strategies

1. Communication may be difficult with patients who are experiencing hallucinations because they may talk out loud to themselves, may make gestures or movements that are sudden and startling, or may accuse you or others of saying or doing things that you know are untrue.
2. Never argue or agree with these false perceptions or accusations because when the patient is in a realistic state of thinking, he or she may remember these events. The patient will think you are untrustworthy yourself and will no longer trust you. Even when patients are not in contact with reality, they know that they are experiencing unique perceptions and sensations. Your agreeing that you hear, feel, or see something that is not real will not make this person feel at ease or self-assured.
3. Most hallucinations are frightening or threatening to the person who is having them.
4. The behavior that you see is in response to these threats and fears. Patients need to know that you and the treatment team are working to keep them safe.
5. They need to know that you do not see, hear, or feel what they are experiencing. Simply state, "I know you think you hear your mother's voice, but I don't," or, " I know that you feel bugs crawling on your skin, but I don't see any bugs on you."
6. Initially, you want to investigate the nature of the hallucinations and help the treatment team understand what the patient is experiencing.
7. Once this has been established, do not continue to focus on the false perceptions and sensations.
8. Instead, help the patient to stay focused on reality and eventually divert the thinking to what is real. You may say something like, "I heard what you are experiencing and it must feel terrible, but I am here to help you think about things that we both know are going on around us. Let's talk about _____."
9. Sometimes, patients are plagued by auditory hallucinations, and they are unable to get the voices out of their heads. Try to help the patient focus on your voice. Say something like, "The voices that you are hearing are making you uncomfortable, so try listening to me instead of these voices."
10. It may sound strange, but sometimes you can help distract the patient from the voices by singing with the patient. Let's face it, you can't sing and listen to voices at the same time.
11. Do not allow the patient who is hallucinating to spend too much time alone. This only gives the patient more time to focus on the voices.
12. Sometimes, the voices may tell patients that they are evil and must die. Patients who hallucinate hostile voices may make attempts to injure, mutilate, or kill themselves because they are acting on the wishes of the hallucinations.
13. At times, people who respond to hallucinations and delusions are threatening to you and others.
14. You must be aware of the person's personal space and keep a distance that is safe for you and the patient. If you get too close or touch the person, you may be perceived as a threat. The person could strike out or hit you because you have invaded his or her personal space.
15. Patients who have paranoid delusions often feel threatened by others. When this is the case, they may threaten to strike staff or other patients. Pay attention to the body language and the verbal messages of people with delusions.
16. When someone who is extremely suspicious of others says, "Get away from me," it is often quite different in tone and intention than the depressed patient who asks to be left alone.
17. If someone who is hallucinating or has delusional thinking says, "Leave me alone," take it seriously. Do not get in this patient's way. Keep a close watch on the patient, but do not attempt to get too close or to explore for reasons.
18. Patients who have delusions of persecution or have paranoid thinking may think that you and the hospital or treatment facility are trying to harm them. They may not eat the food because it could be poisoned. They may refuse medication because they think it is poisoned. They will be argumentative and cannot be persuaded to believe that you want to help them.
19. Do not test the food for this patient. This will only strengthen the belief that even you consider that their delusion is true. Logical thought tells you that if you are willing to eat the food, it must be safe, but this patient's thought process is not logical.
20. Sometimes, you can help this patient to trust the food or medicine by using prepackaged foods and medications.
21. Foods like milk in a carton, canned soda, wrapped sandwiches, and pudding and gelatin in a package are safe to this person. Packaged medications are supplied in unit doses by pharmaceutical companies.
22. Never argue with a delusional thought. Simply state what you believe or know to be true.
23. It is more important to get this patient to say how the delusional thought influences his or her feelings than to argue with the illogical or unreasonable thought process. "So, you think that the food is poisoned. What do you do when you are hungry?" or "You think that the staff wants to kill you. This must be frightening. How can we help you to feel safe?"
24. Always consider your safety and the safety of the patient, other patients, and the staff when a patient is not in contact with reality. The person has a very serious illness that is causing him or her torment and needs your help. You cannot help people if you allow them to hurt you, themselves, or others.
25. Whenever you feel unsafe, other staff and patients probably do too. Let the nurse in charge or supervisor know what you feel.
26. Trust your instincts.

Let's consider another example to which most people can relate.

A Case of Checkout Line Tyranny

You are waiting in the checkout line in the grocery store. A mother and her three-year-old are ahead of you in line. The three-year-old, seeing the notorious candy racks, says, "Mommy, I want candy." The checkout counter candy stand is the stimulus for the child's request (behavior) for a candy bar. The mother responds, "No, I already bought treats for you." The child continues, "Mommy, I want candy! Candy, mom!" Again, the mother calmly replies, "No, I bought treats for you." *"But I want candy!"* The mother is now embarrassed and says, "Pick the candy bar you want."

What did this child learn through this incident about behavior modification?

The child learned that if he screams loudly enough, his mother will give in and buy him a candy bar. The mother reinforced the negative behavior of the screaming child. The child learned that if he screams in public, he can get what he wants. How can this mother reinforce positively and not buy a candy bar that the child doesn't need? Well, before they go shopping, she can tell the toddler, "If you don't ask for a candy bar, I will take you to the playground for a little while after I put the groceries away." Of course, she will have to remind the child of the new reinforcer, or reward, several times throughout the shopping trip. Most important, the child has to find the playground trip as desirable as a candy bar.

This brings us to another important concept of behavior modification, which is finding a new reinforcer to replace the original reinforcer. In the preceding example, the mother may choose the playground as a reinforcer, but if the child doesn't like the swings or monkey bars, the playground will not replace the candy bar. The three-year-old may have wanted to sing a song with the mother because it was the mother's attention and affection that was sought, not the candy bar. It is essential to study and learn the reinforcement that is desired. It is also essential to study and discover the stimulus for the behavior. If grocery stores did not place candy bars on a display rack at the point in the store where shoppers wait and look around, people would not make that impulse purchase. They would forget about the candy bar. Store managers know that the display of candy triggers a response in behavior; that's why the candy display is placed at the checkout area.

If a display of chocolate cake makes you want to eat chocolate cake and you want to resist this temptation, you can avoid the place and the thing of temptation. Of course, this takes willpower. Willpower is the desire to modify a behavior because the reward for modification is stronger or greater than the original reward can offer. Most behavior is "learned." You learned to like chocolate cake because you found that it tasted good and made you feel good. You also learned that the reward of the flavor was no longer the main attraction. It was the actual behavior of eating the cake that you wanted. So, if you want to modify the behavior of eating chocolate cake, then we need to find another behavior that will replace this. This is not easy if you like chocolate!

Types of Reinforcement

Reinforcement can be positive or negative. **Positive reinforcement** is usually considered a reward and is given at different intervals of time. Rewards vary from person to person. Some examples of positive reinforcement are praise, time and attention from a preferred individual, going for a walk, going to the movies, or watching TV. Food is a great reinforcer, especially when teaching someone to cook or to eat. Food should not be withheld, nor should it be used exclusively as a reward. You do not want to add empty, high-calorie foods to the diet of a client to reward desired behavior or completion of tasks. It is most important to find the positive reinforcement or reward that the individual desires. If you choose something that you think is a reward and the individual doesn't really like or desire this reward, you and the client will not be successful in modifying the behavior.

Negative reinforcement is the removal of a response or is no response to a behavior. It is also the application of undesirable reinforcement, like a shock from a probe. You will not apply negative reinforcement of this nature. You may, however, ignore behavior that is undesirable or inappropriate when this is ordered and part of the treatment plan. An example of this is modification of the behavior of a temper tantrum. When a child throws a temper tantrum, someone usually reinforces this behavior by responding to the tantrum. Any attention given for the temper tantrum strengthens this behavior and increases the likelihood of reoccurrence. Usually, parents recognize that the child will not get hurt during the tantrum and they stop responding, ignoring the tantrum. Why should the child throw a temper tantrum if no one responds?

Choosing the schedule and type of reinforcement is often the decision of the treatment team. All members of the team who treat the client must adhere to the behavior-modification program. It is critical for the client to have consistency in the program for it to be successful.

Scheduling Reinforcement

Reinforcement is given immediately, intermittently, or at the end of a specific accomplished task or time period. Positive reinforcement is the type of reinforcement that is typically used. When you are trying to teach a new task or behavior, you would give immediate reinforcement to strengthen the learning of the new behavior. For example, if you are trying to teach a client to brush his teeth, you would teach him one step at a time. And, after each step is completed, you would praise him. This is **immediate reinforcement**. Eventually, you would praise him after completing every two or three steps of the task. This is **intermittent reinforcement**. Once he has learned all of the steps of the task, you would reward or praise him upon completion of the task. This is **end-result reinforcement**.

Understanding Behavior

When we want to modify our behavior or someone else's behavior, first we must study the stimulus, the behavior, and the reinforcement of the behavior before we can attempt to modify it. The process of studying a behavior is called *baselining*. **Baselining** means analyzing the behavior that requires modification. The behavior is studied or analyzed over varied periods of time to examine the stimulus and reinforcement of the particular behavior. Remember that every behavior does not need to be modified. We have behaviors that are harmful, annoying, inappropriate, and undesirable, and others that are positive. Behavior requires modification when it is

- Unhealthy
- Undesirable to the person
- Inappropriate
- Troublesome for the person and others

Some behaviors are just annoying but are not undesired by the individual or harmful or inappropriate. These behaviors may not need modification. You may have a client who counts the number of letters in words. It may be annoying to you and it may be inappropriate in some situations, but is it harmful or unhealthy? Well, it could be if it prevents the client from meaningful social interaction, causes anxiety, or prevents the client from accomplishing required ADLs. Behavior that requires modification is behavior that is unhealthy, harmful, undesired, or socially inappropriate.

Second, behavior is modified when we are teaching new tasks or behaviors. Tasks are taught with a tool

called a *task analysis*. The **task analysis** is a list of steps for a task. This is similar to the list of steps included in patient care procedures that are taught in this text and in your training program. Each task or behavior has steps that are needed to complete the task.

How can you study or baseline a behavior that requires modification? How can you find the stimulus and the reinforcer? Baselining a behavior is a process that takes place over a period of time. The behavior is studied and charted by a few people at different times of the day and week. For example, you may have a resident in a nursing home who screams and curses. You usually work the night shift. This behavior disturbs the sleep of other residents and prevents staff from caring for all residents because they spend so much time quieting this resident. You wonder, "Why does this resident scream? Does this resident scream in the day too? What makes this resident keep screaming?" Well, the staff from days, evenings, and nights would need to study this behavior, or baseline it, to uncover these answers.

When you baseline a behavior, a staff member is assigned to observe the individual's behavior in half-hour increments scheduled over several days. You need to baseline a behavior during day, evening, and night hours on weekdays and weekends. It is important to measure the behavior in early morning, afternoon, evening, and nighttime hours. For example, a resident may scream on Monday mornings and Thursday evenings and Sunday nights. Why? What happens? How frequently does the resident scream? What activities were happening in the nursing home? Who was working or in the presence of the resident? What was the weather?

The Process of Baselining

When behavior is baselined, hours are designated on specific days to study the number of occurrences of the behavior. One staff person observes the resident for a half hour and notes the number of times that the behavior occurs. Another staff person on a different shift notes the time that the resident screams on that shift. This occurs over different days of the week. The occurrences are graphed on a chart, and the greatest number of occurrences indicates the time the behavior is likely to occur. You may notice that the resident does not scream at all during the day and screams occasionally in the late evening hours. But the resident screams most often on the night shift, especially on Friday and Sunday nights. Now, on Friday and Sunday nights, you will baseline the behavior. You will randomly select night shift hours on these nights and count the number of screams. You will also indicate what happens before and after each scream. You will note how the staff responds and what happens before and after each scream.

You use the data or information from the baseline to develop a behavior-modification program. You would find the stimulus that causes the screaming and possibly eliminate the stimulus. Also, you might also discover the reinforcement of the screaming and change or eliminate the reinforcement. Let's imagine that the resident screams on Friday and Sunday nights because the charge nurse on those nights turns off the bedroom night-light after making rounds. It might also be that this resident is frightened by a staff member who works on night shift on Friday and Sunday. Or maybe the staff on these nights spends time in the room with the resident after each screaming episode. This attention reinforces the screaming. You can see that baselining a behavior is useful. You may uncover a solution to a problem that now requires a simple intervention for modification.

Using Behavior Modification to Teach

When you teach a new behavior or task, you use behavior-modification techniques. These techniques are chaining and shaping. **Chaining** is the process of teaching a task step-by-step and linking each step like the links of a chain. Chaining can be forward or backward. Sometimes, you chain forward, and other times backward. You teach the first step first in forward chaining, and the last step first in backward chaining. You use backward chaining when the last step reinforces the behavior or the learning. The last step teaches the client the goal of the task. For example, if you were teaching a client to eat with a fork, you would put the food on the fork and bring it to the client's mouth. Then you would say, "Eat." When the client chews the food and swallows, you praise the behavior: "Good job eating the food." You have provided two types of positive reinforcement: the food itself and the praise for the behavior. You might also use this if you want the client to see the end result first. If you were going to teach a female to set her hair in rollers, you might have her comb her hair when you remove the rollers and praise her for this: "Nice job! You look pretty." She is also re-warded by having a nice hairstyle. When chaining forward or backward, initially you will praise the client after each successful attempt at completing the step of the task analysis. Eventually, you will reward at intervals during the teaching of the task.

Shaping is molding a behavior or teaching the approximate steps of a behavior or task. For example, social interactions are usually shaped, not chained. There are no specific steps for social skills; there are approximate steps that shape or mold this learning.

When you assist a client to shape a behavior, you list the steps of the task or behavior as in a task analysis for chaining. However, when you teach this behavior, you will not use a step-by-step method. You will demonstrate the steps and will assist the client in gaining competence by having him or her repeat the steps in approximately the same way. If you were going to teach a client to meet and greet people, to use public transportation, or to converse with others, you would use the shaping method of teaching behavior or tasks.

Minimental-state Examination

The minimental-state examination is a tool for evaluating the patient's cognitive state and cognitive impairment. The tool consists of eleven questions asked in order and then scored immediately. The ease of this device makes it appropriate for the clinical care associate to use.

Before the test is administered, the patient should be comfortable, and all efforts should be made to reduce anxiety and avoid distractions. Preparation by the clinician provides consistency in administration. For example, in one section, the patient is asked to write a sentence. Using the same sentence provides consistency. Keep in mind that the patient's performance may be influenced by certain factors or barriers, such as the patient's language, culture, ethnicity, religion, and educational level. Examples of the type of questions that are asked and the areas that they assess follow:

- What is the year?   (assesses orientation)
- What is the season?   (assesses orientation)
- Name three objects. (assesses recall)

application to practice

Meeting the needs of clients with mental health disorders can be challenging and exhausting at the same time. Developing skills based on behavioral strategies can eliminate the burnout that health care workers frequently experience. Apply the information you learned in this chapter to respond to each of the following situations.

Learning Activities

Situation 1: You are working in a hospital inpatient psychiatric unit. The nurse asks you to orient a newly admitted patient to the unit. As you show Mr. Jones around the unit and introduce him to the other patients, you notice that he mumbles to himself and does not make eye contact with you. He will not allow you to measure his blood pressure, height, and weight. He says, "Leave me alone. You're not going to touch me. I am the Lord, and you want to see me dead." When you say, "Mr. Jones, I do not want to see you dead. I want to help you," he responds, "The voice of the Holy Spirit has told me that you want me dead." What distortions of thought and perception is Mr. Jones experiencing? What will you report to the nurse?

Author's Explanation: You should tell the nurse what Mr. Jones said and that he refused to have his blood pressure, height, and weight measured. Mr. Jones is probably experiencing auditory hallucinations (the voice of the Holy Spirit) and suspicious thinking ("You want to see me dead;" "Don't touch me"). He is also voicing delusions of grandeur ("I am the Lord").

Situation 2:
How would you approach Mr. Jones based on this situation and information? How would you help to decrease his suspiciousness?

Author's Explanation: You should try to gain his trust slowly by showing him that you are trustworthy with other patients. He will observe your interactions with others and will see that you are not a threat. You should respect his wishes and avoid touching him. Reinforce that you are a staff member and that you want to help him. Do not argue with his delusional thoughts. Provide information in a matter-of-fact tone, and observe him for signs of increasing suspiciousness and fear.

Situation 3:
Mr. Jones refuses to eat the hospital food because he believes it is poison. It has been two days since his admission, and he has had only water. How can you encourage him to eat?

Author's Explanation: You should find out what foods Mr. Jones likes to eat. Also ask him what food he might trust eating. Try offering him a carton of milk or juice and some packages of wrapped crackers. See if he eats these. If he does, contact dietary. Dietary will be able to send his meal trays with prepackaged foods. Remember, do not offer to taste the food to prove it is safe.

Situation 4:
Martha White is a twenty-four-year-old resident of a community living arrangement (CLA); she has been living in this group home for two years. Martha travels every day by public transportation to her vocational workshop, and she takes her medication with minimal supervision. She is learning to cook and do laundry in her residential

program. Her mother visits often and brings her toys, such as dolls. She also washes her clothes. You notice that the mother treats Martha as a small child. She talks "baby talk" and does not encourage her daughter to accomplish household chores. She tells you that Martha is just a child and that she will never be able to function as an adult. You know that Martha has mild mental retardation resulting from Down's syndrome. You are concerned about Martha's treatment plans because each time her mother leaves, it takes a day to get Martha to perform tasks independently again. What should you do?

Author's Explanation: You should discuss your concerns with the manager of the CLA and report your observations. The manager will probably have a rehabilitation treatment team meeting to determine the best approach to this situation.

Situation 5:
The treatment team meets with Martha White and her mother to discuss the goals of the rehabilitation plan. Mrs. White tells the team that she is in full agreement and supports the approaches to help Martha become more independent. Nonetheless, the next time Martha's mother visits, she does her laundry and cleans her room for her. Mrs. White says to you, "I know the staff wants her to do these things for herself, but she's my baby." How will you respond?

Author's Explanation: You should talk with Mrs. White about her feelings regarding Martha's independence. What does she want for Martha? How does she think that doing Martha's chores helps Martha? You should tell her how well Martha does with completing tasks independently and that Martha spends the day following a visit regaining her confidence in performing tasks independently. Ask Mrs. White how you can help her to adjust to Martha's rehabilitation goals. Try to be supportive and to allow Mrs. White to come to the conclusion that Martha will benefit from gaining independence in self-care skills. Do not force the issue, and report this discussion to the house manager. This is not something you can resolve without the support and direction of the team and Martha.

Situation 6:
You are assigned to assist Martha in learning to cook scrambled eggs. This is her favorite Sunday breakfast food. What behavior modification teaching method should you use?

Author's Explanation:

- You should use chaining because this is a task that must begin and end with certain steps.
- You should develop a task analysis for making scrambled eggs.

■ You should consider any safety issues in your instruction.

Situation 7: What are the safety issues?

Author's Explanation: The safety issues include fire safety while using the stove. You should review the steps for turning the stove on and off and for removing a pan from the stove. In addition, you must consider safety regarding Martha's clothing while cooking. Sleeves should not be so wide or long that they come into contact with the burner or the gas flame. To develop your task analysis for cooking scrambled eggs, you should list all of the steps in correct order of completion and then follow your task analysis to be certain all necessary steps are included. When you begin to teach this task, have Martha begin with learning to turn the stove on and off in your first session. Praise her accomplishment; then have her watch you perform the full task. Permit her to ask questions, and in the end, reward her with the plate of scrambled eggs. In your second session, repeat the first session, offering praise. Then have Martha mix the eggs in the bowl. If she knows the next step, permit her to continue. For each step that she completes successfully, offer praise and allow her to continue the task to her current level of ability. Finish the remaining steps and proceed in the same fashion for the next session. Continue chaining until Martha can perform this task safely and independently or with the appropriate level of supervision.

Situation 8: You are working in a community group home with residents who have developmental disabilities. Today, you are assigned to teach Nyles Martin to brush his teeth. Nyles is new to the house. You observe that he has the motor coordination necessary to independently brush his teeth, but you do not know what tasks he can perform already.

Author's Explanation: The most appropriate teaching method would be chaining. Forward or backward chaining can be used. The decision to use forward or backward chaining should be based on Nyles's knowledge and ability to perform any part of the task analysis for tooth brushing. If he is able to turn on the faucet, hold a glass, fill a glass with water, or identify his teeth and tooth brushing equipment, forward chaining would be used. If Nyles is unable to perform or identify any of the above, then backward chaining would be used. Backward chaining would then help him to understand what tooth brushing means before he learns the specific steps that lead to the end result of brushed teeth.

Situation 9: Describe the type and schedule of reinforcement you will use.

Author's Explanation: Develop a task analysis for tooth brushing, and make sure that all necessary steps are listed. You will use this task analysis to teach Nyles. During each teaching session, one step of the task analysis will be taught and reinforced. The task will be completed with your assistance. The teaching sessions should occur at times when one normally brushes teeth. You will reinforce each step learned by offering praise immediately after completion of the step. Immediate reinforcement is necessary when teaching a new task. Each time you assist Nyles in completing the task, offer him praise. Praise is an easy reward to offer, and most individuals enjoy this reinforcement.

Situation 10: What information do you need to know about Nyles before you begin teaching and reinforcing this new task?

Author's Explanation: You will need to learn what reward or reinforcer Nyles wants and is willing to work for. Remember that the reinforcement must be desirable to the learner. It must also be age-appropriate and appropriate to the task that is being taught. For example, a candy bar is not an appropriate reward for tooth brushing. Ask Nyles what he wants as a reward, or allow him to choose a reward from a few options that are within the price limit of the agency. When Nyles learns the entire task, the final or delayed reward is given.

Situation 11: Harry Burns is a fifty-year-old who has been admitted to your mental health inpatient treatment unit. He is diagnosed with major depression. What are the signs and symptoms of major depression?

Author's Explanation: Review "Major Depression" in Chapter 21, and list all of the symptoms.

Situation 12: Mr. Burns is often tearful, awakens early in the morning, eats only bites of his meals, moves very slowly, always has a sad affect, and has difficulty falling asleep. He says very little when you talk to him, and he tells you that he is "a sinner" and doesn't deserve to live. One day, you try to start a conversation with him, and he says, "I don't have anything interesting to say. Just go away." How will you respond?

Author's Explanation: You should let Mr. Burns know that he doesn't have to say anything interesting and that you would like to spend time just getting to know him. You can let him know that it is all right to just sit quietly with you for a while.

Situation 13:
You respond as noted above, and Mr. Burns says nothing in response to the few questions that you ask him. You sit with him for 15 minutes. Then what will you do?

Author's Explanation: You should thank Mr. Burns for sitting with you and tell him when and where you will spend time with him again. You should arrange a specific time to meet and set a goal for how long you will meet.

Situation 14:
You decide that you will meet with him again for 15 minutes at 3 P.M. today. When you return at 3:00 P.M., Mr. Burns is not in the place you agreed to meet. You suspect he is in bed in his room. What do you do?

Author's Explanation: Go to Mr. Burns and tell him that it is 3 P.M. and that you will wait for him in the designated place. Let him know that you will sit there and wait for him. Even if he does not come for your scheduled session, sit and wait for the 15 minutes that you have agreed to spend with him.

Situation 15:
At 3:12 P.M., Mr. Burns comes to the dining room where you are waiting. You offer him a seat, and he sits down and says, "I only came because you wanted me to. And now you have only three minutes to meet with me. What can I tell you in three minutes?" How will you respond? Explain your rationale for this response.

Author's Explanation: You could tell Mr. Burns one of two things. You could tell him that if he wants to talk, you will arrange with another staff person to cover your duties while you spend time with him. This rearrangement of assignments will let Mr. Burns know that you think he is worthy of your time. You could also tell Mr. Burns that the 3 minutes left may be enough time, since that is the amount of time he chose to provide, and that tomorrow you can arrange to spend more time with him. This approach tells Mr. Burns that you realize that he decided on the late arrival and that you are not angry with him. It also lets him know that you are a person of your word, that you adhere to your agreements. Your response should be based on the patient's needs. If he needs limits, set them; if he needs attention for trying, provide it. This issue should have been discussed in the treatment approach to Mr. Burn's care.

Situation 16:
The next day, Mr. Burns arrives early for your meeting. He is talkative and tells you that he is feeling "just great." He tells you, "You are a wonderful counselor, and I am happy that you expressed an interest in me." He says that he is planning to be discharged as soon as possible and that his employer is awaiting his return to the office. During his conversation, he expresses interest in investing in the stock market, and he tells you that he was the vice president of an investment firm. He also reports that he is a lawyer and participated in the O.J. Simpson defense. He tells you that he is planning a trip to the Bahamas and that he has women waiting for him on the islands. He has many thoughts that are expressed rapidly and with pressure. His conversation jumps from one topic to the next. In 15 minutes, he has exhausted you. What do you do with this information?

Author's Explanation: You should get to the nurse in charge stat. Tell the nurse your observations and the content he shared. Let the nurse know about the rapid, pressured speech and the change in his mood and affect. Mr. Burns has ideas of grandeur, and his rapid change in condition is alarming. Mr. Burns may have a bipolar disorder, although his admitting diagnosis was major depression.

Situation 17:
The nurse tells you to place Mr. Burns on every-15-minute checks and to report any other changes in behavior and mood as soon as possible. Why would the nurse tell you to do these checks and to report changes stat?

Author's Explanation: The sudden change in his mood and behavior is not the usual course of improvement for a patient as depressed as Mr. Burns. He could be in a hypomanic state, and this could change to a more pronounced mania with aggressive features. Mr. Burns should be watched closely because this sudden improvement is not a healthy sign.

Situation 18:
Two mornings later, you get a report and find that Mr. Burns's wife visited and told him she wants a divorce. You are also told that he does not work for an investment firm and that he is not a vice president. However, his boss did tell him that he could have his job when he was better. You are told that Mr. Burns is now on a one-to-one observation. You are assigned to do the one-on-one. When you relieve the night shift psychiatric technician, he tells you that Mr. Burns did not sleep, prayed all night, and cried about his "sins." When you say good morning, Mr. Burns does not respond. When the night shift technician leaves, Mr. Burns says, "I am a worthless loser, and I should be dead." How do you

respond? What are the safety precautions of one-on-one observation?

Author's Explanation: You should say, "Tell me about your feeling that you are a worthless loser." Give him time to respond, and tolerate his silence if he does not speak immediately. After he responds, ask him why he thinks he should be dead. Try to find out if he is contemplating suicide. Ask him, "Are you thinking about suicide?" Review Table 22-4, which discusses the one-on-one observation safety precautions.

Situation 19: What will you ask next if he says yes?

Author's Explanation: You should ask Mr. Burns if, in his contemplation of suicide, he has devised a plan. "Since you are thinking about suicide, how have you imagined you would do this?" Tell the nurse in charge about the discussion. Be certain that you have another staff person sit with Mr. Burns when you speak to the nurse in private. If Mr. Burns has a plan, his intentions are quite serious.

Situation 20: Robert Brady is a twenty-five-year-old male who was admitted four days ago as a resident in a group home of your community mental health agency. Mr. Brady seems healthy and capable and is helpful to the staff. Some staff members like him; others think he is untrustworthy. He is a college graduate who recently lost the only job he managed to hold for more than three months. He worked as an accountant for a small firm for six months. He was fired from his job when he was accused of sexual harassment and suspected of drug abuse on the job. Mr. Brady refused to submit to a drug test and slapped his supervisor and ran out of the building. The supervisor pressed charges, and Mr. Brady was ordered by the court to attend mental health outpatient and residential treatment in the community for diagnosis and treatment. His drug screening revealed the presence of cocaine, alcohol, and barbiturates. He has a girlfriend who visits, and she tells staff that he is a liar. She says, "He slaps me around when I won't do what he wants." She also says, "He is so persuasive and appealing that I cannot resist him."

When she leaves one night, he is sad and says, "I only did drugs because I was depressed. She made me do them." What defense mechanism is Mr. Brady using?

Author's Explanation: Mr. Brady is projecting; he is blaming his behavior on someone else.

Situation 21: Mr. Brady does not see that he has any responsibility for his job loss or the problems in his relationship with his girlfriend. In which mental health diagnostic category is this a feature?

Author's Explanation: This is a feature of personality disorders. Often, the problems are identified by those who are involved in relationships with the individual, and the person does not see his or her behavior as a result of personal choices.

Situation 22: Mr. Brady is charming with you. He always tells you how wonderful you are to him. He calls you "the ideal resident counselor" and tells you how all of the other resident counselors ignore him and that they do not have the same integrity as you. What should you do with this information? Why should you be cautious about your response to the praise that Mr. Brady gives to you?

Author's Explanation: You should talk with the group home staff about Mr. Brady's comments. Do not keep his praise and admiration of you to yourself; tell the team. You should realize that you cannot be the only "ideal counselor" and that all of the other staff cannot be unsatisfactory. Whenever you are the *only* object of a client's admiration (in contrast to all others), you should recognize your own need for value and esteem. Do not be caught in the trap of "feeling too special." When this occurs, discussion with the treatment team is essential. A united staff approach is needed. Do not get caught up in the client's manipulations and grant him privileges that are not approved by the team.

Situation 23: The psychiatrist who sees Mr. Brady in the outpatient facility diagnoses borderline personality disorder. He grants Mr. Brady an overnight pass. Mr. Brady goes away for the weekend with his girlfriend. He doesn't return to the group home on Sunday night as scheduled. You report this to the oncoming night shift resident counselor. You are off on Monday and Tuesday, and on your return Wednesday evening, you learn that Mr. Brady did not return until Monday evening. He spent his unemployment check and therefore could not pay his rent.

The treatment team is considering discharging him from the group home if the drug screen results come back positive. Because the court found Mr. Brady to be "mentally ill" and ordered mental health treatment instead of jail time for the assault, the team has to turn his case back to the court. The stipulations of treatment in the group home were that he remain drug-free and abide by all house rules. Before you have time to read the notes in his chart, he approaches you. He is tearful and tells you that he is so happy to see you because "you are the only one who will help me." By the end of your shift, he has convinced you that he should stay in the group home and that he "made a mistake that won't happen ever again." He expresses thoughts of suicide if he should be "thrown out of the group home." "I'll kill myself," he says, "if they want to send me to jail; I need help, not jail." What has happened in your relationship with Mr. Brady?

Author's Explanation: Because of his persuasive style, which appeals to your need to be a helpful and desirable counselor, you have allowed Mr. Brady to manipulate you. The rules of the group home apply to all clients, and he should not be treated differently. This would be unfair to other residents in the house.

Situation 24:
When you tell the other resident counselor on duty about Mr. Brady's thoughts of suicide, he responds, "He's faking; he just wants to stay in the community. Don't take him seriously. He's a typical borderline personality. He would do something just to scare the staff and to stay out of jail." You are concerned about the real possibility of a suicide attempt even if Mr. Brady "just wants to stay out of jail." What should you do about your concern for this client's safety, and how should you respond to his threat?

Author's Explanation: Talk to the other counselor about the seriousness of suicide threats. Ask the counselor to consider his responsibility to the group home residents and to the agency, specifically his accountability and responsibility if something should happen to this resident or any resident who voiced suicidal ideas. Tell the other counselor that you see the need to call the house manager and to report the situation. Also implement a close watch on Mr. Brady. He may simply be threatening to seriously harm himself and may not do anything. However, a person with the diagnosis of borderline personality disorder may attempt self-mutilation to show others his sense of desperation. It would be wise to closely observe Mr. Brady and to document your record of every-15-minute observation. You and the other resident counselor should come to an agreement to do this and should demonstrate concern with a matter-of-fact approach. While you want to ensure Mr. Brady's safety, you do not want to reinforce or enable any manipulative behavior.

Situation 25:
Mrs. Sloan is a fifty-nine-year-old widow of one year. She was admitted to the medical unit with a duodenal ulcer that perforated and resulted in hemorrhage. She is now medically stable and will be discharged within two days. Before hearing about the upcoming discharge, Mrs. Sloan slept a great deal and was lethargic. Now, she is extremely anxious, calls for the nurse very frequently, and pages her physician often. Whenever you pass her room, she calls for you and has numerous requests. Most of the staff on the unit think she is "neurotic," "needy," and "annoying." Staff try to avoid contact with her and respond slowly to her call bell signal. You find that once you go into her room and respond to a request, you inevitably spend at least 15 minutes trying to leave so that you can see to your other patients. Why has Mrs. Sloan's behavior changed? What need could she be expressing by her anxiety and "needy" behavior?

Author's Explanation: Mrs. Sloan was initially too weak from the hemorrhage that resulted from her perforated ulcer to demonstrate her anxiety. Now, she may be trying to tell staff that she is not prepared emotionally to return home. Also, she may not be able to verbalize her fears. In an effort to control her anxiety, she is attempting to keep people close to her. Instead of saying that she is afraid, she manifests her fear with anxious behavior.

Situation 26:
How could you and the staff plan to meet Mrs. Sloan's needs and decrease your feeling of annoyance with her behavior?

Author's Explanation: You should discuss any ideas with Mrs. Sloan's nurse, and the nurse should inform the doctor of her behavior. When you talk with Mrs. Sloan, ask her how she feels about her upcoming discharge. The team should discuss this in her discharge-planning meeting. Any follow-up plans for her care at home should be discussed with Mrs. Sloan. While she is in the hospital, the nursing staff should establish a schedule to attend to Mrs. Sloan's needs. It might be useful to establish a schedule of time intervals when staff will go to Mrs. Sloan's room to meet her needs. If she knows that someone is coming to her room for 10 minutes of every hour, this might make her feel more secure. The more staff members ignore her call bell signals and demonstrate their annoyance, the greater her need for a feeling of safety and security. If the patient's condition warrants more time for interventions, this should determine the frequency and length of time spent with the patient. Often, patients with anxious behavior lead staff to avoid contact with them, and this is not acceptable. This patient needs reassurance and limits set for unreasonable time demands. It is important to tell Mrs. Sloan how you and the staff plan to meet her needs and to reassure her that she will not be abandoned.

Examination Review Questions

1. Anxiety is manifested in all of the following ways *except*
   a. chain-smoking
   b. refusing to talk
   c. hand-wringing
   d. frequent physical complaints

2. A persistent or unreasonable thought that occupies one's thought processes is termed a
   a. ritual
   b. obsession
   c. compulsion
   d. panic

3. If a patient threatens to harm you physically, what should be your next step?
   a. encourage discussion
   b. get help
   c. examine your feelings
   d. set limits

4. What is the *best* response to a depressed patient who refuses to get out of bed?
   a. "What are you feeling right now?"
   b. "What is the worst thing that could happen?"
   c. "Everything will be better soon."
   d. "I know how you feel."

5. When a patient is experiencing an auditory hallucination, which action is *most* appropriate?
   a. trying to hold the patient's hand
   b. agreeing that you hear it too
   c. singing to help distract the patient
   d. arguing with the delusional thought

6. The first step in a behavior-modification plan is analyzing the behavior. This is called
   a. baselining
   b. chaining
   c. shaping
   d. reinforcing

7. Which behavior-modification strategy involves teaching the client the goal of the task or the last step?
   a. forward chaining
   b. backward chaining
   c. positive reinforcement
   d. negative reinforcement

8. If a client talks about committing suicide and asks you not to tell, what should you say?
   a. "I'll keep your secret."
   b. "You can trust me."
   c. "For your safety I must tell."
   d. "Everything will be all right."

9. Clues to suicidal ideation include all of the following *except*
   a. decline in energy
   b. sudden improved mood
   c. making amends
   d. giving away possessions

10. Strategies for helping a client deal with anger include all except
    a. asking questions in a matter-of-fact voice
    b. assuring the client that you are not a threat
    c. setting limits on behavior
    d. recognizing the threats as contrived

The Environment of Care

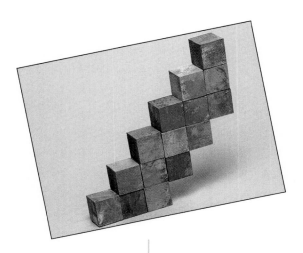

Most people think of the environment as the outdoor world. They use the word *environment* to refer to climate, water, air, animals, and plant life. This natural environment is studied and protected by a government agency called the Environmental Protection Agency (EPA). Today, more than ever before, people around the world are concerned about protecting the environment from the harmful by-products of wasteful, destructive, and thoughtless abuse—theirs and that of the rest of humankind. The fundamental truth is that protecting the environment is everyone's responsibility.

In this unit, you will learn about the psychosocial aspects of health care environments, the need for infection control, and personal safety. Specifically, the security needs related to the patient, resident, and client environments of care and their surrounding community will be discussed. Each care setting presents special considerations of privacy, comfort, safety, and infection control for those who reside in that environment and for those who work there. As a clinical care associate, you should provide considerate, safe care to each individual in whichever environment of care you work.

Chapter 23

Safety and Security Issues in Health Care

Each environment in which care is provided has unique safety, personal space, and security issues. The government and accreditation agencies regulate and assess compliance with established standards for the "environment of care." Nonetheless, it is not possible to regulate and to assess the personal awareness and appreciation for personal space that health care workers should possess. These are not specifically measurable. These are sometimes intangible quality-of-care measures that exemplify excellence. In this chapter, safety issues including body mechanics, infection control, and awareness of threats to security will be discussed.

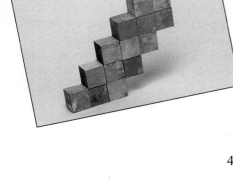

OBJECTIVES

After completing this chapter, you will be able to

1. Discuss the need for personal awareness as it relates to one's safety and security in the various environments of care

2. Describe the cycle of infection

3. Describe the health care worker's role in preventing the spread of infection

4. Describe the standard precautions

5. List and define the three types of isolation

6. List the protective equipment needed for each of the three types of isolation

7. Distinguish the causative agents and mechanisms of disease transmission as they relate to the three types of isolation

8. List the personal safety needs of health care workers in any environment of care

9. Describe the actions of health care workers that are necessary for personal safety and security

10. Define and spell all key terms correctly

	key terms	
airborne isolation precautions	contact isolation precautions	nosocomial
asepsis	droplet isolation precautions	orifices
aseptic technique	environment	pathogens
autoclave	*Escherichia coli (E. coli)*	portal of entry
base of support	gravity	portal of exit
body mechanics	isolation	reservoir
causative agent	method of transmission	r/o (rule out)
Centers for Disease Control and	microorganisms	standard precautions
Prevention (CDC)	midline	susceptible host

The Environment of Care

Consider the meaning of the phrase *the environment of care*. What comes to mind as you reflect on the words **environment** and *care*? Perhaps the most apparent image is a place where one's personal needs are safely and respectfully met by people who care. These are people who consider the individual's need for personal space and comfort and an environment in which the individual's rights are protected.

Your personal awareness is essential to your safety while you work (Figure 23-1). Work in a health care environment requires a significant amount of physical activity. The most frequent injury that health care workers sustain is back injury. The cause is usually a failure to use proper body mechanics. You must use proper body mechanics and infection control measures to protect yourself and your patients. You do not want to injure yourself as you lift, move, push, or pull objects or patients throughout your workday. Your personal awareness and sense of safety will help you to remember to use proper body mechanics and infection control measures.

For those who work in a health care environment, there is always the potential to acquire or to spread infection. Hospitals—and any environment in which one provides care to those who are sick—are rich in infectious microorganisms. When patients acquire an infection during a hospital stay, it is called a **nosocomial** infection. A significant number of patients acquire nosocomial infections. Health care workers are always at risk of contact with microorganisms and become part of the chain of infection.

You should stay on the alert and maintain a watchful eye in the environment of care for your safety and for the safety of your clients. Awareness of the dangers in the community in which you work will help to keep you safe as you travel to and from work. The facility's surveillance system and security officers work more efficiently when you are attentive to potential threats to safety and security in the facility's environment and the surrounding community.

Body Mechanics

Body mechanics is a principle used to describe the way a body moves. There are several concepts that affect body mechanics. The first is gravity. **Gravity** is a force that pulls us down. The distribution of weight of an object and the force of gravity are directly related. This determines the center of gravity, the second concept that affects body mechanics. The third concept is the **base of support**. All objects require a broad base of support to remain in an upright position.

Let's examine a table and some books. Look at the picture of table 1 in Figure 23-2. Where is the center of gravity? It is in the center of the table.

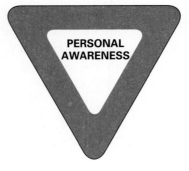

FIGURE 23-1 Personal awareness is essential to your personal safety and that of your patients.

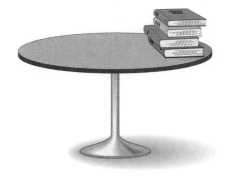

FIGURE 23-2 Table 1.

Look at the base of support. What's wrong with this base? It isn't wide enough. What would happen if books were placed on this table and most of the weight of the books was on the edge? Would the table remain standing? No, it would fall because the center of gravity shifted.

Now let's look at table 2 in Figure 23-3. Where is the center of gravity? It is in the center of the table. Why is table 2 sturdier than table 1? Because table 2 has a broad base of support. Place the same pile of books on the edge of table 2. Would table 2 fall over? Probably not because the books are sitting on a table with a broad base of support.

Our bodies are much like this table. Our center of gravity is our **midline**, that imaginary line that cuts us into two equal halves. Our legs and feet provide our base of support. Therefore, when we stand, our feet should be approximately 8 to 12 inches apart. This broadens our base of support. Distribution of weight should always be close to the midline of our bodies, not on one side, because this alters our center of gravity.

These concepts should be applied to body mechanics and proper body alignment for the patient and for us. Proper body mechanics involves the way we stand, move, reach, lift, push, and pull. There is one other concept that affects body mechanics. Remember the saying "Many hands make light work"? This concept also applies to body mechanics. Many muscles make light work. Use as many muscles as possible to avoid stress and strain of any specific muscles.

Now that these concepts have been addressed, some guidelines for body mechanics need to be established. First, when standing, provide a broad base of support by keeping your feet 8 to 12 inches apart. Keep the center of gravity near the midline of your body by standing erect with your shoulders back and your knees slightly flexed. Use as many muscle groups as possible when moving, lifting, carrying, or pushing an object. For most people, the strongest muscles of the body are the muscles of the legs, especially the quadriceps and hamstrings. Use your arm

and leg muscles to provide the powerhouse work—not the small, weak muscles of the spine. Push an object, rather than pull it. To push it, you can use the weight of your body to move it if necessary. Carry objects near the midline of your body—not to one side. This is why knapsacks are better than shoulder bags. The weight is evenly distributed, close to the body, and near the midline. Always be sure your body is turned in the direction you are moving, and keep your joints slightly flexed so you will not force or twist muscles as you move in a particular direction. Figures 23-4 through 23-9 illustrate good body mechanics.

The principles of body mechanics need to be used at all times, but especially when caring for clients who are weak, immobile, heavy, or larger than you. Back supports are now a requirement for personnel working in long-term care (LTC). Be sure to wear yours. Keep it fastened at the waist. You never know when a problem requiring proper body mechanics will occur. Remember that the back support is not a substitute for proper body mechanics. It is used as extra support and as a reminder to lift without using your back muscles.

The Cycle of Infection

The word **asepsis** means "without infection." **Aseptic technique** is a way of performing skills so that no infection is transmitted. One of the easiest ways to prevent the transmission of germs is handwashing. The hands carry germs and are used for everything. When performed properly, handwashing can prevent infection from spreading. Even if gloves are worn, it is still necessary to wash your hands. Why would this be? Because microbes can penetrate gloves.

Let's focus on the "whys" of handwashing. Infection is caused by **microorganisms** (microbes), organisms that can be seen only with a microscope. Microorganisms are everywhere—on doorknobs, desks, pens, books, faucet handles, and bed linens. It would be impossible to destroy all microorganisms everywhere. Besides, not all microorganisms cause infection. Some are actually helpful, such as those that reside in our intestines. These microbes include the bacteria called *Escherichia coli (E. coli)*, which actually aids in normal elimination. *E. coli* are helpful microbes in the intestines, but they are harmful when they are spread from the bowel to other parts of the body, entering other **orifices** (openings). *E. coli* are a common cause of bladder infections.

Microorganisms that cause infection are called **pathogens** (*patho-* means "disease," and *-gen* means "produce"). Some common pathogens include *streptococcus*, the microorganism that causes strep throat, and *meningococcus*, which causes meningitis.

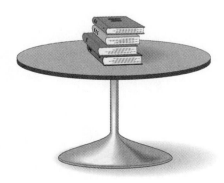

FIGURE 23-3 Table 2.

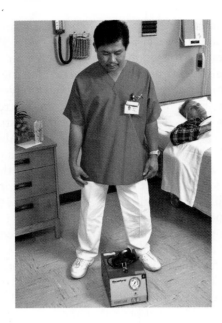

FIGURE 23-4 Stand with your feet 8 to 12 inches apart.

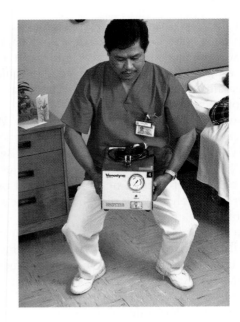

FIGURE 23-5 Use as many muscle groups as possible.

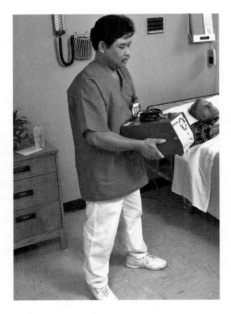

FIGURE 23-6 Carry objects close to your body.

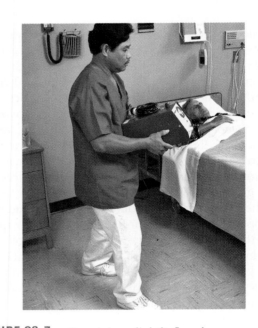

FIGURE 23-7 Keep joints slightly flexed.

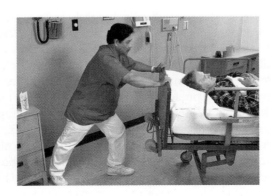

FIGURE 23-8 Push an object, rather than pull it.

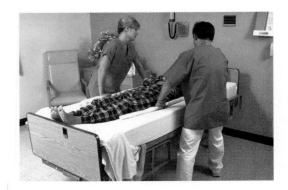

FIGURE 23-9 Keep your body turned in the direction it is moving.

If you can't make your entire environment sterile, then what can you do? Well, always think about the ways in which germs are spread and cause infection. Think of infection as a chain of events (Figure 23-10). The first link in that chain is the microbe, or **causative agent**.

Now, in order for the causative agent to live, certain conditions are required. These conditions—darkness, moisture, and warmth—encourage microbes to thrive. The place microbes grow is the second link of the chain. This place is called the **reservoir**. How many reservoirs, or dark, warm, moist places, can you list?

Microbes grow in favorable conditions, but they require some means of moving or transferring from the reservoir; otherwise, infection won't occur. Therefore, the third chain link is the **method of transmission**. Microbes don't walk or run to infect humans and animals. Somehow, they are carried. The most common method of transmission is by the hands. Other methods are air—droplets in the air—and actual contact with the source of the microbe, the reservoir. The germ that is being transmitted must then enter another living organism or nonliving thing. This brings us to the next chain in the link of infection.

The fourth link in the infection chain is the **portal of entry**. The microbe has to enter the human (or animal) through an opening. The most common opening is the mouth. Other openings include breaks in the skin; the mucous membranes of the eyes, the nose, and the rectum; and the sexual orifices of both male and female. Once inside the body, the microbe has the opportunity to cause infection. The human becomes the host of this microbe.

If the human is not in optimal health or if the organism is particularly tenacious (strong), the host succumbs. Therefore, the fifth link in the infection chain is the **susceptible host**. What makes a human susceptible to disease? We know that lack of rest, lack of exercise, stress, and poor nutrition create an immune system that lacks the weapons it needs to fight back. In addition, certain diseases—AIDS, leukemia, and lymphoma—cause a deficient immune system.

The sixth link in the chain is the **portal of exit**. What goes in must come out. The opening where the microbe exits the host is the portal of exit. Microbes exit through the anus, mouth, nose, urethra, and vagina; these are natural openings of the body. However, wounds, punctures from needles, and any source for drainage of blood or body fluids can be portals of exit. Sometimes, the exit portal is the same as the entry portal, such as a wound that drains pus. Drawing blood from an infected host can also be a portal of exit.

To break the chain of infection, one need only remove one of the links. What happens? The chain is broken. Which chain link is the easiest to break? In many cases, it's the method of transmission. *Handwashing is the single best way to decrease the transfer of germs.* Remember, microbes are everywhere.

The Autoclave

The **autoclave** is a piece of equipment that sterilizes. The method is steam under pressure. It resembles a pressure cooker. Some environments require sterility, some procedures require sterility, and some instruments require sterility. An example of a sterile environment is the operating room. Because the client will have surgical instruments entering a surgically made orifice, it is imperative to maintain a sterile environment. A sterile procedure that the nursing staff performs is urinary bladder catheterization. The catheter that is placed in the bladder is sterile. It is disposable and never reused. A scalpel is an instrument that is sterile, and if it is a reusable scalpel, it is sterilized by an autoclave after use. Dental instruments are sterilized in an autoclave after each use.

Aseptic Technique

Sometimes, sterility is not possible, but prophylactic (preventive) measures can be used to prohibit the introduction of infection. This method is called *aseptic technique* (*a-* means "without," and *septic* refers to infection). Aseptic technique is a method of executing patient procedures without introducing infection. List some procedures that necessitate aseptic technique. A few procedures that require aseptic technique include emptying a Foley catheter and applying a dry dressing.

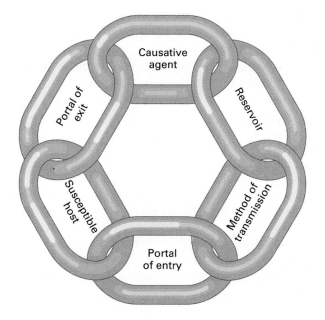

FIGURE 23-10   Chain of infection.

Certain diseases require *quarantine*. This is usually called *isolation*. **Isolation** means the separating, quarantining, or setting apart of a particular patient from all others. This is not a pleasant experience for the person with disease. Imagine how you'd feel if someone isolated you when you were ill and feeling scared. Isolation has been categorized so that the restrictions are related directly to the method of transmission. If the organism is draining from a wound, contact precautions are enforced. Do you have to wear a mask for a draining wound? In almost all cases, the answer is no, except if there is a potential for splashing or spraying blood or body fluids. If the patient has an airborne organism, such as Legionnaires' disease, a respiratory disease that generally affects the lungs, the patient is placed on airborne precautions. Would a mask be necessary? Yes, it would.

CDC Guidelines for Isolation

Standard precautions are the standard, universal, or fundamental infection control measures used by all health care personnel. Standard precautions are a means of reducing the risk of transmitting microorganisms from one person to another.

In 1996, the **Centers for Disease Control and Prevention (CDC)** updated the guidelines for isolation to protect all health care personnel from exposure to infectious diseases and to prevent the spread of nosocomial infections to patients. The new isolation guidelines consist of two tiers. The first and most important tier provides protection from infections transmitted through body fluids. This tier is referred to as *standard precautions*. These precautions are used with *all* patients—no matter what the patient's diagnosis. Most important, these precautions are implemented whether or not the patient is known to have an infectious disease.

The second tier of precautions, according to the CDC guidelines, is known as *transmission-based precautions*. These include

- Airborne isolation precautions
- Droplet isolation precautions
- Contact isolation precautions

These guidelines are designed to provide protection from patients documented or suspected to be carrying or infected with pathogens that require more protection than that provided by standard precautions alone.

Standard Precautions

The CDC's standard precautions are similar to universal precautions—both apply to blood, blood serum, and body fluids that contain blood. How-

Guidelines: Standard Precautions

- Wash your hands before and after patient contact, after removing gloves, and after touching contaminated items or instruments.
- Wear gloves when there is a potential for contact with blood, body fluids, secretions, excretions, or contaminated items. Put on clean gloves before touching mucous membranes and broken skin.
  - Change gloves between tasks on the same patient.
  - Remove gloves promptly and before touching noncontaminated items in the environment.
- Wear mask and eye protection or a face shield to protect the mucous membranes of the eyes, nose, and mouth during procedures and patient care activities that are likely to generate splashes or sprays of blood or body secretions or excretions.
- Wear a gown to protect your skin and prevent the soiling of your clothing during patient care activities and procedures that may splash or spray blood or body secretions or excretions. Remove the gown promptly, and wash your hands.
- Wear gloves when handling patient care equipment that has been contaminated or potentially contaminated with body fluids or blood.
  - Disposable equipment should be discarded in the biohazard trash, and reusable equipment should not be reused until it has been properly sterilized.
- Used linens may be soiled by blood or body fluids and should be handled with gloves.
  - Always check for sharp instruments and needles before handling linens.
  - Do not allow soiled linens to contact clothing.
- Place used needles and other sharp disposable instruments in the sharps container.
  - Never recap needles.
  - Never fill the sharps container more than two-thirds to three-quarters full.

ever, standard precautions are broader because they apply to any moist body substance.

Isolation Precautions

Certain infectious diseases require patient isolation. The CDC has established three categories of isolation for patients with known infectious diseases: *airborne, droplet,* and *contact isolation.*

Airborne Isolation Precautions

Airborne isolation precautions are used to reduce the risk of the transmission of microbes spread through the air. Some of the illnesses that can be spread through the air are tuberculosis (TB), measles, and varicella (chicken pox).

For a number of years, the incidence of TB had dropped substantially. Today, TB is on the rise. Patients who have AIDS are at increased risk for TB because of a weakened immune system. Since the incidence of AIDS has increased, the incidence of TB has increased as well. Patients who may have TB, or patients who are admitted to the hospital with **r/o** (rule out) TB, are placed on airborne isolation. It is safest to place the patient on airborne isolation precautions until tuberculosis is ruled out. If a staff member is exposed to TB, the occupational health nurse or physician will counsel the individual and start a regime of medication to treat the potential infection.

Guidelines: Airborne Isolation Precautions

Follow standard precautions.

In addition:

Patients are placed in a private room with negative air pressure ventilation. This reduces the suspension of microbes in the air for long periods of time. The flow of air is reversed in this type of isolation room; therefore, the air is not mixed with the air in the rest of the environment. Doors and windows must be kept closed.

All personnel and visitors entering the airborne isolation room must wear the N/95 TB respirator. For patients isolated for chicken pox or measles, people immune to the disease may enter the room without a mask. A patient in airborne isolation must remain in the isolation room.

When a patient on airborne isolation leaves the room for essential diagnostic studies, the patient must wear a disposable surgical mask.

The N/95 TB respirator is designed to prevent the microbe that causes TB from entering one's respiratory system. Usually, personnel are "fit-tested" for this type of mask. The fit test is designed to instruct the staff member in the proper application and fit of the mask. If it is not worn properly, it will not protect you.

An "Airborne Isolation" sign must be posted on the patient's door, and TB masks must be kept outside of the door. Usually, a special sticker is placed on the outside of the patient's chart so that staff in the treatment and diagnostic departments will know that the patient is on airborne isolation precautions.

Droplet Isolation Precautions

Droplet isolation precautions are used for patients who have infectious diseases that are spread by the droplet method. This means that the microorganism is spread through sneezing, coughing, or mucous secretions of the respiratory system. The most common infections spread through the droplet method are meningitis, influenza, and respiratory syncytial virus (RSV).

Guidelines: Droplet Isolation Precautions

Follow standard precautions.

In addition:

The patient is assigned to a private room.

A "Droplet Isolation" sign is placed on the patient's door.

Surgical masks are placed outside the patient's room.

Everyone entering the patient's room must wear a mask.

When being transported from the isolation room for essential studies and procedures, the patient must wear a mask.

The patient must wear a surgical mask when leaving the room.

Contact Isolation Precautions

Contact isolation precautions are a method of isolation used when patients have infectious diseases that are spread by the contact method. Most of these infections present a potential for infection to other patients who have compromised immune systems. Staff members in hospitals exposed to these infections may not necessarily become infected, but they may colonize or host the microbes, which are then spread to others through contact. Inanimate objects become contaminated when they are handled by people who have been in contact with the patient who has the infection spread via the contact method of transmission. Some infections spread through contact involve microorganisms that are resistant to antibiotic therapy, such as vancomycin-resistant *enterococcus* (VRE), methicillin-resistant *staphylococcus aureus* (MRSA), and *Clostridium Diffocele (C. Diff)*.

Guidelines: Contact Isolation Precautions

Follow standard precautions.

In addition:

The patient is assigned to a private room.

A "Contact Isolation" sign is placed on the patient's door.

Gloves are placed outside the patient's room.

- Wear gloves when entering the patient's room. Change gloves after contact with infectious material. Remove gloves before leaving the patient's room.
- Wear a gown when entering the patient's room, and remove the gown before leaving the room. Ensure that your clothing does not contact potentially contaminated environmental surfaces to avoid transferring microorganisms to other patients and environments.
- Wash your hands with antimicrobial soap immediately after removing gloves. Do not touch environmental surfaces in the patient's room after washing your hands.

The Care Environment and Personal Security

Health care facilities have established policies and procedures to protect the security of the facility, residents, patients, or clients, and staff. In home care, security is provided by the individual who owns or rents the home or apartment. Police respond to crime in all of these environments of care. You are responsible for adhering to all security procedures and for reporting any potential threats to the security department or the police wherever you work (Figure 23-11). The guidelines provided here deal with basic security measures to protect the health care workers and patients in the care environment as well as personal security measures that you should follow to protect yourself at all times.

Guidelines: Basic Security

- Doors that are locked should not be unlocked or propped open for convenience. Windows should be locked and have privacy shades or curtains.
- In home care environments, lock the doors after you enter, and remind members of the household to relock the doors after they have entered.
- If the home does not have door and window locks or security locks, inform the client and members of the household that these are safety issues that you must report to your supervisor.
- Identification badges must be worn at all times. People entering a hospital or nursing home without ID should be directed to the reception area or security desk for permission to enter the facility.
- In community living arrangements or personal homes, do not open the door for unauthorized people. If someone comes to the door reporting car trouble or personal danger, tell the person

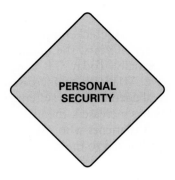

FIGURE 23-11   Personal security measures are your responsibility.

you will call for help. Do call for help, but do not let the person into the home. Teach home care clients and residents of community living arrangements to take these precautions when strangers are at the door.

- Charts should be kept in a designated area and should not be given to anyone who is not authorized to see the medical records. Charts for home care clients should be stored in the agency office. Charts in community living arrangements should be kept in a locked file cabinet in an office that locks.
- Door alarms should never be dismantled. In a nursing home, these door alarms help to protect residents who may wander from the facility. In community living arrangements and private homes, doors and windows may have alarms connected to a private security system.
- Do not allow visitors or vendors to enter through unauthorized or unprotected entrances. Vendors of medical, food, and cleaning supplies and equipment make routine deliveries to hospitals and long-term care facilities. These vendors have access to the facility via specific entrances. Some hospitals provide a temporary pass to vendors. In a private or group home, the client or members of the household will tell you who will be delivering supplies. In community homes, the house manager will know and inform staff of expected deliveries.
- Report any lights that are not working, missing signs, damaged locks, or broken windows.
- Parking lots, stairwells, and entrances should be well lit.
- Residents, patients, and clients should not be permitted to leave the facility with individuals who are not identified as the responsible party or without written and confirmed permission.
- Report any incidents of theft to security or to the local police.
- Do not leave keys to the facilities unattended. Never leave your car or home keys unattended.

- Do not share security alarm codes, access codes, or computer passwords.
- Report any suspicious visitors (visitors who are trying to open locked doors, who are entering unauthorized areas, or who appear to be under the influence of drugs or alcohol) to security.
- Never approach by yourself suspicious visitors or people threatening physical harm or the use of a weapon. Immediately call for help from security or the police. When help arrives, then the individual can be approached.
- Do not carry weapons to work, even if you have a permit to carry a gun. If you carry a gun for personal protection, you must leave the gun with security when you arrive for work.

Guidelines: Personal Security

- Do not carry large sums of cash or credit cards.
- Keep personal belongings locked in a secured area.
- Do not leave the keys in your car.
- Always lock car doors and windows when the car is parked or in operation.
- Do not roll down the window to speak with anyone who approaches your car. If the person needs help, offer to call for him or her.
- Always look in your car before you get in.
- Try to park in a secured parking lot or garage. When you park on the street, try to park in a well-lit area.
- Keep your head up and look at your surroundings as you walk down the street, enter a building, or get into an elevator. If you sense danger, trust your instincts. Do not enter the area, and call for help.
- Women should keep the zipper of their purse or pocketbook closed and should hold the bag close to the body. Men should keep their wallet inside a jacket pocket or in a buttoned pants pocket.
- Never count or show your cash in a public place.
- When you leave your work site, travel outside with coworkers or ask security to escort you to your car. If you are leaving a client's home, ask the client to watch you as you exit. When you leave a community living arrangement, ask another staff member to walk you to your car or to watch you exit the house.
- If you are going to a client's home in a high-crime area, ask the client or household members where to park and where to enter the building.
- Home care agencies will tell staff about the nature of the community in which they must travel. Some agencies have security guards escort staff to and from clients' homes and apartments in high-crime areas.
- If you travel to home care clients with medical supplies in your car, put the medical supplies in the trunk, and lock the car. Even though you are nzot carrying drugs in your supply bag, there are unlawful individuals who will think you have drugs if you are a health care worker.
- Always follow your facility's policies and procedures concerning safety and security.
- Have your car keys in hand ready to unlock your car door when you are exiting a building.

application to practice

Comprehending the principles of body mechanics, infection control, and personal safety and security will reduce the risk of injury to yourself and your patients. Apply these principles to the situations presented here.

Learning Activities

Situation 1: Imagine yourself riding the bus to work. Notice all the things your hands touch. Think of how many other people have touched those same objects or have sneezed and accidentally sprayed the seat that you sat in. Think about the individuals who coughed into their hands and touched the handle of your office when they stopped in to ask a question. Now, you're ready to eat lunch—your sandwich. You're too rushed and don't wash your hands. Do you know how many germs might enter your mouth? Thank goodness your immune system is strong and you are healthy. Those microbes, in most cases, will be destroyed. But if you haven't cared for your health, you could become ill. Some microbes will not be destroyed in spite of your healthy state. Hepatitis A virus is highly infectious, and food handlers who do not wash their hands after using the bathroom can spread this virus to healthy individuals.

Now, go back and identify each link in the chain of infection in this situation.

Author's Explanation: The microbe is the causative agent. The seat, doorknob, and so on, are the reservoirs. The hands are the method of transmission. Your mouth is the portal of entry. You, in less-than-optimal health, are the susceptible host. Your rectum, nose, and mouth are the possible portals of exit.

Situation 2: A hamburger is undercooked. You eat it and develop the infection salmonella, a type of food poisoning. Identify each link in the chain of infection.

Author's Explanation: Salmonella is the causative agent. The hamburger is the reservoir. The method of transmission is eating the burger. The portal of entry is the mouth. The portal of exit is the feces. The susceptible host is you, because you developed the disease.

Situation 3: Chicken pox is a disease caused by the herpes virus varicella. It is an airborne virus. You've never had the disease. Then your son develops the chicken pox, and so do you. Why?

Author's Explanation: Because chicken pox is an airborne virus, contact with an individual who is infected puts you at risk for developing the infection. Also, you are breathing the same air as the patient.

Some lethal viruses can be controlled through vaccines. A vaccination contains the virus that causes the disease. Through the laboratory, it is either killed or weakened, mixed with other liquid products, and then injected into you. Your body stages an attack on this weakened version and stores the strategy in the thymus. Antibodies are then manufactured for future use. When you are reexposed to the causative agent of infection, the strategy is reenacted, and the virus is destroyed by the antibodies. Two vaccines that you probably had as a child are polio and German measles.

In some conditions, the causative agent can be destroyed. Disinfectants, such as Lysol and phenol, kill pathogens. They do *not* destroy *all* microorganisms.

Situation 4: Who is responsible for security and safety in the facility in which you work?

Author's Explanation: You are. Everyone who works in the environment is responsible for security and safety.

Situation 5: You are assigned to help Mr. Jamal to transfer from his bed to a chair. Mr. Jamal is paraplegic and weighs 210 pounds. What principles of body mechanics must you employ to ensure your safety and Mr. Jamal's safety?

Author's Explanation: List the principles of body mechanics. Reread the section "Body Mechanics" if you are unsure.

Examination Review Questions

1. The bite of a tsetse fly causes sleeping sickness. In the chain of infection, it is the
   a. causative agent
   b. reservoir
   c. portal of entry
   d. susceptible host

2. Carrying a shoulder bag defies which body mechanics principle?
   a. base of support
   b. gravity
   c. center of gravity
   d. force of gravity

3. A hospital-acquired infection is
   a. pathogenic
   b. infectious
   c. aseptic
   d. nosocomial

4. The most effective means of breaking the chain of infection is
   a. vaccination
   b. handwashing
   c. isolation
   d. nutrition

5. The airborne organism posing a major health threat due to the increased number of cases is
   a. TB
   b. AIDS
   c. *E. coli*
   d. MRSA

6. Client records should be secured in all of the following areas except
   a. a locked cabinet
   b. the nurse's cabinet
   c. in the home
   d. in the office

7. Which of the following is *not* a personal security precaution?
   a. parking on the street
   b. looking in your car
   c. keeping your head up
   d. traveling with coworkers

8. If a patient has meningitis, in which isolation should he or she be placed?
   a. droplet
   b. airborne
   c. contact
   d. strict

9. Which of the following diseases would *not* require contact precautions?
   a. RSV
   b. VRE
   c. MRSA
   d. *C. diff*

10. For which type of isolation would a gown be required?
    a. strict
    b. droplet
    c. airborne
    d. contact

Chapter 24

The Client's Care Environment

The three settings in which most individuals receive health care are the nursing home or long-term care (LTC) facility, the individual's home, and the hospital. The LTC is the alternative for older adults who are unable to take care of their daily needs and have no caregiver at home. The home is the desired care environment when the individual is able to function with the assistance of caregivers and community resources. When the client requires monitoring or when needed care, equipment, or treatment is not available in the home, then the home is not the best care environment. The hospital is the best care environment when the patient's illness or disease is acute, or short term, or when the patient is undergoing tests.

OBJECTIVES

After completing this chapter, you will be able to

1. Develop an increased awareness of the personal space in the nursing home, private home, and hospital environments of care

2. List and describe the common safety issues for residents in an LTC

3. Describe actions and interventions that the care associate can implement to ensure the safety of LTC residents

4. List some safety hazards in personal home care, and describe actions that the home health assistant can employ to reduce or remove these hazards

5. List the personal safety risks for hospitalized patients, and describe measures to decrease these risks

6. Define and spell all key terms correctly

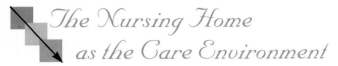
The Nursing Home as the Care Environment

About 5 to 10 percent of older adults in America enter nursing homes or long-term care facilities for care. Some older adults are in LTC facilities for a short time for rehabilitative care; others are there because their condition is such that they are unable to take care of their daily needs and because they have no family members who are able to act as caregivers in a regular home environment.

Most people like to imagine themselves living independently in their own homes throughout their lives. Few look forward to being a resident of a nursing home or of placing a parent or spouse in a nursing home. It is difficult to envision living in a controlled environment, where you eat with strangers and might share a room with a stranger. Embracing this choice is often the "best" or only reasonable alternative. This is definitely the case when individuals are no longer able to care for themselves or when family members who care for a disabled or aging relative can no longer provide nursing and medical care in the home.

Long-term care facilities are perhaps the most regulated industry in American society. The Omnibus Budget Reconciliation Act (OBRA) mandates that individuals who reside in a nursing home receive personal and individualized care, comfort, safety, and residents' rights. Individualized treatment plans and personal choices are ensured. Nursing homes are care environments that provide gentle and sincere quality care to residents. Today, such facilities are staffed with qualified nurses, nurse's aides, social workers, and therapists. However, leaving the comfortable personal space that is home and entering a nursing home can be quite traumatic for both the resident and the resident's family, even if the LTC is a caring environment. Individuals who live in nursing homes or long-term care facilities are referred to as **residents**.

As a care provider in a LTC facility, it is important that you develop an increased awareness of the resident's need for personal space. Always show respect for the resident's personal choices, desires, and needs. The LTC is a health care environment, but it is also the resident's temporary or permanent home. The quality of one's life can only be measured by the person living that life. Do not assume that your interpretation of a "good life" is the same as that of the individuals for whom you provide care. You must include the person in the definition of quality of life. Consider each resident and his or her unique experiences within the social, cultural, and historical perspectives that the individual knew before coming to the LTC and that the resident now knows. Try to empathize with the resident. **Empathy** is the ability to understand or experience another's situation—pain or happiness—through that person's perspective rather than one's own. It is not based on one's own needs or values, as sympathy is. Empathy is free of judgment.

Personal Space in the Nursing Home

There are many measures that long-term care facilities implement to create a homelike and caring environment. Nursing homes generally allow residents to have personal furniture in their room. Recreational and social activities in the facility and trips to the movies, to plays, and to malls are arranged. Residents also spend mealtime together. Family and friends are encouraged to visit often. Family members are invited to attend social activities and seasonal celebrations for residents. Furniture and decorations are attractive. Many residents have pictures of family members and other personal items in their room. They wear their personal clothing instead of hospital gowns and pajamas. The clothes might be laundered by the facility or by family or friends.

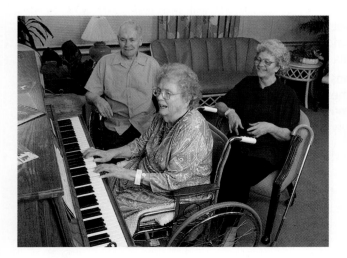

FIGURE 24-1   Many residents enjoy the social interaction available in the nursing home.

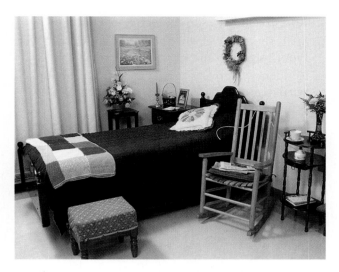

FIGURE 24-2   Typical resident room.

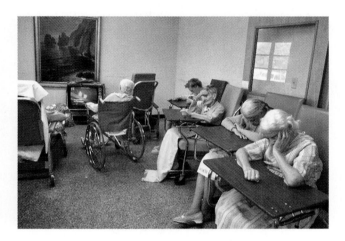

FIGURE 24-3   Residents should not sit alone, be left unattended, and without interaction.

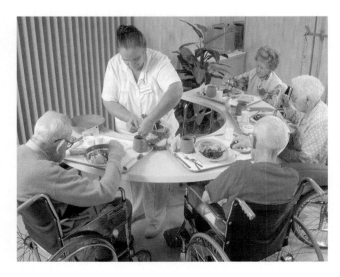

FIGURE 24-4   Residents often find sharing meals with strangers difficult at first.

Helping the Resident Adapt

One of the most important measures of care that you can provide to residents is recognizing the effect that change in the emotional and social living environment may have on them. You must develop an awareness of the residents' former lifestyle, family, home situation, and community setting. It is essential to listen to residents and to provide opportunities to talk about these life issues and events. Learn about residents from the personal stories they tell and the memories they share. When residents are unable to communicate verbally, pay attention to nonverbal behaviors that give clues to their likes and dislikes. Discuss the resident's lifestyle, occupation, and family situation with friends and family who visit. Ask the social worker to provide you with information that will help you to appreciate the life of the person who cannot tell his or her life story. Always treat residents with grace and dignity. Picture the resident who has no available history as someone who cared for others, someone who worked hard, and someone who was fair and giving. Imagine the resident as a child, husband, or mother whom *you* love. Give residents the dignity and respect that everyone has a right to, and perhaps provide that extra bit of sensitivity and attention that you would want given to yourself or to a loved one under the same circumstances.

The work that a care associate performs in an LTC is physically and emotionally challenging. Residents may no longer be self-sufficient. They may be unable to feed or dress themselves, and they may not even remember their own names. Some are demanding; others are generous and always grateful. You may like some residents and dislike others. It is not always easy to be caring and empathic. It is expected that you will treat all people with equal respect. When it is difficult to provide compassion and to show interest, talk with other staff, family, pastors, and friends. Try to remember the motivation and the reason that made you choose this type of work in the first place. If others with whom you work are disinterested and dissatisfied with the work, talk with them about your observations and their reasons for continuing to work in this environment of care. Remember that behavior breeds behavior. Negative and positive attitudes are equally contagious. Support your coworkers in their efforts to improve the residents' quality of life, and ask the facility's administration for support with team-building activities.

Special Safety Issues in the Nursing Home

The regulatory agencies and the laws that govern safety and the provision of care in nursing homes and long-term care facilities are discussed in Chapter 2, "Care Delivery Alternatives." The required safety education and life safety considerations are included in Unit 12, "Emergency Preparedness." In this chapter, we will discuss special issues of resident and personal safety in the nursing home. There are three issues for discussion: falls, restraints, and wandering.

Falls

Residents of long-term care facilities are at considerable risk for falls. Risk factors include

- Age
- Visual impairment
- Unstable gait
- Frailness
- Muscular weakness
- Need for assistive devices
- Beds that are too high
- Toilets that are too low
- Medication side effects
- Confusion
- Unfamiliar environments
- Urgent need to use the bathroom
- Lack of available staff or toileting schedules
- Use of side rails and restraints

Consider the specific risk factors for the residents assigned to you, and follow the guidelines presented here to reduce the risk of falls. Be sure to review the guidelines from time to time to ensure that you are practicing good safety measures to minimize the risk of falls for residents.

Guidelines: Reducing the Risk of Falls

- Rooms should be well-lit, and during bedtime hours adequate lighting should be directed on the floor and in the bathroom.
- Residents should wear their glasses if needed. Check to be sure the lenses are clean and free of smudges.
- Unstable and frail residents should be assisted in walking and in transfers from bed to chair and vice versa.
- Beds should be kept in the lowest possible position.
- Toilet seats should be elevated, and bars or hand rests should be on the toilet or on the wall near the toilet. These measures help the resident to rise from the toilet seat.
- Assistive devices should be the appropriate size. Residents and staff should be instructed in the proper use of walkers and canes.
- Rooms and halls should be free of clutter.
- Spills should be cleaned as soon as noticed. "Wet Floor" signs should be used as needed.
- Residents' footwear should fit well and be supportive. Rubber-soled shoes offer the most protection.
- Medication side effects should be known by the nurse. Preventive measures to counteract these side effects should be instituted.
- Side rails are considered a restraint in a long-term care facility, and residents or responsible parties must sign for the application of side rails. Many residents fall because they try to climb over or between side rails. They are often trying to get out of bed to go to the bathroom or because they are curious about noises they hear outside of the room. Top-half side rails are helpful to residents for security and to assist in mobility in bed.
- Every effort should be made to assist residents in toileting. A toileting schedule, perhaps every two hours, should be established to provide assistance with toileting.
- Some facilities use bed alarms to indicate that a resident who is at risk of falling is moving in bed. The bed alarm is a simple device that clips onto a patient's gown. Be sure the bed alarm is applied correctly to the gown and is activated for proper use.
- Restraints are discouraged as a means of fall prevention. There are as many falls with restraints as without them. In fact, there is a greater incidence of injury with the use of restraints.

Restraints

In today's health care environment, the use of restraints is strongly discouraged. A **restraint** is any device that restricts the movement of the individual or a body part of the individual. A seat belt in a wheelchair and side rails on beds are considered forms of restraints. State inspectors and accreditation surveyors scrutinize medical records closely for sufficient and correct documentation when restraints are used. Figure 24-5 shows examples of soft protective devices. All health care facilities are expected to become restraint-free environments. Most especially, nursing homes and long-term care facilities are moving to restraint-free policies for the management of behaviors that once were considered reason for restraint. There are legal, emotional, physical, and social complications associated with the use of restraints. Residents or responsible parties for the resident must sign a consent form for the use of restraints. *Residents have the right to live restraint-free.* These devices were once considered a protective measure for those who

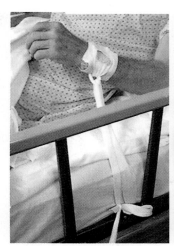
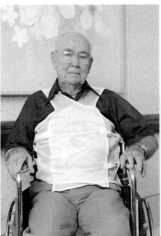
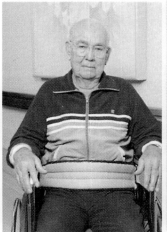
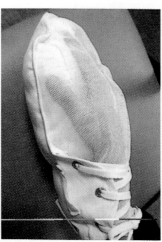

FIGURE 24-5 Soft protective devices: (a) soft limb tie, (b) safety vest, (c) pelvic support, (d) soft cloth mitten.

might fall or might inflict injury to themselves or others. Administrators of long-term care once considered the failure to restrain a resident at risk of falling to be a cause for potential lawsuits. Now, restraints are considered a greater liability when used. Nursing homes are more likely to be sued if restraints are used. Because of restraints, people have died, people have been injured, and people have been humiliated. Some of the complications and hazards associated with the use of restraints are

- Suffocation
- Skin tears
- Incontinence
- Loss of self-esteem
- Depression
- Pneumonia
- Falls
- Broken bones
- Pressure ulcers
- Demineralization of bones
- Atrophy (decreased muscle tone)
- Contractures
- Death

The Food and Drug Administration (FDA) now prints warning labels on restraints that indicate the hazards associated with the use of wrist, waist, and vest restraints. Restraints require a doctor's order that indicates the reason for use. A physician's order for restraints is limited to a period of no more than 24 hours.

Restraint Documentation The documentation of restraint use by the nursing staff is specifically required by law. Documentation must indicate the other measures that were instituted to control the behavior before resorting to restraints. Least restrictive measures must be tried before calling the physician for a restraint order. Additional required documentation includes evidence that the individual was checked every 15 minutes by a staff member, assessed by a nurse every hour, toileted, offered fluids or nourishment every 2 hours, and exercised or walked every 2 hours. In addition, there must be evidence that the resident's position was changed every 2 hours, that the skin was assessed every 2 hours, and that the nurse documented the need for continued use of restraints. The doctor who ordered the restraints must see the patient within the 24-hour period of the written order.

Consider the time involved if you must toilet, exercise, reposition, and provide nutrition or fluids every 2 hours and check the individual's safety every 15 minutes. These tasks will require a significant amount of time from you and the nurse. It would require less staff time and would cause less personal discomfort for the resident if we provided as much attention to preventing the use of restraints. Most long-term care facilities are restraint-free because of the hazards to the residents and the nursing time required to provide care for the person in restraint. *Any* device that restricts freedom of movement is a restraint. If you place a resident in a Geri chair, a chair with an attached tray table, it is considered a restraint. If the tray is attached during a meal for the purpose of feeding, it is not a restraint. Mittens to prevent scratching or removing feeding tubes or indwelling catheters are considered restraints. As stated earlier, side rails are considered restraints. Waist restraints used in wheelchairs are considered restraints. The resident or a responsible party must sign a permission form before this form of restraint may be used.

If a restraint is used, it must be the last alternative available to protect the resident from harm. All of the legal requirements must be met, and the family or responsible party must be notified to give permission. Restraints must be applied properly. If soft wrist or ankle restraints are used, they should not be tied to side rails. You must be able to slip two fingers between the restraint and the resident's wrist or ankle. Vest restraints must be applied with the closed portion of the vest in the back and the crossed V neck in the front. Application with the closed portion (the round neck line) anteriorly is a serious hazard. Residents can suffocate if they attempt to slide free from a vest restraint applied in this fashion. The ties around the abdomen should not be restricting, nor should they interfere with breathing. Any cloth restraint must be tied with a quick release, or slip, knot. Figure 24-6 shows a quick-release knot. This knot allows you to free the person from restraint very quickly. You should be able to pull the ties freely as you would a tourniquet. It is unlawful and unethical to use restraints without permission, a doctor's order, and the required documentation. Restraints hurt people physically and emotionally. The issues of restraints discussed in this section hold true for any health care setting. The exception is in a hospital where there are devices that restrict movement, for example a limb (leg immobilizers). These are considered medical immobilization. Although a device used for medical immobilization is not considered a restraint, the patient must be informed and must give consent.

The procedure for the application of restraints is not included in this textbook.

Wandering

Residents who wander may injure themselves by wandering into unsafe areas, or they might wander off the grounds of the facility. They could be lost, hit by a motor vehicle, or exposed to outdoor elements (extreme cold or heat) for extended periods of time. A resident who is lost is frightened and very vulnerable.

Most long-term care facilities have wander guards on the exit doors. **Wander guards** are door alarms that sound when opened. If a resident opens an internal or external door leading to another area of the facility or outdoors, an alarm is sounded. The alarm will indicate which exit door has been opened. A code can be entered into a keypad so that staff can use these exit doors to get from one area of the facility to another without sounding the alarm. The wander guard should not be disengaged for any purpose.

Residents who wander need to be free to walk in areas visible to staff members. They should not be secluded in their rooms or restrained to prevent wandering. The safety of this resident and others must be ensured. Frequently, other residents will be suspicious of or frightened by a resident who wanders into their rooms. Their privacy is invaded by the resident who wanders into their personal space or who may look at or touch their personal belongings.

Potential Causes of Wandering Residents who wander are often disoriented and suffer from memory loss but generally have good mobility. The cause for the wandering behavior is not always immediately obvious. Staff members should try to determine what causes or prompts certain individuals to wander as soon as it is observed so that the resident can be cared for properly.

Some wandering is goal-directed. The resident is searching for someone or something and may approach others in pursuit of the goal. Another reason is an inexhaustible drive to do things or to remain busy and productive.

Non-goal-directed wandering is aimless wandering in which the person is drawn from one stimulus or activity to another. The individual usually has a short attention span and is in pursuit of something and then is unable to focus his or her attention long enough to follow through.

Underlying Causes of Wandering Unmet physical needs can cause wandering. The individual needs to find the bathroom, to meet hunger or thirst needs, or wants to find a more comfortable, warmer, or quieter place. Boredom, the need to make sense of the environment, fear, stress, and a search for safety and security may also cause wandering behavior. Previous lifestyles and work habits may be causes for some residents to wander. Some people pace when they are anxious. Walking is a means of exercise. Others may have worked in jobs that required extensive walking and active behavior.

The treatment team needs to intervene when wandering behavior interferes with the safety of the

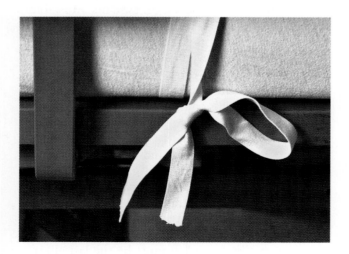

FIGURE 24-6 A quick-release knot.

resident or the comfort of other residents. Not all wandering is unsafe, though.

Guidelines: Techniques to Respond to Wandering

- Gain the resident's trust by talking gently and making eye contact when you approach.
- Describe for the resident what you see and hear him or her doing while wandering. If the individual is looking for someone or says, "I am going home," acknowledge these statements: "You want to go home?" or "Tell me about your home. Where did you live?"
- Try to direct comments at the emotional tone related to the searching. "You miss your home?" or "Tell me about finding your _____. Why do you need _____?"
- Distract the individual. Ask the resident to look at a magazine or to show you family pictures or to listen to music with you.
- Orient the individual to the actual surroundings. Do not force the resident to accept the orienting information if it causes more anxiety and distress.
- Use simple and positive statements to redirect the person. Say, "Come with me to the TV room," instead of saying, "Stop walking into other resident's rooms."
- Walk with the resident for a while and provide orienting information.
- Engage the resident in purposeful behavior to redirect the need to be busy and active. Have the resident walk with you when you make rounds. Ask the resident to help you sort papers, stack supplies, or deliver mail.
- Repeat directions.
- Allow the resident to have some control and sense of freedom.

The Home as the Care Environment

Those who work for a home care agency must be very sensitive to the issue of personal space. As a member of a home care treatment team, you should consider yourself an invited guest in the client's home. You are entering a private dwelling for the purpose of providing care. The individual in the home is entitled to the same rights as a person in a hospital or nursing home. You must have respect for the client's and the family's privacy and personal space. Although you are sent to a client's home to provide care, you should not assume that consent for care is granted. You should not perform any task without first identifying yourself and checking the identity of the client. Always explain the procedure and gain consent. The client and family should know your expected time of arrival, and you should inform them of any delays. It may not be possible to call the client's home because some people cannot afford a telephone. The agency should have a way of contacting the client and of informing the client of scheduled appointments. Sometimes a neighbor or family member who lives close to the client can be contacted by phone.

As a home health assistant, you will enter the homes of clients who are wealthy and clients who are poor (Figure 24-7). Some residences are lovely and clean, and others are unsafe and unsanitary. Always remember that you are there to care for the client and the client's personal space. Some home health agencies also employ homemakers and home health aides/homemakers. You should follow the agency's guidelines regarding the assigned duties for a particular client. Never disrespect a client's environment. The environment may seem unlivable to you, but it is the client's home. Report the condition of the home to your supervisor. There may be resources available to correct safety, security, and sanitation conditions. Nonetheless, these resources can only be employed with the client's permission.

Safety Issues in the Home Care Environment

There are many safety aspects to consider when providing care in the client's home. Inside the home, there may be factors that are general safety issues or issues

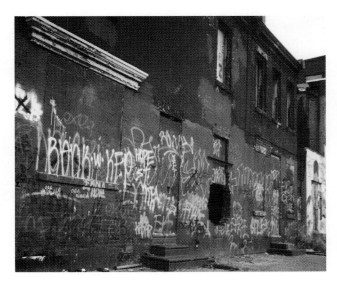

FIGURE 24-7 Some clients live in poor neighborhoods.

that relate only to the client because of the client's age, weakened condition, or illness. The following list gives examples of some general issues you should speak to the client or the family about correcting.

- Gas leaks
- Unlit pilot lights
- Scatter rugs
- Poorly attached stair rails
- Frayed electrical wires or overloaded outlets
- Unkempt pets
- Poor sanitation
- Inadequate utilities
- Faulty heating systems

Potential safety issues for the client might include appropriate handrails for the tub and toilet for the poorly mobile. Visually impaired clients may need additional lighting to help them read food and prescription labels. Observe the way your client functions in his or her home care environment, and recommend improvements that might provide additional comfort or assist your client to cope better.

Remember that dimly lit stairwells and hallways are always a safety issue whether in private homes or in high-rise apartment buildings. Report all obvious safety hazards, such as loose or missing handrails, faulty steps, and structural supports in the home and immediately surrounding the home. In some cases, there may be agencies or community resources in place that can make the necessary repairs. In any event, you are responsible for securing your client's safety and your own.

All home care environments are different on the outside as well as on the inside. If the client's home is in a high-crime area or in a very rural or isolated area, visitation in pairs may be agency policy or it may be prudent to ask someone to accompany you. Often the client will be solicitous of your safety and will remind you to be careful walking to and from your car. Discuss any personal safety concerns you have with your supervisor.

The Hospital as the Care Environment

In the hospital, the patient's environment is referred to frequently as the bedside unit. This consists of the hospital bed, bedside table, overbed table, chair, furniture, and any equipment provided by the hospital for the patient. Some units are a private room, while others are semiprivate with a curtain drawn for privacy (Figure 24-8).

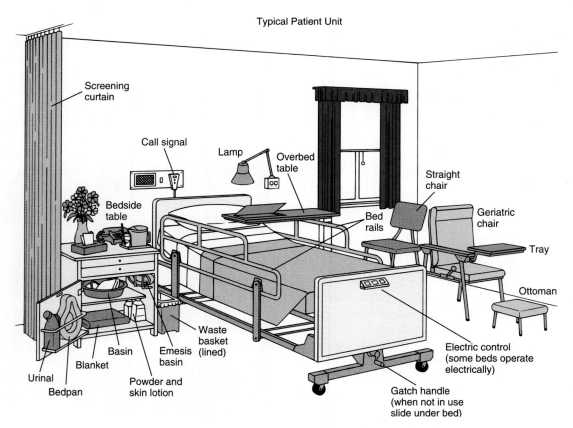

Typical Patient Unit

FIGURE 24-8   Hospital unit.

The organization of the room depends on the amount of equipment that the patient requires. Other factors regarding organization of the bedside unit involve such things as the client's dominant hand, the location of oxygen and suction wall outlets, and the location of electrical outlets for intravenous (IV) pumps. The bedside table provides space for personal items as well as personal care equipment. The wastebasket is another important consideration in room arrangement. Waste containers for biohazard and noninfectious trash are contained within the room. Most hospital rooms have a locked medication bin and a storage area for patient charts. Sharps disposal and glove storage areas are typically installed as a wall unit. As a safety feature, a key is used to unlock the sharps container from the wall unit.

Always be sure that the hospital unit is free of clutter, that spills are quickly cleaned, and that all wastes are removed frequently. Be sure that the unit is free of dust, and that overbed tables are cleaned, especially prior to meals.

The Hospital Experience

The following paragraphs describe what you might encounter upon entering a hospital for care as a patient. You have an arranged room with a curtain that separates you from a stranger. You may be in the greatest pain that you have ever known, you might be told the most devastating news of your life, and the only available privacy is that which can be created by drawing the curtain. Here you are in a strange place where you sleep and eat with a stranger. If you are in an intensive care unit (ICU), it is difficult to detect day from night. It always seems so brightly lit. It seems that the staff never leaves. There is a constant barrage of people in uniform who poke and probe you. You may be unable to speak because you have an endotracheal (ET) tube in place, and this machine they keep calling the *vent* somehow sends an alarm to the nurses who from time to time rush to your bedside. Suddenly, you realize through the haze of medication that the vent is breathing for you. You utter a worried prayer, "Please, help me live through this nightmare, and make sure these nurses respond to the vent alarm. I want to live through this experience!"

Finally, transferred to a "regular" med-surg unit, you find that you share a room with a stranger and that your beds are referred to as *bed A* and *bed B*. You are in bed B. Throughout the day, people in uniforms, scrub suits, and lab coats come and go (Figure 24-9). They enter with a meal, a mop, a needle, a message, or a machine. You didn't ask them to come in; they just arrived. It seems that the person you need or want to see the most for relief or an an-

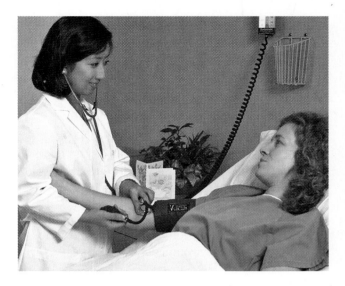

FIGURE 24-9   Blood pressure and other vital signs are measured frequently in the hospital environment.

swer is the most difficult to summon. And you thought that being a patient was "all about you." Suddenly, there are others who are more in need than yourself, but you feel alone and isolated.

Personal Space and Safety in the Hospital

When you provide care in the hospital environment, you soon learn that there is no personal space. Patients may have space to call their own, yet there is nothing "personal" about being a patient in the hospital. It is, in fact, scary for some individuals. It is perhaps the most vulnerable and sick time of anyone's life. Be particularly careful not to disregard patients' rights. It is important to respect the personal space of the patients to whom you provide care. Be empathic. Let your words and actions assure patients that you care about them. Meet patients' needs with interest, dignity, and respect for each individual and for each patient's unique experience.

Hospital environments of care present special considerations for personal space. Always remember that the patient has rights and that these patients' rights were not established without good reason. In a hospital, there are many personnel who enter the patient's room, examine the patient's body and mind, read the chart, and discuss the treatment plan. This can be very frustrating for the patient. The opportunity for error is significant because the number of patients and the number of responsibilities that each staff person must attend to is significant. Regardless of how pressured you feel, you—the clinical care associate—are responsible for giving the right care to the right patient at the right time.

When providing care or traveling from one patient to another, try to be focused. Keep calm and act in an organized and deliberate manner. This will help patients to feel more secure and safe. It will also protect the patient from hurried or careless mistakes you might otherwise make. Clinical care associates care for many patients with varying degrees of illness and disease during an 8-hour shift. Sometimes, it may seem that every patient wants or needs your attention—and always at the same time.

application to practice

Understanding the environment in which you provide care should support your efforts to respect personal space and patients' rights. Use what you have learned in this chapter about caring for individuals—residents, clients, and patients—in different care environments to respond to these situations.

Learning Activities

Situation 1: Emma Sharp is a new resident at Grand Canyon Manor, the nursing home where you work. Emma was discharged from the hospital directly as a permanent placement to your facility. She did not return to her small apartment. She came with no clothes or personal belongings other than the empty purse that she refuses to surrender from her sight even when she is being transferred to the Century Tub. Emma refuses to let anyone near her and has bitten several staff and residents who have come "too close." In her month at Grand Canyon, she has tried to escape from the building numerous times. She has had no visitors since her arrival. Although she was alert on the day of her arrival, she has been confused the last 3 weeks. What do you think is the cause of Emma's confusion?

Author's Explanation: Emma has been yanked from her familiar home environment and has been placed in a strange setting that everyone insists is her new home.

Situation 2: Why does Emma refuse to let her empty purse out of her sight?

Author's Explanation: The purse is the only belonging Emma has retained that she can call hers. As you see it, the purse has no value; to Emma, the purse represents her personal space and the only control she has of her environment.

Situation 3: Why is Emma biting others?

Author's Explanation: Emma lacks trust and feels threatened personally. The transition in her living arrangements occurred so quickly that she did not have adequate time to make a good emotional adjustment.

Situation 4: Emma's roommate, Sarah Blum, approaches you about Emma. Sarah wants Emma moved to another room because Emma keeps taking Sarah's clothes. What should you do?

Author's Explanation: Explain to Sarah that Mrs. Sharp needs much emotional support right now because she is new to the facility. Report the conversation with Mrs. Blum to the nurse in charge.

Situation 5: A team meeting is called to discuss Emma Sharp. Her safety and the safety of others appear to be at risk because Sarah has made several "attempts to escape" and there have been biting incidents involving other residents and staff. Someone brings up restraints. Based on the current guidelines and restraint policies, should restraints be considered as an option?

Author's Explanation: Restraints should not be considered as an option for this resident. Restraints can cause more harm than good. This patient requires a creative approach to reduce wandering and biting. Underlying unmet needs are the real problems that need to be addressed. Providing a safe environment with wander guard alarms or bedside floor padding will improve personal space and safety issues.

Situation 6: Mr. Lightfoot is a ninety-six-year-old home care client with congestive heart failure (CHF) and benign prostatic hypertropy (BPH). He is being seen for a urinary tract infection secondary (UTI 2°) indwelling catheter. Normally, he is alert and oriented. Today, he seems lethargic and disoriented. As you prepare his meal in the kitchen, you notice an unusual smell. What should you do next?

Author's Explanation: Check to see that the pilot lights for the gas range and oven are lit. If one is not lit, and the smell is very pungent, call the home care supervisor at the office for further instructions. It may be necessary to call 911 and to evacuate the patient. If a gas leak is suspected, do not strike a match. To do so may cause an explosion. The gas may be causing Mr. Lightfoot's lethargy and confusion. Open a window for fresh air. Also, do not turn on lights or electrical appliances.

Situation 7: Mrs. Thomson is a forty-four-year-old paraplegic. She lives in a rundown neighborhood. Since the onset of her disability, she has been unable to navigate the steps to the first floor where the kitchen is located. She has no family support and only has one neighbor who checks in on her periodically. The phone in her bedroom upstairs is not by her bedside. The room is cluttered with outdated medications, newspapers, trash, leftover food, and dirty dishes. Twice, the client has fallen and resorted to pulling herself across the floor to the window to yell for help. Name all the unsafe conditions, and state what can be done to resolve each.

Author's Explanation: Mrs. Thomson's room needs some basic housekeeping, and this is part of your scope of practice. Relocation of the phone closer to her bed may require some assistance. Report all the unsafe conditions so that the nurse can evaluate and activate through a physician's order all the disciplines required; these may include a physical therapist and a social worker.

Situation 8: Mr. Wall is a forty-four-year-old truck driver and father of three children. He had a coronary artery bypass graft (CABG) and was treated post-op in ICU for 36 hours. This morning you assist the nurse in his transfer assessment and orientation to your surgical unit. You and the nurse note that he seems hesitant to discuss his discharge needs and family relationships. He asks, "Why do you need to know about my home life? I'm a patient in the hospital, not in the home." The nurse explains that a comprehensive assessment involves discharge planning and that it is important to consider the patient's needs both in the hospital and after discharge.

He then explains that he and his wife separated three weeks before his surgery. He tells you and the nurse that he will need minimal assistance from nursing staff in the hospital or at home. He states, "I can take care of myself. What I really need now is rest and relaxation. I'll call you when I need you."

You assume that Mr. Wall will call you when he needs assistance and that the nurse will direct you in assisting him with specific care needs. Recognizing his need for privacy, you avoid entering his room.

On your 2 P.M. rounds, you look in on Mr. Wall and see him lying on the floor. You enter the room, and he tells you, "I passed out when I was getting up to go to the bathroom. I didn't think this would happen to me."

In the interest of meeting Mr. Wall's request for privacy, what safety issue was neglected?

Author's Explanation: You assumed that the need for privacy superseded safety. A patient who is 36 hours post-op CABG has been in a recumbent position since the start of surgery and has been receiving medications that affect heart rate, rhythm, and blood pressure. Mr. Wall may have experienced orthostatic blood pressure and cardiac output changes when he got out of bed to go to the bathroom.

Situation 9: What instructions should you and the nurse have provided Mr. Wall to ensure his safety without infringing on his privacy?

Author's Explanation: Although the patient's copy of the critical pathway for a CABG would have informed Mr. Wall that he would need assistance with ambulation on day 2 post-op and that he would have his intake and output measured for at least 4 days post-op, you and the nurse should have reinforced these instructions. In this manner, Mr. Wall would have understood the purpose of staff entering his room with frequency to monitor and to assist him.

Examination Review Questions

1. If restraints are applied, how often must they be checked by the nurse?
   a. every 15 minutes   c. every hour
   b. every 2 hours   d. every 24 hours

2. Alternatives to restraints include all of the following *except*
   a. medication   c. wander alarms
   b. floor padding   d. close supervision

3. Reasons for wandering include all of the following *except*
   a. unmet physical needs   c. anxiety
   b. previous lifestyles   d. medication

4. Appropriate measures to control wandering without infringing on personal space include all of the following *except*
    a. distracting the individual
    b. encouraging the resident to assist you
    c. exploring the cause
    d. using a vest guard

5. To reduce the risk of falls, all of the following should be enacted *except*
    a. glasses worn if needed
    b. beds kept in lowest position
    c. toilet seats elevated
    d. Geri chair with tray attached

6. Which of the following is *not* a restraint?
    a. Geri chair   c. side rails
    b. mittens   d. leg immobilizer

7. What should be your response to a wandering patient?
    a. "Stop walking into that room."
    b. "You are here at the nursing home, remember?"
    c. "Come with me, I'll take you home."
    d. "Why don't you help me to deliver the mail?"

8. Complications with restraint use include all of the following *except*
    a. suffocation   c. dementia
    b. atrophy   d. death

9. Cloth restraints must be tied with a _____ knot.
    a. square   c. sailor's
    b. slip   d. quick-release knot

10. Which of these is needed before restraints may be applied?
    a. the nurse's verbal direction
    b. the physician's written order
    c. the family's written consent
    d. a durable attorney document

Essential Procedures and Tasks: Critical Elements and Problem-Solving Tools

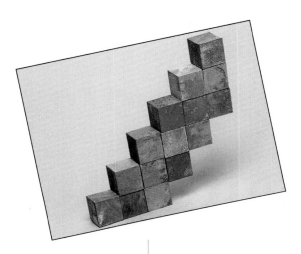

When you think about all the steps that a procedure may have, it can be overwhelming! You may ask, "How can I possibly learn all these procedures and the steps? How can I remember which step comes after which? What if I get mixed up?" Competent job performance is expected, but it is virtually impossible to remember every procedure and every step sequentially. You must be equipped with knowledge and skill to ensure competent performance. You will discover that experience is the best instructor. There will be times, when you are working as a clinical care associate (CCA), that you may need to per-

form the steps out of sequence. There will be times when two or more procedures can be combined and executed simultaneously. Also, keep in mind the importance of critical thinking and problem solving. Procedures may change with new technologies and other advancements—but the basic principles of the procedures will not change. In this unit, you will explore the basic skills every CCA must know. Using the principles of care as a foundation for each skill, you will use the nursing-process approach as a means to structure care delivery.

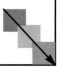

Chapter 25

Essential Procedures and Tasks

Essential Procedures are the fundamental tasks that are performed by unlicensed care assistants. These procedures are performed daily as you assist the nurse in caring for the patient or resident. The nursing process is used to enhance your learning and to help organize care activities. This problem-solving method will also help you think critically. For each procedure, you will assess, plan, implement, and evaluate the situation and your actions.

The principles of time management, safety, patients' rights, outcome-based goal setting, competence, and comfort are incorporated in the nursing-process approach. For each procedure, both the steps that must be performed and problem-solving aspects of the procedure are presented. Remember, rather than memorizing a procedure, keep in mind the outcome, or goal, and use the principles of care to guide your actions.

OBJECTIVES

After completing this chapter, you will be able to

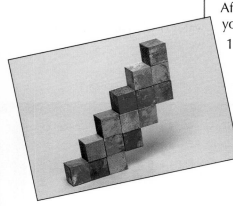

1. List the universal principles of care
2. Describe each principle of care
3. Analyze each principle
4. Apply the principles of care to the essential skills
5. Synthesize a procedure step list using the nursing process
6. Define and spell all key terms correctly

key terms

ACE bandage
active assist
active range-of-motion exercises
aneroid sphygmomanometer
antiembolism stockings
assistance with a tub bath or shower
aural temperature
bathing
bedsores
blood pressure
body alignment
body temperature
buccal
carotid pulse
catheters
clinitest/acetest tablet
closed bed
cold applications
commercially prepared (Fleet) enemas
complete care
crutches
daily weights
decubiti
decubitus ulcers
dentures
diastolic pressure
dorsal lithotomy position
dysphagia
eggcrate mattress
electronic thermometer
emboli
enema

femoral pulse
foot elevators
Fowler's position
fractional urines
gait belt
gel-filled cushions
glass thermometer
handwashing
heart rhythm
heat applications
heel and elbow protectors
height
Hemoccult
impaction
incisal
intake-and-output (I&O)
JOBST stockings
kidney stones
knee-chest position
lingual
mechanical hydraulic lifts
Mercury (Hg)
mercury sphygmomanometer
mobility
mouth care
occupied bed
oil-retention enema
open bed
oral thermometer
ova and parasites (O&P)
partial care
passive range-of-motion exercises
pedal pulse

post-operative (post-op or surgical) bed
pressure sores
pressure ulcers
prone position
pulse
quad cane
radial pulse
rectal thermometer
respirations
saline enema
security thermometer
Sims' position
sitz bath
soapsuds enema (SSE)
sphygmomanometer
sputum
sugar and acetone (S&A)
supine position
surgical stockings
systolic pressure
TED hose
temperature
thermal thermometer
turgor
24-hour urine specimen
tympanic thermometer
unoccupied bed
urine dipstick
vital signs (VS)
walker
water or alternating air mattress
weight

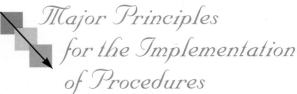

Major Principles for the Implementation of Procedures

There are some major principles that we must include when implementing both essential procedures and tasks and expanded procedures and skills. Let's identify these principles. They are time management, safety, patients' rights, outcome-based goal setting, competence, and comfort.

Time Management

Let's examine the principle of time management (Figure 25-1). Plan and manage your time well. As you probably know, you need to utilize resources in

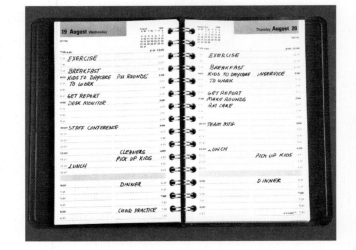

FIGURE 25-1 Plan and manage your time well.

the most efficient manner without sacrifice to the patient. One key way to manage your time is to assess and then plan the procedure carefully. Early in this assessment and planning process you will gather all needed equipment for the procedure. For each procedure, you will need to make sure that the proper equipment is in place and ready to use. Specific equipment is needed for each procedure. A list of equipment is given at the beginning of the procedures described in this chapter. In keeping with the implementation of time management, you should know the basic equipment needed for every procedure. What do you think is included in this group of equipment? If you said nonsterile gloves and handwashing equipment, you are correct.

Safety

Now, let's discuss the principle of safety. Here we are talking about safety as it applies to the execution of skills. Safety must be implemented during the execution of all skills. The implementation of safety may be divided into three categories: safety of the caregiver, safety of the patient, and safety of the equipment.

Safety of the caregiver includes protection against disease and injury. Safety of the caregiver is included in every procedure. Protection against disease involves the implementation of standard precautions using aseptic technique (Figure 25-2). The word *aseptic* means "germfree" and "without infection." Aseptic technique is a way of performing skills so that no infection is transmitted. Since our hands carry germs and our hands are used for almost every-

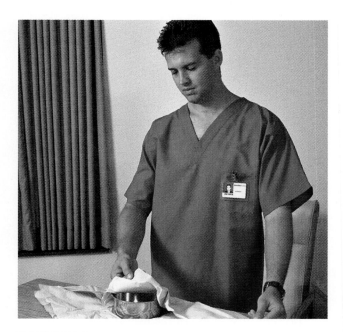

FIGURE 25-2 Some skills require aseptic technique.

thing we do, one of the easiest ways to prevent the transmission of germs is to wash our hands. When performed properly, handwashing can prevent infection from spreading.

Did you know that even when gloves are worn, it is still necessary to wash your hands after removing the gloves? Do you know why this is so? This is so because germs or microbes are everywhere. Although unseen with the naked eye, these germs are found on doorknobs, countertops, clothing, faucets, and so on. Microbes, or microorganisms, grow best in a warm, dark, moist environment. Think about your hands inside a pair of latex gloves. Remember, hands cannot be sterilized. They can only be disinfected to a certain degree. This means there are still germs present on your hands when donning gloves. While your hands are in the gloves, the microbes multiply. So wash your hands before donning and after removing of gloves.

For every skill you perform, you should ask yourself two important questions regarding safety: "Am I using standard precautions? Am I using proper body mechanics?"

Let's think about some of the things involved in proper body mechanics. Proper body mechanics is a way of preventing musculoskeletal injuries. You should be asking yourself the following questions: "Am I wearing my back support? Am I in supportive shoes that also prevent needle injuries? Am I bending and moving correctly? Am I remembering to elevate the bed to the proper working level?"

The next safety principle is safety of the patient. In the hospital setting, you must check the name bracelet of the patient. Do not rely on the patient's response to verbal questioning regarding identity. Be sure you have the right patient for the procedure; one way to be sure is to check the patient's identification bracelet.

Falls are the most common injury to patients. Most of the legal suits against caregivers involve falls. Falls can often be prevented simply by following safety guidelines. Here are some guidelines: Always remain with the patient during a procedure. When appropriate, keep the side rails of the bed in the up position, and keep the bed in the lowest position when you are away from the bedside. Place items that the patient may need when alone within easy reach. Some type of signaling mechanism must be provided so that the patient does not feel trapped in the bed without a means of calling for help. In the hospital, this would be the call button or call signaling device. At home, this might be a bell that the patient can ring.

What do we need to know about safety of the equipment? Examine all equipment that you will use to ensure that it is operating correctly. This means that it has all the necessary parts and that it will allow you to execute the skill safely.

Patients' Rights

Now, let's focus our attention on the principle of patients' rights. In reality, patients' rights represent the purpose of our jobs—respect for the dignity of human life. Patients have the right to privacy. What can you do to ensure privacy? Start by identifying yourself each time you enter the patient's personal space. Remember, you are probably a stranger to the patient, so explain why you have come and what you intend to do. Think about how you would feel if a stranger entered your room at 7:00 A.M., for example, and proceeded to turn down your bed covers and connect the cords of a strange machine to your body without explaining who she is and what is happening! Think about how uncomfortable and frightened you would feel, and this may help you to remember the importance of always identifying yourself to your patient and explaining what you intend to do.

Outcome-Based Goal Setting

Outcome-based goal setting is another important principle in the execution of skills. Generally, the name of the skill is also the goal. Certain skills, such as assisting with range-of-motion exercises, require some specific or special goal setting. Whenever possible, the patient should be involved in goal setting. Including the patient ensures that the patient's rights have not been violated. When setting goals and implementing procedures, keep in mind that things in life do not always happen exactly as we plan. The same holds true for the execution of skills. For example, in the middle of a bed bath, the patient might have an urgent need to use the bedpan. It is an emergency! There's no time to wash your hands. Just don gloves, get the bedpan, and place it properly under the patient.

Competence

For each skill that is performed, both competence and a certain result (the desired outcome) are expected. Consider the following scenario about a painter, and then draw some conclusions and correlations regarding how this scenario relates to your own job and execution of skills. If you hired a painter to paint your bedroom, the desired result would be a completed job accomplished in a competent manner. Can you think of some things that you would expect to be a part of a quality paint job? You might list such things as no spills, no streaks, all appropriate areas painted, furniture protected from paint, no broken items, and total safety of the painter. Your assessment of the quality might be judged by the smooth application of the paint, the proper clean up and storage of equipment, the acceptable placement of furniture in its original position, and so on. In a similar way, as a health care worker, all the skills you perform have a desired outcome, and you are expected to perform them in a competent manner.

Comfort

In all patient care tasks, you must also consider the principle of comfort. Obviously, the comfort of the patient is of the utmost importance. The patient's physical and emotional comfort must be assessed, planned, implemented, and evaluated. You should also be comfortable as you perform your duties. Think about your body mechanics and body alignment before executing all tasks. Keep the bed at a comfortable height for your work, wear comfortable shoes and clothes, and keep patient care equipment within reach of your work site.

If you feel unsure of your actions because you lack skill, experience, or knowledge, get the help you need. Ask for direction or assistance from the nurse.

Always ask the patient about his or her level of comfort. What looks comfortable to you may not be for the patient.

Now that we have discussed the basic principles of time management, safety, patients' rights, outcome-based goal setting, competence, and comfort, you will understand the steps given below. These are steps that should be observed for all procedures. Since these steps are for all procedures, they are not repeated for each individual procedure given in this chapter and Chapter 26, which presents advanced procedures and tasks.

For all procedures, the following steps should be observed:

1. Introduce yourself to the patient.
2. Identify the patient.
3. Explain the procedure to the patient.
4. Provide privacy.
5. Be sure the patient is ready to begin and has consented to being touched if the situation warrants.
6. Follow standard precautions.
7. Use proper body mechanics.
8. Wash your hands before beginning the procedure.
9. Remove and dispose of your gloves (standard precautions) after completing the procedure.
10. Wash your hands after removing the gloves.
11. Dispose of supplies and equipment appropriately.

Basic Hygiene

As a clinical care associate and a health care team member, you are responsible for seeing to patients' daily hygiene and grooming needs. Hygiene includes activities, such as bathing and brushing the teeth, that promote cleanliness and health. Hygiene practices help reduce odors, improve circulation, and make patients more comfortable and relaxed. The routine of bathing and grooming is beneficial to the mind and spirit as well. Hygiene and grooming are basic activities of daily living. Patients in health care facilities usually need some help with these activities. The amount of assistance needed will vary from person to person. While assisting with personal care, maintain the patient's privacy and dignity. You should also encourage patients to do as much for themselves as they can. This promotes independence, self-esteem, and a greater sense of well-being.

Handwashing

Handwashing is the best method for reducing the transfer of germs and therefore for breaking the cycle of infection. The fact that everyone—caregivers and patients—must wash their hands cannot be overemphasized. Since your hands touch so many people and objects, they are a major source of germ transmission.

Handwashing is a simple procedure that offers more protection from microbial invasion than any sophisticated germicide or aerosol disinfectant can offer. However, the procedure must be performed correctly in order to prevent contamination. Use friction plus lukewarm water and soap on all surfaces of the hands, between the fingers, and under the nails to remove surface germs. Friction is used to remove the germs, while the soap helps lift the germs from the skin surface. Use warm water because it is kinder to your hands than hot or cold water and because it is more effective in rinsing the germs and soap from your hands. Then dry your hands thoroughly to prevent chapping. Use lotion or other skin moisturizers sparingly.

You must wash your hands before and after every procedure, even if you wear gloves during the procedure. If your hands become contaminated during a procedure, you must take the time to stop and wash them.

procedure

Handwashing

Assess

Determine when your hands should be washed. Wash your hands immediately before touching any patient.

Plan

Gather required equipment if it is not in place: paper towels, and soap, orange stick or brush. (If you are working in home care, be sure to bring these supplies.)

Implement

1. Turn on the faucet with a paper towel.
2. Discard the towel after adjusting the water temperature.
3. Wet one hand, and dispense liquid soap with the other.
4. Wet the other hand and lather.
5. Scrub all surfaces of your hands, including between your fingers, around your thumbs, and both palms. (Remember the "rule of 10"—10 times each surface.)
6. Use an orange stick or brush to clean under your fingernails.
7. Rinse your hands thoroughly, holding the fingertips downward.
8. Dry your hands completely, using a paper towel. Start at the wrists and dry toward the fingertips.
9. Use a dry paper towel to turn off the faucet.

Evaluate

Evaluate your actions. Did you follow all the steps in the procedure? Did you scrub all surfaces of your hands, including between your fingers, around your thumbs, your palms, and under your nails? Did you wash your hands for the required length of time?

Bedmaking

Some patients are unable to get out of bed due to illness or doctor's orders. You will provide all care for these patients as they lie or sit in bed, including changing the sheets while they are still in bed. It is important to make the bed without wrinkles so that it will be comfortable for the patient. In addition,

wrinkles can restrict circulation and contribute to skin breakdown.

Beds can be made in one of two ways: occupied and unoccupied. An **occupied bed** is made with the patient in the bed. This type of bedmaking should be used only when absolutely necessary (Figure 25-3). An **unoccupied bed** is made when the patient is out of the bed.

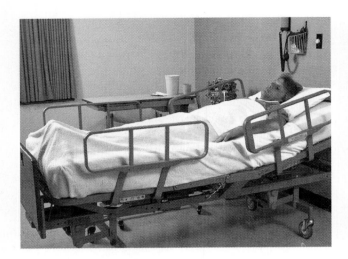

FIGURE 25-3 An occupied bed is made with the patient in the bed.

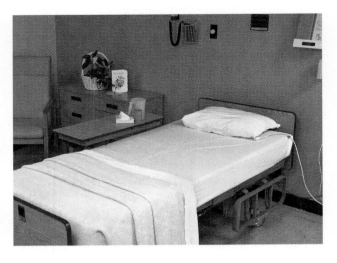

FIGURE 25-4 Unoccupied open bed.

Unoccupied beds are arranged in several different ways; they may be *closed*, *open*, or *postoperative*. You will make a **closed bed** after a patient is discharged from the nursing unit. You will make an **open bed** for a patient who can be out of bed but will be returning to bed soon (Figure 25-4). You will make a **post-operative (post-op or surgical) bed** for a patient who will be arriving from the recovery room on a stretcher (Figure 25-5).

Since many activities will occur in bed, from meals to bedpans, it is important for you to make the bed tight, clean, and wrinkle-free. This will protect the patient's skin from irritation and will be a pleasure enjoyed by the patient.

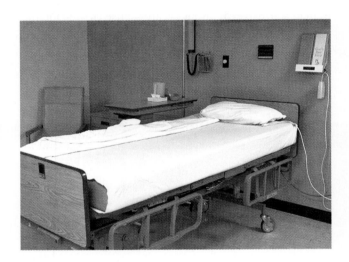

FIGURE 25-5 Surgical bed.

procedure

Bedmaking

Assess

Determine the type of bed that needs to be made for the patient. Should you make a post-op bed, an open bed, a closed bed, or an occupied bed? How will this fit into the type of care the patient needs?

Plan

Gather required equipment: a fitted bottom sheet, two flat sheets, a draw sheet, a pillowcase, and a blanket or spread.

Determine the best time to perform this procedure. When can the patient be out of bed? If the patient is on bed rest, plan to change the bed after the bath.

Implement

1. Raise the bed to a comfortable working height appropriate to proper body mechanics. (Remember to use the principles of safety and comfort.)
2. Pull the sheets tightly, and miter the corners (Figure 25-6).
3. Keep the opposite side rail up if you are making an occupied bed.
4. Monitor the patient's respiratory status, safety, and comfort while making an occupied bed.
5. Complete one side of the bed before moving to the other side.

6. Lower the bed to the lowest level upon completing the linen change.

Evaluate

Evaluate your actions. Did you follow the critical elements of the procedure? Did you complete the procedure independently and in the appropriate time frame?

Evaluate the patient's response. How did the patient tolerate being out of bed? How did the bed patient tolerate the linen change?

Are the side rails raised and patient's call bell within reach?

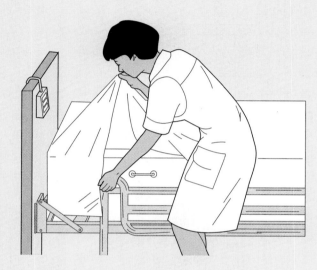

FIGURE 25-6A   Pick up the edge of the sheet at the side of the bed 12 inches from the head of the mattress.

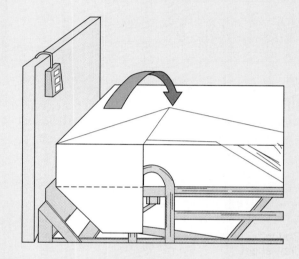

FIGURE 25-6B   Place the triangle (the folded corner) on top of the mattress.

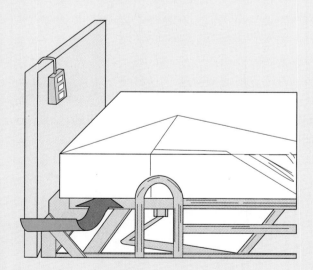

FIGURE 25-6C   Tuck the hanging portion of the sheet under the mattress.

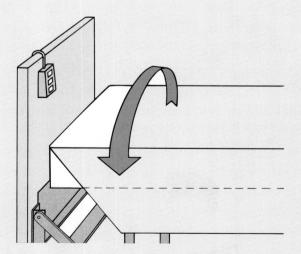

FIGURE 25-6D   While you hold the fold at the edge of the mattress, bring the triangle down over the side of the mattress.

p r o c e d u r e (c o n t i n u e d)

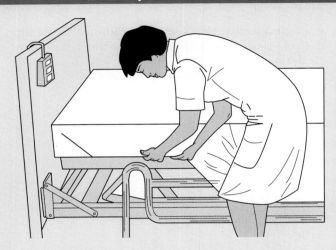

FIGURE 25-6E   Tuck the sheet under the mattress from head to foot. Start at the head and pull toward the foot of the bed as you tuck.

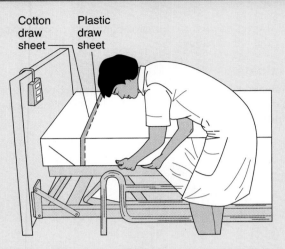

Cotton draw sheet   Plastic draw sheet

FIGURE 25-6F   Fold in half and place the plastic draw sheet 14 inches (the length of your forearm) down from the head of the bed. Tuck it in. Be sure each piece of linen is straight and even as you tuck it in.

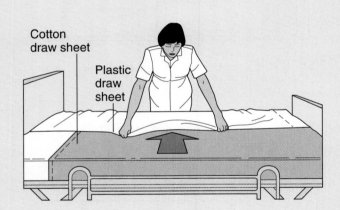

Cotton draw sheet

Plastic draw sheet

FIGURE 25-6G   Fold the top sheet lengthwise and place it on the bed. Place the center fold at the center of the bed from the head to the foot.

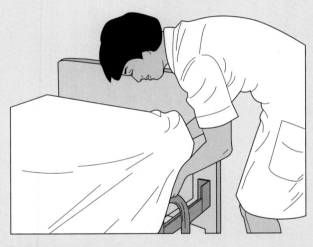

FIGURE 25-6H   Tightly tuck the sheet under at the foot of the bed.

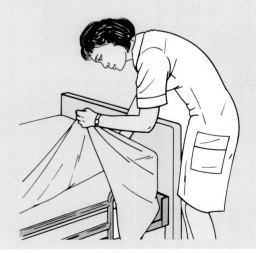

FIGURE 25-6I   Make a mitered corner at the foot of the bed.

Bathing

Bathing is essential to skin integrity and the well-being of the patient. Since bathing involves exposing private areas of the body, perform this procedure with the patient's rights and dignity in mind. Several levels of personal care are recognized. These include *complete care, partial care,* and *assistance with a tub bath or shower.*

Complete care describes the care provided for a patient who must have all personal needs met by a health care worker. This type of care is performed at the bedside and is frequently described as a *bed bath*.

Complete care should be delivered only to those patients who are unable to assist with their own care. Encourage independence at all levels of care.

The term **partial care** indicates that the patient is able to perform some personal hygiene needs independently or with supervision. The patient may need assistance only with washing the back and feet or with washing the lower half of the body.

Assistance with a tub bath or shower is a preparatory skill. The health care worker supervises water temperature, transfers the patient to the shower or tub area, assists the patient in and out of the tub, and assists with some personal hygiene needs.

---

procedure
Bathing

Assess

Determine the type of bath that will be needed for the patient. Will the patient require complete care, partial care, or assistance with a tub bath or shower?

Determine the amount of assistance that will be needed. Is the patient alert and oriented? Will you need assistance to turn or to hold the patient? Is the patient incontinent of bowel or bladder functions?

Determine the appropriate time for the bath. Are any tests or procedures scheduled that require bathing before or after completion? What is the preference of the patient?

Plan

Gather required equipment: towels, washcloths, clean gown, soap, lotion, comb or brush, nail care items, and shaving equipment. Remember that hair and nail care, shaving, and probably skin care will be combined for time management purposes.

If the linens will be changed upon completion of the bath, gather clean linens as well.

Implement
Complete or Partial Care

1. Obtain a basin of bathwater at 105° F.
2. Remove the bedclothes properly.
3. Fold the washcloth into a mitten around your hand.
4. Wash the patient's body in this order: around the eyes, face, neck, ears, arms, chest, abdomen, legs, feet, back, and perineal area.

5. Change the water frequently.
6. Keep the bar of soap out of the bathwater.
7. Use minimal amounts of soap on the washcloth.
8. Expose only the area being washed, keeping the rest of the patient covered.

Tub Bath or Shower

1. Assist the patient to the tub or shower area.
2. Instruct the patient in the use of the call signal.
3. Remain with the patient or check on the patient at frequent intervals.
4. Help the patient to dry off.
5. Assist the patient with dressing.
6. Assist the patient back to the room.

Evaluate

Evaluate your actions. Does the patient look and smell clean?

Evaluate the patient's response. Report any abnormalities of the skin, such as reddened areas, open areas, bruises, or rashes. Report any changes in previously existing skin conditions. Report signs of excessive fatigue, shortness of breath, or complaints of pain during the procedure.

Mouth Care

Mouth care is essential to the health of the patient. Keeping the mouth clean will prevent odors and infection and will increase the patient's comfort and appetite, since many microorganisms enter the body through the mouth and cause disorders that affect the mouth. Some illnesses and medications cause coating or swelling of the tongue. Some medications cause food tastes to be altered. Proper mouth care can enhance the patient's well-being, self-image, and appetite. To keep the teeth healthy for chewing food, you must keep the gums healthy to support the teeth.

Proper mouth care begins with brushing the teeth. Brush all surfaces of the teeth: the **lingual**, or surface nearest the tongue, the **buccal**, or surface nearest the cheek, and the **incisal**, or grinding surface. Use a clean toothbrush with soft bristles. Angle the toothbrush against the tooth and gum line at a 45° angle, and apply light pressure. Use a slight circular motion to massage the surface, moving the toothbrush up on the lower teeth and down on the upper teeth.

Flossing helps clean the surfaces between the teeth (the interproximal surfaces). Many types of floss are available and should be selected according to individual preference. Patients in long-term care (LTC) facilities who are unable to floss may need regular visits from a dentist for cleaning because flossing by aides may not be permitted.

An unconscious patient cannot swallow, so normal brushing techniques cannot be used. Special devices for cleaning the mouth of the unconscious patient are available, such as Toothettes and lemon glycerine swab sticks (Figure 25-7). Similar devices can be made by wrapping a 4-inch-by-4-inch gauze square around a tongue depressor, then soaking it in a solution of 1 part hydrogen peroxide to 4 parts

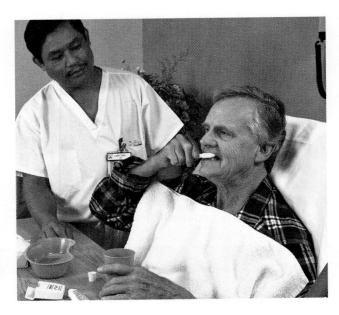

FIGURE 25-8   Mouth care should be performed several times a day.

water. Always be sure the patient's head is turned to the side so gravity will drain secretions away from the throat and out of the mouth.

For the conscious patient who can sit up, you can use a syringe without a needle to irrigate the mouth. Mouth care should be performed several times a day. Most people prefer mouth care before breakfast, after meals, and before bed (Figure 25-8).

Dentures, or artificial teeth, can collect food particles and stains. Dentures must be cleaned at least daily, and they should be removed at night to allow for oxygenation of gum tissue. Dentures are similar to glass: They are sturdy and durable but will break if dropped.

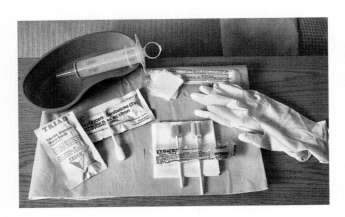

FIGURE 25-7   Mouth care supplies for the unconscious patient.

procedure

Mouth Care

Assess
Determine the special needs of the patient. What is the patient's level of consciousness? Does the patient have full or partial dentures?

Plan
Gather required equipment: towel, toothbrush, toothpaste, glass or cup, emesis basin, tissues, floss, and mouthwash. Gather specialized equipment if needed: denture cup, toothettes, tongue depressor, gauze squares, lemon juice, glycerine or hydrogen peroxide, biohazard bag, and lubricant.

Contact with the mouth requires standard precautions. Gather equipment needed for standard precautions: gloves (mask and eye protection should be used if splashing of body fluids is expected).

Implement

Conscious Patient

1. Raise the head of the bed to a sitting position comfortable for the patient.
2. Place a towel over the patient's chest.
3. Prepare the toothbrush by applying water and toothpaste.
4. Insert the brush carefully in the patient's mouth.
5. Brush all surfaces of the teeth, using short back-and-forth strokes.
6. Brush the inner, outer, and biting surface of each tooth.
7. Offer water to the patient.

procedure (continued)

8. Hold the emesis basin under the chin, telling the patient to expectorate.
9. Help the patient wipe mouth and chin with a tissue.
10. Floss the patient's teeth by stretching an 18-inch piece of floss between the middle fingers of each hand.
11. Stretch the floss further with your thumbs, curve it into a C shape, and gently move it up and down between the teeth.
12. Work from the back of the right side around to the left side.
13. Offer the patient mouthwash after brushing and flossing are completed.

Unconscious Patient

1. Position the patient with the head to one side.
2. Place a towel or underpad on the bed beside the patient's head.
3. Place an emesis basin under the patient's chin.
4. Fold gauze squares around tongue depressors, or use toothettes.
5. Mix glycerine or hydrogen peroxide and lemon juice as described in your facility's policy and procedure manual.
6. Moisten a padded blade or applicator in the lemon juice mixture.
7. Clean the mouth by gently swabbing the teeth, gums, tongue, and roof of mouth.
8. Use an applicator moistened with water or mouthwash to rinse the mouth.
9. Discard used padded blades or applicators in a plastic biohazard bag.
10. Apply lubricant to the patient's lips and tongue.

Assisting a Patient to Brush Teeth

1. Place a towel over the patient's chest.
2. Prepare the toothbrush by applying water and toothpaste.
3. Allow the patient to brush, assisting as needed.
4. Assist with rinsing the mouth by offering water to the patient.
5. Hold the emesis basin under the chin, telling the patient to expectorate.
6. Offer the patient tissue to wipe mouth and chin.
7. Assist with flossing as needed.

Denture Care

Always handle dentures very carefully (Figure 25-9).

1. Obtain the dentures from the patient, placing them in a denture cup.
2. Line the emesis basin or sink with paper towels.
3. Clean the dentures by using warm water and brushing all surfaces.
4. Rinse the dentures in cool water.
5. Place the dentures in cool water in the denture cup if the patient is not going to wear them immediately.

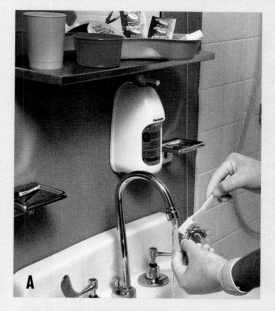

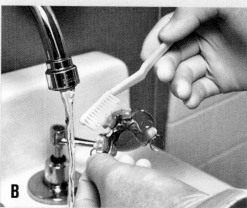

FIGURE 25-9 (a) Denture care materials. (b) Always handle dentures very carefully.

Evaluate

Evaluate your actions. Are the patient's teeth or dentures free from food particles and toothpaste? Evaluate the patient's response. Do the dentures fit properly? Are they in adequate condition? Report any abnormal findings during oral care, such as bleeding gums or dry, cracked lips. Report signs of excessive fatigue or complaints of pain during the procedure.

Read through the following situation, and determine the mouth care needs of Mrs. Ruhll: *Mrs. Ruhll is a cardiac patient receiving heparin, a blood thinner. Prior to hospitalization, she had poor oral hygiene. The nurse informs you at report that Mrs. Ruhll is not to use a toothbrush. Why?* Mrs. Rhull is probably prone to bleeding gums for two reasons: She is taking a blood thinner, and she has a history of poor dental care.

How might Mrs. Rhull's mouth care be modified without sacrificing proper hygiene? Instruct Mrs. Ruhll to rinse with an antiseptic mouthwash. She may use a toothette. The doctor may wish to refer Mrs. Ruhll to a dentist.

Hair Care

Hair is a protective appendage that grows over most parts of the skin. Care of the hair on the head will be discussed in this section. Illness and poor nutrition are directly reflected in the condition of the hair. Therefore, people who are ill have an even greater need for daily hair care than others. Conditions that affect hair care include fever, restrictions on mobility, and disabilities.

Some general guidelines for daily hair care are listed below:

- Follow the patient's preferences when deciding how to style the hair.
- Never cut a patient's hair.
- Brush the hair from the scalp to the ends.
- Use only wide-tooth combs.

The most frequently neglected area of personal grooming for patients is shampooing the hair. This procedure is important for removing dirt and oil, which can trap microorganisms. Hair should be shampooed as frequently as needed for the patient's hair type, diagnosis, and ability to tolerate the procedure. General guidelines for shampooing hair are listed below:

- Perform hair care in the bed or as part of a tub bath or shower, depending on the physician's order.
- Protect the bed if shampooing is to occur in the bed.
- Ensure that water is at a safe and comfortable temperature.
- Use only a small amount of shampoo.

procedure
Hair Care

Assess
Determine where hair care will be given.

If the hair needs to be shampooed, obtain permission to do so. The method for shampooing will depend on the patient's condition and safety needs. Hair can be washed in the shower, in a basin, or using a shampoo board while the patient remains in bed (Figure 25-10).

Plan
Gather required equipment: towel and brush or comb.

Implement
Daily Hair Care Following Shampoo
1. Dry the patient's hair as quickly as possible.

2. Cover the pillow with a towel, if the patient is to remain in bed.
3. Position the patient comfortably.
4. Divide the patient's hair into several sections.
5. Brush and comb all sections of the hair.
6. Arrange the hair according to the patient's preference.

Evaluate
Evaluate your actions. Does the patient's hair look clean, and is it free from tangles?

Evaluate the patient's responses. Report any observations regarding scalp condition or hair loss. Report signs of excessive fatigue or shortness of breath during the procedure.

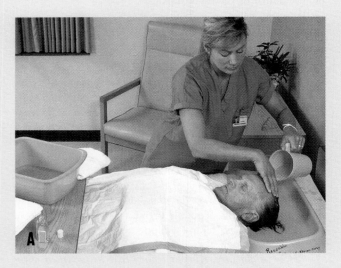
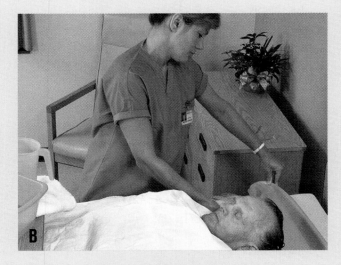

FIGURE 25-10   (a) Obtain permission before shampooing a patient's hair. (b) Hair can be washed while the patient remains in bed.

Nail Care

Different health care facilities have different policies regarding nail care. A general guideline, however, is never to cut a patient's nails. Discuss nail care with the nurse before performing any procedures (Figure 25-11).

Proper foot care is essential, especially for patients with diabetes and poor circulation. Foot care can be performed as part of the bed bath and will help prevent infections and foot odor. Dry the feet well, especially between the toes.

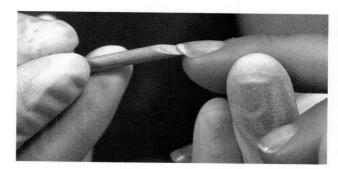

FIGURE 25-11   Follow the policies of your facility regarding nail care.

---

procedure

Nail Care

Assess

Determine the type of nail care that can safely be performed for the patient.

Does the patient have diabetes or vascular disease?

Plan

Gather required equipment: bath basin with warm, soapy water, orange stick, nail file, and lotion.

Combine nail care with the bath or other care activities. For example, administer nail and foot care while the patient is sitting up in a chair. Nails can be soaking while you make the bed, then nail care can be completed.

Implement

1. Soak the patient's nails in soapy water to soften them.
2. Gently push the cuticles back using an orange stick.

3. Carefully clean under nails with the orange stick.
4. File nails straight across, using short strokes, working from the side of the nail to the top.
5. Smooth any rough edges with the smooth side of the nail file.
6. Apply lotion to the patient's hands, including the cuticles.

Evaluate

Evaluate your actions. Do the patient's nails look clean, short, and smooth?

Evaluate the patient's response. Report any abnormal findings, such as redness around the cuticles or thick, discolored nails. Report any complaints of pain during the procedure. Report any evidence of a need for increased attention to nail or foot care.

Shaving

Shaving a male patient's beard is a part of daily personal hygiene. Each patient will have a personal preference for either an electric or a safety razor. If a patient is unable to shave himself using his safety razor, obtain proper authorization before you shave him. A safety razor may be contraindicated due to certain medications or conditions that can cause bleeding or infection.

Before shaving a patient with a safety razor, first warm the beard with a warm, moist washcloth. Then apply shaving cream. As you shave, work with downward strokes, rinsing the razor between each stroke. Hold the skin taut with your free hand.

Always consult with the nurse before helping a patient to shave. As with any procedure, only perform the steps that the patient is unable to do for himself.

---

procedure

Shaving

Assess

Determine which type of razor will be used. If the patient is on anticoagulants, a safety razor cannot be used.

Determine the ability of the patient to assist with the procedure.

Plan

Determine the appropriate time for the patient to shave. Can it be done with other morning care? Does the patient have a preference about the time the procedure is performed? For example, some patients may prefer to

p r o c e d u r e (c o n t i n u e d)

shave before breakfast since that is what they do at home.

Gather required equipment: towel, basin or sink of warm water, washcloth, shaving cream, safety razor, and aftershave lotion *or* preelectric shave and electric razor. Use standard precautions as appropriate.

Implement
Shaving with a Safety Razor

1. Drape the patient's shoulders and chest with a towel.
2. Moisten the beard with a warmed washcloth.
3. Apply shaving cream to a small area.
4. Shave by holding the skin taut, stroking in the direction of hair growth.
5. Shave both cheeks, then the chin, and then the nostril area.

6. Wash remaining shaving cream from the face, then dry.
7. Apply aftershave lotion if desired.

Shaving with an Electric Razor

1. Hold the skin taut.
2. Move the electric razor in a circular or short-stroke motion.
3. Shave both cheeks, then the chin, and then the nostril area.
4. Clean the razor with a razor brush.

Evaluate

Evaluate your actions. Does the patient's face look smooth and free from stubble?

Evaluate the patient's response. Report any abnormalities, such as redness, rashes, or scaling of the facial skin. Report signs of excessive fatigue or shortness of breath during the procedure.

Changing a Patient's Clothing

When you assist a patient to dress and undress, remember the following guidelines:

■ If the patient has a weak or paralyzed limb, always dress the affected limb first. When removing clothing, always undress the unaffected limb first.

■ Encourage the patient to use all assistive devices to promote independence. An example of an assistive device is a long-handled shoehorn.

■ If the patient has a peripheral intravenous (IV) line and no IV gown is available, put the bag and tubing through the arm of the gown first, then put the patient's arm through the gown. In this way, the IV will remain intact.

Skin Care

As you study this chapter, you may also want to refer to Chapter 7, "The Skin." Because the skin is made of cells and cells require nourishment to function in a healthy way, many factors can contribute to skin breakdown. Age, body temperature, diaphoresis (sweating), impaired circulation due to pressure, poor dietary habits, loss of mobility, and loss of sensation all influence the state of the skin. One must assess all these factors to reduce the chances of skin breakdown.

Observe the skin for temperature, color, texture, integrity, and **turgor** (resiliency of the skin). The

skin should feel cool, soft, and slightly moist to the touch. It should not be excessively moist or dry, hot or cold. The skin texture should appear smooth, with good turgor. Normal nail beds and mucous membranes should be pink with good capillary refill.

A variety of conditions can affect the skin. Circulatory impairment and diabetes can cause tissue death. Poor circulation can also change skin color from pink to blue or gray and can change temperature from warm to cold. Nutritional conditions can cause dry, flaky skin or color changes. Certain medications can cause dehydration of the skin. Aging skin loses its elasticity and turgor due to the breakdown of collagen. Redness, rashes, abrasions, wounds, and flaking are all abnormal skin findings. Observe patients' skin for ecchymosis, or bruising, and petechiae, or tiny hemorrhages under the skin. Carefully document any skin conditions that you observe. Include the location and drainage from any wound. Describe any rashes as localized (in one area), generalized (covering large areas of the body), raised, or flat. Describe the lesions as large or small.

Bony prominences are areas of skin where there is little fat to cushion the tissue over the bone (Figure 25-12). These areas are especially prone to skin breakdown. The auricle of the outer ear and the occiput (the back of the head) are examples of bony prominences.

When you provide skin care, you reduce the chances of skin integrity breakdown. Always ob-

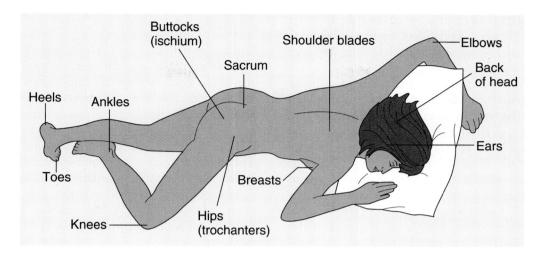

FIGURE 25-12 Check for signs of skin breakdown over bony prominences.

serve the skin carefully and report any abnormalities to the nurse. Follow any nurse's or doctor's orders regarding skin care. Observe the skin over bony prominences frequently. Pay close attention to the occiput, spine, and heels of a bed-bound or paralyzed patient. Pay close attention to the buttocks and coccyx of a patient who sits most of the day. Even an overweight or obese patient can develop pressure sores. Obese patients may develop skin breakdown in skin folds that trap moisture and bacteria or in areas where friction abrades the skin. Re-

port any signs of possible skin breakdown to your supervisor immediately.

A variety of special devices are available to reduce skin pressure. A doctor's order is not required to implement the use of such equipment. An **eggcrate mattress** or wheelchair cushion is designed with an irregular surface to provide airflow. A **water or alternating air mattress** helps prevent pressure areas by redistributing body weight. **Heel and elbow protectors** prevent friction against bed linens (Figure 25-13), and **foot elevators** reduce

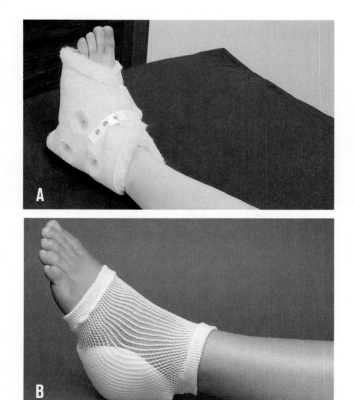

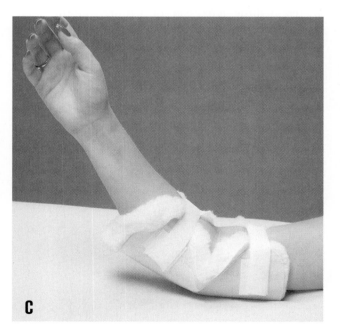

FIGURE 25-13 (a) Heel protector. (b) Elastic mesh heel protector. (c) Elbow protector. Photos courtesy of Posey Company, Arcadia, California.

the opportunities for the heels to rest against the bed, causing pressure. **Gel-filled cushions** simulate the padding of adipose tissue and reduce pressure over bony prominences.

Pressure sores, decubiti, bedsores, decubitus ulcers, and **pressure ulcers** are all terms for skin breakdown. This occurs due to prolonged pressure that causes lack of circulation and oxygenation to the tissue. Did you ever sit in a hard chair for a lengthy period of time? Were your buttocks painful and slightly numb? Maybe you changed positions and rubbed the area to relieve the symptoms. Unfortunately, not all patients are capable of moving or changing positions, and some cannot even feel the symptoms caused by impaired circulation. Left untreated, the lack of circulation causes necrosis, or tissue death, and a bedsore or decubitus ulcer results. The signs of a forming decubitus ulcer are the same as the signs of inflammation: a red, hot, swollen, and tender area. The tenderness may be described as a burning sensation.

Pressure sores can be deceiving. The area of breakdown may appear small on the surface, yet tissue damage may extend down to the bone. Once pressure sores form, they are difficult to heal. The best method of treatment for bedsores is prevention. Patients prone to developing pressure sores are those who are weak, malnourished, or paralyzed or those with impaired circulation. They may have casts, dressings, or bandages that hide the skin beneath. They may be elderly or prone to infections due to diabetes mellitus, leukemia, or acquired immunodeficiency syndrome (AIDS).

Caustic (irritating) agents, such as urine, feces, soaps, lotions, perspiration, and friction can contribute to the development of pressure sores. Even wrinkles in the bed linens can cause skin breakdown. If bedsores develop, treatment will be prescribed by the physician.

Massage

Human touch can have a positive effect on one's sense of comfort. Human touch is required if babies are to develop emotional connections with others. Without it, failure-to-thrive syndrome may occur. Despite this knowledge, adults often neglect touch and its healing properties. Touch has been proven to be an effective alternative for pain management. Therapeutic touch also promotes circulation, which bathes the cell with life-sustaining nutrients.

Massage has risen in popularity in the past ten years. Massage therapy has become an important modality in wellness promotion and a field of health care on its own.

The back, with the spinal cord and its many branches, is an area rich in nerve supply. Therefore, massage is often concentrated on the back. The art of massage is made up of several techniques using different parts of the hand.

The fingers are spread to reach a large surface area. The fingertips are sensitive enough to feel the musculature in the back and to adjust the amount of pressure being applied during the massage. The thumbs are used to reach deeper muscle fibers. Use the sides of each hand to lightly tap the muscles, and use the palms to assist the fingertips.

When performing back massage, begin with your hands at the base of the spine on either side of the spinal column. Use one long stroke to move the fingertips up to the shoulders and back down to the base of the spine. Next, use large circular motions to move the hands up the back and down to the base of the spine (Figure 25-14).

If you are performing massage on elderly patients, keep the following considerations for modification in mind. Aging skin is sensitive and can tear easily. Excessive pressure can cause the bones of patients with osteoporosis to fracture spontaneously.

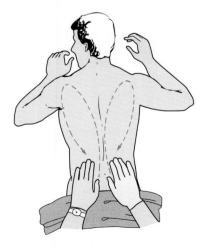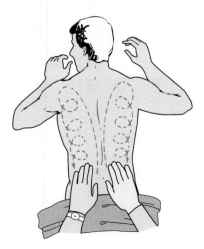

FIGURE 25-14   Provide back rubs to increase circulation and relax the patient.

procedure
Massage

Assess

Determine whether any modifications need to be made for the patient. Are there any areas of skin breakdown? Are there any medical conditions or disabilities that could be aggravated by massage? If the patient has heart disease, has a back injury, or has had surgery, do not perform this procedure.

Plan

Determine when the massage should be given. Can it be incorporated into other care, such as the bath?

Gather required equipment: lotion and a bath blanket. (Avoid using talcum powder or alcohol, which cause drying of the skin.) Use standard precautions as appropriate.

Implement

1. Raise the bed to a comfortable working height in order to use good body mechanics.
2. Assist the patient to a prone or lateral position in proper body alignment.
3. Place your hands, palms down, at the base of the patient's spine.
4. Stroke upward from the buttocks to the shoulders, moving the hands along each side of the backbone.
5. Separate your hands at the patient's neck. Rub in an upward and outward circular motion down over the upper arms, back up the upper arms, across the shoulders and down the back.
6. Using the same circular motions, massage the hips, buttocks, and coccyx.
7. Massage any bony areas using a circular motion.
8. Complete the massage within 4 to 6 minutes.

Evaluate

Evaluate your actions. Is the patient more relaxed and comfortable?

Evaluate the patient's responses. Report any skin abnormalities or muscle tightness. Report signs of excessive fatigue or complaints of pain during the procedure.

The nerves and blood vessels of diabetic patients may be impaired. Patients with paralysis, quadriplegics, paraplegics, and hemiplegics experience loss of some feeling in the back. When in doubt about performing this or any procedure, ask the nurse.

Measuring Skills

Measurements of vital signs, intake and output, and body temperature are taken on patients of health care facilities several times a day. Life-threatening situations are often recognized through these measurements. Accuracy is essential. When performing a measuring skill, you must be accurate in the actual measuring, the reporting, and the recording.

Vital Signs

Vital signs (VS) refer to the measurement of *temperature, pulse, respirations,* and *blood pressure*, which provides valuable information about the vital functions of the body. It is extremely important to be accurate when you measure vital signs. If you report inaccurate readings, the physician could order the wrong treatment for the patient. In order to know what to report immediately, you must be able to recognize abnormal vital sign readings. Generally, vital signs are taken at one time because, although each separate value is important, collective changes indicate significant problems. If a supervisor asks you to "take temps," unless specifically instructed otherwise to include pulse and respirations as well. Should a nurse ask you to take a blood pressure, be sure to include pulse and respirations, too. If the order is to take vital signs, take temperature, pulse, respirations, and blood pressure, abbreviated *T-P-R and BP*.

Temperature

Body temperature is defined as the measurement of the difference between the amount of heat produced and the amount lost by the body. Normal body temperature ranges from 97.6° F to 99.6° F. The *F* stands for "Fahrenheit." **Temperature** is measured with a thermometer. *Glass, electronic,* and *thermal* all are different types of thermometers.

A **glass thermometer** is a fragile tube marked with calibrations that contains an inner core of mercury. **Mercury (Hg)**, a liquid metal, expands as it is heated. When the mercury in the glass tube expands, it moves along the tube (Figure 25-15).

Glass thermometers are available in three types: *oral, rectal,* and *security* (Figure 25-15). **Oral thermometers** are easily recognized by their thin, elongated bulb. An arrow indicates the normal oral temperature of 98.6° F. **Rectal thermometers** are recognized by the red mark at the end of the stem and the rounded bulb. An arrow indicates the normal rectal temperature of 99.6° F. Axillary temperatures average 1° lower than oral temperature. **Security (stubby) thermometers** contain a bulb similar

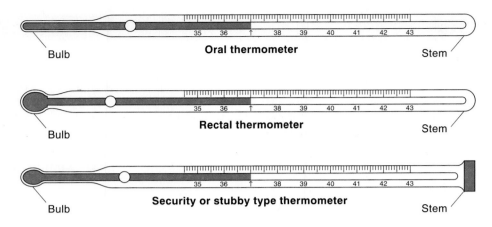

Bulb **Oral thermometer** Stem

Bulb **Rectal thermometer** Stem

Bulb **Security or stubby type thermometer** Stem

Figure 25-15 Three types of tips, or bulbs, on glass thermometers.

to that of a rectal thermometer but are marked the same as an oral thermometer. Security thermometers can be used for axillary, oral, or rectal temperatures.

An **electronic thermometer** is a battery-operated thermometer with an attached probe. The probe can be used to measure oral, rectal, or axillary temperatures, which will appear as a digital readout on the thermometer display screen. The advantages of using an electronic thermometer include avoiding the risks involved with the use of glass and mercury. However, if the battery is not fully charged, the readings will not be accurate. Also, transmission of germs increase with this type of thermometer because it is used on all patients and taken from room to room. A protective sheath covers the probe before it is inserted in a patient's mouth (Figure 25-16).

A **tympanic thermometer** is a type of electronic thermometer that is inserted into the external ear to obtain a digital reading of **aural temperature**. The mechanism of the tympanic thermometer is similar to that of the electronic thermometer. The thermometer must be placed next to the eardrum for an accurate reading; a protective covering is applied to the probe before each use (Figure 25-17).

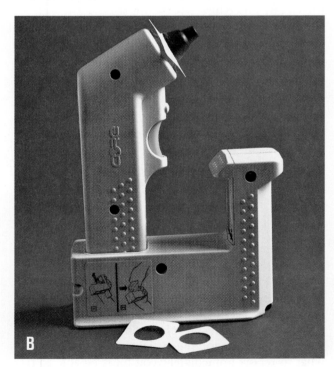

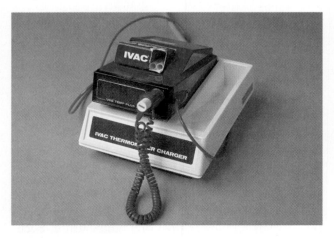

FIGURE 25-16 Electronic digital thermometer.

FIGURE 25-17 (a) A tympanic thermometer is an electronic thermometer that is inserted into the external ear. (b) The thermometer must be placed next to the eardrum for an accurate reading.

procedure

Measuring Oral Temperature Using a Glass Thermometer

Assess

Determine which method to use when taking the patient's temperature. Is the patient able to follow the instructions for using an oral thermometer?

Determine whether the patient has eaten, smoked, chewed gum, or had anything to drink in the past 15 minutes. If so, delay taking the temperature for 15 minutes.

Plan

Gather required equipment: gloves, glass thermometer, thermometer sheath, tissue, disinfecting solution, and pen. Use standard precautions as appropriate.

Implement

1. Rinse the thermometer in cool or tepid water.
2. Read the thermometer. It should register 96° or lower.
3. If needed, shake down the mercury further, holding the stem of the thermometer (use wrist action to shake the thermometer).
4. Put on gloves, and place the thermometer in a sheath.
5. Place the bulb end of the thermometer under the patient's tongue to the right or the left of the base of the tongue.
6. Instruct the patient to hold the thermometer in place with the lips closed. (You may need to assist the patient if he or she is not able to do so alone.)
7. Leave the thermometer in place for 3 to 5 minutes.
8. Remove the thermometer from the mouth.
9. Remove the thermometer sheath, and wipe the thermometer with a tissue.
10. Read the results by turning the thermometer until you can see the mercury line (hold at eye level).
11. Read the results to the nearest tenth of a degree.
12. Place the thermometer in a disinfecting solution.
13. Document the results on the correct form.

Evaluate

What was the patient's temperature?

Did you report abnormal results?

Did you record the results on the flow-sheet or appropriate form?

procedure

Measuring Aural Temperature Using a Tympanic Thermometer

Assess

Determine which mode should be set on the thermometer. Assess any ear conditions or hearing aids that might warrant using one ear versus the other.

Plan

Gather required equipment: electronic tympanic thermometer, probe cover, and pen. Position the patient comfortably and safely to expose the ear to be used.

Implement

1. Remove the thermometer from the case, and attach a probe cover.
2. Grasp the pinna of the ear and pull up and back.
3. Insert the probe.
4. Press the digital button and hold for 1 second (or according to the manufacturer's instructions).
5. Remove the probe, and release the ear.
6. Read the results on the digital screen.
7. Record the reading with a (*T*) following the temperature.

Evaluate

Evaluate your actions. Did the thermometer register an accurate reading?

Evaluate the patient's response. How did the patient tolerate the procedure? As with all temperatures, identify and report any abnormalities.

procedure

Measuring Axillary Temperature Using a Glass Thermometer

Follow the steps for measuring aural temperature, but make these changes:

- Place the bulb of the thermometer under the patient's arm. Be sure that the axilla is dry and that the thermometer is between two skin surfaces, with no clothing in between.
- Have the patient hold the thermometer in place with his or her arm.

- Write (*Ax*) after the temperature reading when documenting an axillary temperature in the chart.

Evaluate

Evaluate your actions. Did the thermometer register an accurate reading?

Evaluate the patient's response. Report a temperature reading above 99° F.

procedure

Measuring Rectal Temperature Using a Glass Thermometer

Assess

Determine whether a rectal temperature is required. Is the patient unable to cooperate with other types of temperature measurement?

Determine whether you will need assistance to take this patient's temperature. Can the patient roll to the side? Can the patient remain on that side without assistance during the procedure?

Plan

Gather required equipment: gloves, rectal glass thermometer, thermometer sheath, lubricant, tissue, disinfecting solution, and pen. Use standard precautions as appropriate.

Implement

1. Rinse the thermometer in cool or tepid water.
2. Read the thermometer. It should register 96° or lower.
3. If needed, shake down the mercury further, holding the stem of the thermometer.
4. Place the thermometer in a sheath, and put on gloves.
5. Apply lubricant to the sheath at the bulb end of the thermometer.

6. Insert the bulb end of the thermometer 1 inch into the rectum.
7. Hold the thermometer in place for 3 minutes, instructing the patient not to change position.
8. Remove the thermometer.
9. Remove the sheath, and wipe the thermometer with a tissue.
10. Read the results by turning the thermometer until the mercury line is seen.
11. Read the results to the nearest two-tenths of a degree.
12. Place the thermometer in a disinfecting solution.
13. Clean and reposition the patient as needed.
14. Document results on the correct form. Write (*R*) after the temperature reading when documenting a rectal temperature in the chart.

Evaluate

Evaluate your actions. Did the thermometer register an accurate reading?

Evaluate the patient's response. Report a temperature reading above 100° F.

A **thermal thermometer** is a heat-sensitive reagent strip. One type is a flat, plastic strip that is placed under the tongue. Heat-sensitive dots change color to indicate the temperature reading. Another type of plastic strip is placed on the forehead, where heat-sensitive squares change colors to indicate the temperature reading (Figure 25-18).

Pulse

Pulse is the wave of oxygenated blood sent through the arteries with each contraction of the heart. Each time the heart contracts, the arteries expand to accommodate this force. The force of this wave of blood can be counted to determine the rate and

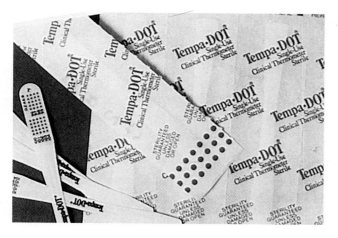

FIGURE 25-18   Chemically treated strips that change color at various temperatures.

rhythm of the heartbeat. Although arteries are buried deep in the body tissues for protection, pulse points are located along various artery routes.

Each pulse point is an important site for determining blood flow to various tissues. For example, the **carotid pulse** is assessed to determine whether the heart is pumping blood to the brain. If no carotid pulse is felt, the heart is in cardiac arrest. The **femoral pulse** is assessed to determine the presence of blood flow to the lower extremities. The **pedal pulse** is measured when the circulatory status of the feet is in question. The most common pulse site, however, is the **radial pulse**, which is located on the lateral or thumb side of the inner wrist.

Listen to different musical scores and feel the beat. It is easy to tap your feet to some songs, but others are harder to follow because the beat changes frequently. A patient's heartbeat is similar to a musical score. This is called **heart rhythm**. Some heartbeats are easy to auscultate (hear) or palpate (feel with the fingertips). The rhythm of the heart can be regular, with beats evenly spaced and occurring at the same intervals, or it can be irregular, with each beat occurring randomly.

Another characteristic of the pulse is its **volume**. Just like the volume on a radio, a pulse can be loud, normal, or very faint. The pulse can be auscultated or palpated to determine the volume. A bounding pulse is one that is loud when auscultated. Palpating a weak or thready pulse is like trying to feel a piece of fine hair under your fingertips.

p r o c e d u r e
Measuring Pulse

Assess
Determine the reason for taking the pulse. Is it part of routine vital signs, or is the patient experiencing a heart problem? What have previous pulse rates been for this patient? Identify a baseline reading.

Plan
Gather required equipment: watch with a second hand and pen.

Implement
1. Position the patient's arm so that it is resting across his or her chest or resting comfortably at the side.
2. Place your index and middle fingers over the radial pulse.
3. Count the beats felt against your fingers for 1 minute (60 seconds).
4. Notice the rhythm and volume of the pulse.
5. Record the results on the appropriate form.

Evaluate
Evaluate your actions. Did you feel and count the pulse for the entire 60 seconds?

Evaluate the patient's response. Report stat a pulse rate that is higher than 100 or less than 60. Report stat a pulse that is weak, thready, bounding, or irregular.

Respirations

Respirations, or the inhaling and exhaling of air, is the third vital sign. Measuring respirations is a simple method of assessing a patient's health status. Oxygen is important to all the cells of the body, and a patient with poor respiratory status has a poor health status. Think of a vacuum cleaner: The stronger the motor, the better the vacuum picks up dirt. If the fan's motor is strong, it will blow out a great volume of air. A healthy respiratory system must be able to draw large amounts of air in and out.

Unlike temperature and pulse, respirations are under conscious and unconscious control. Therefore, it is important that patients are not conscious or aware of your execution of this procedure. When

procedure
Measuring Respirations

Assess

Determine the appropriate time to take respirations. Perform this procedure immediately after counting the pulse, without moving your hand or the patient's arm.

Observe the patient's respirations for one full minute. A respiration is one full breath, both inspiration (breathing in) and expiration (breathing out).

Plan

Gather required equipment: watch with a second hand and pen.

Implement

1. Keep the patient's arm in place across the chest or at the side. Be sure you can see the rise and fall of the chest or the abdominal area.

2. Count the number of respirations in 60 seconds, feeling the rise and fall of the chest.

3. Notice the rhythm and depth of the respirations.

4. Document on the appropriate form.

Evaluate

Evaluate your actions. Were you able to feel or see the respirations for 60 seconds?

Evaluate the patient's response. Report a respiratory rate greater than 20 or less than 12. Report any abnormal findings, such as difficulty breathing, an irregular breathing pattern, or a chest that does not rise equally on both sides during inspiration.

---

patients are aware that you are watching them breathe, conscious breathing patterns may occur. A good time to observe respirations is before or after taking the radial pulse. While your hand is still on the patient's wrist, watch or feel the rise and fall of the chest. Ensure that the patient is relaxed and not talking. Observe the respirations for one full cycle, beginning with the chest rising. One full breath equals one inspiration and one expiration. Count the number of respirations in 60 seconds. Always notice the rhythm and depth (volume) of the respirations.

Blood Pressure

Blood pressure is an indirect measurement of the intermittent force of the blood against the artery walls as the heart contracts and relaxes. Because pressure is present in the blood vessel when the heart both contracts and relaxes, blood pressure is represented by two numbers. When the heart contracts, the vessel pressure increases. This is the **systolic pressure** and is written as the top number of the blood pressure. A certain amount of pressure is always present in the vessels and is measured when the heart relaxes. This is the **diastolic pressure** and is written as the lower number of the blood pressure.

Various internal and external factors can affect blood pressure readings. Internal factors to consider are the age of the patient, the condition of the blood vessels, and the strength of the heart's contractions. If blood vessels are narrowed or hardened, it will cause a rise in blood pressure. This is similar to a narrow straw. The smaller the opening of the straw, the more force it takes to move fluid through the straw. When the inner lumen (opening) of blood vessels is clogged with plaque, the lumen narrows. Then the heart must work harder to force blood through the vessel. If the myocardium (heart muscle) is weakened, the heart cannot contract efficiently. All of these conditions can affect both the systolic and the diastolic blood pressure.

External factors that can affect the blood pressure include rest, exercise, medications, and the patient's position. Blood pressure readings will vary when the patient is lying, sitting, or standing. Altitude may also affect blood pressure.

The normal range for adult systolic pressure is 100 to 140 mm Hg. The normal range for adult diastolic pressure is 60 to 90 mm Hg. The average adult blood pressure is 120/80. A blood pressure that is higher than normal is called *hypertension*. Lower than normal blood pressure is called *hypotension*.

The instrument for measuring blood pressure is called a **sphygmomanometer** (*sphygmo-* means "pulse," *mano-* means "pressure," and *meter-* means "measure"). There are five major components to a sphygmomanometer: the *bulb*, the *cuff*, the *valve*, the *bladder*, and the *manometer* (or *gauge*). Blood pressure can be palpated at the radial site, but it is usually auscultated at the brachial site. A stethoscope is required to auscultate blood pressure. A stethoscope also has several parts: *ear pieces*, *tubing*, a *bell*, and a *diaphragm*.

p r o c e d u r e
Measuring Blood Pressure

Assess

Determine if the patient has any special conditions that limit which arm you use for taking the blood pressure. Is there an intravenous line in the patient's arm? Are there wounds, an atrioventricular (AV) shunt, swelling, pain, or deformities in either arm? Do not take the blood pressure in an arm with any of these conditions. If the patient has had a recent mastectomy, do not take the blood pressure on the side of the surgery.

What have previous blood pressure readings been for this patient? Do you need to measure blood pressure in different positions (lying, standing, or sitting)?

Plan

Gather required equipment: sphygmomanometer, stethoscope, alcohol prep pads, and pen. Be sure to clean the stethoscope earpieces with alcohol, if it is not your stethoscope.

Implement

1. Expose the patient's arm at least 5 inches above the elbow.
2. Support the arm with the palm facing up.
3. Wrap the deflated cuff around the arm above the elbow, with the center of the bladder positioned over the brachial artery.
4. Determine the palpatory systolic pressure by palpating the brachial artery, closing the valve, and pumping up the cuff. When the pulse is no longer felt, this is the palpatory pressure.
5. Release the air from the cuff, and wait 30 seconds.
6. Position the diaphragm of the stethoscope over the brachial pulse site.
7. Close the valve on the bulb and inflate the cuff to 30 mm Hg higher than the palpatory pressure.
8. Release the bulb valve slightly, and let the air escape slowly.
9. When you hear the first sound (and see the first fluctuation of mercury or needle gauge), note the reading on the manometer. This is the systolic pressure.
10. Continue to allow air to escape and watch the manometer or needle gauge.
11. When you hear an abrupt change in sound, note the reading on the manometer. This change can be the absence of any more sounds or a change from clear sounds to muffled or faint sounds. This is the diastolic pressure.
12. Release the remaining air in the cuff by opening the valve completely.
13. Remove the cuff.
14. Record the blood pressure on the appropriate form.

Evaluate

Evaluate your actions. Were you able to hear both the systolic and the diastolic sounds? If you need to recheck or repeat the procedure, wait 1 minute before reapplying the cuff.

Evaluate the patient's response. Immediately report blood pressure readings higher than 140/90 or lower than 100/60.

The two types of sphygmomanometers are *mercury* and *aneroid* (Figure 25-19). The **mercury sphygmomanometer** utilizes a glass cylinder filled with mercury. When the valve is closed and air is pumped into the bladder, mercury is forced up the column. When the valve is released slightly, air escapes. As the air escapes, the bladder deflates, and the mercury descends within the column. An **aneroid sphygmomanometer** works much the same way but utilizes a dial rather than a column of mercury.

In order to measure a patient's blood pressure, you must coordinate what you see with what you hear. As the mercury falls in the glass column, you will begin to hear an auditory pulse. Remember the number where the mercury began to dip, or the needle began to fluctuate, when you hear the first sound. This is the systolic pressure. The fluctuations of the manometer and the auditory pulse will continue and then cease. Finally, when the sounds and fluctuations stop, note the number on the gauge. This is the diastolic pressure.

Intake and Output

Intake and output (I&O) refers to a method of evaluating fluid balance in the body. Fluid balance compares the amount of fluid taken into the body with the amount of fluid excreted by the body. Proper fluid balance is essential for all body cells to perform metabolic functions. The human body is 70 percent fluid. The amount of fluid intake should ap-

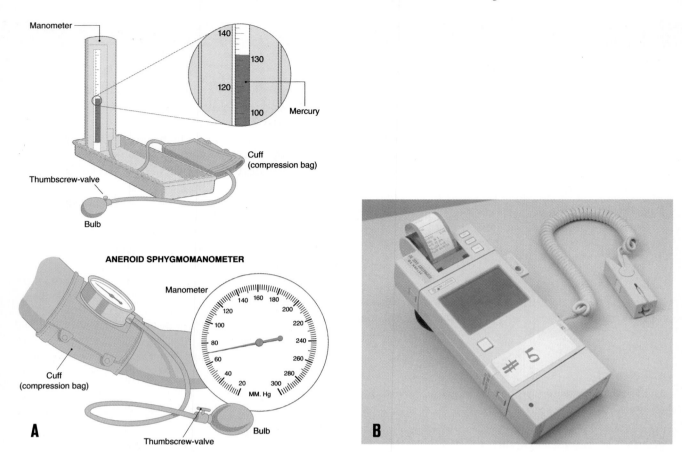

FIGURE 25-19 (a) Two types of blood pressure apparatuses: Mercury sphygmomanometer and aneroid sphygmomanometer. (b) Digital sphygmomanometer and pulse monitor. Place index finger into finger cuff and follow directions to acquire pulse rate and blood pressure.

proximate the amount of fluid output. Another way that can be said is that I = O. What happens if intake is decreased? Initially, output should decrease as well because intake should be equal to or greater than output. If intake increases, what happens to output? Output should increase also. This is part of the homeostatic process.

There are three compartments of fluid in the body: inside the cell, outside the cell, and in the blood. Imagine a wrinkly dry raisin that was once a grape. What happened? The fluid in the tissues was removed. If fluid from each cell is removed, the cells will shrivel. Remember the raisin? What happens if you soak it in water? It plumps again. If it is left too long in the water, it will become mushy. Too much water is just as destructive as too little water. What would happen if you placed the raisins in a strainer and ran water over them? The raisins would soak up

the amount of fluid needed, and the rest of the water would run through the strainer. The kidneys are like the strainer, selectively excreting the excess fluid and impurities.

Fluid is lost through urine, feces, vomitus, sweat, and breathing. Usually, you will measure output of urine. However, if a patient is on strict I&O, you must measure any liquid stool and vomitus.

For intake measurements, you can usually use the facility's chart, which lists in ml or cc the amount of liquid in cups, bowls, etc. Remember that gelatin, ice cream, sherbert, and soup are measurable liquids. Whenever possible, ask patients to inform you of *any* intake or output.

Regulatory mechanisms in our bodies adjust the amount of fluid each cell needs. All the regulatory mechanisms must function properly for fluid balance to be maintained.

procedure
Measuring Intake and Output

Assess

Determine if the patient has any special conditions that will affect the measurement of intake and output. Is the patient incontinent? Is the patient diaphoretic? Are any irrigations being performed?

Determine how to convert ounces to milliliters. It is necessary to know that 1 cubic centimeter (cc) is equal to 1 milliliter (ml) (Figure 25-20).

Plan

Gather required equipment: measuring device, intake and output form, pen, intake and output overbed sign. Use standard precautions as appropriate.

Implement

1. Instruct the patient to write down any fluids taken and report them to you. You should make note of any fluids ingested when you serve and remove meal trays or give the patient fluids. Record your measurements immediately so that you do not forget them.
2. Place an intake and output sign over patient's bed or at the entrance to the patient's room.
3. Measure the amount of all liquids consumed, and record it in milliliters (ml) or cubic centimeters (cc).
4. Instruct the patient to always void into a urinal, bedpan, commode, or measuring device (Figure 25-21).
5. Instruct the patient to dispose of toilet paper in the trash, not in the bedpan or commode.
6. Measure all liquid output and record. This can be in the form of urine, liquid bowel movement, vomitus, or tube or wound drainage.
7. Check intake and output status each hour. Do not wait until the end of the shift.
8. Total the intake and output for your shift, check your math calculations, and record the result in the chart or flow sheet.

Evaluate

Evaluate your actions. Was all liquid intake and output measured and recorded?

Evaluate the patient's response. Did intake match output? Report any gross imbalance between liquid intake and output immediately. Report immediately scanty or no urinary output if the patient has a urinary catheter in place. You should note and report stat no urinary output in a urinary drainage bag. Always note and report the color and clarity of urine. Always report events of vomiting and diarrhea.

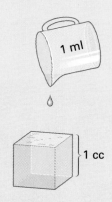

FIGURE 25-20   A 1-centimeter cube will hold 1 milliliter of liquid.

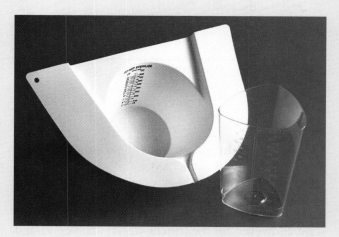

FIGURE 25-21   Types of urine measuring devices.

Height

Height is a linear measurement of the patient. Height and weight are commonly measured using a beam scale. Height can be measured in inches or centimeters. Normally, the measurement is converted to feet and inches when using the English system. The stationary portion of the height bar on the beam scale ascends to a measurement height of 54 inches. How many feet and inches is this? If you said 4 feet, 6 inches, you are correct. Remember, there are 12 inches in each foot. To measure a patient's height beyond 54 inches, raise the sliding bar of the scale above the patient, and gently lower the bar until it rests parallel with the top of the patient's head.

procedure
Measuring Height

Assess

Determine the mobility status of the patient. Will you need assistance to help the patient stand while you measure the height?

Is there a doctor's order for this procedure?

Plan

Gather required equipment: beam scale, pen, and paper.

Determine the best time to measure the patient's height. Can this procedure be performed with the bath or during ambulation to the dayroom, or is there an order to do it stat? Remember to use principles of safety and comfort while performing this procedure.

Implement

1. Raise the height bar.
2. Remove the patient's shoes.
3. Assist the patient onto the scale, facing away from the beam.
4. Instruct the patient to stand erect.
5. Move the measuring bar down carefully to avoid hitting the patient.
6. Position the bar correctly; it should touch the top of the head.
7. Read the measurement in inches.
8. Assist the patient off of the scale and into shoes.
9. Convert the reading to feet and inches (12 inches equal 1 foot).
10. Record the results on the appropriate form.

Evaluate

Evaluate your actions. Were you able to accurately read the measurement in inches and convert it to feet and inches?

Evaluate the patient's response. Report any difficulties in obtaining an accurate height, such as the inability of the patient to stand erect.

Weight

Measuring **weight** is an important assessment tool for determining fluid and nutritional status. **Daily weights** are a good way to detect fluid gain or loss and to evaluate the nutritional status of a malnourished patient. Weights are generally taken on a beam scale. However, for the patient who is unable to stand or balance, weight chairs are available. Weight chairs are operated in the same fashion as the standing scale. Another type of scale is the bed scale (Figure 25-22). This is brought to the bedside as a stretcher would be, but it has a weighing apparatus built in. The bed scale includes four wheels and a hydraulic adjustment.

Patients are weighed on admission and periodically thereafter. The admission measurement is a baseline and is used for comparison with future weights.

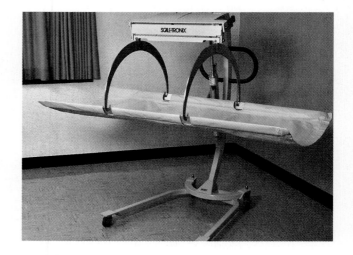

FIGURE 25-22   A bed scale.

procedure
Measuring Weight

Assess

Determine the type of scale you will need based on the mobility of the patient (Figure 25-23). Is the patient able to stand or to transfer with assistance, or is the patient bed-bound? Will you need to use a bed scale, a chair scale, or a standing scale to serve the needs of the patient?

Determine whether you will need assistance to weigh the patient.

What have previous weight readings been for the patient?

Plan

Gather required equipment: the appropriate type of scale, pen, and paper.

Determine when the patient should be weighed. Is this a "daily weight" that should be done before breakfast or at the same time each day?

Since the patient should be in minimal clothing to be weighed, you can combine this procedure with personal care, such as bathing.

Implement

1. Check the scale for balance at 0 pounds.

2. Ask the patient to remove robe, shoes, or slippers. Patients should be weighed wearing only minimal clothing. The same type of clothing should be worn each time the patient is weighed.

3. Help the patient to step onto the scale.

4. Position the patient in the center of the platform, with his or her feet slightly apart.

5. Instruct the patient to stand unassisted.

6. Balance the scale by moving the large and small weights along the beam.

7. Read the patient's weight.

8. Assist the patient off of the scale and back into shoes and robe.

9. Record the weight on the appropriate form.

Evaluate

Evaluate your actions. Were you able to obtain an accurate weight with the patient standing unassisted? Were you able to read the balance scale accurately?

Evaluate the patient's response. Report stat any significant weight gain or loss within a 24-hour period. Report any weight gain or loss compared to previous readings.

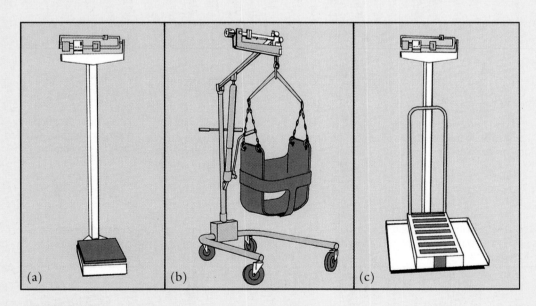

(a)   (b)   (c)

FIGURE 25-23 Types of scales.

Restorative Care Skills

To restore means "to bring back." The term *rehabilitation* is used by physical and occupational therapists, but nurses use the term *restorative care*. Whatever term is used, this care is part of the holistic care approach and includes range-of-motion exercises, ambulation, the use of assistive and adaptive devices (Figure 25-24), transfer techniques, proper positioning of the patient in bed, prosthetics (artificial limbs), and orthotics (braces that support joints and limit movement).

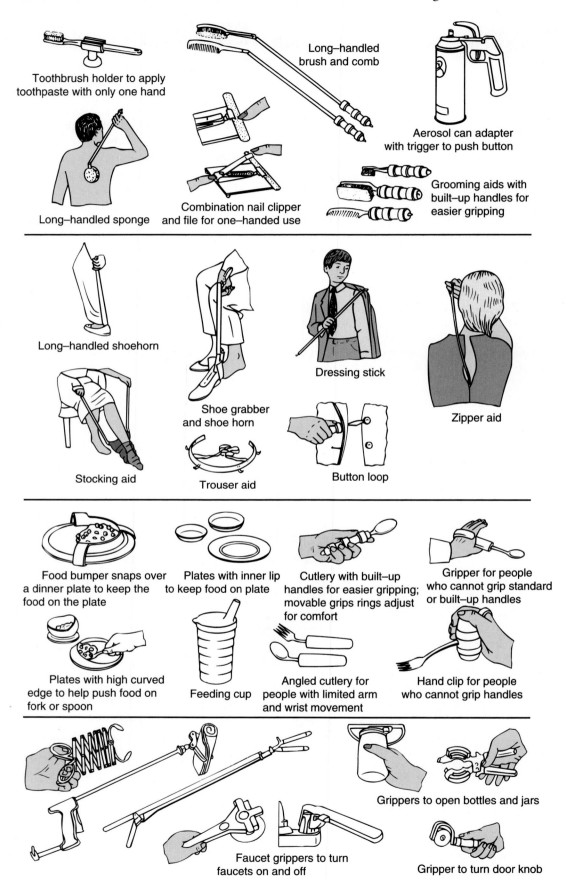

Toothbrush holder to apply toothpaste with only one hand

Long-handled brush and comb

Aerosol can adapter with trigger to push button

Long-handled sponge

Combination nail clipper and file for one-handed use

Grooming aids with built-up handles for easier gripping

Long-handled shoehorn

Shoe grabber and shoe horn

Dressing stick

Zipper aid

Stocking aid

Trouser aid

Button loop

Food bumper snaps over a dinner plate to keep the food on the plate

Plates with inner lip to keep food on plate

Cutlery with built-up handles for easier gripping; movable grips rings adjust for comfort

Gripper for people who cannot grip standard or built-up handles

Plates with high curved edge to help push food on fork or spoon

Feeding cup

Angled cutlery for people with limited arm and wrist movement

Hand clip for people who cannot grip handles

Grippers to open bottles and jars

Faucet grippers to turn faucets on and off

Gripper to turn door knob

FIGURE 25-24   Adaptive devices.

Body Alignment

Body alignment refers to the correct positioning and joint support of the patient's head, spine, and extremities. Body alignment is important whether the patient is in a bed, in a chair, on a stretcher, or ambulating. Just as you practice proper body mechanics and alignment yourself, patients who are confined to bed should be positioned properly. When a patient is lying in the supine position (on the back), evaluate the body alignment while standing at the foot of the bed. Are the head, chest, and trunk in a straight line in the center of the bed? Are the head and upper shoulders supported on the pillow? Is the small of the back supported? Sometimes it is helpful to adjust the lower bed to flex the knees slightly.

When the patient is lying in the lateral (side-lying) position, the head and torso should be in a straight line in the bed (Figure 25-25). The extremities farthest from the body should be supported to prevent internal rotation of the hip and subluxation (partial dislocation) of the shoulder. An adaptation of the lateral position is the Sim's or left lateral position. In this position, the right knee and arm are flexed sharply and supported by pillows. The left leg is slightly flexed.

Proper body alignment is essential for patient comfort and safety. When positioned properly, circulation is promoted to all body parts, reducing muscular aches and pains. Deformities can result from long-term misalignment.

The importance of turning and positioning patients correctly cannot be overemphasized. Proper turning and positioning prevent pressure sores, loosen respiratory secretions (especially post-operatively), and promote comfort.

Turning and Moving a Patient

Some patients will be able to assist in moving and turning themselves. Whenever possible, enlist the patient's help. Always tell the patient what you are going to do. Give the patient clear instructions. Whenever you move a patient with another person, determine and communicate how and when you will move or transfer the patient.

Bed patients who are frail, immobile, or comatose will need to be turned, moved, and positioned every two hours or more frequently if needed. A turning schedule should be posted to ensure consistency in the procedure. To turn laterally,

TOP VIEW

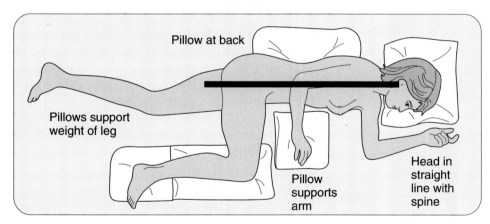

Pillow at back

Pillows support weight of leg

Pillow supports arm

Head in straight line with spine

FRONT VIEW

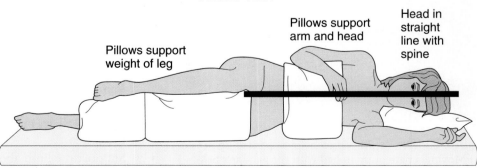

Pillows support weight of leg

Pillows support arm and head

Head in straight line with spine

FIGURE 25-25   Side-lying position.

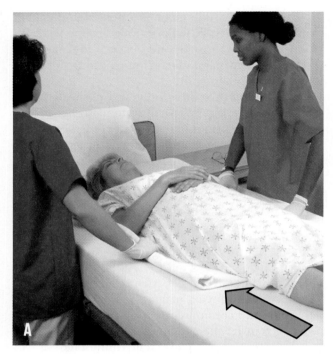

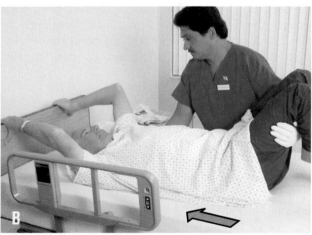

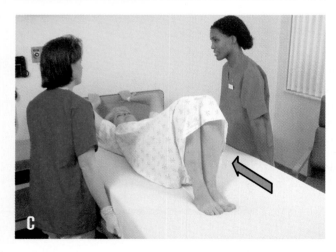

FIGURE 25-26   (a) Moving a helpless patient up in bed.
(b) Moving a patient up in bed with the patient's help.
(c) Patient moving self up in bed.

first move the patient to the edge of the bed by moving the head and shoulders, the torso, and then the lower extremities. In this way, the patient's arms and legs will not hang off of the bed or be forced into the side rails. To maintain proper body alignment, the patient may need to be moved up in bed (Figure 25-26). This is especially true when you are going to elevate the head of the bed.

Range-of-Motion Exercises

It is important in restorative care to keep all of the patient's joints flexible. It is essential to exercise the joints while the patient is confined to bed so that when recovery is complete, the patient will have maximum movement. Exercises of the joints to maintain maximum movement are called *range-of-motion (ROM) exercises*. Since each type of joint moves differently, specific motions are prescribed for each joint type. For example, the ball-and-socket joints of the hip and shoulder have greater range of motion than the elbow, which is a hinge joint.

Review the joints in the musculoskeletal section of this book. Be sure you are familiar with the meanings of the following terms: *abduction, adduction, circumduction, flexion, extension, supination, pronation, inversion,* and *eversion*.

Range-of-motion exercises may be performed by the patient, the nurse, or the patient and the nurse together. **Active range-of-motion exercises** are performed by the patient unassisted. **Passive range-of-motion exercises** are performed by the nurse or clinical care associate when the patient is unable to do so. **Active assist** exercises are done by the nurse with the patient assisting as he or she is able.

Here are some important guidelines to follow when performing range-of-motion exercises:

- Always perform ROM exercises in a logical sequence. Start with the head, and progress from head to toe down one side of the body. Repeat on the other side.
- Always encourage the patient to participate at any level.
- Be gentle. Never force a joint to move beyond its limits or to the point of pain. Stop if the patient complains of pain, and report it to the nurse immediately.
- Never exercise a joint that appears red or swollen. Never exercise a joint that is painful to the touch.
- Support the limb above and below the joint being moved.

procedure

Performing Range-of-Motion Exercises

Assess

Determine the type of range-of-motion exercises appropriate for the patient. Can the patient perform active or active assist ROM exercises, or will passive ROM exercises be most appropriate?

Determine whether a written authorization exists for this procedure.

Plan

Determine when to perform range-of-motion exercises. Can this procedure be incorporated with bathing or turning the patient?

Gather required equipment: bath blanket. Use standard precautions as appropriate.

Implement

1. Loosen the top covers, but do not expose the patient. Use the bath blanket to keep the patient warm (if necessary).
2. Raise the side rail on the far side of the bed.
3. Exercise the neck (Figure 25-27).
4. Hold each extremity to be exercised at the joint (for example, the knee, wrist or elbow).

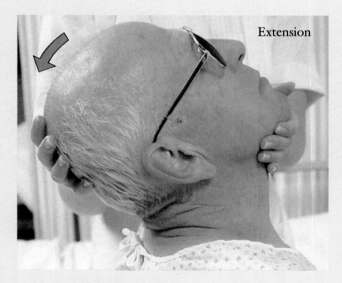
Extension

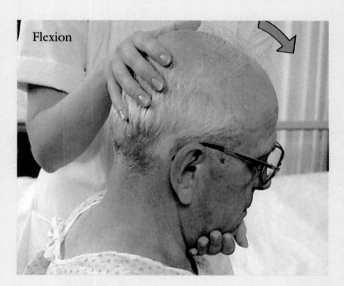
Flexion

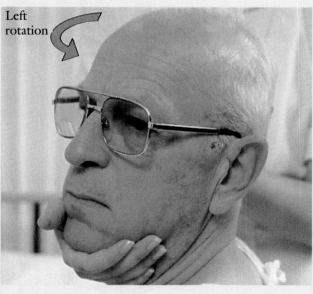
Left rotation

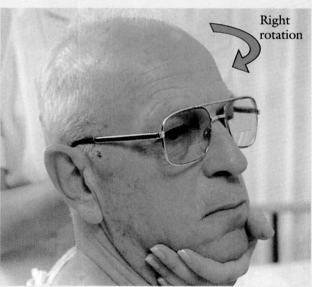
Right rotation

FIGURE 25-27   Exercise the neck.

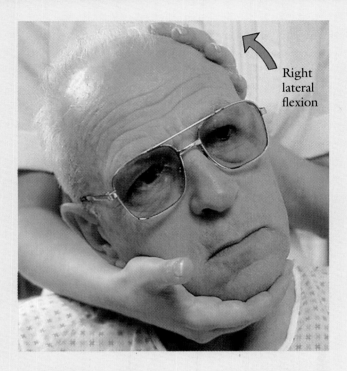

Right lateral flexion

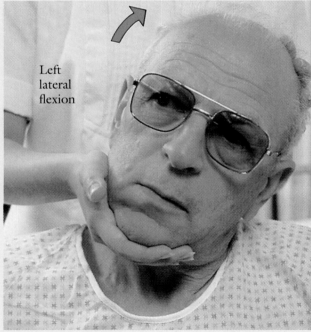

Left lateral flexion

FIGURE 25-27   Exercise the neck. (continued)

5. Exercise the shoulder (Figure 25-28).

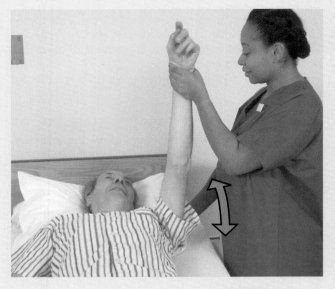

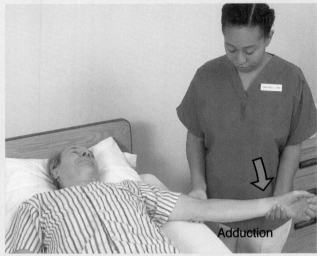

Adduction

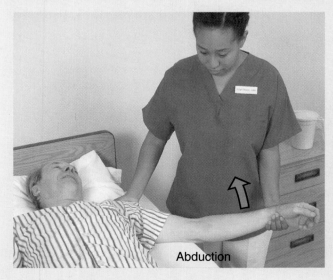

Abduction

FIGURE 25-28   Exercise the shoulders.

p r o c e d u r e   (c o n t i n u e d)

6. Exercise both elbows (Figure 25-29).

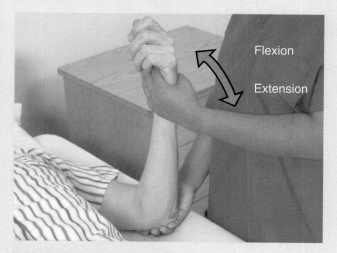

Flexion

Extension

FIGURE 25-29   Exercise the elbows.

7. Exercise both wrists (Figure 25-30).

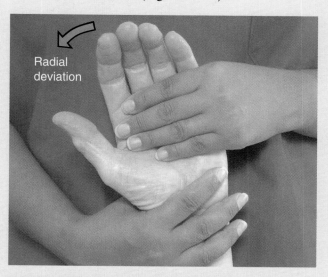

Radial deviation

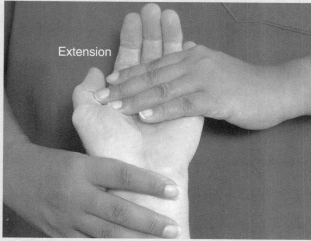

Extension

FIGURE 25-30   Exercise the wrists.

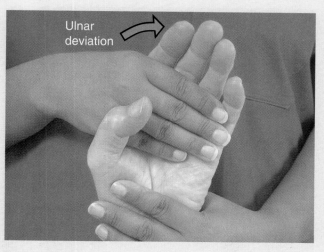

Ulnar deviation

FIGURE 25-30   Exercise the wrists. (continued)

8. Exercise each finger (Figure 25-31).

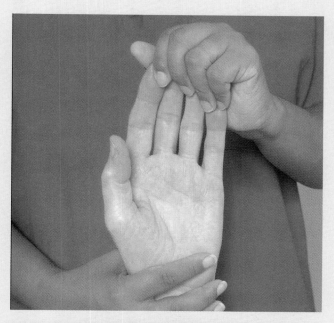

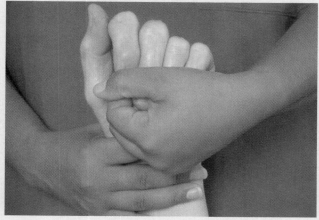

FIGURE 25-31   Exercise the fingers.

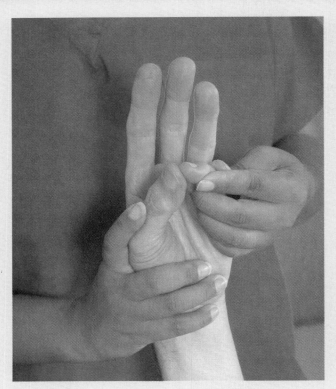

FIGURE 25-31   Exercise the fingers. (continued)

9. Exercise both hips (Figure 25-32).
10. Exercise both knees.

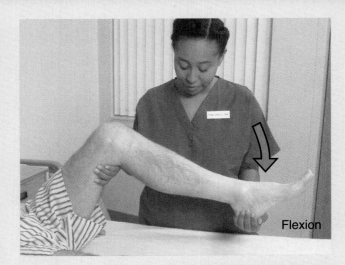

Flexion

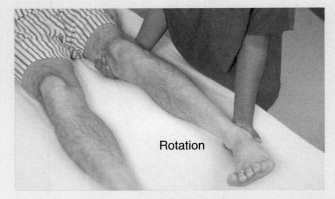

Rotation

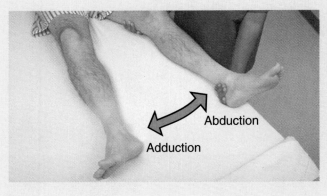

Abduction

Adduction

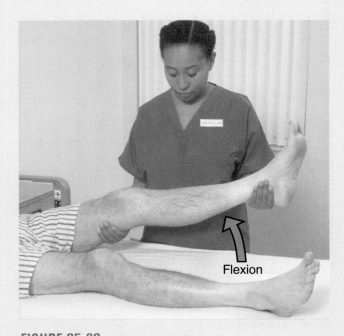

Flexion

FIGURE 25-32   Exercise the hips.

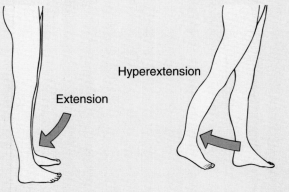

Hyperextension

Extension

FIGURE 25-32   Exercise the hips. (continued)

procedure (continued)

11. Exercise both ankles (Figure 25-33).

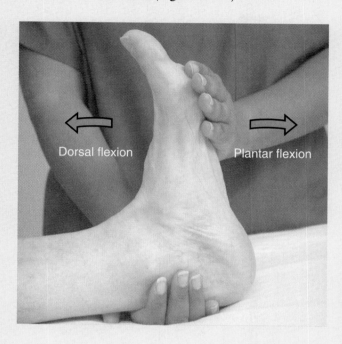

Dorsal flexion   Plantar flexion

12. Exercise each toe (Figure 25-34).

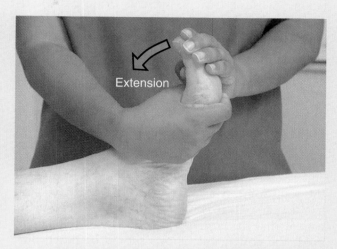

Extension

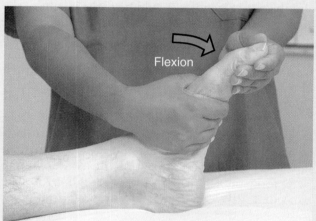

Flexion

FIGURE 25-34   Exercise the toes.

13. Reposition the patient for comfort and safety.
14. Replace the bed covers.

Evaluate

Evaluate your actions. Were you able to move all joints through their full range of motion?

Evaluate the patient's response. Report any complaints of pain and any resistance or difficulty encountered during the exercises.

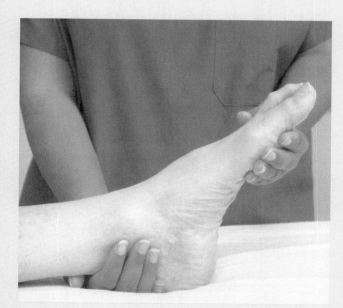

FIGURE 25-33   Exercise the ankles.

Ambulation with Assistive Devices

Patients feel better about themselves when they can perform their own walking or other means of ambulation. Assistive devices, such as crutches, wheelchairs, and walkers, help patients with disabilities to ambulate.

Ambulation with Crutches

Crutches are used to assist in ambulation if an injury to the lower extremities has occurred, but upper-body strength remains intact (Figure 25-35). Crutches may be made of wood or aluminum. They come in many sizes and are adjustable. A rubber tip is in place at the end of each crutch, and foam padding is in place at the top. Some types of crutches have padded grip handles as well. It is imperative to the safety of the patient that the crutches fit properly. As the patient holds the crutch, the elbows should be flexed 30°, and the crutch handles should be at the height of the patient's hip. The top of the crutch should clear the patient's axilla by 2 inches. If the crutch is too tall and the axillary bar does not clear the axilla, permanent brachial nerve damage can occur. If the crutch is too short, the patient will have improper body alignment and will use poor body mechanics.

There are five crutch gaits. They are the *four-point, two-point, three-point, swing-to,* and *swing-through gaits*. In the four-point gait, the patient moves the right crutch forward, then the opposite (left) foot, the left crutch, then the right foot. The two-point gait is actually an advanced four-point gait. In this gait, the right crutch and the left foot advance together, then the left crutch and the right foot advance together. In the three-point gait, the patient advances both crutches, then the affected leg. Body weight is supported with the crutches as the unaffected foot is advanced. The swing-to gait is used generally for weight bearing on one foot only. The unaffected leg and foot bear weight as both crutches are advanced. Then the weight is transferred forward, as both feet swing up to the crutches. The swing-through gait is an advanced modification of the swing-to gait. In this gait, the feet swing through and slightly in front of the crutches. For safety, each crutch should be placed four inches in front and four inches to the side of each foot.

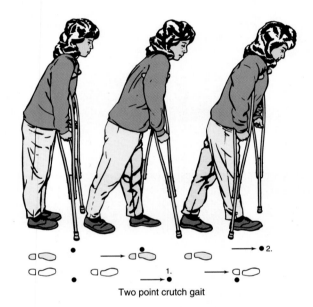

Two point crutch gait

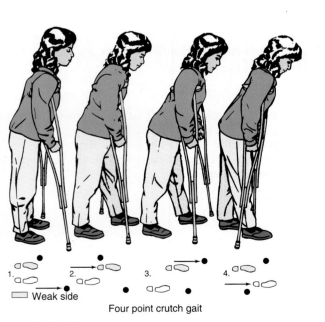

Weak side

Four point crutch gait

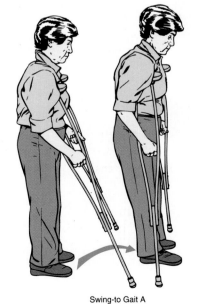

Swing-to Gait A

FIGURE 25-35   Walking with crutches.

procedure
Ambulation with Crutches

Assess

Determine safety needs regarding equipment and footwear. Are the rubber tips and foam padding on the crutches intact? Does the patient have supportive shoes with 1- to 1½-inch heels and nonskid soles?

Determine your own knowledge level. Is there a physician's order for this procedure? Have you been given instructions regarding how to carry out this procedure?

Plan

Gather required equipment: crutches, gait belt, shoes, and robe.

Implement

1. Stand slightly beside and behind the patient.

2. Use a gait belt around the patient's waist for safety.
3. Ensure that the patient does not bear weight on the axillary rest at the top of the crutch.
4. Set realistic distance goals for the patient to ambulate. Do not expect the patient to go too far at one time.
5. Assist the patient to navigate the crutches down stairs using the mnemonic "Good guys go first."

Evaluate

Evaluate your actions. Was the patient steady and safe on the crutches?

Evaluate the patient's actions. Report the distance the patient walked and any complaints of pain or difficulty. Report the type of gait the patient used.

Ambulation with a Gait Belt

A **gait belt** or ambulation belt is used in conjunction with assistive devices to steady the patient and help prevent falls (Figure 25-36). The gait belt is placed around the patient's waist and held posteriorly. Always stand slightly behind and to the side of the patient when assisting with or supervising ambulation. If the patient starts to fall and you are unable to steady him or her, ease the patient to the floor. This will help prevent serious injury to the patient. Assure frightened or weak patients that they are safe (Figure 25-37).

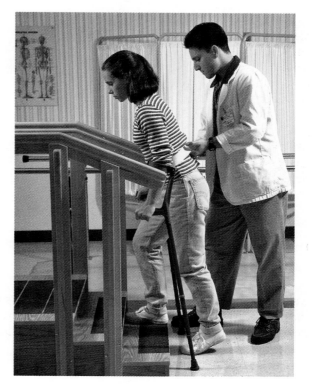

FIGURE 25-37 Stand slightly behind and to the side of the patient when assisting with ambulation.

Ambulation with a Walker

A **walker** is an assistive device used for the ambulation of patients who have full upper-body functioning but whose legs are weak and unsteady. The walker provides a broad base of support with its four legs. The patient must use the walker properly to be safe. The walker should be lifted, never rocked. Instruct the patient to lift all four legs and advance the

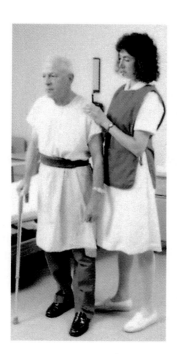

FIGURE 25-36 Patient wearing a gait belt.

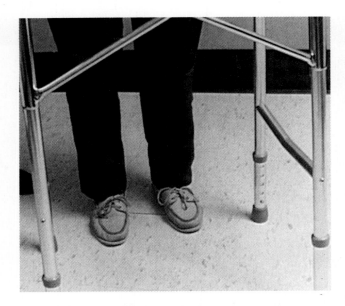

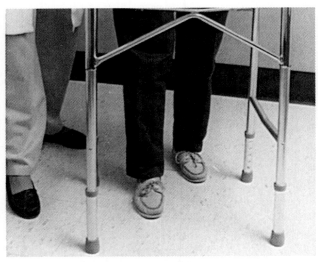

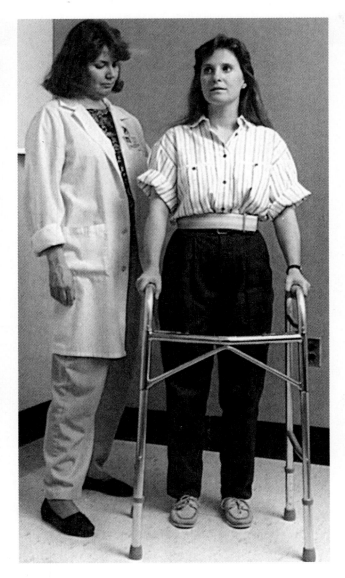

FIGURE 25-38   Walking with a walker.

walker. Instruct the patient to advance the walker so that the rear legs of the walker are in front of the patient's toes. Then the patient should walk into the open area of the walker (Figure 25-38).

Ambulation with a Quad Cane

If the patient is weak or paralyzed on one side, a **quad cane** with a four-prong base may be used. The cane should be held on the unaffected side. The common gait used with a quad cane is to advance the cane with the weakened leg to support the weight of the body.

Transfers

Mobility is essential to restorative care. The goal of mobility is ambulation, but that may not be a realistic goal for some patients. Instead, the goal of sitting up in a chair may be appropriate. Moving the patient out of bed to a chair increases circulation, helps promote lung expansion, stimulates the senses, and encourages progress. This change of position also improves eating, digestion, and elimination processes.

A bedside chair with arms is appropriate for weak patients. Special chairs are available for patients with special needs. Examples of special chairs are wheelchairs, geriatric chairs, recliners, and lift chairs. Whatever chair is used, follow these guidelines for transferring a patient to a chair:

- Lock the brakes on the chair.
- Ensure safety.
- Use leg supports as needed.
- Always secure the correct chair for the patient.

procedure
Ambulation with a Quad Cane

Assess

Determine the patient's level of knowledge and ability. Which gait was the patient taught to use by the therapist? Does the patient require more supervision than you are able to provide?

Determine your own knowledge level. Is there a physician's order for this procedure? Are you comfortable performing this skill?

Determine safety needs regarding equipment and footwear. Are the rubber suction tips on each foot of the cane intact? Does the patient have walking shoes with low, broad heels and nonskid soles?

Determine the fit of the cane. Does it reach the top of the femur? Follow agency protocol regarding adjustments.

Plan

Gather required equipment: quad cane, shoes, and robe.

Implement

Assist the patient with the gait ordered.

Common Gait

1. Move the cane and the weak or affected foot forward, keeping the cane fairly close to the body to prevent leaning.

2. Transfer body weight forward to the cane.
3. Move the strong or unaffected foot forward.
4. When negotiating stairs, remember "Good guys go first."
5. Record all required information on the chart.

Alternative Gait

1. Move the cane forward.
2. Move the weak or affected leg forward to the level of the cane.
3. Move the strong or unaffected leg forward ahead of the cane.
4. When negotiating stairs, remember "Good guys go first."
5. Record all required information on the chart.

Evaluate

Evaluate your actions. Was the patient steady and safe using the cane?

Did you record the date, time, type of cane used, distance walked, any problems encountered, and any complaints by the patient?

Evaluate the patient's response. Report the distance the patient walked and any complaints of pain or difficulty. Report any problems stat.

procedure
Transfers

Assess

Determine the transfer needs of the patient. What is the patient's size? Can one person safely transfer the patient? What functional limitations must be considered? Is there weakness or paralysis on one side? How has this patient been transferred previously?

Determine the patient's ability to sit up. Is the patient elderly or very weak? Is this the patient's first time out of bed?

Plan

Determine which is the patient's dominant, or unaffected, side. This will help you to plan for the patient to assist in the transfer.

Gather required equipment: robe, slippers or shoes, chair or wheelchair, safety belt, and blanket for lap covering. Use standard precautions as appropriate.

Request assistance if needed.

Implement

1. Place the chair or wheelchair next to the bed near the dominant, or unaffected, side of the patient.

2. Ensure that the bed is at its lowest level.
3. Remove the bedcovers.
4. Turn the patient onto one side.
5. Instruct the patient to use the elbow and forearm to push up from the bed as you assist him or her to a sitting position.
6. Assist the patient to sit on the side of the bed.
7. Observe for diaphoresis, change in skin color, or complaints of dizziness. If any of these occur, help the patient to lie back down, and report to the nurse.
8. Check the pulse if the patient is elderly, very weak, or getting out of bed for the first time.
9. Assist the patient with robe and slippers.
10. Assist the patient to the edge of the bed, so that the patient's feet can touch the floor.
11. Instruct the patient to place his or her arms on your shoulders as you place your hands at the patient's waist.
12. Instruct the patient to stand upright and pivot on the count of three.

13. Ask the patient to repeat the instructions back to you. Correct any misunderstandings.

14. Count to three and assist the patient to stand and pivot, with the patient's back to the chair (Figure 25-39).

15. Instruct the patient to reach for the arm of the chair as you lower the patient into the chair.

16. Secure the safety belt, and cover the patient with the blanket, ensuring that it does not touch the floor.

17. Arrange the patient's personal items within reach, including the call light and telephone.

18. Check on the patient at intervals for any signs of distress, such as diaphoresis, change in skin color, or complaints of pain or dizziness.

19. Record all required information on the patient's chart or flowchart.

Evaluate

Evaluate your actions. Were you able to transfer the patient smoothly and safely? Did you record the procedure, the length of time the patient was out of bed, and any problems the patient had tolerating the procedure?

Evaluate the patient's response. Report any diaphoresis, change in skin color, or complaints of pain or dizziness immediately.

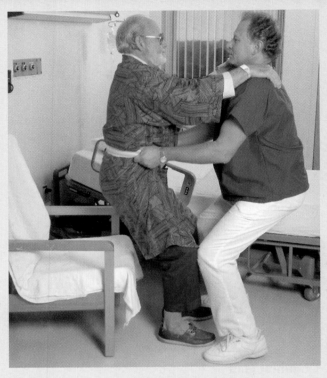

FIGURE 25-39   The use of proper body mechanics during transfers will help you avoid fatigue and injury.

Transfer with a Mechanical Lift

Mechanical hydraulic lifts are devices used to move patients who are unable to tolerate usual transfer techniques. These patients may be unable to bear weight or may be too heavy for other transferring methods. Two types of mechanical lifts are the *Hoyer lift* and the *Versa lift*. Some long-term care facilities require the use of mechanical lifts for *all* transfers (Figure 25-40).

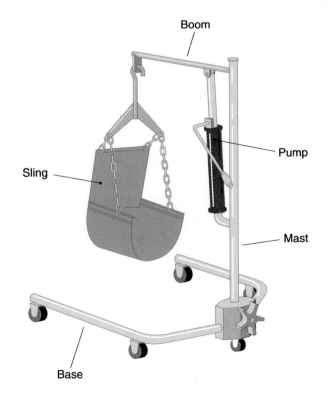

FIGURE 25-40   Mechanical lift.

procedure

Transfer with a Mechanical Lift

Assess

Determine if the equipment is safe. Does the locking mechanism work correctly? Is the canvas sling intact? Does the lift work correctly overall?

Determine the knowledge level of the patient. Does the patient understand the procedure? Can the patient cooperate during the transfer?

Plan

Enlist the help of another health care worker. A mechanical lift should always be operated with two caregivers present.

Gather required equipment: lift, canvas sling, and chains with hooks. Use standard precautions as appropriate.

Implement

1. Position the lift over the bed or chair.
2. Lock the base of the lift.
3. Place the canvas sling under the patient.
4. Attach the chair hooks to the back and the seat on each side of the sling.
5. Pump the jack until the patient's buttocks are no longer touching the bed or chair.
6. Release the base locking mechanism to move the lift.
7. Align the patient correctly over the bed or chair.
8. Lock the base of the lift.
9. Slowly open the release valve to gently lower the patient onto the bed or chair.
10. Remove the canvas sling from beneath the patient.
11. Realign the patient in a safe, comfortable position.

Evaluate

Evaluate your actions. Was the patient transferred in the lift smoothly and safely?

Evaluate the patient's response. Report any complaints of discomfort or any difficulties performing the procedure.

Should a patient fall when being transferred with a lift, follow these guidelines:

- Do not move the patient.
- Call for the nurse stat.
- Remain with the patient.
- Check the patient's vital signs.
- If the patient is able to answer, ask if he or she is experiencing any pain.
- Record all required information on an incident report with the help of the nurse.

Specimen-Collection Skills

A specimen is a sample or small amount of body fluid. A specimen can be tested using some simple tests on the nursing unit, or more extensive tests can be performed in the lab. These tests can provide information about the state of the patient's health. Specimens can be obtained from urine, stool, and sputum (mucus from the lungs).

Urine Specimens

Because urine is a filtration of blood, urine tests can provide a good deal of information about an individual's state of health. Urine specimens can be collected using clean technique or sterile technique.

Collecting Urine Specimens by Clean Technique

To collect a urine specimen by clean technique, first obtain a sterile urine container. Instruct the patient to void in a clean bedpan or in the specimen cup if he or she is able to do so. Obtain 120 cc of urine, then cap the container. This is an adequate amount for a clean specimen.

Tests Performed on Urine Specimens Obtained by Clean Technique   A variety of tests can be performed on specimens obtained by clean technique. The most common are urinalysis and testing for sugar and acetone (S&A). A urinalysis (U/A) is a thorough exam of the urine contents and is performed in a laboratory. The specimen container must be labeled legibly, completely, and accurately (Figure 25-41). Never place the label on the lid. Why? Because when the lid is removed, the sample is no longer identifiable.

Sugar and acetone (S&A) should not be present in normal urine. If a diabetic's blood sugar is high, sugar may appear in the urine. In the diabetic patient, if sugar cannot be metabolized as a fuel source, the body will resort to burning fat for fuel. When the body is using fat for fuel, the by-product is acetone. Sometimes, S&As are called **fractional urines** because they are documented as a fraction (S/A).

Urine tests for sugar and acetone are rarely done since blood tests for glucose are most accurate and

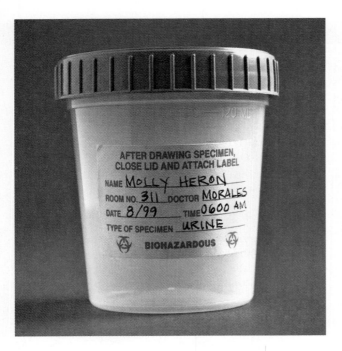

FIGURE 25-41   Specimen labeling must be legible, complete, and accurate.

acetest tablet, test tube, eyedropper, water, and a paper towel. This is a two-part test. To test for sugar, place ten drops of water and five drops of urine in the test tube. Without touching the tablet, drop one clinitest tablet into the test tube and wait 30 seconds while the reaction takes place. Gently swirl the contents, and compare it to the color chart. A negative result will be indicated by blue contents in the test tube. Remember that a chemical reaction occurs inside the test tube; because of this, heat is produced. Do not touch the bottom of the test tube for your own safety. Next, place an acetest tablet onto a paper towel. Release one drop of urine onto the tablet. Wait 10 seconds. Read the results by comparing the color change of the tablet to the acetest chart. No color change indicates a negative result.

The second method of testing for the presence of sugar and acetone is the dipstick method. Different pharmaceutical companies manufacture this product by trade names such as Clinistix, Dipstix, and Ketodiastix. The procedure for using these dipsticks is similar, but there are slight variations. Take a reagent strip from the cylinder container. Dip the stick into the urine sample until the reagent makes contact with the urine. Remove the stick and tap it to remove excess urine. Wait the appropriate time to read the results against the color chart on the outside of the cylinder. Record the results. Always check expiration dates when using reagent tests, and read the instructional information that accompanies each brand.

easy to perform. However, if you are asked to perform an S&A test, it is important that you know the steps to follow. Sugar and acetone can be detected by the **clinitest/acetest tablet** method or the use of a **urine dipstick**. The clinitest/acetest method requires the following equipment: clinitest tablet,

procedure
Collecting a Urine Specimen

Assess
Determine the type of urine test ordered. Do you need to obtain the urine using the clean-catch method, or just obtain a simple specimen for urinalysis?

Determine the patient's toileting status. Will the patient need assistance to the bathroom or bedside commode? Does the patient have a catheter? Determine the patient's understanding of the procedure. Secure patient assistance whenever possible.

Plan
Gather required equipment: gloves, graduate, clean-catch or urinalysis specimen container (Figure 25-42), label, pen, and transport bag. Use standard precautions.

Implement
Obtaining a Specimen for Urinalysis
1. Assist the patient to use the bedpan or urinal, or to void into the specimen container.

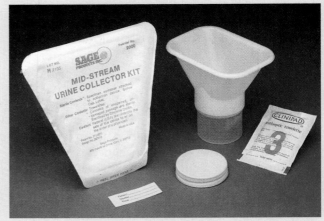

FIGURE 25-42   Midstream urine collection kit.

2. Pour urine from the bedpan or urinal into a graduate to measure and record the amount.

p r o c e d u r e (c o n t i n u e d)

3. Pour 30 cc of urine into a specimen container, and cover it with the lid.
4. Wash and dry the outside of the specimen container.
5. Complete the information required for the label, and apply it to the container.
6. Place the container in a plastic transport bag.
7. Take the specimen to the lab or to the appropriate location for lab pickup.
8. Document in the appropriate place on the chart that the specimen was obtained.

Obtaining a Clean-Catch Midstream Urine Specimen

1. Instruct the patient to cleanse the genital area, or cleanse the area yourself if the patient is unable to do so.
2. Remove the lid from the sterile container without contaminating it.

3. Instruct the patient to begin to void. (If the patient is on intake and output, be sure the urine is voided into a container so it can be measured.)
4. Catch the urine in a sterile container after the patient has voided a small amount.
5. Instruct the patient to finish voiding after the specimen is collected.
6. Place the sterile cap on the container immediately without contaminating the container or the cap.
7. Place the container in a plastic transport bag.
8. Take the specimen to the lab or to the appropriate location for lab pickup.
9. Document in the appropriate place on the chart that the specimen was obtained.

Evaluate

Evaluate your actions. Did you collect the specimen correctly without contamination?

Evaluate the patient's response. Report any abnormal color or odor or the presence of sediment in the urine.

p r o c e d u r e

Collecting an Infant Urine Specimen

Assess

Check the genital area for cleanliness. Ensure that all fecal material has been cleansed, since it will contaminate the urine specimen.

Plan

Gather required equipment: gloves, urine collector, specimen container, label, pen, and transport bag. Use standard precautions.

Implement

1. Remove the infant's diaper.
2. Remove the protective strip from the adhesive on the urine collection bag.
3. Apply the adhesive area to the skin around the male's penis or the female's vulva. Do not place over rectum (Figure 25-43).
4. Reapply the diaper.
5. Check the collection bag for urine every 30 minutes.
6. Once the infant has voided, carefully remove the urine collector.
7. Wash and dry the diaper area, and replace the diaper.
8. Transfer the urine from the collection bag into the specimen container, and cover it immediately.

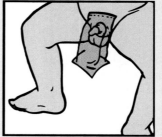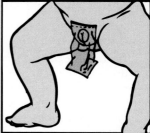

FIGURE 25-43   Placement of infant urine specimen collection bags.

9. Complete and apply the label to specimen container.
10. Place the container in a plastic transport bag.
11. Take the specimen to the lab or to the appropriate location for lab pickup.
12. Document in the appropriate place on the chart that the specimen was obtained.

Evaluate

Evaluate your actions. Did you collect the specimen correctly without contamination?

Evaluate the patient's response. Report any abnormal color or odor or the presence of sediment in the urine.

Collecting a 24-Hour Urine Specimen

A **24-hour urine specimen** is ordered for many different reasons. It is important to follow these guidelines to ensure the accuracy of the test. First, obtain from the lab a 24-hour urine collection container with any needed chemicals inside. Store the container properly during the 24-hour period. In most situations, the container must be kept on ice. This is done by filling a wash basin with ice and placing the collection container inside it, much like sodas in an ice chest. Place signs in the patient's bathroom near the toilet and by the bedside to indicate that a 24-hour urine specimen is in progress. Anyone who assists the patient with toileting will know to save the specimen. Begin the test by asking the patient to void. Mark the 24-hour test sheet to begin with this time. Discard this specimen. Each time the patient voids during the next 24 hours, examine and measure the urine, then pour it into the collection container. Record the time and amount on the test sheet. Continue this collection until the 24-hour period ends. If the patient must void in a bedpan, take care that no toilet paper enters the specimen. It is also important to keep the specimen from being contaminated with feces.

procedure

Collecting a 24-Hour Urine Specimen

Assess

Determine the appropriate method for collecting the urine specimen. When is the best time to begin the test? Does the patient understand the instructions to assist with the test? Do you need to review the procedure before you begin?

Plan

Gather required equipment: gloves, two signs, 24-hour specimen container, container for ice, ice, intake-and-output record, and pen. Use standard precautions.

Implement

1. Instruct the patient to void, then discard the voided urine. (If the patient is on intake and output, be sure to record the amount voided.)
2. Note the time the patient voided. This will be the beginning time of the 24-hour test.
3. Place signs marked with the beginning and ending times of the test in appropriate locations.
4. Pour all urine voided within the 24-hour period into the special specimen container, which has been placed on ice.
5. Instruct the patient to void when the 24-hour period is at an end.
6. Pour the final urine into the 24-hour specimen container.
7. Remove the signs.
8. Label the 24-hour specimen container, and transport it to the lab or to the appropriate location for lab pickup.
9. Document in the appropriate place on the chart that the specimen was obtained.

Evaluate

Evaluate your actions. Was all urine collected during the 24-hour period?

Evaluate the patient's response. Report any abnormalities of color or smell of the urine.

Ensure that the patient is safe and comfortable before leaving the bedside.

Straining Urine

Urine must be strained if renal calculi (**kidney stones**) are suspected. It is imperative to perform this procedure accurately because when a kidney stone is passed, the course of treatment changes. Use a paper urine strainer to strain all urine saved by the patient. Pour the urine through the filter, and save any residue as a specimen. Record and report any sediment or residue remaining in the filter.

Collecting Stool Specimens

Stool specimens or samples may be ordered to detect abnormalities of the intestines. Two common stool tests are the **Hemoccult test** and the **ova and parasites (O&P)** test. The Hemoccult test is ordered to detect occult blood (*hemo-* means "blood," and *occult* means "hidden"). Bleeding may occur along the digestive tract in small amounts not visible to the naked eye.

procedure
Straining Urine

Assess

Determine whether any obstacles exist in implementing this procedure. Is the patient incontinent? Do you need to review the steps in the procedure?

Plan

Gather required equipment: gloves, disposable strainer, sign, intake-and-output record, and pen. Use standard precautions.

Implement

1. Instruct the patient to void only into a bedpan, urinal, bedside commode, or urine-measuring device.
2. Instruct the patient to notify the nursing staff each time urine is voided.
3. Carefully pour the urine from the receptacle through the disposable strainer (Figure 25-44).
4. Inspect the strainer for any sediment, especially anything that resembles gravel, sand, or irregularly surfaced sand stones.
5. Save any sediment found in the strainer, and notify the nurse.
6. Record the amount of urine on the intake-and-output record.

Evaluate

Evaluate your actions. Did you strain all of the urine for sediment?

Evaluate the patient's response. Report any abnormalities of urine color or odor as well as any sediment found in the strainer.

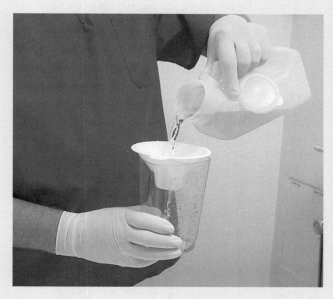

FIGURE 25-44 Pour the urine through the strainer.

procedure
Collecting a Stool Specimen for Occult Blood

Assess

Determine the patient's toileting status. Will the patient need assistance to the bedside commode or bathroom? Is the patient incontinent? Will you need assistance to perform this procedure?

Plan

Gather required equipment: gloves, bed pan, Hemoccult slide packet (Figure 25-45), paper towel, applicator, biohazard bag, developing solution, pen, and transport bag. Use standard precautions.

Implement

1. Instruct the patient to notify you when the urge to defecate is felt.
2. Collect the specimen in the bedpan.

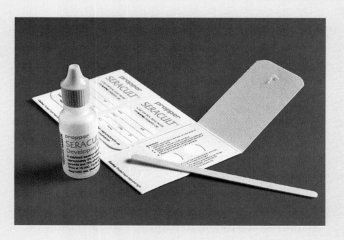

FIGURE 25-45 Hemoccult slide packet.

p r o c e d u r e   (c o n t i n u e d)

3. Take the specimen to the dirty utility room (or the patient's bathroom).
4. Place Hemoccult slide packet on top of a paper towel.
5. Open the front cover or flap of the packet.
6. Use the applicator to smear a small amount of stool on the correct area of the slide.
7. Discard the applicator in the biohazard bag.
8. For a guiac test, place the correct amount of developing solution on the guiac paper.
9. Wait for the specified amount of time, then read and record the results.
10. Close the cover or flap of the packet.
11. Place the packet in the transport bag, and take it to the lab or to the appropriate location for lab pickup.

Evaluate

Evaluate your actions. Did the paper around the specimen change color when the developer was applied?

Evaluate the patient's response. Report any abnormal findings, such as positive color changes on the Hemoccult slide or abnormal color, consistency, or odor of feces.

Collecting a Stool Specimen for Ova and Parasites Test

A test for ova and parasites is a test to detect worms and their eggs. Pinworms, tapeworms, and hookworms are all parasites. A *parasite* is an organism that obtains its nourishment from another organism. Parasites may live in or on another living being. *Ova* is the term for eggs. This test must be performed on a fresh stool specimen, not one that has been refrigerated.

Collecting Sputum Specimens

Sputum is a secretion from the lower *respiratory tree*, a term used to describe the bronchial tubes and lungs. Sputum is produced in response to bronchial or lung irritation. Such a response by the body may or may not be due to an infection. Noninfected sputum is white or clear. Infected sputum is yellow, green, bloody, or blood-tinged. Because sputum is viscous (thick, sticky, or glutinous), it may be difficult to expectorate (cough up from the lungs). Encourage the patient to drink warm fluids to help moisten and loosen bronchial secretions. Plan to obtain a sputum specimen early in the morning before the patient has anything to eat or drink and before the patient has brushed his or her teeth. The first morning specimen will contain the largest number of microbes or cells needed for laboratory tests. Assist the patient to sit in high Fowler's position. Instruct the patient to inhale and exhale deeply twice. Instead of the third exhalation, instruct the patient to cough. The cough should raise sputum into the mouth. Instruct the patient to spit it directly into the specimen container. Do not use sputum that has been expectorated into a tissue. As with any specimen, wear gloves and avoid contaminating the specimen container. Sputum tests can detect the presence of chronic lung diseases, cancer, tuberculosis (TB), and pneumonia.

p r o c e d u r e

Collecting a Stool Specimen for Ova and Parasites Test

Assess

Determine the toileting status of the patient. Will the patient need assistance to the bedside commode or bathroom? Is the patient incontinent? Will you need assistance to perform this procedure?

Plan

Gather required equipment: gloves, bedpan, tongue blades, specimen container, biohazard bag, label, pen, and transport bag. Use standard precautions.

Implement

1. Instruct the patient to notify you when the urge to defecate is felt.
2. Collect the specimen in the bedpan.
3. Take the specimen to the dirty utility room (or the patient's bathroom).
4. Use tongue blades to transfer the stool specimen from the bedpan to the specimen container.
5. Discard the tongue blades in the biohazard bag.
6. Place the lid on the specimen container, and label it.
7. Place the specimen container in the plastic transport bag, and seal it.
8. Take the specimen to the lab or to the appropriate location for lab pickup.
9. Document in the appropriate place on the chart that the specimen was obtained.

Evaluate

Evaluate your actions. Did you collect the stool specimen correctly, free from urine contamination?

Evaluate the patient's response. Report any abnormalities of the stool, especially the presence of mucus or blood.

procedure
Collecting a Sputum Specimen

Assess

Determine the best time to obtain the specimen. Which shift can best get an early morning specimen? Will you need an N–95 TB respiratory mask or a standard face mask? Will you need protective eyewear or a gown to ensure your safety?

Determine the patient's ability to understand and cooperate with the procedure.

Determine your own knowledge of the procedure. Do you need to review the procedure? Can you give correct instructions to the patient?

Plan

Gather required equipment: gloves, sterile specimen cup, label, pen, and transport bag. Stand to the side of the patient to avoid being contaminated when the patient coughs. Use standard precautions.

Implement

1. Place the patient in high Fowler's position.
2. Unwrap the sterile specimen cup.
3. Hold the sterile specimen cup near the patient's mouth.
4. Instruct the patient to take three deep breaths and to cough on the third expiration.
5. Instruct the patient to expectorate directly into the specimen cup.
6. Place the lid on the cup without contaminating it, and attach the completed label.
7. Place the specimen cup in the plastic transport bag, and seal it.
8. Take the specimen to the lab or to the appropriate location for lab pickup.
9. Document in the appropriate place on the chart that the specimen was obtained.

Evaluate

Evaluate your actions. Was the specimen obtained from the lungs and not the mouth?

Evaluate the patient's response. Report any green, yellow, brown, blood-tinged, or blood-streaked sputum stat. Report thick, sticky, or stringy sputum.

Collecting Throat Cultures

Throat and wound cultures can be taken using a culture kit. This kit contains a cotton-tipped applicator and a test tube filled with nutrient broth.

procedure
Collecting a Throat Culture

Assess

Determine the patient's ability to cooperate with the procedure. It the patient alert? Is the patient able to hold the mouth open while the culture is taken? Will you need assistance to perform this procedure?

Determine your own knowledge level. Is there a written order for the procedure? Do you need to review the procedure? Have you performed this procedure before? Do you remember the principles of sterile technique? This is a sterile procedure, and accurate results are essential for the correct treatment to be prescribed.

Plan

Gather required equipment: gloves, culture kit, penlight, tongue depressor, label, pen, and transport bag. Use standard precautions.

Implement

1. Open the culture kit (Figure 25-46) without contaminating the contents.

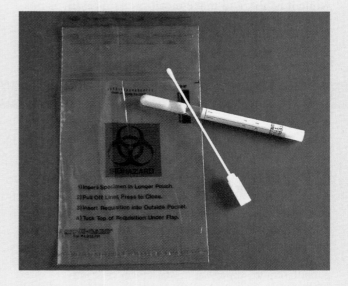

FIGURE 25-46   Culture kit.

p r o c e d u r e (c o n t i n u e d)

2. Instruct the patient to open the mouth as widely as possible.
3. Examine the throat quickly using the penlight.
4. Hold the tongue down with a tongue depressor held in one hand, and hold the sterile swab in the other hand.
5. Ask the patient to say "Ah," which will lower the tongue.
6. Quickly insert the swab into the back of the throat, and slide it over at least two areas, especially any areas with obvious secretions.
7. Remove the swab and tongue depressor from the patient's mouth.
8. Carefully open the test tube, and insert the cotton-tipped swab without contaminating it.

9. Replace the lid, and label the specimen.
10. Place the specimen container in the transport bag.
11. Take the specimen to the lab or to the appropriate location for lab pickup.
12. Reposition the patient for comfort and safety.
13. Document in the appropriate place on the chart that the specimen was obtained.

Evaluate

Evaluate your actions. Did you take the culture from at least two areas of the throat?

Evaluate the patient's response. Report any unusual observations of the patient's throat or any complaints of pain during the procedure.

Nutrition Skills

Nutrition, as stated in Unit 6, is essential to healthy body cells. The body needs protein to rebuild and repair cells, and it needs carbohydrates for energy to heal. In addition, fat functions to cushion the major organs.

Feeding a Patient

Meals are normally a time for socialization and pleasure. Mealtimes for patients in a health care institution should be made pleasant and special. Individuals who have difficulty swallowing or chewing may become frustrated at mealtime. Patients who have poor appetites or dysfunctional digestive tracts may be discouraged when it is time to eat. Always serve food while it is hot, and make mealtime as pleasant as possible. Remove any bedpans, emesis basins, or urinals from the eating area. Always be sure that each tray is served to the correct patient.

Encourage patients to be as independent as possible during mealtime, but assist with feeding as needed. Some patients may be too weak to feed themselves. Others may have **dysphagia** (difficulty swallowing) or be restricted by physician's orders so that they are unable to feed themselves. Patients with arthritis or paralysis of the hands will require assistance with meals. Patients with cognitive impairments such as Alzheimer's disease may need verbal reminders to swallow. If a patient is visually impaired, set up the tray so that the food placement corresponds to a clock. Never put hot liquids at the six o'clock space. This will prevent a visually impaired patient from accidentally being burned.

As you feed patients, allow time for chewing, swallowing, and settling of food before the next bite. Do not rush the patient during a meal. It is very important to supervise dysphagia patients during mealtime to prevent choking.

p r o c e d u r e
Feeding a Patient

Assess

Determine the required preparation for meals. How much time is needed to assist the patient with cleaning teeth or dentures? How much time is needed to assist the patient with toileting?

Does the patient require transportation to a dining area?

Determine the feeding needs of the patient. Does the patient require supervision, assistance, or complete care? What is the patient's diet?

Plan

Ensure that the patient is prepared for the meal (face and hands have been washed, oral hygiene has been performed, and the patient has been to the bathroom if needed).

Ensure that the bedside area is cleared and clean. Determine the patient's diet order. Know if patient is on a calorie count.

Gather required equipment: patient's tray with sugar, salt, straws, and condiments (condiments may be limited or withheld due to special diet orders); napkin or towel. Use standard precautions as appropriate.

procedure (continued)

Implement

1. Place the tray on the over-bed table.
2. Position a napkin or towel under the patient's chin.
3. Assist the patient as needed by cutting meat, opening cartons, and buttering bread.
4. Test the temperature of hot liquids or foods on your wrist.
5. Use a separate straw for each liquid.
6. Place a small amount of food on the spoon, and identify it for the patient.
7. Feed the patient from the tip of the spoon, holding it at a right angle to the patient's mouth.
8. Allow time for the patient to chew the food.
9. Alternate giving the patient liquids and solids.
10. Wipe the patient's mouth periodically.
11. Encourage the patient to eat as much as possible.
12. Provide conversation as appropriate.
13. Measure and record liquid intake if the patient is on intake and output.
14. Record the percentage of food eaten from the tray.
15. Position the patient for comfort and safety before leaving the bedside.

Evaluate

Evaluate the patient's response. Was the patient able to chew and swallow all foods on the tray? Were there foods that the patient disliked or could not eat on the tray? Report any difficulty the patient experienced while being fed. If the patient is on a calorie count, record the percentage of each food or fluid ingested.

Basic Elimination Skills

Elimination of waste products from the body is a normal and necessary process. Some of your patients, however, may have conditions that interfere with normal elimination. Other patients may be confined to bed and unable to get to the bathroom. Whatever the particular situation, you will need to assist the patient in meeting his or her elimination needs. Some patients will require assistance with toileting, whereas others will require more specialized care.

Assisting with a Bedpan

Some patients may not be able to take care of their own toileting needs. If patients are weak or confined to bed, you will need to assist them. Bed-confined patients use a bedpan for toileting. Most patients can use regular bedpans. Patients who cannot move (because they are in a cast or in traction, for example) may need to use a fracture pan. Bedpans are usually made of plastic.

procedure
Assisting with a Bedpan

Assess

Determine the patient's ability to assist with the procedure. Does the patient have any disabilities or mobility problems? Will you need assistance to get the patient on and off of the bedpan?

Determine any special needs to consider. Is this an emergency need? Is the patient being bowel- or bladder-trained? Does the patient have any skin problems, such as reddened areas or an open sacral area? What type of bedpan should be used?

Plan

Gather required equipment: gloves, bedpan, toilet paper, washcloth, and soap. Use standard precautions.

Implement

1. Instruct the patient to flex the knees and place weight on the feet (Figure 25-47A).
2. Establish a signal, and when ready, give the signal.

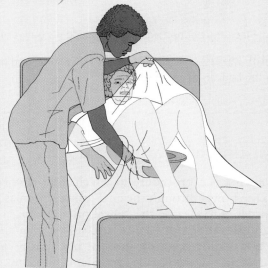

A Slide the bedpan under the resident's buttocks.

FIGURE 25-47A Instruct the patient to flex the knees and place weight on the feet.

p r o c e d u r e   (c o n t i n u e d)

3. Raise the patient's hips with your hand under the small of the patient's back, and slide the bedpan into place.

Alternate Method for Placing Bedpan

Turn the patient to the side, position the bedpan over the buttocks, and holding the bedpan in place, turn the patient onto his or her back (Figure 25-47B).

4. Correctly support the patient on the bedpan (Figure 25-47C).
5. Provide the call signal and toilet paper.
6. Provide privacy.
7. Answer the call signal immediately.
8. Correctly remove the bedpan and cover with a paper towel.

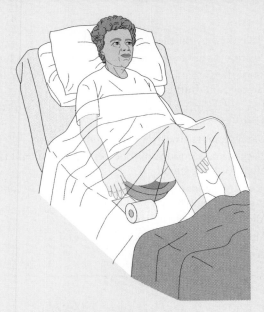

C Adjust the head of the bed so that the resident is in a sitting position.

FIGURE 25-47C Correctly support the patient on the bedpan.

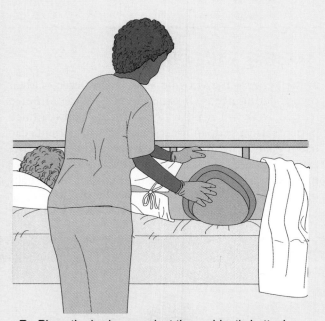

B Place the bedpan against the resident's buttocks

FIGURE 25-47B Turn the patient to the side, and position the bedpan over the buttocks.

9. Place the covered bedpan on a chair while you assist the patient with cleaning the genital area.
10. Dispose of bedpan contents, remembering to measure liquid output if the patient is on intake and output.

Evaluate

Evaluate your actions. Were you able to place and remove the bedpan without difficulty?

Evaluate the patient's response. Report any abnormalities of urine or stool. Report any significant complaints of pain or discomfort during the procedure.

Assisting with an Enema

An **enema** is a procedure in which fluid is injected into the bowel through the anal orifice. Enemas may be ordered to cleanse the bowel prior to surgery or diagnostic studies or to evacuate stool remaining in the bowel due to constipation or **impaction** (hardened stool). Occasionally, an enema is given as a medicinal treatment to return normal flora to the bowel. Enemas may be commercially prepared, or they may be prepared just before use. State regula-

tions may limit or prohibit an unlicensed caregiver's administering an enema in long-term care. A doctor's order is required for any enema.

Commercially prepared enemas are sometimes called **Fleet enemas** after the first manufacturer (Figure 25-48). Enemas of this type contain a small quantity of fluid and come in two forms: **saline** and **oil-retention enemas**. Oil-retention enemas are used to soften feces so they can be evacuated. *Retention* means "to hold in," and these enemas must be held by the patient long enough for the oil to soften the fecal matter.

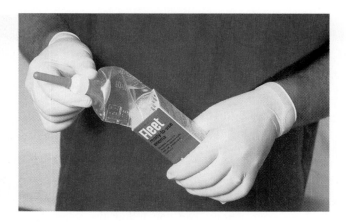

FIGURE 25-48   Commercially prepared enema.

A **soapsuds enema (SSE)** must be prepared manually. An enema kit is needed for this purpose. An enema kit contains a disposable bag or bucket, tubing with a clamp, and a mild soap such as castile (Figure 25-49). Soapsuds enemas are administered with caution because they can be very irritating to the bowel. General guidelines for preparing a soapsuds enema are to mix one packet of liquid enema soap with 1,000 cc of warm water. The water should be at 105° F.

Place the patient in Sim's (left lateral) position to prevent injury during the enema. Always use a water-soluble lubricant jelly to lubricate the tip of the tubing before inserting it into the anal orifice.

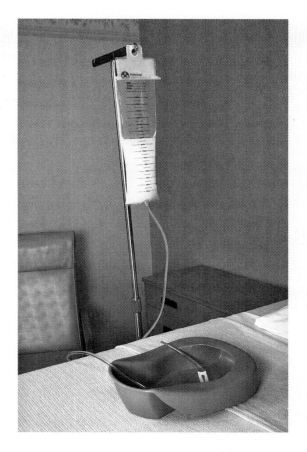

FIGURE 25-49   For certain types of enemas, an enema kit is needed.

procedure
Assisting with an Enema

Assess
Determine the patient's ability to assist with the procedure. Will the patient need to use the bedpan, a commode, or the bathroom? What is the mobility status of the patient? Will you need assistance to perform this procedure?

Plan
Gather required equipment: gloves, enema kit, bed protector, bath blanket, lubricating jelly, and pen. Use standard precautions.

Implement
Administering a Soapsuds Enema
1. Prepare the enema solution, and expel all air in the tubing.
2. Place the bed protector under the patient's buttocks.
3. Assist the patient to Sim's position.
4. Drape the bath blanket to cover the patient, but fold it back to expose the anal area.
5. Lift the buttock to expose the anus.
6. Insert the lubricated tip of the enema tubing 2 to 4 inches into the rectum. If resistance is met, do *not* force the tubing. Remove and report the situation.
7. Instruct the patient to relax and breathe deeply.
8. Open the clamp to allow the solution to flow.
9. Raise the enema container 12 inches above the anus to obtain a slow flow.
10. Clamp the tubing when all of the solution, but not air, has entered the rectum.
11. Encourage the patient to retain the enema solution for 5 to 10 minutes.
12. Position the patient on a bedpan, or assist the patient to the bathroom.
13. Record and report the results of the enema.

Administering a Disposable Enema

Follow steps 2 through 7 for soapsuds enema, then

8. Squeeze the enema container to push the solution through the tip.
9. Squeeze the container in a spiral fashion to expel all of the solution.
10. Hold the container at an angle to avoid introducing air bubbles.
11. Encourage the patient to retain the enema solution for 5 to 10 minutes.
12. Position the patient on a bedpan, or assist the patient to the bathroom.
13. Record and report the results of the enema.

Administering an Oil-Retention Enema

Follow steps 2 through 7 for soapsuds enema, then

8. Squeeze the container to push the oil to the tip.
9. Coil the container to expel all of the solution.
10. Encourage the patient to retain the enema solution for at least 5 to 10 minutes.
11. Position the patient on a bedpan, or assist the patient to the bathroom.
12. Record and report the results of the enema.

Evaluate

Evaluate your actions. Did you follow the steps of the procedure?

Evaluate the patient's reactions. Report any complaints of pain during the procedure. Report any abnormalities in the enema return, such as blood or mucus in the stool. Report and record the amount, color, and consistency of the enema return.

Catheter Care

Catheters are flexible tubes used to drain fluids from the body. Urinary catheters are inserted through the urethra into the bladder to drain urine. Sterile technique is required because the urinary system is a sterile system and connects directly to the blood supply. If microorganisms are introduced, major damage to the kidneys, such as nephritis, can result. The microorganisms could also enter the bloodstream and cause septicemia.

Catheter care is a vital component of quality care. Catheter care involves special cleaning procedures for the genital area of the patient with an indwelling catheter. Each facility has policies regarding the procedure and frequency of catheter care.

When you care for a patient with an indwelling catheter, follow these general guidelines.

- Keep the tubing free from kinks, with excess tubing coiled on the bed. This allows the urine to flow by gravity into the drainage bag.
- Always keep the drainage bag below the level of the bladder to prevent the return of the urine into the bladder.
- Do not place the drainage bag on the floor or in the patient's lap.
- Be alert for patient complaints of pain, burning, or urges to urinate.
- If permitted, encourage the patient to drink plenty of fluids.
- Observe the color, odor, amount, and clarity of the urine.

- Hang the collection bag on the side of the bed facing the door for easy observation. Never hang the bag from the side rail. Instead, use the bed frame to attach the bag to the bed (Figure 25-50).
- Some patients may use a leg bag instead of a drainage bag, especially if the patient is ambulatory or usually dresses in pants. Whatever type of drainage bag is used, always use a leg strap or tape the catheter tubing to the patient's thigh to prevent movement of the catheter.

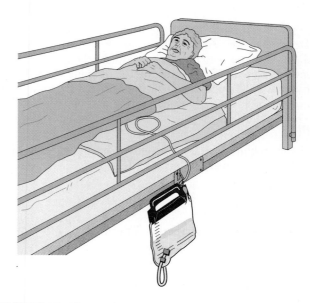

FIGURE 25-50   Use the bed frame to attach the catheter collection bag.

procedure

Catheter Care

Assess

Determine your own knowledge level. Is there a written order for the procedure? Do you need to review the procedure?

Determine the best time to perform the procedure. Can this procedure be performed with personal care?

Determine any special considerations for performing the procedure.

Plan

Gather required equipment: gloves and catheter care kit *or* washcloth, towel, soap, and water. Use standard precautions.

Plan to preserve the patient's right to privacy when performing this procedure.

Implement

1. Employ standard precautions.
2. Explain the procedure to the patient.
3. Handle the catheter and drainage bag gently.
4. Cleanse around the catheter insertion site. For males, retract the foreskin and cleanse in a circular motion from the insertion site outward. For females, clean the perineal area from front to back.
5. Clean the catheter by starting at the insertion site and wiping the tubing in the direction away from the patient.
6. Record the procedure and your observations on the appropriate chart form.

Evaluate

Evaluate your actions. Did you clean the area in such a way as to prevent contamination? Is the catheter patent (unobstructed) and flowing?

Evaluate the patient's response. Report any complaints of pain during the procedure. Report any leakage or drainage around the catheter urinary meatus.

Special Applications and Preps

Often patients will need care in the application or use of special items, such as stockings, bandages, a specialty bath, or an application of heat or cold. Also, frequently special preparations are needed for patients preparing for surgery. It is important that you know and implement these skills properly.

Heat and Cold Applications

Heat applications are used as a treatment to promote healing by increasing oxygen and nutrient delivery to the tissues. This treatment may also be used to ease inflammatory pain caused by blood vessel congestion.

Heat applications can be classified as dry or moist. Dry applications do not contain any water; dry applications include heat lamps, Aqua-K pads, and electric heating pads. Moist applications include warm soaks, warm compresses, moist heating pads, sitz baths, and tub baths.

Cold applications are used to reduce swelling, fever, and pain, since cold constricts blood vessels. Cold applications are also classified as dry or moist. Dry applications include a hypothermia blanket, ice packs/collars, and a commercial cold pack unit. Moist applications include cold compresses, cool wet packs, and cool soaks.

Heat and cold applications are most effective when applied for 20 minutes. After that length of time, the temperature of the treatment begins to change. Physicians order these types of treatments, so always follow the written order.

Sitz Baths

A **sitz bath** is a procedure designed to soak the perineal area in water without immersing the patient in a full tub of water. Portable sitz baths are convenient, plastic, disposable units that the patient can use once he or she understands the procedure (Figure 25-51). Because the sitz bath bag is similar to an enema bag, it can be used to deliver medicated liquids as well as tap water.

Sitz baths are ordered after vaginal and rectal surgery to promote healing of wounds and to prevent infections. A sitz bath can also be ordered as a comfort measure for the patient with hemorrhoids.

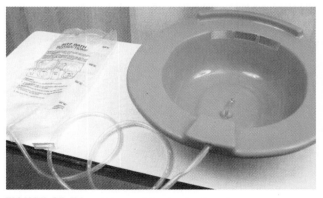

FIGURE 25-51 Disposable sitz bath unit.

p r o c e d u r e
Assisting with a Sitz Bath

Assess

Determine the type of equipment available. Will the patient be using a tub, chair, or portable unit?

Determine the needs of the patient. What is the patient's mobility level? Will you need assistance to perform this procedure? During the 20-minute procedure, can you leave the patient alone with instructions to use the call light if you are needed?

Plan

Gather required equipment: towels, robe, slippers, and portable sitz unit if appropriate. Use standard precautions.

Some patients, especially maternity patients with portable units, may prefer to be given instructions and left to function independently.

Implement
Using a Sitz Chair or Tub

1. Set the temperature at 105° F.
2. Fill the chair or tub with the appropriate amount of water.
3. Plug in the electrical cord.
4. Place a towel in the bottom of the chair or tub to prevent slipping.
5. Assist the patient to a comfortable position with the perineal area in the water.

6. Cover exposed parts of the body.
7. Continue the procedure for 20 minutes or as ordered.
8. Record the procedure on the appropriate form.

Using a Portable Sitz Unit

1. Place the sitz unit on a commode or toilet seat.
2. Connect the tubing to the sitz unit, and clamp.
3. Position the tubing so that the holes are facing inside the sitz unit.
4. Fill the bag with water at a temperature of 110° F to 115° F.
5. Assist the patient to a comfortable position with the perineal area in the water.
6. Cover exposed parts of the body.
7. Continue the procedure for 20 minutes or as ordered.
8. Record the procedure on the appropriate form.

Evaluate

Evaluate your actions. Was the bath the correct temperature and duration?

Evaluate the patient's response. Did the bath soothe the patient's discomfort? Report any complaints of pain or discomfort during the procedure. Report the patient's response to the therapy. Report the patient's level of participation.

Preparing a Patient for an Exam

Occasionally, examinations and procedures are performed at the bedside. You may need to prepare the patient for a respiratory, gynecological, endoscopic, rectal, or spinal exam. Certain exams require specific positions (Figures 25-52 through 25-59).

Sim's position or the left lateral position is used for rectal exams and procedures. **Fowler's position** may be used during respiratory exams. The **dorsal lithotomy** position is used for gynecological and urethral exams and procedures. The **knee-chest position** may be an alternative to Sim's position, depending on the patient's mobility. The **supine** (horizontal recumbent) **position** may be used for abdominal exams and procedures. The **prone position** is used for spinal exams and procedures.

Fowler's position is generally a bed position. This position is expressed as Fowler's and semi-Fowler's, and the degrees of elevation are noted. This position assists the patient with respiratory problems to breath more easily. It is also the position used for enteral feedings.

Always know the position patients are permitted to use before changing the level of the head or the foot of the bed. Know the types of patient positions for the various types of examinations. Assist the patient, and ensure safety, comfort, and privacy.

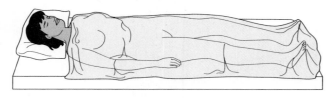

FIGURE 25-52 Horizontal recumbent position (supine position).

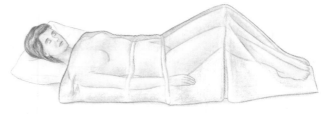

FIGURE 25-53 Dorsal recumbent position.

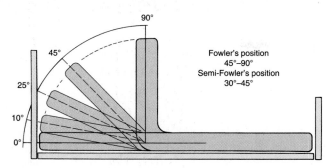

FIGURE 25-54   Fowler's position.

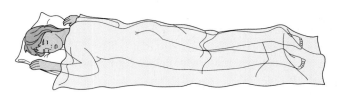

FIGURE 25-57   Prone position.

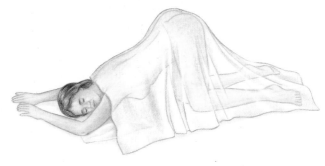

FIGURE 25-55   Knee-chest position.

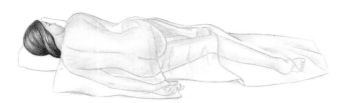

FIGURE 25-58   Left Sim's position.

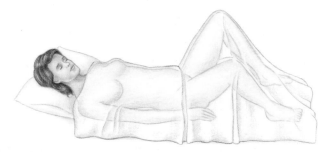

FIGURE 25-56   Dorsal lithotomy position.

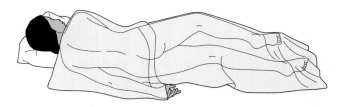

FIGURE 25-59   Left lateral position.

procedure

Preparing a Patient for an Exam

Assess

Determine the doctor's needs for the procedure. In what position should you place the patient? (If you are unsure, ask the nurse for help.) What equipment will be needed for this procedure or exam?

Determine the patient's needs for the procedure. What is the patient's level of mobility? Will you need assistance during this procedure? What is the patient's knowledge level regarding the exam or procedure?

Plan

Gather required equipment: gloves, bath blanket, sheet or drape, pillows, and any specialized equipment needed. Use standard precautions.

Arrange for the patient's privacy.

Implement

1. Raise the level of the bed, and lower the side rails.

p r o c e d u r e (c o n t i n u e d)

2. Assist the patient into the correct position, and check body alignment.

3. Drape the patient with a bath blanket, sheet, or disposable drape.

4. Raise the side rails.

5. Remain with the patient as long as the bed is elevated. If you must leave before the physician is ready, lower the bed.

6. Assist the physician as necessary, or alert the nurse that the physician is ready for assistance.

7. Upon completion of the exam, assist the patient to a comfortable and safe position.

8. Lower the bed, and raise the side rails.

9. Remove the drape, and return the bedcovers.

10. Record the procedure on the appropriate form.

Evaluate

Evaluate your actions. Was the patient in the proper position and draped correctly for the procedure? Did you remove any biohazardous wastes or soiled linens?

Evaluate the patient's response. Report any complaints of discomfort or pain. Report any unusual observations.

Applying Support/Therapeutic Hose

In daily life, women wear pantyhose, thigh-high stockings, and knee-high stockings. Most men wear either calf-, knee-, or ankle-high socks. Most people are familiar with support hose or stockings. However, the stockings discussed in this section are therapeutic stockings or hose. These hose are available in more than thirty-two sizes and two lengths: knee-high and thigh-high (Figure 25-60). Measurements for therapeutic hose must be accurate for the hose to fit.

Follow these guidelines when you measure a patient for therapeutic hose. For knee highs, measure around the ankle and around the largest part of the calf. Then measure from the bottom of the heel to the back of the knee. For thigh-high hose, measure around the ankle, around the widest part of the calf, and around the widest part of the thigh. Then mea-

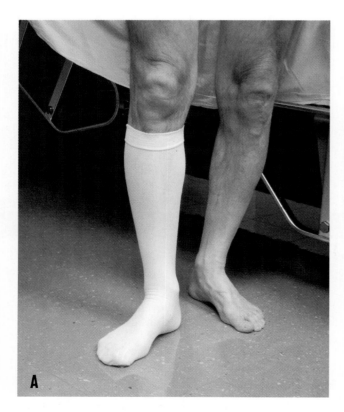

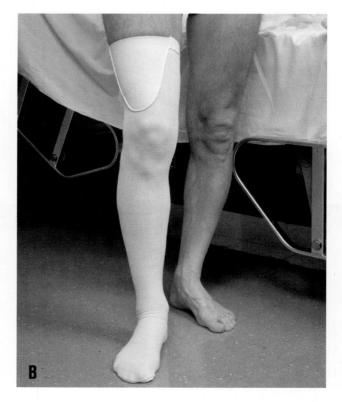

FIGURE 25-60   (a) Knee-high stockings. (b) Full-length, or thigh-high, stockings.

procedure
Applying Elastic Support Hose

Assess

Determine what steps are needed to obtain support hose. If this is a new order, the patient must be measured for size, and the stockings must be ordered. Unless the order is stat, the stockings can be applied when they arrive from the pharmacy. If this is not a new order, you will reapply the patient's stockings after performing personal care and before the patient gets out of bed.

Determine the patient's needs for this procedure. Can the patient assist with applying the stockings? Will you need someone to support the patient's legs while you apply the stockings?

Plan

Gather required equipment: new stockings from the pharmacy or stockings removed during personal care.

Implement

1. Turn the hose so that the smooth side is out.
2. Slide the foot and heel of the stocking onto the patient's foot.
3. Position the heel of the stocking on the patient's heel.
4. Pull the stocking over the patient's foot and ankle with a gentle motion.
5. Ease the stocking up the patient's leg, avoiding stretching the stocking.
6. Remove wrinkles from the stocking by using the palms of your hands to smooth them out.
7. Pull the toe forward slightly.

Evaluate

Evaluate your actions. Were you able to apply the stockings without causing discomfort to the patient? Are the stockings free from wrinkles?

Evaluate the patient's response. Report any complaints of pain or discomfort during the procedure. Report any abnormalities, such as discoloration of the skin, temperature changes of the skin, and swelling of the feet, ankles, or legs.

---

sure from the bottom of the heel to the top of the thigh.

Therapeutic hose may be called by several names, all meaning the same thing. Sometimes they are called **antiembolism stockings** (*anti*- means "against," and *embolism* literally means "a condition of traveling blood clots"). Sometimes they are called **TED hose** or **JOBST stockings**, which are brand names, or **surgical stockings** since they are used to prevent post-operative circulatory complications.

Because these stockings help prevent traveling blood clots, or **emboli**, they are worn whenever venostasis might occur. Name some situations in which venostasis might occur. If you thought of patients on prolonged bedrest, patients recovering from major surgery, and patients with thrombophlebitis, you are correct.

Therapeutic stockings are applied differently than regular stockings, so follow the procedure carefully.

Applying ACE Bandages

An **ACE bandage** is an elastic wrap that provides external support and pressure. These wraps are primarily used to support a joint after a musculoskeletal injury. They can also be used to compress the veins to

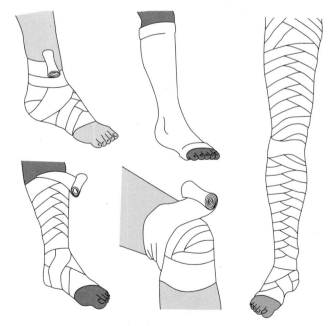

FIGURE 25-61 Elastic bandages, sometimes called *Ace bandages*.

promote venous return. ACE wraps come in a variety of widths (Figure 25-61). As with any elastic device, these wraps can lose stretch after repeated use. Discard any ACE bandage that has lost its elasticity.

procedure

Applying ACE Bandages

Assess

Determine the size and number of ACE bandages needed. Where is the ACE wrap to be applied? What is the size of the patient?

Determine the needs of the patient for this procedure. What is the condition of the skin beneath the wrap? Would clips or tape be the best way to fasten the wrap, or would a Velcro ACE be the best choice?

Plan

Determine the best time to perform the procedure. Can the wraps be removed during personal care? If so, the best time to rewrap the bandages is after personal care and before the patient gets out of bed.

Gather required equipment: clean, rolled ACE wraps; clips, pins, or tape. Use standard precautions as appropriate.

Implement

1. Expose the area to be wrapped with the ACE bandage.
2. Extend and support the joint.
3. Begin the wrap at the distal end of the part, on the anterior surface.
4. Wrap twice around to secure the end of the ACE bandage.
5. Continue to wrap while unrolling the bandage.
6. With each wrap, overlap the edge of the ACE approximately one-half of its width.
7. Wrap snugly and keep even, light pressure on the body part, leaving fingers and toes exposed for circulatory checks.
8. Overlap the ends of each ACE bandage if you are using more than one.
9. Secure the end with clips, pins, or tape.

Evaluate

Evaluate your actions. Is the wrap on snugly but loose enough so that capillary refill is adequate? Is the exposed skin of the body part warm with normal color? Does the patient say that the wrap is comfortable and not too tight or loose?

Evaluate the patient's response. Inquire about any numbness, tingling, or loss of feeling or sensation. Report any abnormalities of the wrapped area, such as edema, discoloration, or signs of infection. Report any signs and symptoms of circulatory impairment, such as cyanosis, coolness of skin distal to the wrap, and complaints of numbness or lack of sensation, movement, or feeling.

Preoperative Shaving

The skin must be shaved before surgery because hair is a harbor for microorganisms, which can enter the surgical incision. An area much larger than the incisional site is prepped to ensure that all hair near the site has been removed. See Figures 25-62 through 25-68; examine these visuals carefully.

What can you notice about the areas to be shaved? The area may involve sensitive tissue around the genitals which could cause the patient embarrassment during the prep. Shaving these areas may require extra care to avoid nicking the skin. Razor nicks compound the problem of infection risk.

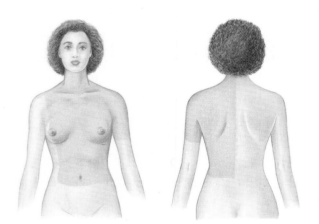

FIGURE 25-62   Prep for breast surgery. Shave from the nipple line of the unaffected side to the middle of the patient's back on the affected side. On the affected side, shave from the chin down to the umbilicus (navel), the axilla (armpit), and part of the upper arm.

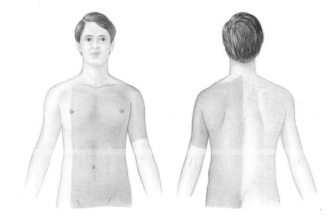

FIGURE 25-63   Chest prep for thoracic surgery. Shave the area extending from the nipple of the unaffected side, across the chest area of the affected side, and across the back, from the top of the shoulders down to the pubic hair.

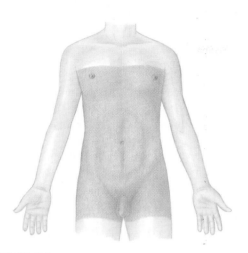

FIGURE 25-64 Abdominal prep. Shave from the nipple line on male patients and from below the breasts on female patients down to and including the pubic area. Shave the width of this area to each side of the body.

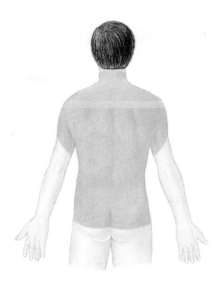

FIGURE 25-66 Back prep. Shave the patient's entire back from the hairline on the neck down to the middle of the buttocks, including the axillary area.

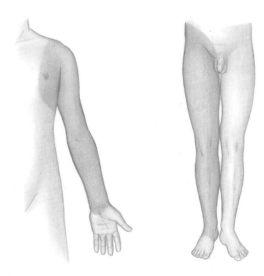

FIGURE 25-65 Prep for surgery of an extremity (arm or leg). If a joint such as an elbow or knee is going to be operated on, shave up to the next joint above and down to the next joint below. For example, if the patient's elbow is going to be operated on, shave the entire arm from the shoulder down to the wrist. If an area between joints is going to be operated on, shave the entire area, including the joints above and below. Shave all around an arm or a leg.

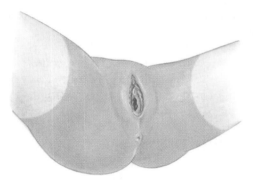

FIGURE 25-67 Vaginal prep, or the preparation of the genital area of female patients.

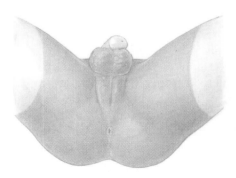

FIGURE 25-68 Scrotal prep, or the preparation of the genital area of male patients.

procedure
Preoperative Shaving

Assess

Determine the needs of the patient for this procedure. Has the patient been seen by the surgeon or anesthesiologist? When is the surgery? What area needs to be shaved?

Plan

Gather required equipment: gloves, shave kit, cotton gauze, cotton-tipped applicator, basin, towel, and bath blanket. Use standard precautions.

Implement

1. Position the light source to thoroughly illuminate the area to be shaved.
2. Don gloves.
3. Identify the area to be shaved, and begin the procedure proximally.
4. Apply soap to a small area, and hold the skin taut.
5. Shave in the direction of hair growth.
6. Rinse the razor, and rub it across the gauze to remove hairs.
7. Continue to shave in this manner until the entire area has been prepped.
8. Clean the umbilicus with a cotton-tipped applicator if the abdomen is being shaved.
9. Check the area with the light source, and remove any remaining hairs.
10. Wash, rinse, and dry the entire area.

Evaluate

Evaluate your actions. Has *all* hair been removed from the shaved area? Use the light source to check this carefully. Was the patient nicked during the procedure? If so, report it immediately.

Evaluate the patient's response. Report any complaints of pain or discomfort during the procedure.

---

application to practice

As you have learned, when implementing procedures, there are some major principles that must be included. These major principles are time management, safety, patients' rights, outcome-based goal setting, competence, and comfort. Based on your learning from this chapter, respond to the following situations.

Learning Activities

Situation 1: Mrs. Kief is a ninety-year-old patient who has diabetes mellitus and is blind. She recently had a left radical mastectomy. You are required to check her blood pressure twice this shift. In assessing and planning personal care for this patient, what factors should be considered?

Author's Explanation: The patient has diabetes; therefore, you should pay close attention to her skin and nails. The podiatrist should cut this patient's toenails. Since the patient is blind, there will be special safety considerations. Arrange care items and meals so they are easily accessible to Mrs. Kief. Because of the left mastectomy, use only the right arm for measuring blood pressure and for phlebotomy.

You should also determine the patient's mobility status and the type of assistance she needs to perform activities of daily living (ADLs). Investigate the diet and any special procedures or studies ordered for this day.

Situation 2: Mr. Tobar is a seventy-five-year-old resident on the dementia unit of the nursing home where you work. He is a new resident in your assignment. He has just been transferred from the hospital after being treated with C. Diff. This is the information that you are given in morning report:

Incontinent of urine and stool.

Temperature 101° F at 6:00 A.M.

Vital signs at 9:00 A.M.

Daily weight this A.M.

Recreation activity at 9:00 A.M.

Bath in the Century Tub.

What plans should be made for Mr. Tobar's morning care? To manage your time well, you should assemble all supplies before you enter Mr. Tobar's room. He should be on contact precautions; therefore, you will need gown and gloves. You should plan to complete his morning care before any recreation activities.

What should you assess in this situation?

Author's Explanation: Since Mr. Tobar is incontinent of urine and stool and he has a bowel infection (C. Diff.), he should not be put into the Century Tub for a bath. This tub is used by other residents. Mr. Tobar has an infection of the bowels, and he could be incontinent in the tub. You should determine from the nurse the temperature that needs to be reported because he was febrile at 6:00 A.M. You should assess his ability to participate in completing ADLs and eating. You should observe the condition of the skin in his perineal area since he is incontinent. Report any findings to the nurse. If he is febrile at 9:00 A.M., you should check with the nurse about participation in recreation activities. The facility may also have a policy that prevents a resident on contact precautions from joining in community meals and activities.

What principles of patient care should be considered as you perform Mr. Tobar's morning care? In each of the tasks that you implement for Mr. Tobar, consider safety, asepsis, time management, patients' rights, comfort, and goal-based outcomes.

Situation 3: Mr. Taglieb is a resident who suffers from dementia, and he is frequently confused and agitated. The nurse instructs you to take his temperature stat. What should you assess and plan for in this situation?

Author's Explanation: You should assess Mr. Taglieb's ability to cooperate with the task of temperature measurement. Since the resident is frequently confused and agitated, the aural method of temperature is probably safest. You should plan to obtain the tympanic thermometer and probe protectors and take the temperature stat. Report the results immediately to the nurse.

Situation 4: You are working the evening shift on a surgical patient care unit. Your assignment includes the following tasks, which must be completed for a fresh post-op patient. Using the principle of time management, organize and prioritize the tasks listed below. Rate the tasks from 1 to 5 (1 is the most important, and 5 the least):

Instruct patient on use of incentive spirometer _____, stat vital signs _____, change gown and bottom sheet (patient has been bleeding) _____, 12-lead ECG _____, venous blood sample for CBC and Chem 7 _____.

Author's Explanation: Stat vital signs <u>1</u>____, 12-lead ECG <u>2</u>____, venous blood sample for CBC and Chem 7 <u>3</u>____, change gown and bottom sheet (patient has been bleeding) <u>4</u>____, instruct patient on use of incentive spirometer <u>5</u>____.

Situation 5: Ms. Nuygen is a resident who has left hemiplagia and aphasia. She requires assistance with wheelchair transfers. Her restorative nursing care goals include ambulation with a quad cane. Today she is to walk 20 feet. She is to wear a sling on her left arm and a brace with shoe attached on her left leg.

As part of the assessment for transfers, what factor should you consider? In planning for transfer to wheelchair, what factor should you consider?

Author's Explanation: The patient's understanding of the transfer procedure is important. Consider her aphasia when you determine her understanding of transfers. She may be able to show you how she transfers from bed to chair, and so on.

For wheelchair transfers, the placement of the wheelchair relative to the bed and Ms. Nuygen's dominant or unaffected side is important. The wheelchair should be positioned so that Ms. Nuygen can lead with her right side.

Examination Review Questions

1. Bathing includes all of the following *except*
   a. complete care
   b. partial care
   c. assistance with shower
   d. Assistance with transfer

2. Which factor does *not* contribute to skin breakdown?
   a. poor nutrition
   b. elevated temperature
   c. improved circulation
   d. impaired sensation

3. The device that prevents skin breakdown through the intermittent redistribution of body weight is the
   a. air mattress
   b. heel protector
   c. eggcrate mattress
   d. wheelchair cushion

4. Another term for pressure ulcer is
   a. decubitus
   b. petechiae
   c. edema
   d. diaphoresis

5. Which thermometer measures temperature in the ear canal?
   a. rectal
   b. oral
   c. aural
   d. axillary

6. Which pulse point is used in the measurement of blood pressure?
   a. radial
   b. brachial
   c. carotid
   d. pedal

7. Blood pressure is usually measured by _____ with the stethoscope.
   a. percussion
   b. auscultation
   c. palpation
   d. observation

8. If intake is less than output, what will occur?
   a. edema
   b. emesis
   c. dehydration
   d. homeostasis

9. The body position in which patients are positioned on their back is called
   a. lateral
   b. supine
   c. prone
   d. Fowler's

10. On which side should a quad cane be held?
    a. unaffected
    b. affected
    c. left
    d. right

u n i t   1 1

Advanced or Expanded Procedures and Tasks: Critical Elements and Problem-Solving Tools

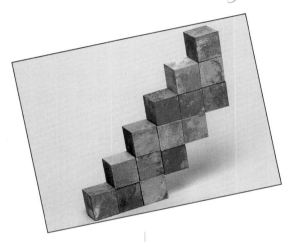

Today, caregivers need a broad range of skills and techniques to care for patients and to meet their needs. This unit includes advanced and expanded skills that require knowledge of such topics as aseptic technique as well as knowledge of basic anatomy and physiology. Many of the skills included in this unit require a physician's order or are intended to be implemented following an institution's written protocol for care. Each of the skills requires attention to the patient's response to the procedure. Sometimes, unpredictable patient responses or outcomes require additional skills and intervention by a nurse or physician.

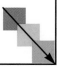

Chapter 26

Advanced or Expanded Procedures and Tasks

In this chapter, you will learn some advanced or expanded skills that you might perform as a clinical care associate in certain care environments. Each state stipulates which skills an unlicensed caregiver can perform. In some health facilities, caregivers perform all the skills described in this chapter, plus additional skills based on training and demonstration of competence. For your safety and that of your patient, never perform a task or skill that you have not been deemed competent and been given permission to perform. Your understanding of the major principles for implementing all patient care tasks is essential to safe performance.

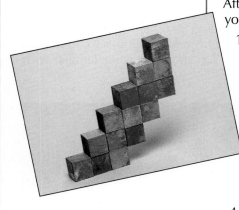

OBJECTIVES

After completing this chapter, you will be able to

1. Differentiate between straight and indwelling catheterization
2. Identify the principles of care and the procedural steps for performing tube feedings
3. Explain how the electrocardiogram traces pictures of heart activity
4. Identify the principles of care and the procedural steps for recording a twelve-lead electrocardiogram
5. Distinguish between the types of dressings and describe the procedure for applying each type
6. Identify the different types of stomas and the variations in the care of each stoma
7. Identify the principles of care and the procedural steps for performing ostomy care
8. Identify the principles of care and the procedural steps for performing respiratory care
9. Identify the principles of care and the procedural steps for performing phlebotomy
10. Identify the principles of care and the procedural steps for performing bedside blood glucose monitoring
11. Describe the principles of care and the procedural steps for performing oral suctioning

key terms

aspirate	indwelling catheter	premature ventricular contraction
aspiration pneumonia	infusion pump	(PVC)
bolus method	IVAC pump	pulse oximetry
catheterization	multichannel ECG machine	residual
catheterization kit	nasal cannula	single-channel ECG machine
colostomy	normal sinus rhythm	straight catheterization
continuous method	oral suction catheter or Yankeur	stylus
Duoderm dressing	ostomy care	suctioning
ECG paper	oxisensor	Tegaderm dressing
expectorate	percussion	telemetry technician
face mask	percutaneous endoscopic	three-way Foley catheter
Foley	gastrostomy (PEG)	total parenteral nutrition (TPN)
French gauge	phlebotomy	urometer
gastrostomy tube (GT)	pneumatic (intermittent) pressure	urostomy
ileostomy	stockings	V leads
incentive spirometer (IS)	precordial	wet-to-dry dressing

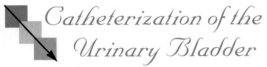

Catheterization of the Urinary Bladder

Catheterization is the insertion of a sterile tube into the urinary bladder. There are two different types of catheterization procedures. A **straight catheterization** is performed to remove urine remaining in the bladder after voiding (called residual urine), to intermittently empty the bladder when a person is unable to void voluntarily, and to obtain a sterile urine specimen. When an **indwelling catheter** is used, the purpose of the procedure is to insert and leave in place a sterile tube that will continuously drain urine from the bladder. An indwelling catheter might be ordered for conditions that require continuous monitoring of urinary output or as a result of surgical procedures performed in the abdominal and pelvic cavities.

Inserting a Catheter

Indwelling and straight catheterization procedures require the same application of principles and techniques. When you insert an indwelling catheter, you will inflate a small, attached balloon that keeps the tube from slipping out of the bladder. You will also connect an indwelling catheter to a drainage device or urine-collection bag. A straight catheter is removed after the urine is drained from the bladder into a measuring device.

Often, people refer to the indwelling catheter as a **Foley**. A Foley is actually a type of catheter. It is a flexible rubber tube with openings and an inflatable balloon near the tip and two or three ports (connection areas) at the distal end. A **three-way Foley catheter** is used for continuous irrigation and drainage of the bladder. After a surgical procedure involving the urinary bladder, the bladder is irrigated continuously with a saline or antibiotic solution. A three-way catheter is usually inserted while the patient is in the operating room. Typically, you would insert a Foley catheter with only two ports at the distal end of the tube. This is called a *two-way Foley* (Figure 26-1).

Foley catheters come in various sizes. They are sized using a **French gauge**. Foleys come in 14-, 16-, 18-, 20-, and 22-gauge French sizes. This measurement reflects the width of the lumen of the catheter. The amount of fluid that can be held by the inflatable balloon is also part of the size of a catheter. These can range from 5 cc balloons to 30 cc balloons (Figure 26-2). You should become familiar with the

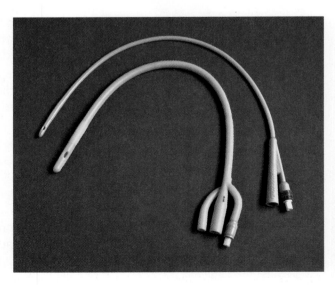

FIGURE 26-1 Two-way and three-way Foley catheters.

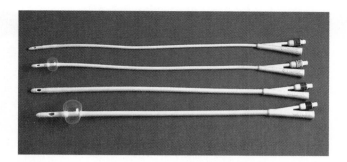

FIGURE 26-2 Catheters of various sizes.

types of supplies stocked by your facility. You also need to know your institution's policies and procedures regarding urinary catheterization. These will vary from one facility to the next.

A **catheterization kit** is a prepackaged collection of supplies needed for inserting a catheter using sterile technique. There are two types of kits: *straight catheterization kits* and *indwelling catheterization kits*. It is important to choose the correct kit when you gather supplies for this procedure. The indwelling catheterization kit contains a drape for the patient, a bed protector, a specimen container with a label, cotton balls, forceps, lubricant, Betadine, and a syringe filled with sterile water. All of these items are packaged in a sterile plastic container. The straight catheterization kit contains all of the same items except for the syringe. Instead, a straight catheter is included in the kit. Some kits also contain a pair of sterile gloves.

A **urometer** is a special measuring device that is attached to some urinary drainage bags. It is used to provide accurate and frequent measurement of urine output.

procedure
Inserting a Catheter

Assess

Determine the information needed to perform this procedure. Determine the catheter and supplies needed. What size catheter is needed for this patient? Is this a straight catheterization? If so, what type? (To drain the bladder or to obtain a sterile urine specimen?) Or is this order for an indwelling catheter? If so, are you inserting a new catheter or changing a catheter that is due to be removed and replaced? Determine the correct size catheter and the correct type of catheter kit.

Determine the patient's needs during this procedure. What is the patient's mobility status? Will you need assistance during the procedure? Female patients must be placed in the lithotomy position, and male patients must be placed in the supine position. Both sexes must be able to remain still during the procedure.

Do you need to be supervised while you perform this procedure?

Plan

Determine the best time to perform the procedure. If the patient's perineal area is not clean, it must be cleaned before the procedure. Be aware that this procedure may take up to 30 minutes, depending on your skill and the patient's condition.

Gather required equipment: two catheterization kits, extra pair of sterile gloves, two catheters, measuring device, and biohazard bag. (Two catheterization kits and two catheters are needed in case sterile technique is broken. If so, the assistant won't need to leave the room to get a new kit or a new catheter.) Check the date on sterile supplies to ensure that they are not outdated. If you are inserting an indwelling catheter, you will also need a uri-

nary collection bag. Use standard precautions. Check with the nurse to see if a urometer is needed.

Determine whether you need to obtain a urine specimen while performing this procedure.

Determine whether modifications are needed for this patient. If a female patient is unable to assume the lithotomy position, can the Sim's position be used?

Implement
Catheterizing a Female

1. Follow the principles of sterile technique while performing this procedure.
2. Position the patient, and provide for her comfort and privacy.
3. Arrange the lighting so that it is adequate for illuminating the genitalia.
4. Raise the bed to a comfortable working level, keeping the opposite side rail raised.
5. Open one catheterization kit without contaminating the contents, and bring it to the bed.
6. Remove the underpad from the kit, and place it under the patient's buttocks, with the plastic side toward the bed.
7. Carefully remove the sterile wrapper of the kit, and use it to create a sterile field.
8. Don the sterile gloves (Figure 26-3).
9. Place the plastic tray between the patient's legs or as close to the genitalia as possible.
10. Open the Betadine solution, and pour it over the cotton balls.
11. Open the lubricant package, and lubricate the catheter from the tip to 3 to 4 inches along the tube.

procedure (continued)

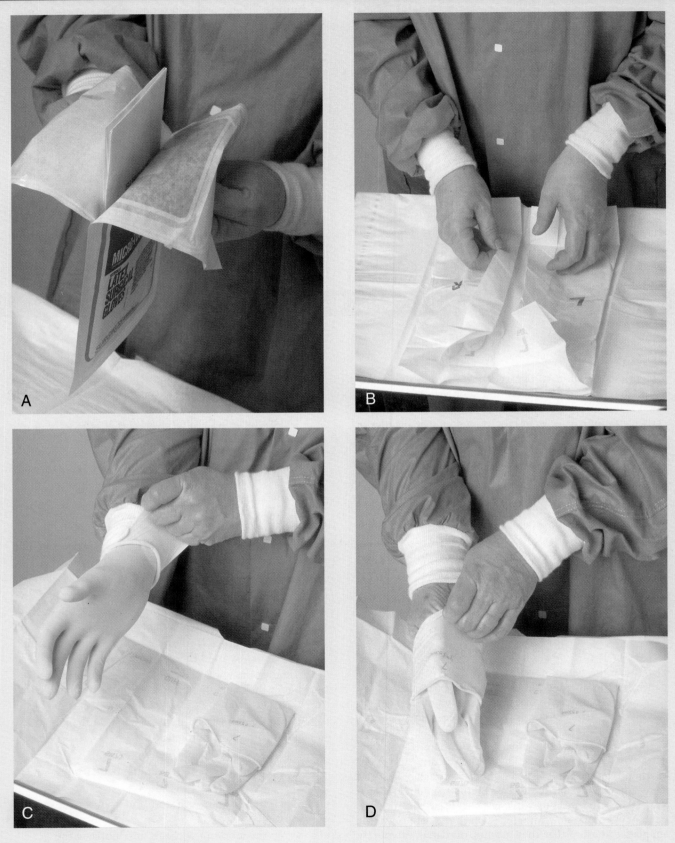

FIGURE 26-3 Applying sterile gloves.

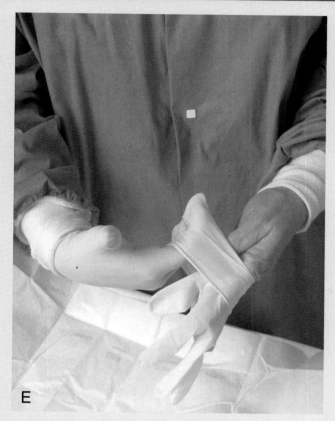

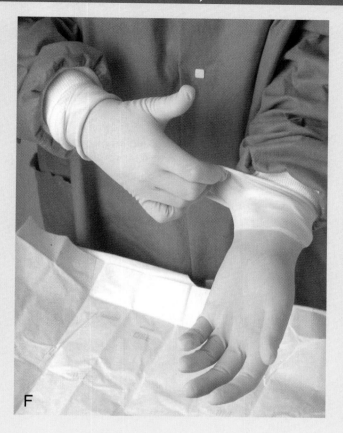

E

F

FIGURE 26-3   Applying sterile gloves. (continued)

12. Separate the labia with your nondominant hand, and expose the urinary meatus. Your nondominant hand is now *contaminated* and must remain in place throughout the procedure.

13. Use the forceps to pick up a Betadine-soaked cotton ball.

14. Use one cotton ball to wipe in a circular motion around the urethral meatus, then discard it.

15. Use another cotton ball to wipe one side of the labia from top to bottom, then discard it.

16. Use a third cotton ball to wipe the other side of the labia, then discard it.

17. Using only your sterile (dominant) hand, place the sterile drape around the genitalia.

18. Place the distal end of the catheter in the sterile plastic tray.

19. Using your sterile (dominant) hand, gently insert the catheter about 2 inches into the urinary meatus, instructing the patient to take a deep breath as you do so.

20. Observe the flow of urine out of the catheter, and drain the bladder of all urine.

21. If this is an indwelling catheter, inject the appropriate amount of sterile water into the balloon through the balloon port.

22. Pull back gently on the catheter to ensure that it is secured in the bladder.

23. Connect the urine-collection bag to the open end of the catheter.

24. Hang the collection bag below the level of the bladder.

25. Place a leg strap on the patient's thigh, and secure the catheter tubing to the leg strap.

26. Dispose of all biohazard trash appropriately.

27. Collect a urine specimen. It may be needed.

28. Reposition the patient for comfort and safety.

29. Document the procedure on the appropriate form.

Catheterizing a Male

1. Follow the principles of sterile technique while performing this procedure.

2. Position the patient, and provide for his comfort and privacy.

3. Arrange the lighting so that it is adequate for illuminating the genitalia.

4. Raise the bed to a comfortable working level, keeping the opposite side rail raised.

5. Open the catheterization kit without contaminating the contents, and bring it to the bed.

6. Remove the underpad from the kit, and place it under the patient's buttocks, with the plastic side toward the bed.

7. Carefully remove the sterile wrapper of the kit, and use it to create a sterile field.

8. Don the sterile gloves.

9. Place the plastic tray between the patient's legs or as close to the genitalia as possible.

10. Open the Betadine solution, and pour it over the cotton balls.

11. Open the lubricant package, and lubricate the catheter from the tip to 5 to 6 inches along the tube.

12. Grasp the penis with your nondominant hand, and hold it at a 90° angle to the patient's body. Your nondominant hand is now *contaminated* and must remain in place throughout the procedure.

13. Retract the foreskin of an uncircumcised patient to expose the urethral meatus.

14. Use the forceps to pick up a Betadine-soaked cotton ball.

15. Use one cotton ball to wipe in a circular motion around the urethral meatus, then discard it.

16. Use another cotton ball to wipe in a circular motion around the urethral meatus, then discard it.

17. Place the sterile drape around the genitalia by bringing the penis through the opening in the drape. Hold the penis upright and taut.

18. Have a sterile collection container between patient's thighs.

19. Using your sterile (dominant) hand, gently insert the catheter about 6 inches into the urinary meatus, instructing the patient to take a deep breath as you do so.

20. Continue to insert the catheter until urine flows out through the catheter.

21. Observe the flow of urine out of the catheter, and drain the bladder of all urine.

22. If this is an indwelling catheter, inject the appropriate amount of sterile water into the balloon through the balloon port.

23. Pull back gently on the catheter to ensure that it is secured in the bladder.

24. Connect the urine-collection bag to the open end of the catheter.

25. Hang the collection bag below the level of the bladder.

26. Place a leg strap on the patient's thigh, and secure the catheter tubing to the leg strap.

27. Dispose of all biohazard trash appropriately.

28. Collect a urine specimen. It may be needed.

29. Reposition the patient for comfort and safety.

30. Document the procedure on the appropriate form.

Evaluate

Evaluate your actions. Did you use sterile technique at all times? What can you do to be more efficient the next time you perform this procedure? What do you need to learn about the procedure or about anatomy to make this easier the next time? Did you measure the output and record it appropriately? Did you label the urine specimen and send it to the lab?

Evaluate the patient's response. Report any complaints of pain during the procedure. Report any bleeding or difficulty during the procedure.

Evaluate your charting. Did you record the size of the catheter used? Did you record the color, clarity, and quantity of urine obtained? Did you record that a urine specimen was obtained and sent to the lab?

If you encounter difficulty obtaining urine flow when catheterizing a female patient, you have probably put the catheter in the vagina. Should this occur, here are some steps to follow:

1. Leave the catheter in the vagina.

2. Open another sterile catheter. (If you cannot do this with one hand, remove your gloves and then put on a new pair of sterile gloves.)

3. Lubricate the new catheter.

4. Gently insert the catheter above the vaginal orifice.

If you have difficulty advancing the catheter 6 inches in the male urethra, here are some steps to follow:

1. If you meet resistance, pull the tubing back a little, and readjust the angle of the penis.

2. Tilt the penis away from the body, and insert the tubing gently.

3. If the catheter does not advance, tilt the penis toward the body, and advance the tubing.

4. Never force the catheter against resistance.

Removing an Indwelling Catheter

An indwelling catheter is removed because it is no longer needed or because it needs to be changed. Different institutions have varying policies on the length of time an indwelling catheter may remain in place. Follow the policy guidelines of your institution regarding standard catheter changes. Some medical conditions require that a patient have an indwelling catheter indefinitely. The longer a person has an indwelling catheter, the greater the chance of developing an infection due to the presence of a foreign object in the body. Also, the extended presence of a catheter increases the size of the meatus, which can cause leaking of urine around the tube. In that case, a larger catheter must be used.

When you remove a catheter, you will use clean, rather than sterile, technique. Standard precautions must be followed.

p r o c e d u r e

Removing an Indwelling Catheter

Assess

Determine the reason for removing the catheter. Has the doctor ordered the catheter discontinued? Or, according to your institution's guidelines, has the standard length of time for an indwelling catheter expired? Will you be inserting another catheter after the removal of this one?

Plan

Gather required equipment: gloves, bed protector, 10 cc syringe, and biohazard bag. Use standard precautions.

Determine whether the tip of the catheter is to be sent to the lab for culture. If so, obtain a sterile container and a label.

Determine whether you need any other instructions to perform this procedure. Check with the nurse for guidance.

Implement

1. Position the patient on his or her back, providing for comfort and safety.
2. Raise the bed to a comfortable working height.
3. Remove any leg strap or tape from the patient and the catheter.
4. Place the bed protector between the patient's legs.
5. Insert the syringe into the side port of the distal end of the catheter tubing.
6. Withdraw 5 to 10 cc of fluid. (Check the plastic cap on the port for the amount of fluid required to inflate the balloon.)
7. Gently pull the catheter from the meatus until the entire tube is removed. It may help the patient to relax by taking a panting breath.
8. Clean the perineum or penis.
9. Reposition the patient for comfort and safety.
10. Inspect the catheter to be sure that all parts have been removed.
11. Package the catheter to be sent to the lab, if required, or discard it in the biohazard trash.
12. Measure the urine in the collection bag, and discard it in the toilet.
13. Record the amount of urine on the intake-and-output record.
14. Record the procedure on the appropriate form.

Evaluate

Evaluate your actions. Did you completely empty the balloon of fluid? Did the catheter slide out easily? Did you label any specimens and send them to the lab?

Evaluate the patient's response. Report the procedure to the nurse, along with the condition of the catheter. Report any patient complaints of pain or discomfort during the procedure.

Once a catheter has been removed, it is very important that you continue to observe the patient's urinary status. Here are some steps to follow:

1. Note the time of the next urination; measure and document the amount, color, and clarity of the urine.
2. Report any patient complaints of burning, hesitation in starting a stream of urine, dribbling, or incontinence of urine.

Gastrostomy Tubes: Tube Feedings, Irrigation, and Aspiration of Residual Feeding

Sometimes, patients are unable to swallow or chew food, and they require an alternate feeding method. This type of feeding is called an *enteral feeding method*. Patients may have a nasogastric (NG) tube or a gastrostomy tube in place for alternate methods of feeding. An NG tube is placed through the nose and is advanced to the stomach (Figure 26-4). This tube is inserted by the nurse or doctor. It is a temporary method of feeding. The NG tube can also be used to remove stomach contents. It is not used simultaneously for emptying the stomach and for feeding. When used to remove stomach contents, the patient is NPO. The tube is connected to suction to "pump" the stomach contents. A nurse will usually be assigned to perform NG tube feedings. The nurse's assessment of the patient and the functioning of the NG tube is required.

A **gastrostomy tube (GT)** is used to place liquid nutrition or formula directly into the stomach. A GT is used to provide nutrition for the patient who is unable to eat or drink through the mouth. Examples of situations that might require a GT are a patient on a ventilator for an extended period or a patient who cannot swallow food or fluids. The GT is placed in the stomach through a puncture site or surgical incision using an endoscope. A gastrostomy tube inserted by the puncture method is called a **percutaneous endoscopic gastrostomy (PEG)** tube (Figure 26-5). Usually, the PEG is located on the left side of the abdomen just below the ribs. The

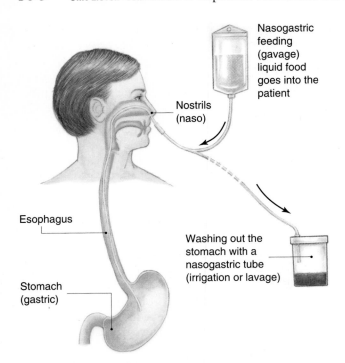

Nasogastric feeding (gavage) liquid food goes into the patient

Nostrils (naso)

Esophagus

Washing out the stomach with a nasogastric tube (irrigation or lavage)

Stomach (gastric)

FIGURE 26-4   Nasogastric tubes.

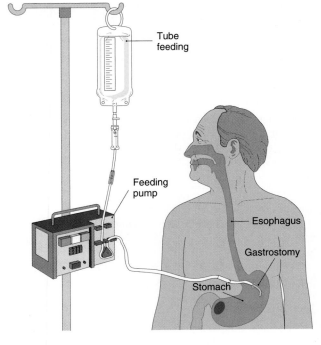

Tube feeding

Feeding pump

Esophagus

Gastrostomy

Stomach

FIGURE 26-5   Gastrostomy (PEG) tube feeding.

insertion site is generally covered with a piece of gauze for a few days after placement of the tube. The area around the insertion site should be monitored for redness, swelling, drainage, and pain. Report any of these signs to the nurse. If the tube appears to have slipped out of place, notify the nurse immediately.

When a PEG tube is first placed, the nurse will perform the initial feedings and flushes as well as aspiration for residual feeding. This is done so that the nurse can assess the patient's response to the placement of the tube and his or her tolerance of the tube feedings.

It is very important that the PEG tube remain patent (unclogged). To prevent clogging, the tube must be irrigated or flushed with water at regular intervals. When the patient is receiving bolus feedings, the tube is flushed after each feeding. When the patient is on continuous feedings or is not receiving any feedings, the tube must be flushed every 8 hours.

The doctor will order the type, amount, rate, and frequency of the tube feedings to be given. Commercially prepared feedings, such as Ensure and Sustical, are provided for the patient by either the dietary department or the pharmacy. These canned formulas are expensive but have a long shelf life and do not require refrigeration. Some facilities prepare tube-feeding formulas. These formulas must be refrigerated and expire after 24 hours. Such feedings

are packaged in a carton or plastic bag with tubing attached. In some situations, the physician may order dilution of the feeding solution to determine how well the patient will tolerate it. The order may be for one-half strength or three-fourths strength. The formula will be diluted by the dietary department. You should not dilute the feeding yourself.

Tube feedings can be administered in two different ways. The **bolus method** involves three or four feedings during a 24-hour period. The prescribed type and amount of formula is instilled in the PEG tube using a large syringe. The plunger of a 50 cc syringe is removed, and the tip of the syringe is inserted into the PEG tube. The formula is poured into the hollow syringe and moved into the PEG tube by gravity. Never use the plunger in a syringe to push formula into a PEG tube. The **continuous method** involves a small amount of feeding continuously instilled in the PEG tube. An **infusion pump** or controller is used to regulate the drip rate of the liquid feeding. One brand name you might hear is the **IVAC pump**. With this method, the formula is poured into a plastic bag, similar to an intravenous bag with tubing attached. The tubing is then threaded through the pump, which controls the rate of infusion. Do not allow formula to remain in the plastic bag for more than 8 hours. When you add formula to a bag, do not pour in any more than a 6- to 8-hour supply.

Before administering a tube feeding by either method, you must always aspirate for residual feeding. (To **aspirate** means "to withdraw by force," and **residual** means "left over.") Residual feeding refers to any tube feeding formula that remains in the stomach and may not be digested. To aspirate for residual feeding, insert the tip of a syringe into the PEG tube and pull back on the plunger. You must then measure the amount of the undigested nutritional supplement and gastric juices obtained.

Before administering a bolus tube feeding, you must check to see if any of the previous tube feeding still remains in the stomach. If the patient is on a continuous feeding pump, it is expected that some residual will be in the stomach. However, you must measure the amount found in the stomach. The physician will usually specify an amount of residual stomach contents that indicates the need to withhold the next feeding. If no order is written,

the general rule is that an aspirated amount of 150 cc or more indicates the need to withhold the next feeding. Notify the nurse stat if the amount of residual exceeds these limits. When that much residual is found in the stomach, either the supplement is not being digested or there is an obstruction preventing the formula from moving to the small intestine.

You might aspirate for residual and withdraw only gastric juices, with no formula present. In this case, the feeding is being completely digested. Replace the gastric secretions by pushing them back into the PEG tube. These secretions contain important acid, enzymes, and electrolytes.

Never start a feeding without first checking for residual. Overfilling the stomach with feeding can *endanger* the patient. A large amount of residual

p r o c e d u r e
Aspiration of Residual Stomach Contents

Assess

Determine the amount of the last residual recorded. Check the chart or intake-and-output record for this information.

Determine the condition of the PEG tube and site. Look at the skin around the site, checking for any drainage, irritation, or redness. Check the tube for any signs of dislocation.

Plan

Gather required equipment: nonsterile gloves, bed protector, 50 cc syringe, and measuring container. Use standard precautions. (Irrigation trays and large syringe should be changed every 48 hours or according to your institution's policy).

For effective time management, perform this procedure immediately before administering a tube feeding. However, you may be directed to perform this procedure as a separate task.

Implement

1. Position the patient for comfort and safety, with the head of the bed elevated in semi-Fowler's position or with the patient sitting in a chair.
2. Place the bed protector under the PEG tube.
3. Remove the clamp from the PEG tube, and keep it within easy reach.
4. Insert the tip of the syringe into the tube.
5. Pull back on the plunger, and withdraw the stomach contents.

6. When the syringe fills to 40 cc, place the contents in the measuring container.
7. Repeat steps 5 and 6 until you have aspirated all of the stomach contents.
8. Measure the total amount of aspirated stomach contents.
9. If the aspirated stomach contents equals 150 cc or more, reclamp the tube and notify the nurse. Do not proceed.
10. If the contents equals less than 150 cc, record the measured amount, then remove the plunger from the syringe.
11. Reinsert the tip of the syringe into the PEG tube.
12. Reinstill the gastric contents by pouring them into the hollow syringe.
13. Allow the contents to drain by gravity back into the PEG tube.
14. Proceed with the tube feeding.

Evaluate

Evaluate your performance. Did you maintain a clean environment? Did you record the amount of residual contents? Is your patient safe and comfortable?

Evaluate the patient's response. Report a residual of 150 cc or more. Report the results of the procedure and the condition of the patient to the nurse.

If the PEG tube is not secure or appears to be slipping, do not aspirate stomach contents. Notify the nurse immediately.

in the stomach plus an added new feeding can cause the backflow of stomach contents into the esophagus and can cause vomiting. The patient can easily aspirate the vomit or backflow into the lungs, causing **aspiration pneumonia**. This condition is *life-threatening*. Patients most at risk for aspiration pneumonia are those who are nonresponsive, are unable to communicate, or must lie flat because of a physician's order.

Patients receiving a tube feeding should be kept in semi-Fowler's position whenever any feeding is in progress. Patients on continuous tube feedings must be in this position at all times. The purpose of elevating the head of the bed is to prevent aspiration. If you must lower the head of the bed at any time during a feeding, first stop the infusion pump or the bolus.

Record the amount of water used for flushing the tube and the amount of formula given on the patient's intake-and-output record. When the nurse gives medication through the PEG and flushes the tube, the amount will be recorded.

procedure
Bolus PEG Feeding

Assess

Determine the type and amount of feeding to give. Check the most recent order for this information. Check for residual stomach contents. Follow the general rule for residual, or check for a specific order regarding the amount of residual that indicates the need to withhold the scheduled feeding. Check the expiration date on the formula.

Determine the condition of the PEG tube and site. Look at the skin around the site, checking for any drainage, irritation, or redness. Check the tube for any signs of dislocation.

Plan

Gather required equipment: nonsterile gloves, bed protector, 50 cc catheter-tip syringe, measuring container, prescribed formula, irrigation tray, and tap water. If the dressing around the PEG needs to be changed, you will also need a gauze pad and tape. Use standard precautions. (Irrigation trays and large syringe should be changed every 48 hours or according to your institution's policy.)

Determine the amount of time this procedure will take, and ensure that your other patients have no immediate needs. Allow the patient to use the bathroom or wash his or her hands before you begin.

Implement

1. Position the patient for comfort and safety, with the head of the bed elevated in semi-Fowler's position or with the patient sitting in a chair.
2. Place the bed protector under the PEG tube.
3. Remove the clamp from the PEG tube.
4. Aspirate and measure residual stomach contents, then reinstill the aspirated fluid.
5. Remove the plunger from the syringe.
6. Insert the tip of the syringe into the end of the PEG tube.
7. Slowly fill the syringe with feeding formula.
8. Continue to refill the syringe until the prescribed amount is given.
9. Flush the tube with the prescribed amount of water, usually 30 cc.
10. Remove the syringe.
11. Clamp the PEG tube.
12. Record the procedure on the appropriate form.

Evaluate

Evaluate your performance. Did you keep the head of the bed elevated at all times? Did you accurately measure the residual stomach contents? Did you know whether to withhold the scheduled feeding?

Evaluate the patient's response. Report any complaints of pain or fullness during the procedure. Report any diarrhea, vomiting, or bloating that the patient experiences. Report any redness, pain, or irritation of the skin at the PEG insertion site.

If you experience a problem during a bolus feeding, here are some guidelines to follow:

1. If the formula does not flow easily into the PEG tube, try raising the height of the syringe.
2. If the patient complains of pain or vomits, stop the tube feeding immediately.
3. If water runs out of the tube when you flush after the bolus feeding, hold it in an upright position to promote better flow.

procedure
Continuous Gastrostomy Feeding with a Pump

Assess

The nurse will determine the appropriateness of continuing the tube feeding. What is the appearance and amount of aspirated residual stomach contents? Will you proceed with the feeding based on the amount of aspirated contents?

Determine the type and amount of feeding to give. Check the most recent order for this information. Check the expiration date of the formula.

Determine the condition of the PEG tube and site. Look at the skin around the site, checking for any drainage, irritation, or redness. Check the tube for any signs of dislocation.

Determine the availability of a clean, properly functioning pump.

Plan

Gather required equipment: nonsterile gloves, bed protector, 50 cc syringe, measuring device, prescribed formula, bag with tubing, clamp, pump (IVAC), irrigation tray, and water. If the dressing around the PEG needs to be changed, you will also need a gauze pad and tape. Use standard precautions. (Irrigation trays and large syringe should be changed every 48 hours or according to your institution's policy.)

Determine the amount of time this procedure will take, and ensure that your other patients have no immediate needs.

You should complete this procedure in conjunction with the aspiration of residual stomach contents and the irrigation of the PEG tube.

Implement

Removing the Used Tubing and Formula Bag and Starting a New Bag

1. Position the patient for comfort and safety, with the head of the bed elevated in semi-Fowler's position or with the patient sitting in a chair.
2. Place the bed protector under the PEG tube.
3. Hang the new bag of formula on the IV pole.
4. Fill the length of the new tubing with formula to prime the tubing.
5. Do not fill the drip chamber more than one-fourth full.
6. Close the roller clamp on the tubing.
7. Place the pump on HOLD.
8. Close the roller clamp on the used tubing, and open the pump door.
9. Remove the used tubing from the pump.
10. Disconnect the used tubing from the PEG tube, discarding the bag and tubing in the biohazard trash.
11. Connect the new tubing to the PEG tube.

12. Insert the drip chamber into the chamber holder on the pump.
13. Position the tubing around the wheel or fingers of the pump and the latch.
14. Close the latch.
15. Secure the tubing within the guide, located below the wheel or fingers.
16. Close the pump door.
17. Open the roller clamp on the tubing.
18. Read the display in the VOLUME INFUSED window on the pump.
19. Clear the VOLUME INFUSED display.
20. Press RUN.
21. Read the display in the RATE window on the pump.
22. Set the pump to the desired cc rate, or consult with the nurse for instructions.
23. Mark the tags with the date and time of the tubing change, initial the tags, and attach them to the tubing and formula bag.
24. Remain at the bedside for a short time to ensure that the pump is working correctly.

Refilling a Formula Bag without Changing the Tubing or Bag

1. Press the RUN/HOLD button on the pump. The word HOLD will flash.
2. Remove the bag from the IV pole, and fill it with the required amount of feeding.
3. Read and note the VOLUME INFUSED.
4. Press the RUN/HOLD button again to resume the feeding.
5. Remain at the bedside for a short time to ensure that the pump is working correctly.

Hanging a Bag of Prefilled Formula without Changing the Tubing

1. Press the RUN/HOLD button on the pump. The word HOLD will flash.
2. Turn the bag of formula upside down, and spike it with the tubing that remains in the pump. Then hang the bag on the IV pole.
3. Read and note the VOLUME INFUSED.
4. Press the RUN/HOLD button again to resume the feeding.
5. Remain at the bedside for a short time to ensure that the pump is working correctly.

After 2 minutes on HOLD, an alarm will sound to remind you that the pump is on hold. If you need more time, press the RUN/HOLD button again.

Always check the date on the tubing in the pump. If it indicates that it has been longer than 48 hours since the tubing was changed, do *not* spike the bag. Instead, change the tubing as described in the earlier procedure.

Evaluate

Evaluate your actions. Did you manipulate the pump correctly? Is the correct flow rate displayed in the RATE window? Did you record the AMOUNT INFUSED on the intake-and-output sheet? Is the patient in semi-Fowler's position or sitting in a chair?

Evaluate the patient's response. Report any complaints of discomfort during the procedure. Report any redness, irritation, drainage, or pain at the insertion site.

A Note about Feeding Pumps

Each facility purchases the brand of pump that its products committee or the purchaser chooses. Each brand of pump has unique features. Most pumps operate using the same principles and have similar features, but the displays, signals, latches, and sensors are different in appearance. Never assume that because you have used one brand of pump, you are competent to use another brand.

You will have opportunities for learning to operate feeding pumps. If your facility changes brands, you will be instructed on the use of the new pumps. You must learn how to operate and troubleshoot all mechanical devices before using them on patients. Practice opportunities will be provided when the pump is *not* attached to a patient. Attend in-service workshops, read the available literature, and seek supervision before you use any new pump or mechanical device.

The Twelve-Lead Electrocardiogram

An electrocardiogram (ECG) records the electrical activity of the heart. Twelve leads allow twelve different views of the heart's activity. Each lead reveals a different aspect of the heart's electrical system. Three leads can be used to produce a *rhythm strip*. This provides a quick picture of the overall heart rhythm. This type of ECG is used in emergency situations and to continuously monitor the heart's rhythm.

A twelve-lead ECG is performed when the doctor needs to look at all views of the heart's rate and rhythm. A nurse can determine abnormalities of cardiac rate and rhythm and can assess the patient's cardiac status, but a cardiologist must interpret the twelve-lead ECG to give a diagnosis.

As a clinical care associate, you will not be expected to interpret an ECG. However, you should know how a normal heart rhythm would appear on a tracing. This pattern, with the conduction system of the heart firing in the predicted sequence, is called **normal sinus rhythm**. You will also be expected to recognize a technically accurate ECG.

Review the anatomy and physiology of the heart in Chapter 11, "The Cardiovascular System." Pay special attention to the electrical activity and structures of the heart. Figure 26-6 shows a normal waveform. Each wave represents a specific segment of the electrical stimulation and relaxation of the heart muscle.

P wave = atrial depolarization
QRS wave = ventricular depolarization
T wave = ventricular repolarization

Some hospitals employ **telemetry technicians** whose job is to continuously observe the cardiac activity of patients attached to cardiac monitors. The monitoring station is located in one room of the hospital, which may be many floors away from the patients being monitored. In many hospitals, these technicians are cross-trained to perform additional tasks. One technician may monitor several patients' cardiac activity by constantly watching ongoing rhythm strips displayed on a computer screen. When changes occur in a patient's heart rate or rhythm, the telemetry technician will call the nursing unit with this information.

You may be asked to check a patient on telemetry (remote cardiac monitoring) when a technician calls to report a problem. First, check the patient's status. Is the patient having any pain? Is the patient moving around? Next, check to be sure the electrodes and wires are correctly attached to the patient and the telemetry unit. Sometimes, the wires become disconnected from the patient's chest. The telemetry technician will call immediately if he or she is unable to view the patient's cardiac status. If a patient has a lethal dysrhythmia, the telemetry technician will call a *code blue*.

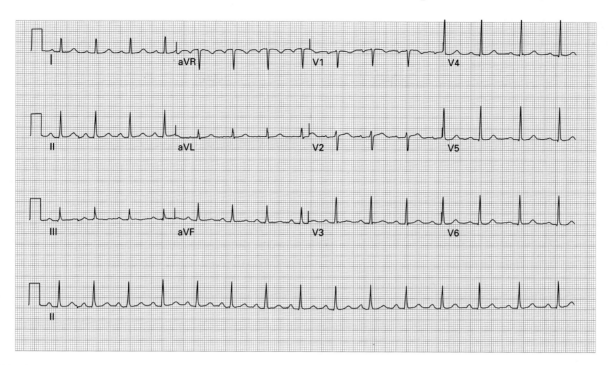

FIGURE 26-6   Normal waveform.

ECG Machines

An electrocardiograph is an instrument used to record the heart's electrical activity. A **multichannel ECG machine** is capable of recording all twelve views of the heart simultaneously and is the most common machine. The **single-channel ECG machine** records each of the twelve leads individually. It is rarely used today. It has been replaced by the more efficient and accurate multichannel machines.

A variety of manufacturers produce multichannel machines, and each brand has its own unique features. You must become familiar with the particular features of the machine used at your facility. The following text discusses the general principles and common features of the multichannel ECG machine. It is important to follow the procedural steps to obtain a tracing that is technically correct so that the physician can accurately interpret the ECG.

Each brand of ECG machine, though different, operates on the same principles. A large cable connects the machine to the patient. The cable splits into ten marked wire extensions. Each extension attaches to a specific place on the patient's body (Figure 26-7). Electrode gel or a self-sticking electrode disk is used on the body to promote adequate conduction of the body's electrical impulses.

Another part of the ECG machine is the **stylus**, which is the pen-tipped point that transcribes thermally the electrical message transmitted from the heart. A complex is the tracing of the heart's electrical activity during one heartbeat. The **ECG paper** is specially coated to accommodate the stylus and mark appropriately. The vertical lines on the paper serve to measure the amplitude, or height, of the complex. The horizontal lines serve to measure the speed, or rate, of the heart.

Each small block on the ECG paper measures 0.04 seconds. Each large block measures 0.2 seconds. Therefore, five large blocks are equal to 1 second, and fifteen large blocks are equal to 3 seconds. Three seconds of the graph paper represents 3 seconds of the heart's activity.

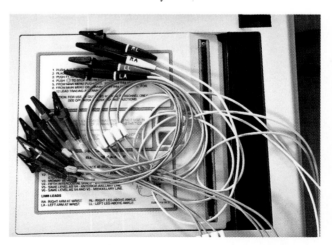

FIGURE 26-7   ECG leads.

Limb Lead Placement

The central cable of the ECG machine splits into ten marked wire extensions. When you look at those ten wires, you will see four of them marked and color-coded in the following way:

LL—red
LA—black
RL—green
RA—white

These are the "limb leads" and will be applied to the left leg (LL), left arm (LA), right leg (RL), and right arm (RA). The color codes are universal for all ECG machines. Before you attach the limb leads to the patient, you must prepare the skin. Make sure that the skin is clean and dry. If the patient is sweating, cleanse the area with an alcohol pad and dry it before placing the leads. Good skin contact is essential to produce a clear tracing. You may have to shave a patient who has a great deal of limb or chest hair in order to provide good skin contact. Only shave the specific areas of lead placement.

When placing the limb leads, always place them as far from the heart as possible, over the fleshy areas of the wrists and ankles, not over bone (Figure 26-8).

The limb leads must be placed symmetrically. Place the leads in the same area on each arm and each leg. If you must move a lead because of a dressing or amputation on one limb, then position the lead on the opposite limb at the same point on the limb. When you attach the right leg lead to a patient who has had an above-the-knee amputation, for example, you must attach the lead in an area of the thigh. This means that you must place the left leg lead on the left thigh, not the left lower leg.

Be certain to place the leads on the correct side of the patient's body. Most ECG machines will give a message indicating incorrect lead placement. One quick test for correct limb lead placement is to look at lead 1. If the QRS complex is upright, then the limb leads have been placed correctly. If the QRS complex is upside down, check limb leads for correct placement.

Chest Lead Placement

The other six wires splitting off from the central cable are called the **precordial** chest or **V leads**. These wires are numbered V1 through V6, and each has a specific placement on the patient's chest (Figure 26-9). You must remember the anatomical landmarks to place the V leads correctly. In order for the ECG to be accurate, the chest leads must be placed in these exact positions (Figure 26-10 and Figure 26-11):

- V1 is placed on the fourth intercostal space to the right of the sternum.
- V2 is placed on the fourth intercostal space to the left of the sternum.
- V4 is the next to be placed. *Look at Figure 26-9. On which intercostal space is V4 placed?* V4 is placed on the fifth intercostal space in the mid-clavicular line.
- V3 is placed next, midway between V4 and V2.

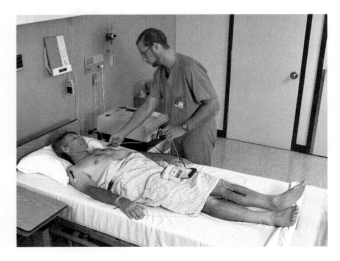

FIGURE 26-8 Limb lead placement.

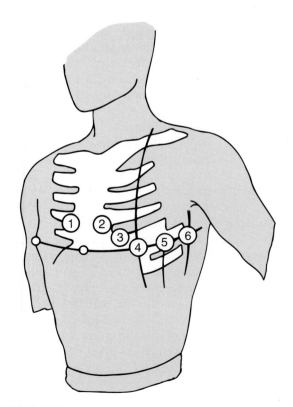

FIGURE 26-9 Chest or V-lead placement.

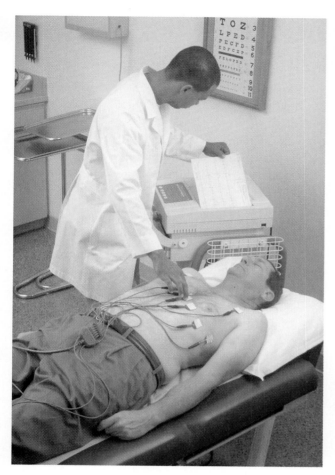

FIGURE 26-10 Clinical care associate performing an ECG on a patient.

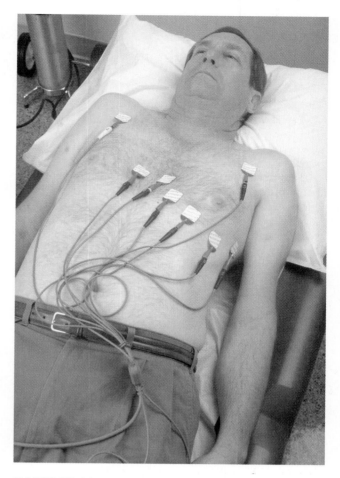

FIGURE 26-11 Correct lead placement is important.

▪ V5 is placed on the fifth intercostal space anterior axilla.

▪ V6 is placed on the fifth intercostal space midaxilla. *If V5 and V6 are on the same intercostal space, why is V6 positioned on a higher plane than V5?* Due to the anatomy of the ribs descending from vertebral attachment, the ribs are higher laterally than anteriorly. Therefore, the intercostal spaces are also higher laterally than anteriorly.

To locate these anatomical landmarks, you must feel and count the intercostal spaces. It will be necessary to look at the chest to approximate the middle of the left clavicle and the axillary markings. To place the V1 and V2 leads, you must feel the borders of the sternum. When placing leads on a female patient with large breasts, it may be necessary to lift the left breast to place the V3 and V4 leads. It may also be necessary to move the left breast away from the axillary area to correctly place leads V5 and V6.

If a chest dressing is in place that prevents the placement of a V lead, discuss with the nurse the proper action to take. If you cannot place a V lead,

place the lead wire on a pillow on the patient's chest to reduce artifact on the tracing. Be sure to indicate on the ECG recording the reason for a blank V lead.

Entering Patient Information

Multichannel ECG machines will "prompt" you to enter patient information or data. This enables the computer to store ECGs for specific patients. The following information is requested most often:

New patient? Yes or No.

Push the keyboard button to indicate YES. Otherwise, this ECG will be recorded as belonging to the previous patient.

Patient last name?

Type in the patient's last name, and push the ENTER key.

Patient first name?

Type in the patient's first name, and push the ENTER key.

p r o c e d u r e

Twelve-Lead ECG

Assess

Determine the type of ECG ordered. Is this a routine ECG or a stat ECG? If this is stat, run the twelve-lead ECG, and then enter any patient data required after you have performed and saved the ECG. Always save the data for editing at a later time.

Determine the needs of the patient. Is the patient in discomfort or cold? Does the patient have a tremor? Is the patient sweating? Does the patient have excessive hair on the limbs or chest? Does the patient have more important needs that must be met before performing this procedure?

Determine any equipment needs. Is the ECG machine operating correctly? Is a diskette in the cart, paper in place, lead wires intact?

Plan

Gather required equipment: ECG cart with tracing paper and diskette, electrical outlet with no other cords plugged in, alcohol pads, and tabs or conduction devices. Use standard precautions as appropriate.

Manage your time to complete stat ECGs first, then complete other ordered ECGs in time for the diskette to be available to be downloaded into the main cardiology computer.

Implement

1. Position the patient for privacy and comfort, with the level of the bed at a comfortable working height.

2. Clean the areas of skin where the leads will be placed.
3. Attach limb leads.
4. Attach chest or V leads.
5. Enter all required patient data.
6. Push the RUN 12 LEAD button on the keypad.
7. Examine the tracing for technical accuracy. Correct any technical problems. Rerun the ECG if needed.
8. Review the recorded information to ensure that all patient data are correct. Edit the data if needed.
9. Remove all leads and electrode "tabs."
10. Clean any remaining conduction gel from the patient's chest and limbs.
11. Reposition the patient for comfort and safety.
12. Unplug the ECG cart/machine, and return it to the storage area.
13. Give the nurse the temporary copy of the ECG.

Evaluate

Evaluate your actions. Is the tracing technically accurate and readable? Is all patient data accurate?

Evaluate the patient's response. Report any complaints of pain or discomfort. Report any concerns regarding a dysrhythmia.

Patient age?
Use the numerical keypad to enter the patient's age.

Patient medical record number?
Type the medical record number for this patient. This is usually a six- or eight-digit number. Double check the medical record number for accuracy.

Male? Female?
Type the correct response, or strike the key that indicates male or female.

Patient race?
Type the correct response, or strike the key that indicates the patient's race.

Weight?
Enter the patient's weight, using the numerical keypad.

Height?
Enter the patient's height in inches, using the numerical keypad.

Systolic blood pressure?
Enter the most recent systolic blood pressure, using the numerical keypad.

Diastolic blood pressure?
Enter the most recent diastolic blood pressure, using the numerical keypad.

Physician?
Enter the requesting doctor's name or the attending physician's name.

Technician's number or initials?
Enter your number or initials. Some facilities give everyone a code number, and some require staff initials.

Technical Quality of the ECG Tracing

Here are some ways to correct the contributing factors of poor-quality tracings.

1. Are the complexes in lead 1 upright? If not, check limb leads for correct placement.
2. Does the ECG look like it was drawn with a fine ballpoint pen? If not, check the following:
   ▪ Does the patient have a tremor of the limbs? When a patient has a tremor, it is usually the

distal areas that shake. Move the limb leads to the proximal area of the limbs. You can place the limb leads near the hips and clavicles. This helps reduce artifact. Limb leads for the arms are placed on the trunk of the body near the shoulder area.

- Did the cables or lead wires move during the procedure?
- Check the electrode tabs or lead conduction devices for skin contact. Poor skin contact due to sweat or hair will cause artifact.
- Be sure the clips that attach to the electrode tabs or to conduction devices are securely clipped to the metal end of the tabs. Poor connections will cause artifact (Figure 26-12).
- Be sure the patient is warm and comfortable. A cold, shivering patient will result in artifact.
- Check the outlet used for the ECG machine. No other equipment should use the same outlet. This will cause 60-cycle interference, which looks like ink was spilled on the ECG paper (Figure 26-13). If it is necessary to unplug other equipment to free up an outlet for the ECG machine, check with the nurse first. Pumps and controllers used for feedings and IVs can be unplugged for a time and still operate using battery power.

3. Do all the complexes on the ECG originate from a straight baseline? Is the baseline as straight as a ruler's edge? The baseline for all of the complexes should be on the same line of the graph paper. When the baseline moves up and down along the paper, it is called a *wandering baseline* (Figure 26-14).

- Check the patient for movement. The patient must lie still while the ECG is running, usually about 1 minute.
- Check the patient's respirations. If the patient is breathing heavily, coughing, sneezing, or laughing, it will cause the baseline to jump. Wait for the coughing, sneezing, or laughing to stop. Then rerecord the ECG.

Troubleshooting the ECG Machine

The LCD screen on the computer keyboard will display messages that indicate a problem during the recording of an ECG. Again, each brand of ECG machine is a little bit different, but some messages are fairly universal.

No Acquisition

If you get this message, check the cable that connects the lead wires to the cart. Usually, all of the

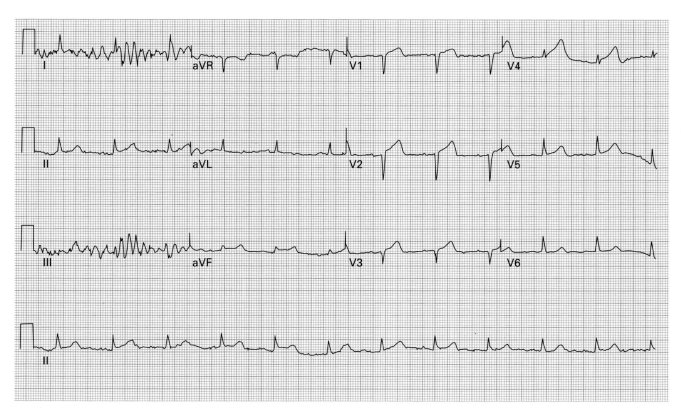

FIGURE 26-12   Artifact.

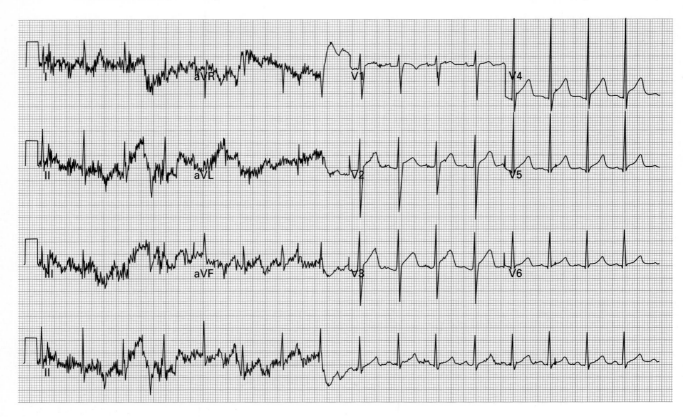

FIGURE 26-13 60-cycle electrical interference.

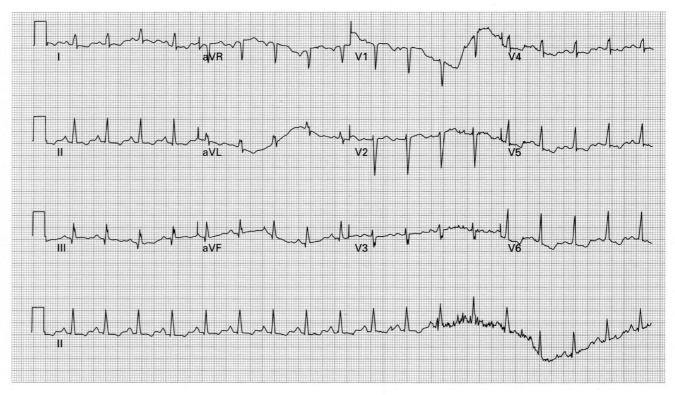

FIGURE 26-14 Wandering baseline.

lead wires are attached to the cart with a plastic clamp like a telephone jack.

Lead Not Attached

When you get this message, push the STOP button on the keyboard. Check the clamp and lead wire connection for the lead or leads that are indicated in the message. Once you have ensured proper connection, push the RUN 12 LEAD button to record the ECG.

Disk or Diskette Error

If you get this message, check that a disk is in the ECG cart. Insert a disk if none is in place. The ECG you record will be downloaded into the main computer. Then the cardiologists can access the ECG for review and interpretation. If no diskette is available on the ECG cart, follow your institution's policy to obtain a new diskette.

Problem-Solving Exercise

Read each of the following situations, then indicate the actions that you would take to resolve the problem.

Your patient, Mr. Oleg, is post-op coronary artery bypass graft (CABG) and is experiencing chest pain. A stat ECG is ordered. He has a dressing that prevents exact placement of V1 and V2 leads.

If you can lift the edges of the tape securing the dressing, then place V1 and V2 as close as possible to the exact locations needed. If you cannot lift the tape or get close to the correct anatomical landmarks, place the lead wires for V1 and V2 on a pillow, and run the ECG. Tell the nurse or doctor the reason these leads were not recorded on the tracing.

Mr. James is complaining of severe chest pain. When you attempt to perform a stat ECG, the display window reads "Check placement of V6."

Push the STOP button on the keypad. Check the electrode tab for skin contact, and check the clamp of the V6 wire for contact. Push the RUN 12 LEAD button on the keypad. If you continue to get the error message, override it by pushing the RUN 12 LEAD button again. This is a stat ECG, and you may need to run it without V6 if you cannot solve the problem immediately.

Mr. Paul is a seventy-two-year-old patient with Parkinson's disease. You notice the presence of artifact on the ECG graph paper.

Try moving the limb lead conduction devices or electrode tabs as close to the patient's trunk as possible. This will reduce artifact caused by the tremor in his hands and feet. Then rerun the ECG.

Mrs. Mark has a right below-the-knee amputation. You are asked to perform a twelve-lead ECG.

Since this patient has had her right leg amputated, you must place the right leg electrode tab or conduction device above the amputation. You must be sure that the left leg lead is placed symmetrically with that of the right leg.

The display window reads "Lead V4 and V5 disconnected."

Push the STOP button on the keypad. Check the connections of the lead wires and the skin contact of the electrode tabs. Also check the clamps of the lead wires. Again, push the RUN 12 LEAD button to run the ECG.

Dressings

Dressings are used to protect wounds and surgical incisions from infection, to promote wound healing, and to prevent further skin breakdown. There are numerous types of dressings (Figure 26-15). Nurses change dressings that cover IVs, surgical incisions, and wounds that require the application of medications because of the need to assess these wounds. This includes dressings over infected wounds, decubitus ulcers, and stasis ulcers. The first dressing change after a surgery is often done by the surgeon.

As a clinical care associate, you will apply and change nonsterile dressings, Tegaderm and Duoderm dressings, and wet-to-dry dressings.

Tegaderm Dressings

A **Tegaderm dressing** is a clear adhesive shield that protects the wound from water and potential irritants. Because it is transparent, the site can be observed without removing the dressing. These types of dressings can remain in place for 24 to 48 hours. Your facility will have a policy regarding the length of time such dressings may be left in place.

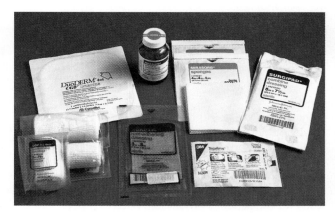

FIGURE 26-15   Various types of dressings.

p r o c e d u r e
Applying a Tegaderm Dressing

Assess

Determine the size and type of dressing needed. Where is the Tegaderm dressing to be applied? What size is the existing dressing, incision, or wound?

Determine the condition of the incision or wound. Is there any sign of redness, swelling, drainage, pain, or warmth around the incision or wound? If so, notify the nurse so he or she can assess the site.

Determine the needs of the patient. Is the patient comfortable and ready for you to proceed? Have you provided for the patient's privacy and safety?

Plan

Gather required supplies: two pairs of nonsterile gloves, washcloth, soap and water, Tegaderm dressing of the correct size, and biohazard waste receptacle. Use standard precautions.

Determine the best time to perform this procedure. Can it best be done before or after the bath?

Implement

1. Position the patient for comfort and safety, with the bed at a comfortable working height.
2. Remove the existing Tegaderm dressing by holding the skin taut and gradually pulling the dressing away. This will prevent skin tears and discomfort. Discard the used dressing.
3. Remove your gloves, and wash your hands. Apply clean gloves.
4. Gently cleanse the skin around the site with soap and water, then pat dry. Do not touch the incision unless you are instructed to cleanse the site or wound.
5. Peel open the Tegaderm package.
6. Write the date and time of the dressing change on the Tegaderm with a ballpoint pen.
7. Peel the window frame from the top surface of the Tegaderm.
8. Center the Tegaderm over the wound.
9. Gradually remove the paper backing from the Tegaderm as you adhere the dressing to the site.
10. Smooth the dressing in place, making sure that all edges are firmly adhered.
11. Assist the patient to a comfortable and safe position.
12. Record the time and type of dressing change on the correct form.

Evaluate

Evaluate your actions. Has the nurse assessed the site if needed? Is the Tegaderm the proper size and centered over the wound? Is it free of wrinkles and adhering to the skin?

Evaluate the patient's response. Report any complaints of pain or discomfort during the procedure. Report the dressing change to the nurse.

Duoderm Dressings

Duoderm dressings are wafer-type dressings that provide a protective "second skin" for wounds. These dressings are designed to protect initial skin breakdown, such as that associated with stage 1 and stage 2 pressure wounds. Duoderm dressings seal the wound or irritated area from further breakdown caused by pressure and irritation. This type of dressing can be left in place for 48 to 72 hours. Your facility will have a policy regarding the length of time such dressings may be left in place.

---

p r o c e d u r e
Applying a Duoderm Dressing

Assess

Determine the size and type of dressing needed. Where is the Duoderm dressing to be applied? What size is the existing dressing or wound?

Determine the condition of the wound.

Determine the needs of the patient. Is the patient comfortable and ready for you to proceed? Have you provided for the patient's privacy and safety?

Plan

Gather required equipment: two pairs of nonsterile gloves, washcloth, soap and water, Duoderm dressing of the correct size, and biohazard waste receptacle. Use standard precautions.

Arrange for the nurse to be present to assess the wound when the current Duoderm dressing is removed.

p r o c e d u r e (c o n t i n u e d)

Determine the best time to perform this procedure. Can it best be done before or after the bath?

Implement

1. Position the patient for comfort and safety, with the bed at a comfortable working height.
2. Remove the existing Duoderm dressing by holding the skin taut and gradually pulling the dressing away.
3. Dispose of the old dressing and gloves, then wash your hands. Put on clean gloves.
4. Clean the surrounding area of the skin with soap and water. Pat dry.
5. Allow time for the nurse to assess the wound and surrounding skin area.
6. Open the packaging of the Duoderm dressing.
7. Apply the Duoderm smoothly and firmly to the site.
8. Hold your hand on the Duoderm for approximately 30 seconds to mold the wafer dressing to the skin. Note: The heat of your hand helps to adhere this dressing firmly in place.
9. Assist the patient to a comfortable and safe position.
10. Record the time and type of dressing change on the correct form.

Evaluate

Evaluate your actions. Is the Duoderm the proper size and centered over the wound? Is it adhering to the skin?

Evaluate the patient's response. Report any complaints of pain or discomfort during the procedure.

Wet-to-Dry Dressings

A **wet-to-dry dressing** is used to promote wound healing. When this type of dressing is used, the inner gauze is allowed to dry before removal. When the dried gauze is removed, necrotic, unhealthy tissue tears away from the wound as well. With such "dead" tissue removed, circulation to the wound improves, allowing healing to occur.

Current theories of wound healing do not support the need for the inner gauze to dry completely. In fact, many wound specialists now believe that the trauma of tearing away the dry dressing causes a greater opportunity for infection to occur. Follow the policy of your institution regarding whether to allow the inner gauze to dry completely or not. Such dressings are ordered to be changed every 4, 6, or 8 hours.

When a wet-to-dry dressing change is performed, normal saline is usually the solution ordered for soaking the inner gauze. The size and depth of the wound will determine the type of inner gauze used. For wounds that are deep but small in circumference, a strip of narrow, long gauze material is needed. One brand name for this type of gauze is Nugauze. For wounds that are wider in circumference and level with the skin surface, 4-inch-by-4-inch gauze squares (4-by-4s) or 2-inch-by-2-inch gauze squares (2-by-2s) are required. A wound that is wide in circumference and deep below the skin surface requires rolled gauze for packing into the wound. One brand name for this type of gauze is Kling.

After the saline-soaked gauze is applied to the wound, a dry gauze covering is applied over it and taped in place using a crisscross taping method. The best tape choice is an allergen-free tape, such as Transpore. Silk tape can cause irritation and tearing of the skin because it is nonporous. The adhesive used on silk tape can be irritating to the skin.

It is important to follow some rules of asepsis and sterile technique regarding the use of normal saline solution. When you open a new bottle of saline, write the date and time it was opened on the label. Most institutions allow a bottle of saline for irrigation to be used for 24 hours. Always check the date and time to be sure the saline has not become outdated. If no date and time is written on an opened bottle, do not use the solution. Instead, get a new bottle.

When you remove the lid of the saline bottle, keep the open end of the bottle cap facing upward. If the open end is placed down, it will become contaminated with microbes from the surface on which it is placed. Then these microbes will be transferred to the saline bottle.

When you pour the saline onto the gauze, do not touch the bottle to the gauze. This will prevent contamination of the gauze with microbes from the saline bottle.

p r o c e d u r e

Applying a Wet-to-Dry Dressing

Assess

Determine the size and type of dressing materials needed. What type of dressing is currently on the wound? Discuss with the nurse the appropriate dressing materials to use.

Determine the needs of the patient. This type of dressing change can be painful for the patient. Discuss the patient's pain medication schedule with the nurse before performing this procedure. Schedule the dressing change for after the patient has received pain medication.

Plan

Gather required supplies: two pairs of nonsterile gloves, sterile gloves (if required), nonallergenic tape, type and amount of gauze needed, sterile normal saline for irrigation, and a biohazard waste receptacle. You may also need a bed protector and an irrigation basin or tray. Use standard precautions.

Discuss with the nurse whether you will need to use sterile gloves when applying the new wet dressing.

Arrange for the nurse to be present to assess the wound when the current dressing is removed.

Implement

1. Position the patient for comfort and safety, with the bed at a comfortable working height.
2. Remove the current dressing, including the inner gauze. Discard the dressing and your gloves in the biohazard waste container.
3. Allow time for the nurse to assess the wound.
4. Open the package of gauze roll or squares.
5. Tear or cut four strips of tape to the correct size to tape the edges of the dressing in "window frame" fashion.
6. Pour enough saline over the gauze to fully wet all layers of the gauze.
7. Apply clean or sterile gloves as directed.
8. Cover or pack the wound with the wet gauze. If you are packing the wound, gently fill it completely with the gauze, but do not force the wound edges.
9. Cover the wet dressing with dry gauze, and secure it with tape in "window frame" fashion.
10. Assist the patient to a position of comfort and safety.
11. Record the time and type of dressing change on the appropriate form.

Evaluate

Evaluate your actions. Did you maintain clean or sterile technique as directed? Was the gauze wet through all the layers? Is the dressing taped in place correctly?

Evaluate the patient's response. Report any complaints by the patient during the procedure. Report any difficulty in packing or dressing the wound.

Ostomy Care

Ostomy care involves caring for a patient who has a surgical stoma. A stoma is an opening on the abdomen for the elimination of stool or urine. You may see different types of ostomies. A **colostomy** results from surgically opening the large intestine and forming a stoma (hole) of colon tissue on the surface of the abdomen. The consistency of the stool passed through a colostomy will usually be pasty to formed. An **ileostomy** is created by opening the last part of the small intestine, the ileum, and forming a stoma of ileal tissue on the surface of the abdomen. The consistency of the stool passed through an ileostomy will be liquid to pasty. A **urostomy** is an opening created for the passage of urine. The stoma is formed by surgically looping the ureter through the ileum. The urostomy stoma on the abdomen is smaller than the colostomy or ileostomy stoma (Figure 26-16).

A person might require an ostomy because of a birth defect, cancer, ulcerative intestinal disorders, or an accident or trauma to the intestines or the bladder. Most often, ostomies are permanent procedures, and the person will need to wear an ostomy appliance for life. Occasionally, such procedures are temporary. Some conditions of the intestines or bladder, such as ulceration or trauma, may heal with time. The ostomy allows the organ to remain inactive while it heals.

As you can imagine, the patient who undergoes this type of surgery has many emotional needs. The patient must cope with the original diagnosis, the alteration of normal elimination functions, and a change in body image. When you care for a patient who has an ostomy appliance, you must be especially concerned with your reaction to the patient, the stoma, and the ostomy appliance. The patient may be self-conscious about the need for assistance with such a private bodily function. The patient may also feel unattractive due to the stoma and appliance. The possibility of odor or leakage from the appliance can also cause the patient to become isolated.

Initial postoperative ostomy care should be performed by the nurse or enterostomal nurse specialist. The assessment, plan of care, and evaluation steps must be performed by the nurse. Your responsibilities

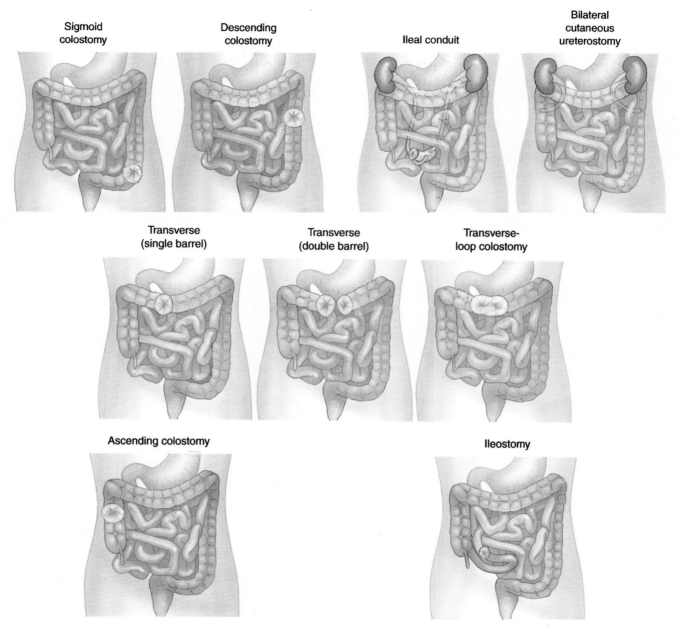

FIGURE 26-16 Types of ostomies and position of the stoma.

in care will involve observation and care of the stoma and the surrounding skin, as well as emptying and changing the appliance. Patients will be taught by the nurse, doctor, or enterostomal therapist to care for their own ostomies. However, patients with new ostomies and patients who are too ill to perform their own care will need your compassionate assistance.

Ostomy appliances are routinely changed every three to four days. In addition, the appliance is changed anytime leaking occurs. An ostomy appliance must be emptied when it is one-third full of urine, stool, or gas. A urostomy appliance will collect urine slowly and constantly, so you must check frequently to determine when it should be emptied.

The amount, frequency, and type of food and fluid intake will affect the consistency and frequency of stool elimination. Patients with a colostomy have more predictable times for stool elimination than those who have an ileostomy. Ileostomy appliances need to be emptied more frequently than colostomy appliances because the stool is more liquid and is eliminated more frequently. The hospital dietitian will assist the patient in choosing a diet that is nutritious and does not cause increased intestinal gas.

Plan to empty or change the patient's ostomy appliance well before or after mealtimes. Be aware that eating will increase peristalsis, which will cause stool to pass into the ostomy appliance.

All stomas should be pink in color and should appear raised above the skin surface of the abdomen. Any problems with leaking around the stoma or the ostomy appliance should be immediately reported to the nurse. The skin around the stoma can be irritated easily by the acid and enzymes in the urine or stool. Careful attention to skin care and proper appliance fit are essential. The skin around the stoma can be irritated by removing the appliance. The skin care you will be expected to perform includes cleansing the area around the stoma with soap and water, then gently drying the skin. Always report any signs of irritation to the nurse.

Many appliances have a deodorant sealed into the plastic. These types of appliances should not be washed because the deodorant can be washed out. A variety of manufacturers produce appliances and ostomy supplies. The surgeon or enterostomal nurse will determine the size and type of appliance appropriate for each patient. Decisions regarding the need for additional adhesives or skin care products will also be determined by the enterostomal nurse.

p r o c e d u r e

Emptying the Ostomy Appliance

Assess

Determine the condition of the ostomy appliance. Is it adhering firmly to the skin? What type of clamp is used to close the pouch? Is it one-third full? Is the urine or stool normal in appearance?

Determine the condition of the skin. Is the skin around the appliance red, irritated, or open? Is any stool or urine leaking onto the skin?

Determine the patient's needs during the procedure. What is the patient's emotional response to the ostomy? To what extent is the patient participating in the care procedure?

Plan

Gather required equipment: gloves, bed protector, measuring container, toilet tissue, washbasin with warm water and soap, washcloth, and towel. Use standard precautions.

Determine the best time to perform this procedure. Can it be combined with other care, such as the bath? Is it time for a meal to be served?

Implement

1. Position the patient for comfort and safety, raising the bed to a comfortable working height.
2. Place the bed protector under the ostomy appliance.
3. Lift the end of the ostomy pouch upright, and remove the clamp. Save the clamp.

4. Empty the contents of the pouch into the measuring container, and note the amount. If the stool is pasty or formed, gently press the pouch from the top to the end to expel the contents.
5. Clean the end of the pouch and the clamp with toilet tissue. It may be necessary to wash the clamp with soap and water before reapplying.
6. Cuff the end of the colostomy or ileostomy pouch by double-folding the end over the clamp.
7. Secure the clamp.
   Note: Urostomy pouches are emptied through a port by opening the cap. Drain the urine into the measuring container, and replace the cap.
8. Wash and dry the skin of the abdomen near the ostomy appliance.
9. Reposition the patient for comfort and safety.
10. Record the procedure on the appropriate chart form.

Evaluate

Evaluate your actions. Is the ostomy area clean and dry? Is the appliance end cuffed and clamped or capped? Did you remember to measure the output and record it on the intake-and-output record?

Evaluate the patient's response. Report any complaints of discomfort. Report the unusual appearance of urine or stool. Report the patient's participation in and emotional response to the procedure.

p r o c e d u r e

Changing the Ostomy Appliance

Assess

Determine the size and type of appliance needed.

Determine the condition of the skin. Is the skin around the stoma red, irritated, or open? Is any stool or urine leaking onto the skin? Is the stoma pink and elevated? Is there any evidence of bleeding? Arrange for the nurse to assess any skin abnormalities.

Determine the patient's needs during the procedure. What is the patient's emotional response to the ostomy? To what extent is the patient participating in the care procedure?

Plan

Gather required supplies: gloves; bed protector; new ostomy appliance; measuring container; toilet tissue; washbasin with warm water and soap; washcloth; any supplemental paste, powders, or adhesives (if ordered); towel; gauze pads; and biohazard waste receptacle. Use standard precautions.

Determine the best time to perform this procedure. Can it be combined with other care, such as the bath? Is it time for a meal to be served?

Implement

1. Position the patient for comfort and safety, with the bed elevated to a comfortable working height.
2. Place the bed protector under the ostomy appliance.
3. Remove the paper backing on the new appliance.
4. Note the consistency and color of the contents of the current appliance before emptying and measuring it.
5. Remove the appliance from the skin, and remove the clamp from the appliance. Clean and save the clamp or port and cap.
6. Discard the used appliance in the biohazard waste container.
7. Wash the skin and the stoma, then pat dry.
8. Allow time for the nurse to observe the skin and stoma, if needed.
9. Center the appliance over the stoma, and apply it to the skin. Ask the nurse whether a skin prep is to be used.
10. Smooth any wrinkles in the appliance and adhesive backing.
11. If an elastic waist belt is used, secure it to the appliance, ensuring that it does not constrict the skin.
12. Cuff and clamp the appliance, or attach the port and cap, then close securely.
13. Record the procedure on the appropriate form.

Evaluate

Evaluate your actions. Is the appliance securely adhering to the skin? Is the clamp or cap in place? Did you remember to measure and record the output from the old appliance?

Evaluate the patient's response. Report any complaints of pain or discomfort during the procedure. Report the unusual appearance of urine or stool. Report the patient's participation in and emotional response to the procedure. Report the condition of the stoma.

Respiratory Care

Oxygen Therapy

During your work as a clinical care associate, you will care for patients who require oxygen therapy. The amount of oxygen and the delivery method will be prescribed by the physician. You will need to be knowledgeable about delivery methods and safety issues regarding oxygen therapy.

Oxygen is supplied in the hospital either through a wall outlet or in a green oxygen tank (Figure 26-17). Oxygen can be supplied from the wall or tank to the patient in several ways. The following information is about two of the most basic methods.

A **nasal cannula** is the most common and the simplest way to deliver oxygen. The cannula is a hollow tube with prongs attached. The prongs are placed in the patient's nose, and the tubing is hooked behind the ears and under the chin (Figure 26-18). Tubing that is too tight can cause irritation to the skin around the nose and ears. Oxygen is odorless and tasteless, so the patient wearing a nasal cannula can smell, eat, and talk normally. The patient should be instructed to breathe through the

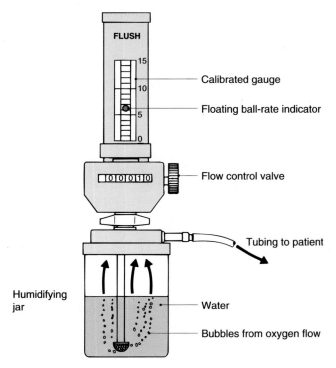

FIGURE 26-17   Oxygen-delivery system.

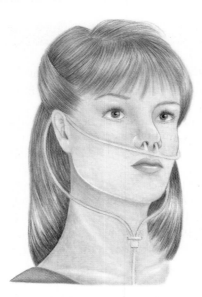

FIGURE 26-18   The tubing of cannulas is flexible.

nose rather than the mouth in order to get the most benefit from this delivery method. Oxygen does cause dryness of the mucous membranes of the mouth and nose, therefore extra care should be given to prevent problems from this drying effect.

The other oxygen-delivery method is the **face mask**. Different types of masks deliver different percentages of oxygen. The mask fits over the nose and the mouth, so it must be removed to allow the patient to eat and drink. Elastic straps secured behind the ears hold the mask in place. If the elastic is too tight, it will cause skin irritation around the ears. Some patients may complain that the oxygen mask feels "suffocating." Remind the patient to breathe normally and reassure him or her that suffocation is not possible. Again, skin and mouth care are necessary to combat the effects of dryness due to oxygen therapy.

The safe administration of oxygen is extremely important. Place a sign on the patient's door that says, "Oxygen in use: No open flames." Instruct patients on oxygen to avoid the use of electric razors and hair dryers for fire safety reasons. *Never* change the oxygen flowmeter setting from the prescribed liter flow. Tanks must *always* be secured to a holding device because of the danger of a tank or canister falling over.

procedure
Applying a Nasal Cannula

Assess

Determine the prescribed liter flow of oxygen. Is the flowmeter set at the correct amount? If not, notify the nurse or respiratory therapist. Is the patient keeping the cannula in place? Is all equipment working properly? Are the nasal prongs free from secretions? Is the tubing free from food or other substances?

Determine the condition of the skin and mucous membranes. Are the nose and mouth in need of lubricant? Is mouth and skin care being given every 2 hours? Are there reddened areas of skin around the nose, mouth, or ears? What is the color of the skin, lips, mucous membranes, and nail beds?

Plan

Gather required equipment: nasal cannula and mouth and skin care supplies (if needed). Use standard precautions as appropriate.

Determine the best time to perform this procedure. Can it be combined with mouth, nose, and skin care? Is this patient in need of oxygen promptly?

Implement

1. Place the two prongs of the cannula into the patient's nostrils, with the prongs curving inward following the curve of the nose and with the tab in the upward position.
2. Position the tubing behind and over the ears.
3. Gently secure the cannula by adjusting the slide under the chin.
4. Securely attach the distal end of the tubing to the oxygen output adapter.

Evaluate

Evaluate your actions. Do the nasal prongs curve inward and downward? Does the tubing fit around the chin and behind the ears?

Evaluate the patient's response. Report any patient questions, concerns, or complaints of discomfort. Report the completion of the procedure to the nurse.

procedure
Applying a Face Mask

Assess

Determine the condition of the current face mask. Is it in need of change? What type of face mask is ordered?

Determine the prescribed liter flow of oxygen. Is the flowmeter set at the correct amount? If not, notify the nurse or respiratory therapist. Is the patient keeping the mask in place? Is all equipment working properly? Is the tubing free from food or other substances?

Determine the condition of the skin and mucous membranes. Are the nose and mouth in need of lubricant? Is mouth and skin care being given every 2 hours? Are there reddened areas of skin around the nose, mouth, or ears? What is the color of the skin, lips, mucous membranes, and nail beds?

Plan

Gather required equipment: face mask and mouth and skin care supplies (if needed). Use standard precautions as appropriate.

Determine the best time to perform this procedure. Can it be combined with mouth, nose, and skin care? Is this patient in need of oxygen promptly?

Implement

1. Gently place the face mask over the patient's face, covering the mouth and nose.
2. Slip the loosened elastic straps over the patient's head, and position them above the ears.
3. Pull the ends of the elastic straps to create a snug fit.
4. Adjust the metal nosepiece to fit the patient's face.

Evaluate

Evaluate your actions. Does the face mask fit over the nose and mouth? Is the elastic adjusted for a snug fit? Is there any indication that the elastic is too tight, constricting the skin?

Evaluate the patient's response. Report any questions, concerns, or complaints of discomfort. Report the completion of the procedure to the nurse.

Patients on oxygen therapy require special attention to mouth and skin care. Lubricate the nose, and give oral care every 2 hours. Use a non-oil-based lubricant. Observe the skin around the mouth, nose, chin, and ears for signs of irritation. Remind patients to keep the cannula or mask in place at all times in order to receive the prescribed oxygen amount. Observe the skin, lips, and nail beds for cyanosis or excessive redness. If the patient is receiving too little oxygen, cyanosis can result. If too much oxygen is being delivered, excessive redness will result. Report any changes in color or breathing immediately.

A nurse, respiratory technician, or respiratory therapist will set the oxygen flowmeter to the prescribed liters of oxygen. Because this is actually a prescription, it must be administered by a licensed professional. However, you will need to know the amount of liter flow prescribed and the method of delivery for the patients in your care. You may also be asked to prepare the equipment for oxygen delivery. At times, you may transport patients who are receiving oxygen therapy.

Pulse Oximetry

Pulse oximetry is used to monitor a patient's respiratory status. This technology uses light to measure the saturation of oxygen in the patient's circulating blood. The **pulse oximeter** is used routinely in the operating room and intensive care settings to continuously monitor the saturation of oxygen (SaO_2) (Figure 26-19). A nurse or respiratory therapist will set the oximeter to alarm when the SaO_2 falls above or below prescribed limits. When the alarm sounds, the nurse will assess the patient.

In general nursing care areas, this procedure is performed at scheduled intervals to measure the

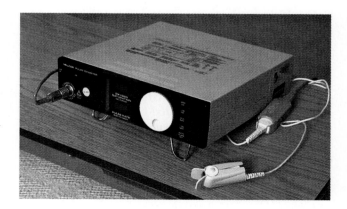

FIGURE 26-19 Pulse oximeter.

p r o c e d u r e

Measuring SaO₂ Using a Pulse Oximeter

Assess

Determine the appropriate sensor site. Do you need to remove any nail polish or other substance that will interfere with the reading?

Determine previous readings. Are previous pulse oximetry readings recorded on the data sheet? What is the range of the previous readings?

Plan

Gather required equipment: alcohol pad, oxisensor, oximeter, and nonallergenic tape (if continuous monitoring is ordered).

Determine the best time to perform this procedure. Is the measurement ordered at a specific time interval? Is this a stat measurement? Is this an order for continuous pulse oximetry?

Implement

1. Clean the patient's finger with alcohol, and allow it to dry.
2. Connect the oxisensor to the patient cable, then connect the cable to the oximeter.
3. Plug the oximeter into a grounded 100 to 120 alternating current (AC) outlet.
4. Place the light-emitting portion of the oxisensor against the nail bed, with the alignment marks properly positioned.
5. Turn on the oximeter. You will hear a beep with each detected pulse.
6. When the number or value stabilizes, note the number on the oximeter display.
7. Record the oximeter reading on the appropriate form.
8. Return the oximeter to the storage area, but leave the oxisensor at the bedside.

Evaluate

Evaluate your actions. Were all cables hooked up correctly? Was the oxisensor positioned correctly? Were you able to obtain an oximetry measurement?

Evaluate the patient's response. Report the value to the nurse. Report any difficulty in obtaining the measurement. Report any patient complaints of discomfort or difficulty breathing.

If you experience difficulty obtaining an oximetry reading, here are some guidelines to follow:

- If the alarm is sounding, go to the patient and check the site. Be sure that all cables are attached correctly and that the oxisensor is attached to the patient.
- If all connections are secured and the alarm is still sounding, call for the nurse stat.
- If the oximetry value has changed since the last measurement was read, determine the size of the change. Report any increase greater than 15 percent. Report any value that has decreased since the last reading. (Oximetry values will change as the patient's condition changes.)

---

effectiveness of oxygen therapy or to determine the patient's need for oxygen therapy. A light-sensitive device, called an **oxisensor**, is placed on the patient's index finger. In small children, a toe or earlobe may be used. The vascular areas of the nail beds and the earlobes are the preferred sites for measuring the SaO₂. If the patient is wearing nail polish, it must be removed before obtaining an SaO₂ measurement.

Incentive Spirometry

An **incentive spirometer (IS)** is a device that measures the volume of air inhaled by the patient (Figure 26-20). Incentive spirometry is ordered for post-op and immobile patients (Figure 26-21). By using the IS to take deep breaths, the patient helps prevent respiratory complications during recovery. The air sacs, or alveoli, in the lungs can collapse, hampering gas exchange and allowing secretions to accumulate in the lungs. The patients who are especially susceptible to alveoli collapse are those with decreased mobility or pain, those suffering the residual effects of anesthesia, and those on pain medication. This type of medication can decrease the depth and rate of respirations. Patients with these types of conditions must cough, deep-breathe, and use incentive spirometry to prevent pneumonia and other respiratory complications.

The volume goal for inspirations is determined by the respiratory therapist or by doctor's order. The IS will also measure the progress made by the patient with each successive inspiration. You will need to remind patients to use the incentive spirometer at least hourly. Cues to help people remember include timing the activity with TV commercial breaks or radio news breaks. Family members can also help remind patients to use IS, cough, and deep-breathe. Sometimes, a patient does not cooperate in these procedures because they cause pain. Encourage the patient to splint any incisional areas with a pillow during breathing exercises or IS. If the pain is more generalized, encourage the patient to request pain medication.

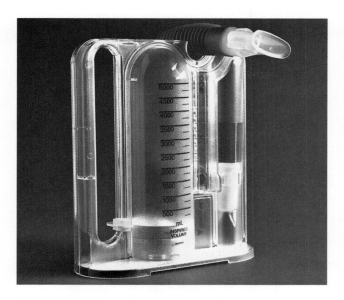

FIGURE 26-20   Incentive spirometer.

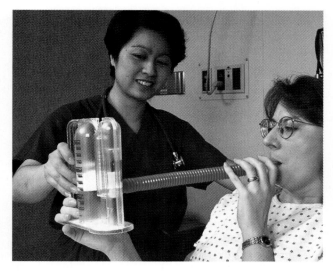

FIGURE 26-21   Use of the incentive spirometer helps prevent respiratory complications during recovery.

procedure
Assisting with an Incentive Spirometry

Assess
Determine the patient's abilities. Can the patient sit upright or tolerate elevation of the head of the bed? What is the patient's level of pain? Does the patient understand how to use the IS?

Plan
Gather required equipment: incentive spirometer, tissues, and emesis basin or sputum specimen container. (After IS is performed, the patient usually coughs up mucus suitable for a sputum specimen if one is ordered.) Use standard precautions.

Determine the best time to instruct the patient on IS. Is the patient comfortable and able to listen? Is the patient able to understand and follow the instructions? Are there easy cues to help the patient remember to use IS every hour?

Implement
1. Position the patient in an upright position if possible.
2. Instruct the patient to exhale normally.
3. Place the mouthpiece between the patient's lips. Instruct him or her to close the mouth tightly around the mouthpiece.
4. Ask the patient to inhale slowly and deeply through the mouth, as if using a straw.
5. Note the level to which the ball inside the cylinder rises. This is the maximum volume of air.
6. Instruct the patient to hold this inspiration for 3 seconds.
7. Remove the mouthpiece, and instruct the patient to slowly and fully exhale through the mouth.
8. Instruct the patient to repeat steps 2 through 7. This should be done 5 to 10 times each hour.
9. Record the procedure on the appropriate chart form.

Evaluate
Evaluate your actions. Did the patient fully understand the instructions? Did you note the maximum volume of inspired air?

Evaluate the patient's response. Did the patient experience any dizziness or fatigue? Did the patient produce any mucus from the cough? What was the color and consistency of any sputum produced? Report the results and your observations to the nurse.

Oral Suctioning

Suctioning is the process of withdrawing secretions or fluids from the airway with a catheter. These secretions can accumulate in the upper airway after surgery or when the patient is immobile. The patient may not be able to **expectorate** (cough up) the secretions adequately due to weakness or due to an excessive amount of secretions. Therefore, the fluids accumulate in the mouth.

As an unlicensed caregiver, you should only perform *oral* suctioning. Tracheal suctioning is a procedure that requires a nurse's assessment and problem-solving ability. Some states have guidelines that allow unlicensed personnel to perform other types of suctioning, such as tracheal suctioning. In many cases, patients who have had oral surgery or ear, nose, or throat procedures perform oral suctioning themselves after instruction by the nurse or surgeon.

An **oral suction (Yankeur) catheter** is a plastic tube with a thick grip for easy use (Figure 26-22). Oral suctioning is not a sterile procedure, so the catheter or Yankeur is kept clean and is used only for one patient. Always follow standard precautions when performing suctioning. You will suction only the inside of the mouth. Use care not to insert the suction catheter so far into the mouth that the patient gags or vomits. Insertion of a Yankeur too far into the mouth can cause trauma to the delicate tissues of the oral pharynx. Suction catheters must be replaced according to facility policy. Rinse the inside of the catheter with normal saline for irrigation. You can do this by inserting the catheter into a basin of normal saline and engaging the suction source. This will wash viscous secretions into the collection canister. Rinse with water and dry the catheter after each use.

The source of suction will be either a portable suction machine or suction piped through the wall (wall suction). A collection container is connected to the suction source. This is a graduated plastic cylinder that contains an inner, removable liner. When full, the liner is removed and discarded in a biohazard waste container.

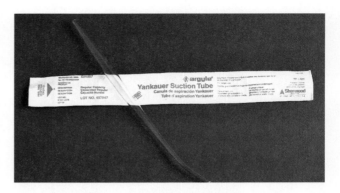

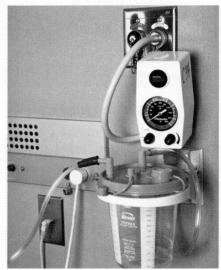

FIGURE 26-22 An oral suction catheter is also called a Yankeur catheter. Top: Yankeur catheter. Bottom: Wall suction.

procedure
Performing Oral Suctioning

Assess

Determine the need for oral suctioning. Are fluids or secretions present in the mouth? Is the patient unable to expectorate the secretions?

Determine the patient's needs during the procedure. Is the patient able to perform the procedure independently? Is the patient unconscious? If so, place the patient in the lateral position for suctioning. If the patient is alert, use semi-Fowler's position.

Determine the status of the equipment. Is the collection container full? Is the suction source working properly?

Plan

Gather required equipment: nonsterile gloves, oral suction catheter (Yankeur), suction machine or wall suction access, suction-collection canister, normal saline for irrigation, irrigation tray, tissues, and mouth care supplies. Use standard precautions. Note: If the patient has had oral surgery, you will need to follow specific orders for mouth care.

Implement

1. Connect the suction catheter to the suction-collection canister, and activate the suction.

2. Pour approximately 50 cc of saline into the irrigation tray.

3. Test the suction source for proper function by placing the catheter in the irrigation tray. Saline should move through the catheter and into the suction-collection canister.

p r o c e d u r e (c o n t i n u e d)

4. Insert the catheter into the anterior portion of the patient's mouth, being careful of the tongue and any areas of suture or injury.

5. Remove secretions by moving the catheter about in the mouth, continuing to suction until all secretions are removed.

6. Provide mouth care.

7. Clean the suction catheter, and place it in a clean location. (The original packaging can be saved for this purpose.)

8. Reposition the patient for comfort and safety.

Evaluate

Evaluate your actions. Were you able to clear the mouth of secretions? Were you able to avoid any areas of injury or oral sutures? Did you clean the catheter and store it appropriately? Did you note the color, amount, and condition of the secretions?

Evaluate the patient's response. Report any complaints of discomfort during the procedure. Report any change in the color or consistency of the secretions. Report all observations of the condition of the mouth.

Percussion

Percussion is a respiratory care procedure that is performed to loosen mucous secretions in the lungs by consistently and rhythmically moving cupped hands against the exterior chest wall overlying the lungs. The name of the procedure comes from the musical term *percussion*, referring to instruments that are struck, such as the drums. The drummer uses precise motions to produce a specific sound, just as one who performs percussion to the chest wall uses precise motions.

The purpose of percussion is to dislodge mucous secretions adhering within the lungs. It is usually performed by a nurse or respiratory therapist. It is most commonly performed in conjunction with postural drainage, a procedure in which the patient assumes specific positions designed to promote drainage of bronchial and lung secretions. Because the patient's head is positioned lower than the chest during postural drainage, changes in blood pressure and air flow can occur. Therefore, an unlicensed or untrained health care worker should never perform percussion in combination with postural drainage. The patient's response to these procedures can be unpredictable, so the patient must be assessed throughout the therapy. A professional must implement adaptations to the procedure if the patient experiences any untoward effects.

As a clinical care associate, you may be asked to perform percussion for patients who are at risk for accumulating lung secretions. When these secretions accumulate, the patient can develop bronchial infections or pneumonia. If you are asked to perform this procedure, you must be competent to do so. Because patients may have unpredictable responses and the person performing the procedure must react quickly, this task can only be delegated to those who will be able to react appropriately.

When you perform percussion, it is expected and desirable for the patient to expectorate sputum. If the patient is coughing excessively, stop the procedure and notify the nurse. When percussion is performed properly, the sound heard will be a rhythmic, muted beating, like the sound of a drum. If a slapping sound is heard, or if the patient's skin is turning red, the procedure is being performed incorrectly. This entire procedure will take about 15 minutes and can be very tiring for your arms. The patient should be placed in a lateral position while one side of the posterior chest wall is percussed from the inferior to the superior area of the back. Percussion on one side is usually completed in 5 to 8 minutes. Then the patient is given a rest period and instructed to cough. Next, the other side is percussed in the same manner (Figure 26-23).

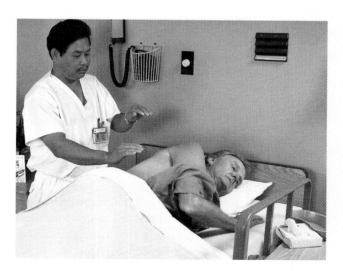

FIGURE 26-23   Percussion on one side is usually completed in 5 to 8 minutes.

p r o c e d u r e
Performing Percussion

Assess

Determine the patient's needs during this procedure. Can the patient safely be placed in a flat, side-lying position?

Determine the precautions you will need. If the patient has tuberculosis (TB), you will need a TB particulate respirator (N-95). If the patient has a respiratory infection, you may need a face mask.

Plan

Gather required equipment: nonsterile gloves, tissues, emesis basin, and sputum specimen container, if ordered. A bed protector may be required if the patient cannot expectorate into an emesis basin. Use standard precautions.

Gather supplies for mouth care to be given after this procedure.

Determine the best time to complete this procedure. Is this treatment scheduled to be done at a specific time? Have you been directed by a nurse or respiratory therapist to perform percussion now? You will need at least 10 to 15 minutes of uninterrupted time to perform this procedure.

Implement

1. Raise the bed to a comfortable working height.
2. Place the patient in a side-lying position, with the head of the bed flat.
3. Place a towel or gown over the patient's back to protect the skin and prevent chilling.
4. Percuss, with your hands cupped, on one side of the patient's back, beginning at the distal end of the thorax.
5. Gradually move your hands upward to the uppermost portion of the back on this side.

Note: It may be easier to imagine the posterior, lateral aspect of the thorax in quarters. Spend at least 2 minutes in each quarter.

6. Encourage the patient to cough and expectorate secretions.
7. Allow the patient to rest for at least 2 minutes as you relax your arms and hands.
8. Position the patient on the opposite side, and repeat the procedure.
9. Obtain a specimen if required.
10. Perform or assist with mouth care.
11. Reposition the patient for comfort and safety.

Evaluate

Evaluate your actions. Did you stop the procedure if the patient complained of shortness of breath or pain? Did you stop if the patient coughed excessively? Did you use cupped hands to avoid causing slapping sounds or redness to the patient's skin? Did you observe the sputum for color, amount, and condition? Are your fingernails short to prevent injury to the patient?

Evaluate the patient's response. Report any difficulties during the procedure, such as complaints of shortness of breath, pain, or excessive coughing. Report the patient's response to the treatment and the amount and color of the sputum produced.

Always stop percussion if the patient complains of pain or shortness of breath. Stop the procedure if the patient coughs excessively. Stop the procedure if you are unsure of the patient's response.

Phlebotomy

The word **phlebotomy** literally means "opening into a vein." Phlebotomy involves puncturing a vein (venipuncture) and is performed to obtain a venous blood sample for laboratory analysis. To perform this procedure, you must be constantly aware of your safety and the safety of the patient, and you must be able to think critically and solve problems.

No one enjoys having blood drawn. Many patients dread the sight of a health care worker arriving to perform this procedure. Patients fear pain during and after the procedure. Some patients may even faint or feel dizzy as blood enters the collection tube. To feel confident performing this procedure, you will require a great deal of practice. Your first phlebotomy experiences will involve the use of a manikin arm. This training arm is designed with rubber tubes to simulate veins and red liquid to simulate blood. Only after you become proficient at phlebotomy on the training arm will you attempt to perform venipuncture on a real person.

Types of Specimens

Venous blood is examined under a microscope for chemical and cellular components. This information will be useful to the doctor in assessing the patient's condition. Different types of tests will require different types of patient preparation.

One type of test performed on venous blood is a blood culture. This test is ordered to identify the microorganisms causing infection in the blood, so the site for venipuncture must be prepared in a specific way to promote asepsis. Some laboratory studies require the patient to be "fasting," which means that the venipuncture is performed in the early morning before the patient eats. Other studies require that the blood collection tube be protected from light. When an ionized calcium test is performed, for example, the blood collection tube must be covered with aluminum foil or carbon paper to block out light.

Blood specimens are sent to a variety of specialized laboratories for study. Some of the particular labs include chemistry, microbiology, pathology, blood bank, and hematology.

Phlebotomy Needles

The gauge of a needle indicates the width of the lumen of the needle. Phlebotomy needles range in gauge from 18 to 22. The bevel is the opening of the needle (Figure 26-24). Needle lengths range from ½ to 1½ inches. You will choose a needle to use based on the size of the patient's vein, the procedure ordered, and the supplies in stock.

Vacutainer needles are straight needles. Butterfly and shamrock needles are made with a protective sleeve to pull over the used needle, which helps prevent needle sticks (Figure 26-25). Never recap a used needle. Discard any used needle or sharp directly into the "sharps" biohazard waste container.

Vacutainer Tubes

Blood collection tubes, or Vacutainer tubes, are made with a vacuum that will draw the blood into the test tube. This vacuum will be present only if the rubber top on the tube has not been punctured and only if the tube has not expired. Always check expiration dates on tubes to ensure proper vacuum. Once you push the needle through the rubber top on the tube, the vacuum is activated. If blood does not go into the tube for some reason, that tube will not be usable again, as the vacuum has escaped.

Each blood test requires a tube with a specific-color stopper, and a specific order must be followed when drawing more than one tube of blood. When multiple tubes are drawn during a single venipuncture, tubes without additives should be drawn before tubes with additives. This will help prevent any pos-

sible contamination of additives. The order for drawing is as follows:

Order of Blood Draw		
Order	Color of Top	Diagnostic or Additive
First		Blood culture bottles
Second	Red	Nonadditive
Third	Blue	Coagulant or citrate
Fourth	Red or tiger	SST/serum separator tube
Fifth	Green	Heparin
Sixth	Lavender	EDTA-K3
Seventh	Gray	Oxalate/fluoride

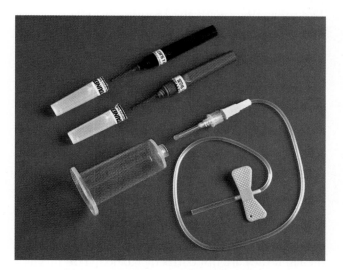

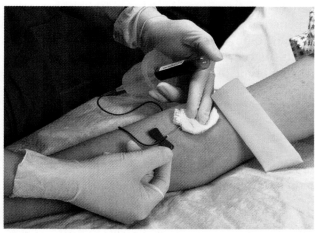

FIGURE 26-25 Butterfly and shamrock needles have a protective sleeve to pull over the used needle. This type of needle helps prevent needle sticks.

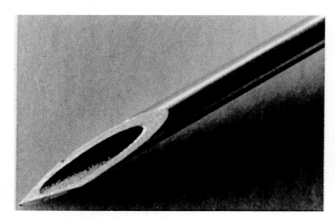

FIGURE 26-24 The bevel is the opening of the needle.

Some blood collection tubes have an added solution, such as an anticoagulant or preservative, in the tube. (See chart on previous page.) Gently invert these tubes once they are filled to mix the additive with the venous blood. It is necessary to prevent natural blood clotting to perform certain lab studies, such as a complete blood count (CBC). Some collection tubes contain serum separators, which divide the formed blood cells from the serum, or liquid portion of the blood.

Always review the required protocol for obtaining blood specimens: the tubes required, the time to obtain the specimen, and any special procedures to follow. Most institutions use laboratory requisitions that indicate the color of the tube to use and any special procedures required.

Labeling Blood Specimens

Today, most health care facilities provide computerized, preprinted labels that adhere to the Vacutainer. This label identifies the patient and the specimen. The tube, along with the requisition form, is taken to the lab.

The label includes the patient's full name, medical record number, and room number. The requisition form is stamped with the patient's identification plate and indicates the type of blood testing to be performed. The labeled tube and requisition are placed in a sealed plastic bag and sent to the lab.

Blood Bank Specimens

Most institutions have very specific protocols for blood bank specimens. Such specimens are ordered to provide for necessary or potentially needed blood transfusions. Blood bank specimens are refused by the lab if they are not correctly labeled. This means a patient will be traumatized by another phlebotomy experience if you do not follow instructions *exactly*. Usually, blood bank specimens require handwritten labels that include the phlebotomist's name, the date and time of collection, and his or her signature. The tests ordered are "type and cross," "type and screen," or "type, cross, and screen." These tests are ordered most often for patients who are scheduled for surgery or who require blood transfusions. Review Chapter 11 on the anatomy and physiology of the circulatory system to refresh your memory about blood types.

If errors occur in labeling blood bank specimens, the results are grave. Blood transfusion reactions can cause death. It is imperative to pay close attention to detail when obtaining any blood specimen, especially blood bank specimens.

Approaching the Patient

You must perform certain steps when approaching the patient for venipuncture. First, identify the patient by checking the name bracelet. Then ask the patient to state his or her first and last name.

Next, gain the patient's confidence. Tell the patient what you are about to do, and reassure the patient to relieve apprehension.

Positioning the Patient

There are two reasons for positioning the patient before performing venipuncture. One is to provide ready access to the vein to be entered, and the other is to place yourself in a comfortable working position to increase your chance of success.

The Bed Patient

If the patient is in bed, reposition him or her so that the arm to be used is at the edge of the bed. Place your equipment on the overbed table or nightstand—never on the bed. Position the table so the equipment is readily available to you, but not in danger of being upset by the patient.

The Ambulatory Patient

Ask the patient to sit near a small table. If no table is available, position the patient so the arm can be placed across the bed. Place a small pillow or rolled towel under the patient's arm to support it in an extended position. *Never* attempt to perform a venipuncture on a standing patient. If fainting occurs, the standing patient might collapse suddenly.

Position the patient's arm so that you have adequate lighting and a full view of the arm from the hand to the biceps area.

Applying the Tourniquet

To apply a tourniquet correctly, first slide it under the patient's forearm about midway between the antecubital space and the biceps muscle. Position the tourniquet so that the ends are equal in length. Take care not to pinch the skin. Keep the tourniquet lying flat as you cross, wrap, and loop the ends. Grasp one end of the tourniquet and cross it over the other, then fold it under and pull it through. Pull it again to tighten the tourniquet (Figure 26-26). Keep the ends of the tourniquet close to the skin as you apply it.

To release the tourniquet, pull upward on one end. The tying method is designed to allow for quick release. The tourniquet should *never* be tied in a knot.

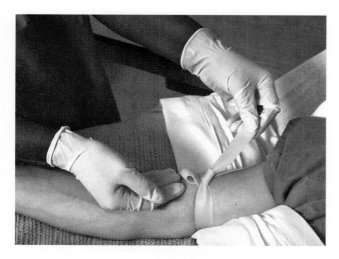

FIGURE 26-26 Tying the tourniquet.

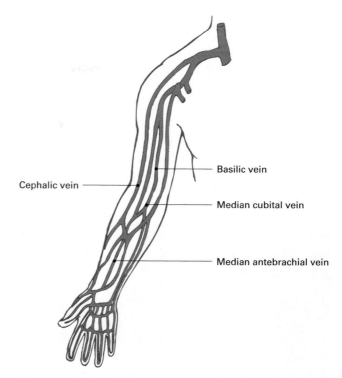

FIGURE 26-27 Anatomy of an arm for venipuncture.

Cephalic vein

Basilic vein

Median cubital vein

Median antebrachial vein

Vein Inspection

In general, arm veins are preferred for venipuncture. If the arms are bandaged, sore, or have been punctured repeatedly, it may be necessary to use the veins in the hands. Figure 26-27 shows the veins of the forearm. The most common vein used for venipuncture is the median vein. Often, the patient will be able to tell you which vein is accessed most easily. Occasionally, arm veins are thrombosed due to IV procedures. This means that clots have formed and blood no longer flows through the veins. Thrombosed veins are firm, discolored, and tender. Do not attempt venipuncture in a thrombosed vein. You will also need to choose another site if hematoma or phlebitis (inflammation of a vein) is present. If you are uncertain about vein selection, notify the nurse for assistance.

Selecting a Vein

- First, inspect the area you plan to use. You may be able to see the blue, slightly raised surface of the vein. In obese people, the vein is more difficult to see.
- Palpate, or feel, the veins. Apply the tourniquet about midway between the elbow and shoulder, then ask the patient to make a fist and pump it open and closed. This pumps blood into the vein, making it larger and more visible.
- Apply the tourniquet with enough tension to compress the vein but not the artery. Compressing an artery would halt blood flow to the area.
- Always palpate for the vein, even when it is easily seen. In this way, you will be able to feel deeper, unseen veins. The vein will feel like an elastic tube that "gives" under the pressure of your finger. Arteries pulsate, so you must be certain that

the structure is not pulsating. Never use arteriovenous shunts or fistulas for venipuncture.

- If the vein feels like a cord, do not use it for venipuncture. This vein has been used repeatedly for IVs and venipuncture, and it will be difficult to draw blood from a cordlike vein.
- To better visualize a vein, massage over the vein area two or three times from wrist to elbow, using the index and middle finger. A warm compress to the site will also cause the vein to dilate and be more visible.
- If you have difficulty finding a vein, examine the other arm. Veins in one arm may be larger than those of the other arm.
- A patient who has had many venipunctures may be able to tell you where the best vein can be found.

Performing the Venipuncture

- If the tourniquet has been in place for more than a minute while you search for a vein, release it for 1 to 2 minutes, then reapply. Prolonged obstruction of blood flow can cause changes in some test results.
- Visualize and palpate the veins in the antecubital space. Choose the vein you feel the best. It is necessary that you feel the vein's structure before venipuncture.

- Scrub the area for venipuncture, using an alcohol pad. If you accidentally touch the skin you have cleaned, reclean the area.
- The use of the vacuum blood collection tube is illustrated in Figure 26-28.
- Place the tube into the Vacutainer holder (Figure 26-29) with the label side down so that you can see the blood enter the tube.
- "Fix" the vein you have chosen to use by placing the thumb of your nondominant hand about 1 inch below the intended puncture site. Press down on the arm while pulling the skin toward the patient's hand to stretch the skin and hold the vein taut.
- Introduce the needle with the bevel up. The needle should line up with the direction of the vein, at a 15° angle from the skin. You will feel a slight "give" as the needle enters the vein. Once the needle enters, release the anchored thumb.
- Hold your index finger along the hub of the needle braced against the patient's arm. If the patient moves, your finger and the needle will move with the patient.

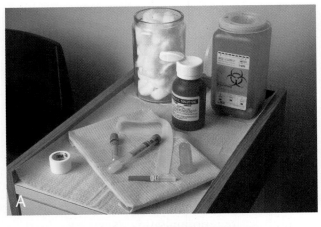

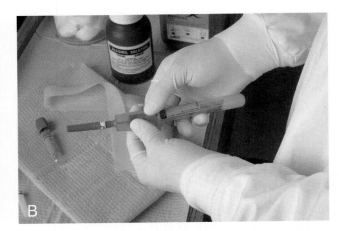

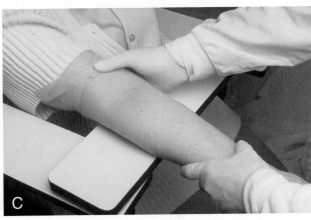

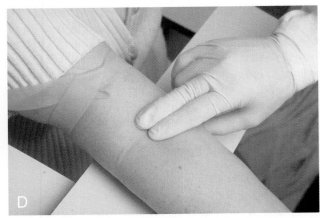

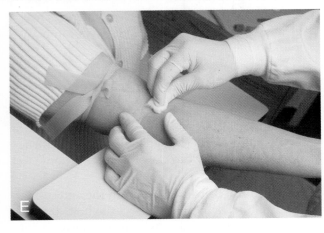

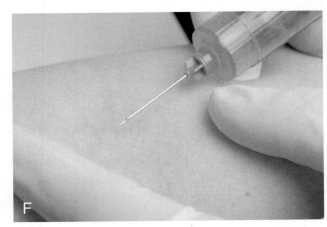

FIGURE 26-28   Drawing blood with a Vacutainer.

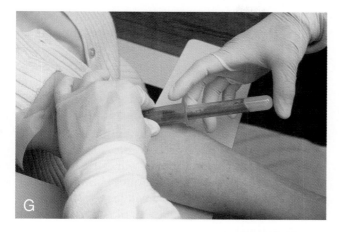

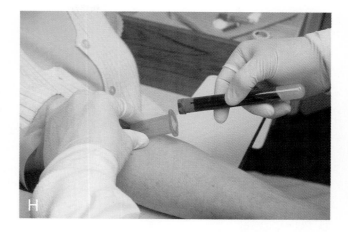

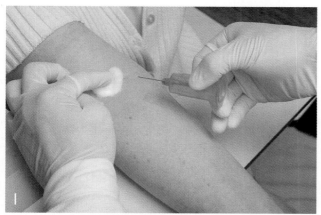

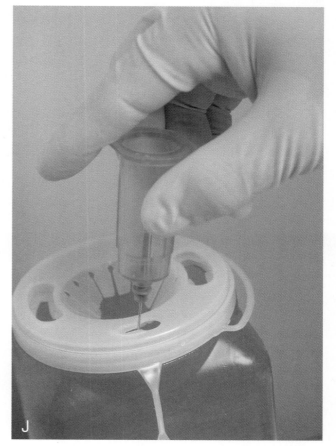

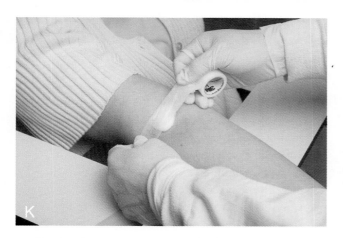

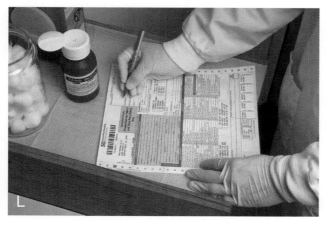

FIGURE 26-28 Drawing blood with a Vacutainer.
(continued)

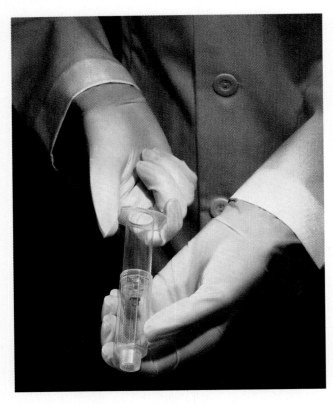

FIGURE 26-29   Vacutainer brand safety lock needle holder.

- Push the Vacutainer tube into the holder so that the other end of the needle punctures the rubber top.

- If you are filling only one tube, release the tourniquet as soon as the blood begins to flow. If you are filling multiple tubes, release the tourniquet as soon as blood begins to flow into the last tube.

- After releasing the tourniquet and filling the last tube, gently withdraw the needle. Jerking the needle rapidly from the vein will cause injury. If you fail to release the tourniquet before withdrawing the needle, blood will flow from the needle wound into the tissues of the arm, causing a hematoma.

- Place a sterile gauze pad over the needle puncture, and apply pressure. Instruct the patient to keep the arm extended in a straight position while applying pressure for at least 3 minutes. Use this time to label the specimens and clean the area. Instruct the patient not to bend the arm. This will keep the needle puncture wound open and cause hematoma. If the patient cannot hold the gauze pad, you should hold it for at least 2 minutes.

- Place an elastic bandage (Band-Aid) over the site after the bleeding has stopped.

procedure

Performing Venipuncture to Obtain a Venous Blood Sample

Assess

Determine the type of specimen to be collected. What tubes will be needed? What special procedures must you follow? In what order should the tubes be filled?

Determine the condition of the patient. What contraindications exist for vein selection? What size and type of needle will you use? Is the patient apprehensive?

Plan

Gather required equipment: nonsterile gloves, tourniquet, alcohol pads, two needles, Vacutainer holder, correct number and color of tubes, 2-inch-by-2-inch sterile gauze pads, Band-Aid, labels for tubes, lab requisition forms, sharps waste container, and a biohazard waste container. If a blood culture is to be drawn, you will also need betadine preps, blood culture bottles, hemostat, tape, and a butterfly or shamrock needle with tubing. Use standard precautions.

Determine the appropriate time to perform the procedure. Does the patient need to be fasting? Do any other time protocols exist?

Arrange to have all supplies in close proximity to your work site.

Implement

1. Position the patient for comfort and safety. Position yourself in a comfortable working posture.
2. Apply the tourniquet.
3. Select the appropriate vein.
4. Clean the site with alcohol, and allow it to dry.
5. Assemble the needle, Vacutainer holder, and collection tube or tubes.
6. Enter the vein smoothly and gently with the bevel of the needle facing up and the vein "fixed."
7. Push the tube into the Vacutainer holder so that the needle penetrates the rubber top.
8. Collect the correct amount of blood for the tube or tubes.
9. Change tubes without moving the needle in the vein.
10. Remove the tourniquet as blood flows into the last tube.
11. Pull the top of the Vacutainer tube free from the needle.
12. Withdraw the needle with the Vacutainer holder attached.

procedure (continued)

13. Place a 2-inch-by-2-inch gauze over the puncture site, and apply pressure for 2 to 3 minutes.
14. Discard the needle into the sharps container (Figure 26-30).
15. Place a Band-Aid over the puncture site after the bleeding stops.
16. Fix the labels to the tubes.
17. Place the tubes and the requisitions in the plastic bag.
18. Reposition the patient for comfort and safety.
19. Record the procedure on the appropriate form.

Evaluate

Evaluate your actions. Were you able to locate a suitable vein? Did you "fix" the vein? Did you insert the needle tip all the way into the vein? Did you insert the needle with the bevel up? Did you obtain all ordered tubes? Did you apply pressure over the site for the appropriate length of time?

Evaluate the patient's response. Report any complaints of discomfort or any complications of the procedure. Report any difficulty in obtaining the blood sample.

If any of the following problems occur, here are some guidelines to follow:

1. The patient becomes faint or faints during the procedure.
   - If the patient feels faint and you are almost finished drawing the samples, try to complete the procedure to prevent having to repeat venipuncture at a later time. Reassure and calm the patient.
   - If the patient faints, stop the procedure. Call for assistance, and do not leave the patient. If a patient sitting in a chair faints, stand in front of the patient and place his or her head between the knees. Keep your hands on the patient's shoulders to prevent him or her from falling. If a bed patient faints, remove the pillows from beneath the head and place them under the feet to promote blood flow to the head.
2. The needle is inserted but no blood is flowing.
   - Try gently advancing or retracting the needle to adjust the position in the vein. Remove the collection tube, and try another in case the tube has lost its vacuum.
   - The most common errors a beginner makes are these: failure to "fix" the vein, failure to insert the needle tip all the way into the vein, and failure to insert the needle with the bevel up.
   - If none of these measures are successful, stop the procedure. Do not move the needle to search for the vein. *Never* attempt venipuncture more than twice! If you are unable to obtain blood, get someone else who is accomplished at venipuncture to perform the procedure. If the patient has fragile skin and has numerous venipunctures, you may wish to try only once before asking for help.
3. You draw blood from the wrong patient.
   - Tell the nurse promptly what has happened. Perhaps this patient has lab studies ordered and the samples can be used.
   - If not, you will need to assist the nurse in completing an incident report. You also need to apologize to the patient.
   - Report the error to the lab if the tubes have already been delivered. Determine which tubes still need to be drawn to complete the original order.
4. You stick yourself with a used needle.
   - Wash the site immediately. Use an antibacterial soap, and wash for at least 2 minutes.
   - Report the incident promptly to the nurse.
   - Follow the policy of your facility for reporting and follow-up care. Your options will be explained to you.
   - Complete an incident report.
5. The patient has a fistula or shunt used for hemodialysis or has had a mastectomy.
   - Select a vein in the unaffected arm. *Never* perform venipuncture or measure blood pressure in the affected arm.
   - Place a sign above the patient's bed that identifies the affected arm and the procedures to avoid if no sign is currently in place.
6. A blood transfusion is in progress.
   - Do not draw a complete blood count until 1 hour after the transfusion is finished.
   - Inform the nurse of the reason for the delay.
7. An IV is infusing.
   - Select a vein in the opposite arm for phlebotomy if possible. If you are unable to locate a desirable vein, discuss the situation with the nurse before performing venipuncture below the IV site.

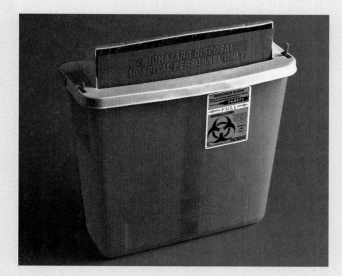

FIGURE 26-30 Always discard used needles in the sharps container.

Capillary Blood Glucose Measurements

Blood glucose levels are monitored for several reasons. When a patient has diabetes mellitus, periodic measurements of blood glucose levels are done to assess the effectiveness of insulin therapy, oral hypoglycemic medications, or diet therapy. Often, patients with diabetes monitor their blood glucose at home, using a glucose meter (glucometer). Other patients who require blood glucose monitoring are those receiving high doses of steroid medications and those receiving **total parenteral nutrition (TPN)**, also called *hyperalimentation*. Total parenteral nutrition solutions contain high levels of dextrose, a sugar similar to glucose.

Blood glucose can be measured in venous or capillary blood. Since frequent testing is done, capillary blood is generally used because it is easiest to obtain. The critical elements or steps for using glucometers will not be presented here. Since there are a variety of glucose meters on the market, the brands used will vary in homes, hospitals, and physician's offices. Although the brands vary, the underlying principles are the same. Each glucometer has specific features of operation, and each has some type of quality-monitoring system. While it may be impossible to remember the specifics of each monitoring instrument, it is possible to learn the principles for collecting capillary glucose specimens and for operating glucometers.

Principles of Glucose Meters

Glucose meters measure blood glucose when capillary blood is dropped on a glucose test strip placed in the meter (Figure 26-31). Glucose test strips are designed to fit specific brands of glucose meters (Figure 26-32).

Asepsis

When a glucose meter is used by and for just one patient in his or her home, infection-control issues are not critical. The only blood contact would be with the patient's own blood so the blood sample can be applied directly to the test strip.

In a hospital or office setting, the principles of infection control and aseptic technique are critical. One glucose meter may be used for numerous patients. A health care worker will obtain and measure the blood sample, so standard precautions must be followed. The blood sample must be applied indirectly to the test strip. In this setting, the health care worker will perform a fingerstick procedure and ex-

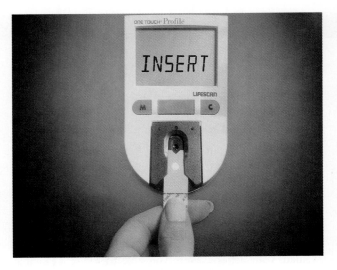

FIGURE 26-31A Press POWER, and insert the strip into the meter. Photo courtesy of Johnson & Johnson.

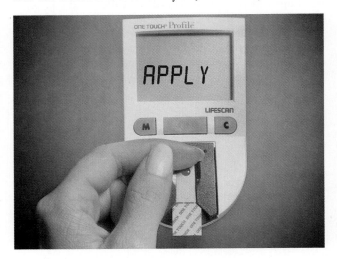

FIGURE 26-31B If the meter is used at home for individual use, apply the blood sample directly to the strip. Photo courtesy of Johnson & Johnson.

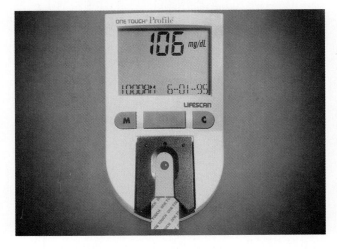

FIGURE 26-31C Wait a short time for the results to appear on the blood glucose meter. Photo courtesy of Johnson & Johnson.

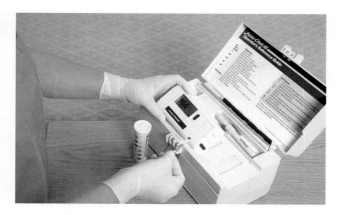

FIGURE 26-32   This Accu Check™ meter measures the level of glucose in a blood sample.

press the blood sample into a collection tube (Figure 26-33). A drop of blood from the collection tube is placed on the test strip.

Quality Control

Whether it is used in a home or a hospital, the glucose meter must be monitored for quality control. The procedure for conducting quality control varies with different brands, but the principles are the same. The glucometer must be checked for accuracy in reading

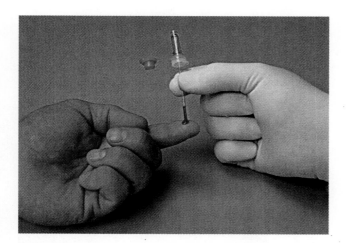

FIGURE 26-33   A fingerstick is useful for obtaining small amounts of blood.

high and low glucose levels. Solutions of concentrated and dilute glucose are used when testing the range of the meter. The solutions are applied in the same manner as a blood sample, though the meter recognizes it as a test solution rather than blood.

In hospitals, quality control is performed at least every 24 hours. Most meters have a warning message informing the user to "do Q.C."

Operating a Glucose Meter

Each glucose meter has a small display screen that presents directions for each step of the procedure. The meter will prompt you to clean the test strip holding area, insert the test strip, and apply the blood sample. Then the meter will display the blood glucose measurement. Most glucometers will prompt you if there is not enough blood on the strip, if the test strip is out-of-date, or if a quality-monitoring check is needed.

Glucose meters are designed to be "user-friendly"; that is, they provide the user with clear messages regarding performance of and problems with the procedure. Protect glucose meters from extreme temperatures. Anytime a glucose meter is dropped, it will prompt you to perform quality-control monitoring.

Clean the test strip holding areas with soap and water, not alcohol. Glucose meters use light waves to read the blood sample. Using alcohol to clean the meter causes "clouding" or streaking of the light-sensitive area, which will affect the accuracy of the readings.

Capillary Blood Specimens

The most common sites for obtaining a capillary blood specimen in an adult are the fingers. Occasionally, the earlobe is used. For newborns and infants, the heel may be used. Common terms used to describe capillary blood specimens are *fingerstick* and *heelstick*. A lancet is used to puncture the skin. It is important to know how different lancets are used to prevent needle-stick injuries. Some lancets retract automatically after use to prevent such injuries. One large drop of blood is all that is required for blood glucose testing.

p r o c e d u r e

Obtaining a Capillary Blood Specimen

Assess

Determine the last blood glucose reading. Does this patient often run high or low?

Plan

Determine the correct time to perform this procedure. Is this glucose measurement scheduled to be done at a certain time? Is this a stat order?

p r o c e d u r e   (c o n t i n u e d)

Gather required supplies: nonsterile gloves, alcohol pads, lancet, capillary tube, glucose meter, test strips, 2-inch-by-2-inch gauze, and Band-Aid. Use standard precautions.

Determine the correct order for performing the procedure. Does this brand of glucose meter require that the test strip be in place before or after you apply the sample?

Implement

1. Clean the patient's finger with the alcohol pad, and allow it to dry or dry with gauze pad. (Any residual alcohol can affect the glucose reading.)

2. Grasp the selected finger firmly, squeezing or milking the finger to promote blood flow to the fingertip. This creates a tourniquet effect, trapping the blood in the fingertip.

or

Milk the finger from the second knuckle to the fingertip to ensure adequate blood supply for the procedure.

3. Place the end of the lancet firmly against the fingertip, and puncture the skin.

4. Squeeze the fingertip to obtain a large, hanging drop of blood.

5. Place the open end of the capillary tube in the drop of blood.

6. Create suction by placing your finger over the end of the capillary tube or by squeezing the bulb on the capillary tube.

7. Maintain constant suction to avoid drawing air bubbles into the capillary tube.

8. Fill the capillary tube completely with blood.

9. Drop the blood sample onto the test strip by releasing the suction.

10. Apply Band Aid if needed.

11. Wait for the glucose meter to finish the measurement.

Evaluate

Evaluate your actions. Were you able to obtain a large drop of blood from the fingerstick? Were you able to fill the capillary tube with blood, avoiding air bubbles? Did you release the suction and drop the blood sample onto the test strip? Did you receive any error messages from the glucometer?

Evaluate the patient's response. Report the glucose reading to the nurse. Report any difficulties with the fingerstick procedure or the glucometer function.

Pneumatic Hose

Pneumatic (intermittent) pressure stockings are ordered by the physician for selected post-operative patients to prevent the complication of deep vein thrombosis (DVT). Certain surgical procedures, such as hip, abdominal, and thoracic surgeries, place the patient at risk for clot formation in the veins of the pelvis and lower extremities. An extreme danger of clot formation in the lower extremities is presented by pulmonary embolism, a clot that moves from the legs to the lungs. Pneumatic hose are used in addition to elastic stockings (TEDs) to increase the return of venous blood from the lower extremities to the heart. Pneumatic pressure stockings are for single patient use and will not be reused on other patients (Figure 26-34).

The hose are connected to a pump that exerts intermittent pressure against the muscles of the lower legs. The pressure begins at the ankles and moves up to the thighs in an intermittent, wavelike pattern. Generally, the patient wears elastic hose beneath the pneumatic hose. The pump is set at the ordered pressure setting, usually between 40 millimeters of mercury (mm Hg) and 20 mm Hg. The pump plugs into a wall outlet. Plastic tubing con-

nects the pump to the hose. The hose contain a plastic bladder that is inflated and deflated by the pump. This intermittent pressure helps to increase the blood flow from the lower extremities to the heart. It is this action that helps prevent blood clots from forming in the legs. Pneumatic hose should fit the leg securely, but not tightly. If the hose are too tight, the stagnation of venous blood may result.

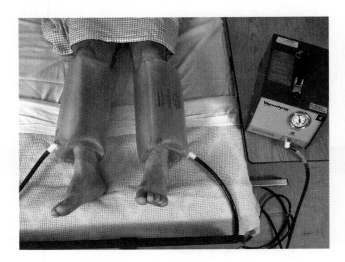

FIGURE 26-34   Pneumatic pressure stockings.

procedure
Applying Pneumatic Hose

Assess

Determine the specific orders for this patient. What is the ordered or established pressure setting? Will the hose be applied to both legs? Are elastic stockings to be worn underneath the pneumatic hose?

Determine the condition of the patient's legs and feet. Are there any wounds or skin irritation? If so, notify the nurse. Are the legs and feet pale, reddened, cold, hot, or discolored in any way? If so, notify the nurse for assessment before applying the hose.

Determine the functioning of the equipment. Is the pump working correctly? Is the outlet to be used adequate? Are the plastic bladders inflating and deflating appropriately?

Plan

Gather required supplies: single-patient-use prepackaged pneumatic hose, flow pump, and elastic hose (if ordered). Use standard precautions as appropriate.

Determine the appropriate time to perform this procedure. When are the hose to be applied? When are they to be removed or discontinued?

Implement

1. Plug in the flow pump.
2. Remove the hose from the bag. The hose can be used on either leg.
3. Unfold the hose, and position the square portion behind the patient's knee. This will be labeled in some manner.
4. Wrap the hose snugly around the leg, ensuring that the inflatable bladder is directly behind the patient's calf and thigh.
5. Secure the fastener tabs in the calf section first, then those in the thigh section.
6. Repeat steps 3 through 5 for the other leg.
7. Attach the hose to the air tubing using the snap connector. You will hear a click when it is securely connected.
8. Attach the tubing to the flow pump. You will hear a click when it is securely connected.
9. Set the pump pressure regulator to the ordered setting or to the manufacturer's recommended pressure setting.
10. Turn on the flow pump. The ON/OFF switch will be illuminated in the ON position.
11. Remain with the patient for at least 5 minutes.
12. Remove the hose, and notify the nurse if the patient complains of pain, numbness, or tingling in the legs.
13. Record the procedure on the appropriate chart form.

Evaluate

Evaluate your actions. Did you apply elastic hose beneath the pneumatic hose if ordered? Did you apply the pneumatic hose correctly? Did you set the pressure at the ordered or recommended amount?

Evaluate the patient's response. Report to the nurse stat any changes in the sensation or temperature of the patient's legs, feet, or toes. Report the application of the hose and the patient's response.

---

application to practice

Perhaps all, or maybe some, of the procedures and information you have studied in this chapter are new to you. If so, you will want to use the material in this chapter as a resource for additional study and review. Now that you have completed your initial study of the chapter, use what you have learned about advanced or expanded procedures and patient care to consider the situations presented here.

Learning Activities

Situation 1: Mr. Simmons has a PEG tube through which he receives bolus feedings. What should you assess before you begin the tube feeding?

Author's Explanation: You should determine the type and amount of feeding to be given. You should also determine the amount of residual stomach contents that can be withdrawn before you have to withhold the scheduled feeding.

Situation 2: You withdraw 180 cc of residual stomach contents. What is your plan?

Author's Explanation: Tell the nurse immediately. This is a large amount of residual. You should not start a new feeding with a residual greater than 150 cc. Await direction from the nurse.

Situation 3: Mrs. Marks has four lab studies ordered this morning. She is a patient who receives outpatient dialysis treatment, and has an atrioventricular (AV) shunt in her left arm. You need to draw blood now. What should you include in the preprocedure assessment?

Author's Explanation: See what lab studies are ordered. What color tubes are needed? Check the condition of the veins in Mrs. Marks' right arm. Determine the patient's readiness for the procedure.

Situation 4: What do you need to plan?

Author's Explanation: Prepare the patient. Gather all necessary equipment. Review the "order of the draw" to determine which color tube must be drawn first, second, and so on. Choose the best vein in the right arm. Ensure the safety and comfort of yourself and the patient. If lab studies are ordered stat, do these now.

Situation 5: Mr. Haab is a seventy-nine-year-old male who has chronic obstructive pulmonary disease (COPD). He was admitted yesterday in congestive heart failure (CHF), and he has pneumonia. You are assigned to do an ECG stat because of chest pain. You must also perform a pulse oximetry (OX) and perform chest percussion, cough and deep breathe (PT). What task will you do first, and why?

Author's Explanation: Do the ECG first because the patient is having chest pain and it is ordered stat.

Situation 6: The ECG has a significant amount of artifact. What do you plan to do?

Author's Explanation: Check Mr. Haab for muscle tremors. Ask the patient if he is cold. Determine if he is shivering. Move the limb leads closer to the trunk of the body, and rerun the ECG.

Situation 7: You complete the pulse OX, and it is 89. Pulse OX was last measured two hours ago, and it was 98. What do you do?

Author's Explanation: Report the results immediately to the nurse. This is a significant decrease in oxygen saturation.

Situation 8: During chest PT, Mr. Haab begins to cough uncontrollably. What do you do?

Author's Explanation: Stop the percussion. See if his cough is productive. If he is in distress, call for the nurse from the bedside.

Situation 9: Mr. Glover has been diagnosed with Crohn's disease. Yesterday, he arrived on your unit post-op after having an ileostomy. You are assigned to perform A.M. care for this patient. In report, you are given the following information:

▪ Assist with ADLs
▪ Vital signs q. 4h
▪ Clear liquid diet
▪ OOB to chair with assistance
▪ Empty ostomy appliance p.r.n.

How do you plan to proceed with his care this morning?

Author's Explanation: Assess, plan, implement, and evaluate all patient care tasks using the major principles of care.

Time management: Determine when the patient wants a bath, when vital signs were last measured, when he wants to eat his clear liquid breakfast, and when he wants to get out of bed to the chair.

Outcome based goal setting: Check the ileostomy appliance to see if it is full. Ask the nurse if you need to measure and record the output from the ostomy appliance.

Comfort: If the patient is in any pain, ask the nurse if he can have any pain medicine. Be sure the patient is painfree before you proceed with care. Keep the bed at a comfortable working level while you assist with care. Remember that the patient may be afraid to look at his stoma and ileostomy appliance. The patient may be embarrassed, angry, or sad about this surgery.

Safety: Determine how much assistance Mr. Glover will need with transfer to a chair. Return the bed to the lowest level after completing care tasks. Keep the call bell within easy reach. Remember to wear gloves when you empty the ostomy appliance and to wash your hands as needed. Keep the skin area around the ileostomy clean and dry. Observe the color, shape, and size of the stoma. Report any complaints of discomfort and any bleeding from the operative site.

Competence: If you have never emptied an ostomy appliance before, you should tell the nurse and ask to observe the nurse before you do this independently. If the patient has questions about the stoma or the care of the ostomy appliance, refer the questions to the nurse. If the patient allows, stay in the room while the enterostomal therapist teaches Mr. Glover about the care of the stoma and the ostomy appliance. Report any vital sign measurements that are not within the normal range.

Patients' rights. Provide for privacy, and be sensitive to the patient's need to be treated with dignity and respect. Identify yourself and the patient before you proceed with any care measures. Explain any care tasks before you perform them.

Examination Review Questions

1. Which catheter would be used for continuous irrigation?
   a. three-way c. French
   b. two-way d. straight

2. Which tube provides continuous feeding through the stomach?
   a. PEG c. residual
   b. IVAC d. TPN

3. It is imperative to check proper placement of feeding tubes to prevent
   a. gastric distension
   b. aspiration pneumonia
   c. bowel obstruction
   d. pulmonary embolism

4. Which wave of the ECG denotes atrial contraction?
   a. P c. R
   b. Q d. T

5. Which clear adhesive dressing protects wounds from water and irritants?
   a. Tegaderm c. wet-to-dry
   b. Duoderm d. microspore

6. Which ostomy will have the most predictable times for stool elimination?
   a. ileostomy c. ureterostomy
   b. colostomy d. ileoconduit

7. A pulse is used to measure
   a. PAO_2 c. O_2 saturation
   b. $PACO_2$ d. air volume

8. Which respiratory care procedure loosens mucous secretions in the lungs?
   a. percussion c. spirometry
   b. suctioning d. oximetry

9. Which blood collection tube contains heparin?
   a. red c. gray
   b. blue d. green

10. A patient with which of the following is *not* a candidate for capillary blood glucose measurements?
    a. diabetes mellitus
    b. high steroid dosages
    c. hyperalimentation
    d. pulmonary embolism

Emergency Preparedness

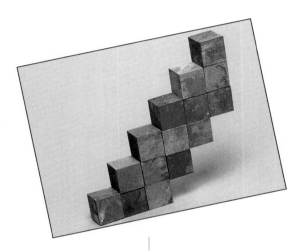

This unit will introduce you to the observation and intervention skills used by the clinical care associate (CCA) in emergencies. Identification and quick response to an emergency are essential for safe practice in any health care setting. Some emergency situations presented in this unit involve the condition of the patient, such as shock and seizure. Other emergencies involve the patient, the staff, and the facility, such as fire.

Chapter 27

Clinical and Environmental Emergencies

When you work in a health care setting, you should always be prepared for potential emergencies. You must always know and fulfill your role in preventing, detecting, and assisting in emergencies. Most emergency situations require extreme tightening of time management and problem-solving skills. Acting swiftly and effectively, you can save a life. Teamwork is important when performing all the actions necessary to save lives. What is your role? Your immediate recognition of life-threatening emergencies is of the utmost importance.

OBJECTIVES

After completing this chapter, you will be able to

1. Explain the clinical care associate's role in responding to a seizure
2. Identify the signs and symptoms of shock
3. Explain the ABCs of CPR
4. List the measures you will use for a choking victim
5. Describe the signs and symptoms of cardiac arrest
6. Describe your role in fire, electrical, biohazard, and hazardous material safety
7. Define the acronym *RACE*
8. Explain the meaning of disaster preparedness
9. List the steps that you would take if there were a bomb threat
10. List and describe the five sections of an MSDS
11. Define and spell all key terms correctly

k e y   t e r m s

biohazard	Heimlich maneuver	seizure
cardiac arrest	Jacksonian seizures	septic shock
cardiopulmonary resuscitation	Material Safety Data Sheets	shock
(CPR)	(MSDS)	temporal lobe epilepsy
epilepsy	partial seizure	triage
generalized seizure	petit mal seizures	
grand mal seizures	psychomotor seizures	

Seizures

A **seizure** is a condition in which there are electrical disturbances in the brain. Seizure activity can be compared to an overloaded circuit or a circuit breaker that receives too much voltage. In addition, a seizure can be compared to a television set that stores extra electricity within it although the power source to the TV is in the off position.

A seizure is not a disease. **Epilepsy** is a disorder in which the primary symptom is seizures or convulsions. Epilepsy can result from any type of trauma to the brain (for example, fever or a blow to the head). Some people have a family history of epilepsy. Other people develop seizures with no known history of head trauma and no family history of seizures.

Seizures are classified by two major categories: partial or generalized. The difference is whether all of the cerebrum is involved (**generalized seizure**) or only one part is involved (**partial seizure**). Generalized seizures include *grand mal* and *petit mal seizures*. Partial seizures include *Jacksonian seizures* and *psychomotor seizures*. Other types of seizures are classified under these two major categories, but these are the commonly occurring types.

Petit Mal Seizures

Petit mal seizures are small seizures whose symptoms may include staring, "fading out" for a few seconds, or rapid blinking of the eyelids (*petit* means "little" or "small"; *mal* is Latin for "bad"). There is a momentary "electrical storm" in brain functioning. Often, petit mal seizures are not detectable because the symptoms are not dramatic and the seizures are brief. This type of seizure is found typically in children and not in adults.

The victim may have as many as one hundred or as few as one petit mal seizure a day. Each seizure may last for only 10 to 30 seconds. It may appear as though the victim is just "staring into space." There are no emergency interventions required. It is imperative, however, to observe the time of the seizure and to ensure the victim's safety.

For a child, these seizures can be very serious if they interfere with learning or play activities. If the child has frequent petit mal seizures in the classroom, then he or she will be unable to pay attention to the learning activities. In play, the danger is physical safety. Loss of consciousness while riding a bike or skating in the street could result in serious accidents.

Grand Mal Seizures

The type of seizure that involves emergency intervention is grand mal (*grand* means "big" or "large," and *mal* means "bad"). **Grand mal seizures** are full-blown seizures that involve four phases: *aura, tonic, clonic,* and *sleep.* The aura, or first phase, may or may not be experienced by an individual. This phase involves a premonition of the senses that something is about to occur. Some individuals have an aura that increases hearing or visual acuity. In others, it is a heightened smell or taste. Still others describe it as using all senses.

The second stage is the tonic phase. In this stage, the individual loses consciousness and falls to the ground. All the muscles become tight or rigid. It is in this phase that the victim's jaw will close and lock. No muscle can be moved.

The third stage is the clonic phase. During this phase, the muscles, now charged with electrical impulses, release the energy by a rhythmic rocking and shaking. The head bangs into the ground, and all extremities alternately contract and relax. Because the bowel and bladder are controlled by sphincter muscles, the alternate contraction and relaxation of these muscles may cause incontinence. In addition, since swallowing is a conscious movement, saliva collects at the back of the pharynx. As the patient breathes and air is forced over the saliva, frothing of the mouth may occur. This is similar to what happens when air is blown into a straw that is immersed in water.

Once the energy has been released and the electrical impulses have been discharged, the patient usually falls asleep. The sleep phase is the fourth and final phase. This is an exhausting experience for the body. Grand mal seizures can last 1 to 5 minutes. Any seizure that lasts longer than 5 minutes is life-threatening.

Assisting the Patient Having a Grand Mal Seizure

Remember two important ideas in all procedures: safety and comfort. Let's examine safety first. What steps ensure the safety of the patient?

1. Call for help from the nurse stat.
2. Move furniture out of the way to protect the patient.
3. Place a pillow or other support under the patient's head.
4. Loosen tight clothing.
5. Monitor respiratory status.
6. Turn the patient's head to the side if possible.
7. Stay with the patient.
8. Protect the limbs from injury.
9. Report the events you witnessed to the nurse.

What steps should be taken to ensure your own safety?

1. Do not try to restrain the patient.
2. Follow the Centers for Disease Control and Prevention (CDC) guidelines for handling blood and body fluids.
3. Do not attempt to open the airway by putting your fingers in the patient's mouth. This could injure the patient and you.

Comfort measures for the patient include

1. Loosening clothing
2. Providing emotional support following the seizure
3. Assisting in cleaning the patient if there has been any incontinence of urine or feces

Never restrain the person because the force of the restraint against the contracting muscles could cause injury to you and to the patient. Make no attempt to open the airway or to prevent the tongue from being swallowed. The tongue cannot be swallowed, and putting your fingers or other objects into the victim's mouth could cause injury to you or the patient.

Jacksonian seizures involve one side of the body. The person remains conscious and the "march" of tensing and jerking muscles is visible as it moves up one side of the body. There is nothing that you can do to interrupt the event. Stay with the person and protect him or her from injury.

Psychomotor seizures are varied in the appearance of the seizure activity. This type of seizure is the result of temporal lobe malfunction. It is called **temporal lobe epilepsy**. These seizures take several forms: "epileptic furor," "running fits," and repetition of senseless activity (for example, buttoning and unbuttoning a shirt). These seizures involve loss of consciousness. Epileptic furor is rare and is displayed by events of violent anger that are brief and unprovoked. Running fits are rare also and involve running that is brief and not directed to a goal or destination. The only thing that you can do to assist the individual is to protect him or her from harm. You would not know what was happening to the person with psychomotor seizures unless you were told that this is the nature of the seizure activity.

Shock

Shock is not a disease but a warning signal that the body is in grave danger. It is the "fire alarm" of the body. When the body is confronted with a perceived life-threatening situation, the autonomic nervous system (ANS) is signaled to redirect blood flow. Blood from the extremities is directed to the organs of the abdominal cavity. This pooling of blood creates a drop in blood pressure. The body's hurrying to redirect blood flow creates an increased pulse. The necessity for increased oxygen is like the mad rush to the grocery store to stock up on supplies before a major snowstorm. The respiratory rate increases.

Initially, the patient in shock presents with a decrease in blood pressure and an increase in pulse and respirations. In addition, the patient will feel weak, will feel sweaty, and will need to lie down. This autonomic response to a drop in blood pressure actually forces the person to a horizontal position. The horizontal position helps blood flow to the brain, so that the heart need not work against gravity. In an emergency, the body's "red alert" is signaled. The response is to become weak and fall to a horizontal position. This enables the free flow of blood to vital organs. For example, if your car's transmission is not functioning, the roads best traveled are flat roads that do not require uphill navigation. The same principle holds true for the body.

Many things can cause shock, such as (1) low blood volume (hypovolemia) due to the loss of large amounts of blood, (2) myocardial infarction, and (3) trauma to the body tissues due to a motor vehicle

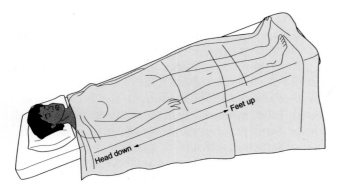

FIGURE 27-1   Trendelenburg position.

accident. Massive infection and adverse reactions to medications can cause shock known as **septic shock**.

The clinical care associate's role in the treatment of shock consists of the following principles of care:

Safety of the Patient

1. Stay with the person and call for help stat.
2. Cover the patient with a warm blanket.
3. Give nothing by mouth (NPO) because of the potential loss of consciousness. The person could vomit and aspirate the stomach contents.
4. Elevate the legs or place the patient in the Trendelenburg position to help with blood flow to the brain and heart (Figure 27-1).
5. Monitor the patient's vital signs, especially pulse, blood pressure, and respirations.
6. When someone is in shock, it is difficult to hear the blood pressure or palpate a peripheral pulse. You will need to feel for the carotid pulse. If you are in a setting with a sphygmomanometer, you can use the palpation method to obtain a systolic blood pressure (BP) reading. The BP you report is "__ palpable."

Loss of Consciousness

Loss of consciousness can result from many body traumas. Some causes are shock, seizure, complete airway obstruction, hyperglycemia, hypoglycemia, and head injury. If you discover a person who appears to be unconscious, you must first determine unresponsiveness. How do you determine whether someone is responsive? Shake the person and shout, "Can you hear me? Can you hear me?" Do not shake an infant. Tap the feet and shout, "Baby, baby," or something similar. Then you must call for help. Activate the Emergency Medical System (EMS) or call a CODE, depending on your employment setting. The most important action you can take with an unconscious adult is to notify emergency services personnel who will determine the cause of unconsciousness and treat the victim.

Cardiopulmonary Resuscitation (CPR)

In an emergency, certain ranking priorities exist that mandate sequential intervention. Simply stated, A must be performed before B, and B must be performed before C.

The ABCs of Emergency Care

A = airway
B = breathing
C = circulation

The most important functions of the body are supplying air, breathing the air, and circulating oxygen via the blood.

Airway

Without an open airway, the most vital substance of life is missing—oxygen! So, in an emergency, after determining and responding to unconsciousness, the first thing you evaluate is A for *airway*. Airway is the maintenance of an open passageway for air to flow freely to the lungs. Open the airway, and look, listen, and feel. Sometimes, the only emergency intervention you need to perform is to open the airway. If the person is unconscious, the muscles of the throat relax, the tongue folds back in the mouth, and the airway is obstructed. Use the head tilt–chin lift maneuver to open the airway. This pulls the tongue forward. Airway obstruction is caused by the relaxation of the tongue and throat muscles. The other most common cause of airway obstruction is a foreign object in the throat. Food is the typical culprit.

Breathing

The second step is B—check for *breathing*. Is the chest rising and falling? Can you hear or feel breath being exhaled through the mouth or nose? Use the head tilt–chin lift maneuver to maintain the airway. Place your cheek next to the person's face, with your head turned in the direction of the person's chest. Now, look, listen, and feel for breathing.

If the person is not breathing, you need to breathe for him or her. Now, make a tight seal over the victim's mouth with your mouth, and pinch the nose. Give one breath, and watch for a rise on the chest. If the breath was not successful, reposition the head and give another breath. Give two successful breaths before checking the carotid pulse. Note: The use of a one-way valve mask for artificial breathing is ideal and recommended.

Circulation

The third step is C for *circulation*. Is the heart pumping blood? Remember, in an emergency, palpate the carotid pulse. In an infant, palpate the brachial pulse. If there is no pulse, circulation must be provided. Feel the carotid pulse for 5 to 10 seconds. If no pulse is present, locate the site for chest compressions. Feel along the rib cage to the center of the chest, and locate the xiphoid process. Place two fingers on the xiphoid process and the heel of the opposite hand next to these two fingers. This will mark your position for chest compressions on the adult chest. Place the hand that located the xiphoid process on top of the other hand. Give fifteen chest compressions. Depress the chest approximately 1½ to 2 inches.

It is just as important to check the circulatory system. Has the system remained a closed one? Is the client bleeding? If a major vessel has been damaged and blood loss is occurring, this must be treated stat. The system must be closed before the air that is being taken in can travel to all organs. The system works through pressure. Pressure requires a certain amount of blood volume. Apply pressure to the site of bleeding. A car will not ride well with a major leak in the tire, even if the engine runs. The tire requires a certain amount of pressure, as it is a closed system. When the tire springs a leak, air is expelled, and the tire deflates. To add air is futile if the leak is not repaired.

If breathing and circulation are not present, **cardiopulmonary resuscitation (CPR)** is initiated. Figure 27-2 depicts the procedure for one-rescuer CPR. Remember, in unconscious adult victims, the most important thing that you can do is activate the EMS or call a CODE if you are in a medical setting. When an adult's heart ceases to function, the adult requires the medications and electrical stimulation of the heart with equipment only the EMS or CODE team can provide.

FIGURE 27-2 One-rescuer CPR.

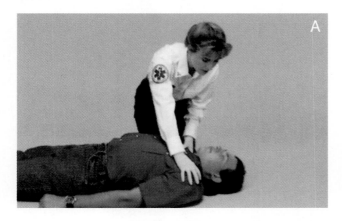

(a) Establish unresponsiveness, and activate the EMS.

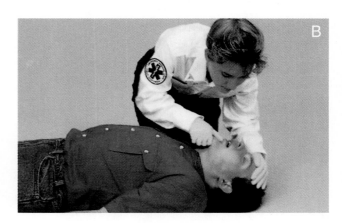

(b) Open the airway using the head tilt-chin maneuver.

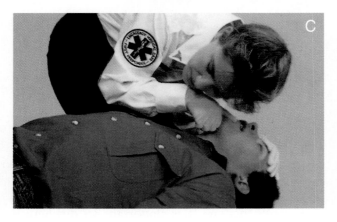

(c) Look, listen, and feel for breathing. If there is no breathing . . .

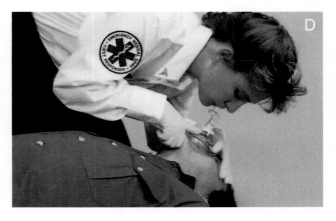

(d) Ventilate twice.

FIGURE 27-2 One-rescuer CPR. (continued)

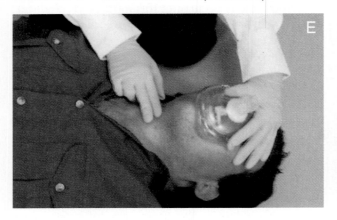

(e) Establish pulselessness—feel the carotid pulse for 5 to 10 seconds. If there is no pulse . . .

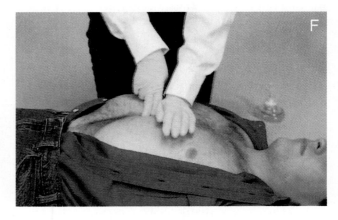

(f) Locate the site for chest compression.

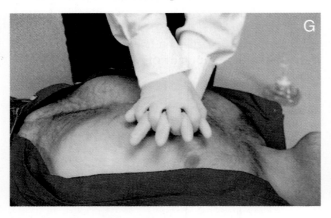

(g) Position hands—use the heel of the hands; keep fingers off the chest.

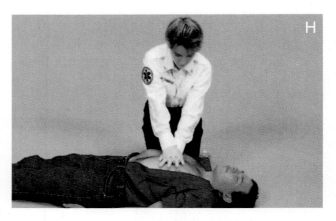

(h) Give fifteen chest compressions, depressing the chest 1½ to 2 inches.

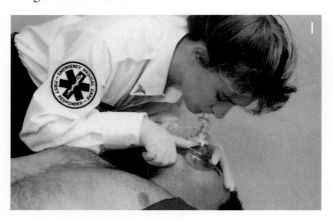

(i) Repeat the cycle of two breaths and fifteen compressions.

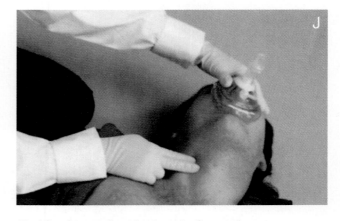

(j) After four cycles, check again for a pulse.

Choking

When the epiglottis fails to seal the lower respiratory tract in the act of swallowing, food or fluid may enter the trachea. In addition, stomach contents may be regurgitated into the pharynx and be aspi-rated, or sucked into the lower respiratory tree, during the breathing process. In either case, choking occurs. Choking may produce partial or complete airway obstruction. It is important to distinguish between the two because intervention is different for each.

Whenever a person is choking, always ask, "Can you speak?" If the victim can cough, speak, or make sounds, the airway is obstructed partially. In this case, be sure the victim is sitting in high Fowler's position. If the victim must be supine, turn the victim or the victim's head to a left lateral or Sims' position. Do not perform any physical interventions. To do so may force the substance further down the respiratory tree. Observe the person and permit him or her to cough to try to clear the partial obstruction.

The cardinal signs of complete airway obstruction are the inability to speak and clutching at the throat. If the patient cannot make any sounds and is unable to cough, a complete airway obstruction is present. *Immediate* physical intervention is essential.

The Heimlich Maneuver

The **Heimlich maneuver** is the most notable intervention technique for removing an airway obstruction from a choking victim. For effectiveness and prevention of other complications, it must be performed correctly.

Heimlich Maneuver

1. Stand behind the person.
2. Encircle your arms around the victim's torso.
3. Using your dominant hand, make a fist with your thumb held straight and inside your fist.
4. Locate the space between the umbilicus and the xiphoid process.
5. Place your fist against the abdominal area located in step 4.
6. Cap the hand held in a fist with the other hand.
7. With one swift inward and upward movement, thrust the abdominal area. This uses the air in the lower respiratory tree below the area of obstruction to force the contents blocking the airway to move up the airway and out the mouth.
8. Repeat this maneuver until the obstruction is cleared or the person becomes unconscious.

If the conscious choking victim becomes unconscious and falls to the ground, follow the measures listed below to help clear an obstructed airway.

Obstructed Airway—Unconscious Adult

If you have been helping a conscious choking adult who becomes unconscious and begins to fall to the ground, ease the person to the ground to avoid head injury. Activate the EMS or call a CODE, then return to the victim (Figure 27-3).

Clearing the Airway—Adult

1. Open the airway, using the head tilt–chin lift maneuver.
2. Use the finger sweep technique to remove any object that may have dislodged in falling to the ground.
3. Attempt to ventilate (give one breath). If the object moved in the fall, the air passageway may now be free.
4. If unsuccessful in the first ventilation, reposition the head and attempt a second ventilation.
5. If unsuccessful, begin abdominal thrusts:
   a. Straddle the victim.
   b. Place the heel of one hand between the umbilicus and the xiphoid process.
   c. Place the heel of the other hand on top of that hand.
   d. Give five upward and inward thrusts.
   e. Return to the victim's head.
   f. Finger-sweep the mouth.
   g. Attempt to ventilate.
6. Repeat steps 5a to 5d.
7. Repeat steps 5e to 5g.
8. Continue the same cycle until you can ventilate the victim successfully or the victim breathes spontaneously.
9. If you can ventilate successfully, give a second breath.
10. Check for a pulse. If a pulse is present and the person does not breath spontaneously, continue rescue breathing.
11. Rescue breathing for an adult is one breath every 5 seconds or twelve breaths per minute.

Cardiac Arrest

Cardiac arrest means that the heart has ceased to beat. Cardiac arrest can result from

- Lethal dysrhythmias
- Respiratory arrest
- Myocardial infarction
- Electrical shock
- Hypovolemia
- Electrolyte imbalance

Cardiac arrest requires swift intervention. The ABCs of emergency care and CPR must be carried out immediately.

In an acute setting, a CODE must be called stat. The crash cart, filled with defibrillator, airways, Ambu bags, and medications, is brought to the patient's room. In the community, 911 or EMS must

FIGURE 27-3   Clearing the airway—adult.

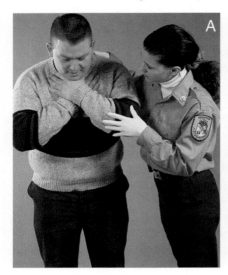

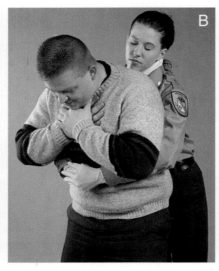

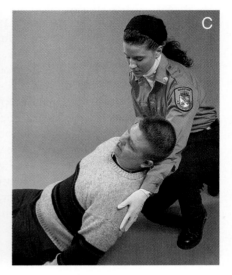

(a) Recognize that the patient is choking. Ask, "Are you choking?"

(b) Position yourself to perform the Heimlich maneuver.

(c) If the patient becomes weak or unconscious, assist him or her to the floor.

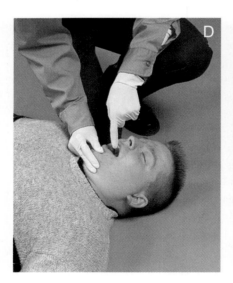

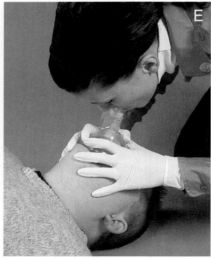

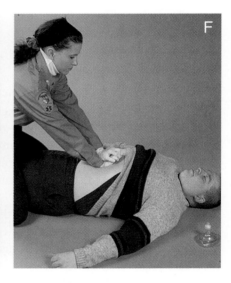

(d) Perform a finger sweep.

(e) Open the airway and attempt to ventilate. If this fails, reposition the head and try again. If you are not successful . . .

(f) Perform the five abdominal thrusts and repeat the cycle until the obstruction is relieved.

be activated stat so that the ambulance can bring the necessary life-sustaining equipment to the victim.

Cardiac arrest may occur suddenly or may provide warnings. The signs and symptoms of an emerging cardiac arrest include

- Crushing chest pain
- Epigastric distress (heartburn)
- Profuse sweating
- Radiating pains in the neck or arm
- Pallor
- Cyanosis
- Weakness

Fire Safety

As in any emergency, fire safety requires an action plan predetermined before the disaster strikes. Each institution has its own fire safety and evacuation plan. Therefore, it is imperative that all staff members participate in fire drills or in-service training re-

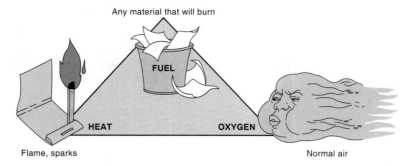

FIGURE 27-4 Oxygen, heat, and fuel are necessary to start a fire.

garding the evacuation plan. In your orientation to a facility, always note the location of fire extinguishers, fire evacuation routes, and any code or fire alarm system for the institution.

To promote fire prevention and swift intervention, it is important to understand fire concepts. There are three elements necessary to start a fire: *oxygen*, *heat*, and *fuel* (Figure 27-4). Taking away at least one of these elements will put out the fire.

Fire Extinguishers

There are three categories of fuel. These are *wood, paper, and cloth*; *gas, oil, cooking fats, and burning liquids*; and *electrical*. Each fuel source requires a different approach for extinguishing the fire. Fire extinguishers have been developed and are manufactured according to the fuels that cause fires. Therefore, there are three classes of extinguishers: A, B, and C.

Fire extinguishers marked *A* contain pressurized water. Which type of fire would they extinguish? They are made for paper, wood, and cloth fires.

Fire extinguishers labeled *B* contain carbon dioxide (CO_2). B extinguishers are used for gas, oil, cooking fats, and burning liquids. Carbon dioxide smothers the flame, but in doing so, it leaves a powdery white residue that can be dangerous if inhaled. It is irritating to the skin, eyes, and mucous membranes.

Class C extinguishers are made from a dry chemical such as potassium bicarbonate or potassium chloride. Their use is limited to electrical fires.

Combination extinguishers labeled *ABC* can be used on all classes of fire. These contain a graphite chemical. As you know, graphite substances are also used to make pencils. This extinguisher leaves a residue that can be irritating to the mucous membranes and skin.

RACE

As with any emergency, remaining calm is extremely important. Remembering the acronym *RACE* and what it stands for is essential (Figure 27-5).

RACE

R = Rescue or remove.
A = Alarm.
C = Contain the fire.
E = Extinguish or evacuate.

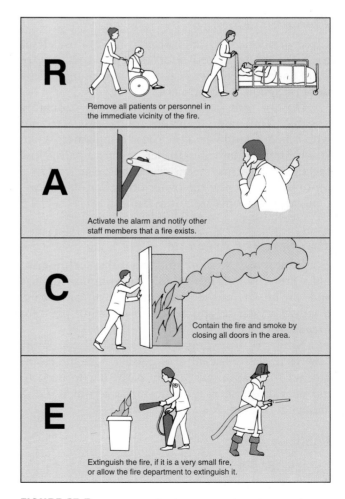

FIGURE 27-5 In case of a fire, remember the word *RACE* and what it stands for.

Rescue or Remove

If you discover a fire, you should remove everyone in danger from the room with the fire and consider your personal safety in the rescue. Cover faces with a wet towel if smoke is evident. You will not help anyone if you endanger yourself.

1. Ambulatory patients and visitors should be directed to the nearest safe area or fire tower.
2. Patients in bed should be removed from the room with the fire.
3. Call for help, and inform staff in the area.

Alarm

Pull the nearest fire alarm, and dial the hospital's extension for fire to inform the operator of the exact location. In many hospitals, a fire bell code is posted to indicate the location. The bell code tells everyone where the fire is located, and then the hospital operator indicates the location over the loudspeaker. If you are in the community, call the fire rescue or 911.

Contain the Fire

Close all doors. Clear all hallways. Do not use elevators. Touch any closed doors with the back side of your hand to feel for heat before opening. If the door or handle is hot, do not open it.

Do not turn on lights. Remove bed patients if possible. You may be unable to remove a patient who is bed-bound when the room is in flames. When you cannot use an extinguisher to clear a path, close the door. This may seem cruel, but you may save more lives by swiftly removing other bed-bound patients whose rooms are not in flames.

Extinguish or Evacuate

Evacuation may be more important than extinguishing a fire. You may not be able to extinguish the fire and remain safe at the same time. If you cannot extinguish, evacuate and follow the facility plan for evacuation.

Never try to extinguish a fire unless you know how to properly use an extinguisher. Use the extinguisher to clear an evacuation path. If you need to use an extinguisher, remember the acronym *PASS* and what it stands for.

PASS

P = Pull the pin.
A = Aim at the base of the fire.
S = Squeeze the handles together.
S = Sweep from side to side.

Know the location of fire exits. Know the location of any horizontal ramps to adjacent buildings. Do not use elevators in an evacuation. Evacuate the area under the directions of the fire marshall. Horizontal relocation methods are used to move people in the area of fire to a place across from the area of fire. Horizontal evacuation methods are used to move people to another fire compartment for safety. Fire-resistant doors seal off an area for at least an hour.

Staff Responsibilities for Fire Safety

- Know the evacuation routes in your area.
- Know where the fire alarms are located in your work area.
- Remember where the fire hose or extinguishers are found.
- Identify the fire bell code that shows the location of the fire. (Most large institutions use a bell system to indicate the location of the fire.)
- Never prop open fire doors.

Electrical Safety

Electrical safety helps to prevent shock, electrocution, and fires. In health care settings, especially hospitals, electricity powers a vast array of equipment for patient life support, treatment, and care. In operating rooms and intensive care units, the reliance on electricity is acute. However, all patient areas are equipped with many electrical devices, such as beds and call signals. Electrical safety is the responsibility of all staff. The following is a list of electrical safety precautions.

Electrical Safety Precautions

- Check all outlets before using them.
- Report any cracked, broken, or chipped outlets.
- Have all new electrical equipment or the patient's personal equipment checked by the biomedical/clinical engineering department before it is used.
- Before using any new electrical equipment, read or receive instructions.
- Inspect any electrical device before using it.
- Make sure the ground plug is present.
- Make sure the prongs are not bent or missing.
- Check for nicked, frayed, or damaged cords. The insulation of the cord should be smooth along the length of the cord.
- Remove power cords by pulling the plug from the outlet. Never pull on the cord.

- Never use adapters or extension cords.
- Never use electrical devices where there is water or moisture near the equipment or outlet.
- Always be certain that your hands are dry before plugging in an electrical device.
- Never stack things on or behind electrical equipment that can interfere with the proper ventilation of the device.
- If you notice a burning smell or unusual odor from equipment, remove the power cord from the outlet and have the equipment checked by qualified staff.
- Keep electrical equipment as far away as possible from the patient's bedside.
- Be sure the power switch is off before plugging equipment into an outlet.
- Remove any patient connections from the equipment before unplugging.

Disaster Plans

The forces of nature impose their threat to the safety and well-being of all. Tornadoes, hurricanes, and floods have been known to destroy lives, homes, and even towns. Natural disasters can create havoc in a health care setting. Hospitals must be staffed and ready to help patients and incoming disaster victims. Hospitals have an internal disaster plan to manage the staffing needs that result from disasters that prevent staff from leaving or getting to the hospital. Your hospital will also have an external disaster plan. External disasters result from train and bus crashes or any situation that results in many accident victims who will come to your hospital for care.

During a disaster, personnel, equipment, and the facility's needs are prioritized. This type of prioritizing is called **triage**. Patients are triaged accordingly: from the most life-threatening conditions to the least serious or non-life-threatening conditions.

You should know the names that your institution has assigned to indicate internal and external disasters. You must know where the disaster manual or policies are located and what they include. You must know what your responsibilities are and where you report for disaster assignments. Preparedness is essential in a disaster. Drills should be held periodically to ensure the readiness of the staff and the facility for potential disasters.

Bomb Threats

Bomb threats are another serious concern. Any bomb threat should be taken seriously. All mea-sures should be taken to promote the safety and the comfort of the patients. You should follow your facility's policy and procedures for responding to a bomb threat. If you receive a telephone call and the caller tells you that there is a bomb on the grounds or in the facility, try to keep the caller on the phone for as long as possible. Write down everything the caller says. Alert someone to call security personnel to the phone. Find out where the bomb is located. Ask where the caller is located and who is calling.

The security department will contact the local police, and a bomb squad will check the facility. Any information that you can give to security or to the police is vital. The instructions of the security officers and the police will determine whether evacuation is necessary.

Biohazardous Wastes

Any blood product, body fluid, or item contaminated with blood or body fluids is a **biohazard** (*bio-* means "life," and *hazard* means "danger" or "peril"). This includes dirty needles, dressings, bedpans and other bedside equipment, surgical equipment, waste containers, and linens. Any time you have been exposed to a biohazard, it must be reported immediately. An incident report must be completed for your protection and for the safety of the institution. Prevention is very important. Of course, prevention is the best measure to deal with biohazardous materials. When you are exposed to a biohazard, you must report it immediately.

All blood and body fluids must be treated as though contaminated with lethal organisms and must be handled according to the CDC guidelines. Bags marked with the biohazard symbol should be used for all disposable products contaminated with blood and body fluids. These bags are usually red, or they may be marked with a red biohazard symbol. Biohazardous trash is separated from regular trash. Although not disposable, contaminated linens must be bagged in yellow biohazard bags to protect central supply workers. Figure 27-6 depicts several types of waste and biohazard containers.

You will need to be certain that biohazard trash bags are in the designated trash receptacles. Be sure that sharps containers are not overfilled. When full, follow the policy for disposal of sharps containers. Never stuff a used sharp into these containers when they are full. Most needle sticks are the result of overfilled sharps containers. All used sharps must be put into these containers. Never recap a used needle. Make certain that gloves are available in treatment and care areas.

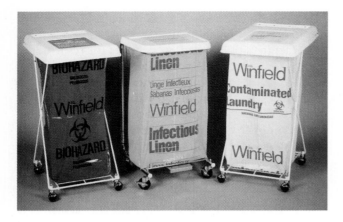

FIGURE 27-6 Examples of waste and biohazardous waste containers.

Hazardous Materials

Every day, you are exposed to hazardous materials (HAZMATS). They have become so common that it is easy to forget to take special precautions. Hazardous materials include acids, alcohol-containing products, peroxide, correction fluid, chemotherapy agents, and mercury. There are two sources of information about HAZMATS. These are (1) the *product label*, which gives warnings and identifies the materials contained in the product (Figures 27-7 and 27-8), and (2) *Material Safety Data Sheets* (Figure 27-9).

Material Safety Data Sheets (MSDSs) are provided by the manufacturer or distributor to give comprehensive information about the hazardous product. There are five sections of the MSDS: chemical hazards, physical hazards, health hazards, control measures, and emergency first aid. The chemical hazards section includes information about the chemical ingredients. The physical hazards section will be helpful. This section explains the potential for fire, explosion, reactions with chemicals, and toxic fumes. The health hazards section details adverse health effects that may result from improper handling. Look for key words to identify the hazards. Some key words are *irritant*, *toxin*, and *carcinogen*. The control measures section recommends protective equipment such as gloves, gowns, hoods, masks, goggles, or respirator. Always use the correct protective equipment. Finally, the MSDS has an emergency first aid section. This describes the first aid steps that could prevent serious or permanent injury.

Your role as a clinical care associate is to

▪ Know where the MSDS are kept.

▪ Read all labels before using products, and always use the correct protective equipment.

EMERGENCY GUIDE—HAZARD SIGNALS

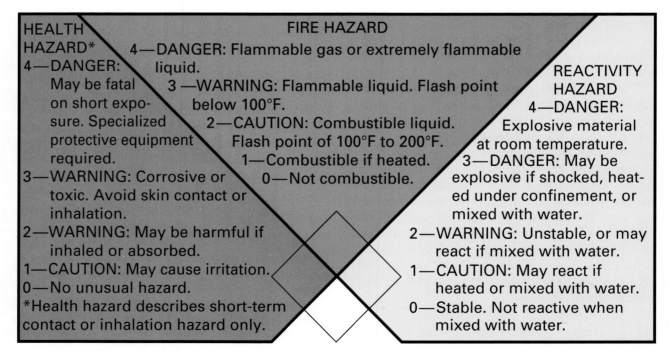

HEALTH HAZARD*
4—DANGER: May be fatal on short exposure. Specialized protective equipment required.
3—WARNING: Corrosive or toxic. Avoid skin contact or inhalation.
2—WARNING: May be harmful if inhaled or absorbed.
1—CAUTION: May cause irritation.
0—No unusual hazard.
*Health hazard describes short-term contact or inhalation hazard only.

FIRE HAZARD
4—DANGER: Flammable gas or extremely flammable liquid.
3—WARNING: Flammable liquid. Flash point below 100°F.
2—CAUTION: Combustible liquid. Flash point of 100°F to 200°F.
1—Combustible if heated.
0—Not combustible.

REACTIVITY HAZARD
4—DANGER: Explosive material at room temperature.
3—DANGER: May be explosive if shocked, heated under confinement, or mixed with water.
2—WARNING: Unstable, or may react if mixed with water.
1—CAUTION: May react if heated or mixed with water.
0—Stable. Not reactive when mixed with water.

FIGURE 27-7 Hazardous material signals.

Hazardous Materials Warning Labels

DOMESTIC LABELING

EXPLOSIVE A 1	EXPLOSIVE B 1	EXPLOSIVE C 1	BLASTING AGENT 1	POISON GAS 2	FLAMMABLE GAS 2	NON-FLAMMABLE GAS 2
CHLORINE 2	OXYGEN 2	FLAMMABLE LIQUID 3	FLAMMABLE SOLID 4	DANGEROUS WHEN WET 4	OXIDIZER 5.1	ORGANIC PEROXIDE 5.2
POISON 6	IRRITANT 6	(Infectious Substance) 6	RADIOACTIVE I 7	RADIOACTIVE II 7	RADIOACTIVE III 7	CORROSIVE 8

General Guidelines on Use of Labels
(CFR, Title 49, Transportation, Parts 100-177)

- Labels illustrated above are normally for *domestic shipments.* However, some air carriers *may* require the use of International Civil Aviation Organization (ICAO) labels.
- Domestic Warning Labels *may* display UN Class Number, Division Number (and Compatibility Group for Explosives only) [Sec. 172.407(g)].
- Any person who offers a hazardous material for transportation MUST label the package, if required [Sec. 172.400(a)].
- The Hazardous Materials Tables, Sec. 172.101 and 172.102, identify the proper label(s) for the hazardous materials listed.

- Label(s), when required, must be printed on or affixed to the surface of the package near the proper shipping name [Sec. 172.406(a)].
- When two or more different labels are required, display them next to each other [Sec. 172.406(c)].
- Labels may be affixed to packages (even when not required by regulations) provided each label represents a hazard of the material in the package [Sec. 172.401].

**Check the Appropriate Regulations
Domestic or International Shipment**

Additional Markings and Labels

HANDLING LABELS

DANGER
Cargo Aircraft Only
172.402(b)

CAUTION
Bung Label
172.402(e)

ORM-E
172.316

INNER PACKAGES
COMPLY WITH
PRESCRIBED
SPECIFICATIONS
173.25(a)(4)

↑↑   ↑↑   Package
Orientation
Markings
172.312(a)(c)

Fumigation
173.9

EMPTY
173.427

Here are a few additional markings and labels pertaining to the transport of hazardous materials. The section number shown with each item refers to the appropriate section in the HMR. The Hazardous Materials Tables, Section 172.101 and 172.102, identify the proper shipping name, hazard class, identification number, required label(s) and packaging sections.

Poisonous Materials

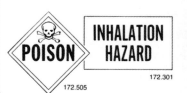

POISON
172.505

INHALATION
HAZARD
172.301

Materials which meet the inhalation toxicity criteria specified in Section 173.3a(b)(2), have additional "communication standards" prescribed by the HMR. First, the words "Poison-Inhalation Hazard" must be entered on the shipping paper, as required by Section 172.203(k)(4), for any primary capacity units with a capacity greater than one liter. Second, packages of 110 gallons or less capacity must be marked "Inhalation Hazard" in accordance with Section 172.301(a). Lastly, transport vehicles, freight containers and portable tanks subject to the shipping paper requirements contained in Section 172.203(k)(4) must be placarded with POISON placards in addition to the placards required by Section 172.504. For additional information and exceptions to these communication requirements, see the referenced sections in the HMR.

Keep a copy of the DOT Emergency Response Guidebook handy!

FIGURE 27-8 Hazardous labels.

Material Safety Data Sheet

May be used to comply with OSHA's Hazard Communication Standard, 29 CFR 1910.1200. Standard must be consulted for specific requirements.

U.S. Department of Labor

Occupational Safety and Health Administration (Non-Mandatory Form)
Form Approved
OMB No. 1218-0072

Identity (As Used on Label and List)

Note: Blank spaces are not permitted. If any item is not applicable, or no information is available, the space must be marked to indicate that.

Section I

Manufacturer's Name	Emergency Telephone Number
Address (Number, Street, City, and ZIP Code)	Telephone Number for Information
	Date Prepared
	Signature of Preparer *(optional)*

Section II–Hazardous Ingredients/Identity Information

Hazardous Components (Specific Chemical Identity; Common Name(s))	OSHA PEL	ACGIH TLV	Other Limits Recommended	% *(optional)*

Section III–Physical/Chemical Characteristics

Boiling Point		Specific Gravity (H$_2$O =1)	
Vapor Pressure (mm Hg)		Melting Point	
Vapor Density (AIR = 1)		Evaporation Rate (Butyl Acetate = 1)	

Solubility in Water

Appearance and Odor

Section IV–Fire and Explosion Hazard Data

Flash Point (Method Used)		Flammable Limits	LEL	UEL

Extinguishing Media

Special Fire Fighting Procedures

Unusual Fire and Explosion Hazards

(Reproduce locally)   OSHA 174, Sept. 1985

FIGURE 27-9 Material Safety Data Sheets.

Section V–Reactivity Data

Stability	Unstable	Conditions to Avoid	
	Stable		

Incompatibility *(Materials to Avoid)*

Hazardous Decomposition or Byproducts

Hazardous	May Occur	Conditions to Avoid	
Polymerization	Will Not Occur		

Section VI–Health Hazard Data

Route(s) of Entry:	Inhalation?	Skin?	Ingestion?

Health Hazards (Acute and Chronic)

Carcinogenicity:	NTP?	IARC Monographs?	OSHA Regulated?

Signs and Symptoms of Exposure

Medical Conditions Generally Aggravated by Exposure

Emergency and First Aid Procedures

Section VII–Precautions for Safe Handling and Use

Steps to Be Taken in Case Material is Released or Spilled

Waste Disposal Method

Precautions to Be Taken in Handling and Storing

Other Precautions

Section VIII–Control Measures

Respiratory Protection (Specify Type)

Ventilation	Local Exhaust	Special	
	Mechanical (General)	Other	
Protective Gloves		Eye Protection	

Other Protective Clothing or Equipment

Work/Hygienic Practices

U.S.G.P.O.: 1986-491-529/45775

FIGURE 27-9 Material Safety Data Sheets. (continued)

application to practice

Emergencies can be personal, patient-related, or environmental. Emergency preparedness is exactly that—knowing your facility's policies and procedures and feeling competent to respond quickly when an emergency arises. Apply what you learned in this chapter to the following situations.

Learning Activities

Situation 1: Mr. Cohn, an eighty-eight-year-old homebound client, is being followed post–myocardial infarction (MI). Following A.M. care, Mr. Cohn complains of dizziness and, in seconds, loses consciousness. What is your first response?

Author's Explanation: Be sure Mr. Cohn is in a safe position in bed or on the floor. If you shake him and shout and he does not respond, you must activate the EMS. Return to the victim, continue the ABCs, and determine if CPR is needed. When the ambulance arrives, you will give the emergency personnel a complete and concise report of the event.

Situation 2: Upon assessment of Mr. Cohn, you observe that he is not breathing. What is your next step? How did you determine the absence of breathing?

Author's Explanation: After opening the airway, no air exchange was felt and the rise and fall of the chest were absent. You should administer two breaths with the rescue mask you keep handy in your CCA bag.

Situation 3: You are able to give Mr. Cohn two effective breaths. What is your next step?

Author's Explanation: Check the carotid pulse for circulatory status. Count the number of beats for 10 seconds.

Situation 4: Mr. Cohn has no carotid pulse. What intervention is next?

Author's Explanation: Initiate chest compressions. Since you are alone, fifteen compressions should be administered. Take time to ensure proper placement of your hands and correct depth (1 to 2 inches) for each compression. Follow the fifteen compressions with two artificial breaths. Complete four cycles of fifteen compressions and two breaths, and check for a pulse. Continue this until the ambulance arrives. If at any time there is a return of cardiac status or breathing, stop CPR and take Mr. Cohn's vital signs. Careful monitoring is essential. When the ambulance arrives, be sure to report the time of the event and all of the steps you took.

Situation 5: When the ambulance arrives at 9:40 A.M., you say that the patient became unconscious after A.M. care, which was at 9:31 in the morning. You initiated CPR at 9:33 A.M. From what emergency condition did the patient suffer? Was CPR initiated before brain damage could occur?

Author's Explanation: Mr. Cohn suffered a cardiac arrest. CPR was initiated within 2 minutes of the onset. Since you initiated CPR so quickly, hopefully brain damage will not occur. There is no absolute time frame in which to predict the occurrence of brain damage. Many factors need to be considered.

Situation 6: John Rocket is your assigned patient on the neurology service. He has a history of petit mal seizures. Recently, he has had many petit mal seizures. You are transferring him into a chair to eat his lunch, and he says to you, "I smell bread baking." He then lets out a cry and begins to fall to the floor. What do you do?

Author's Explanation: Help ease him to the floor, and call out for help. Stay with him and monitor him.

Situation 7: John begins to have jerking motions of his arms and legs; his head is in danger of banging the floor. He has frothy saliva coming from his mouth, and his lips are turning blue. What actions will you take?

Author's Explanation: Protect his head from injury. Remove any furniture that he could bang with his limbs. You should try to turn his head to the side. Try to remove any excess saliva by wiping it away with a cloth. Loosen any tight clothing. Note the time the event began and when it ended.

Situation 8: The nurse arrives, and you describe the details of the event. The nurse asks if there was any warning sign, or aura. Was there?

Author's Explanation: John Rocket reported an unusual sensory experience; he smelled bread baking. This was probably his olfactory aura.

Situation 9: The nurse asks what you think just occurred. You and the nurse return John to bed and find that he has been incontinent of urine. He says he has a headache and wants to sleep. What interventions will you take now?

Author's Explanation: You tell the nurse that you think the patient had a grand mal seizure. You should wash and change John's pajamas since he was incontinent of urine. Take his vital signs. Allow him to sleep, and frequently check on him. Be sure to raise the side rails. If John Rocket sustained any injuries from the event, you and the nurse should complete an incident report.

Situation 10: Mrs. Denlinger is a sixty-eight-year-old who is being followed at home following a compression fracture of L₅ secondary to osteoporosis. She also suffers from chronic obstructive pulmonary disease (COPD). This morning while she is eating her breakfast, she begins to cough. Her face is bright red, and she is struggling. What should you do?

Author's Explanation: Be sure Mrs. Denlinger is sitting in a high Fowler's position. Stay with her and remain calm. Do not provide any physical intervention techniques at this time. If she can cough, she may effectively raise the obstruction on her own. Assistance may force the foreign object further down her respiratory tree.

Situation 11: Mrs. Denlinger coughs until she is blue, and then she is no longer coughing. She is making no sounds at all. What is your next strategy? From what type of airway obstruction is Mrs. Denlinger suffering?

Author's Explanation: Mrs. Denlinger now has a complete airway obstruction. If she can stand, stand her up. From behind, encircle your arms about her torso. Perform the Heimlich maneuver. If Mrs. Denlinger does not respond immediately, call 911. Repeat the Heimlich maneuver again. Monitor the client closely for the foreign substance in her mouth. If the client is able, have her remove it with her fingers. Remember the CDC guidelines regarding body fluids.

Situation 12: Mrs. Denlinger passes out on the floor of the kitchen. She does not appear to be breathing. What is your next plan of action?

Author's Explanation: Call the EMS because she has lost consciousness. Do abdominal thrusts. Follow the steps for obstructed airway of an unconscious adult victim.

Situation 13: Henry Prezuski is a resident in your community residential rehabilitation (CRR) facility. He is found smoking in his bedroom. The resident counselor tells him to put out the cigarette. He should smoke in the designated area on the ground floor of the house. An hour later, you smell smoke coming from upstairs. Other residents are sleeping in their bedrooms. You find that Mr. Prezuski's room is in flames, and smoke is coming into the hallway. You last saw Mr. P. in the kitchen, eating a sandwich. What is your first action? What acronym should you call to mind immediately to help you to respond?

Author's Explanation: RACE: *Remove* all patients from their rooms and send them outside the house. Sound the *alarm*—activate the fire emergency number by dialing 911 to report the fire, and give the address of the CRR. *Contain* the fire—close all the doors on that floor. *Extinguish* the fire, if it is very small, or allow the fire department to do so. Also (and this is a big also) make sure all residents have been evacuated from the house. Take a head count of all house staff and residents while you are outside the building. Await further instructions from the fire department.

Situation 14: While you are changing bed linens, you are stuck with a needle that was in the linens. To what risk have you been exposed, and what should you do?

Author's Explanation: You have been exposed to a biohazard. Immediately wash the area with antibacterial soap and water. Inform the nurse in charge stat. Report to Occupational Medicine stat. Complete an incident report, and follow the directions or recommendations of the doctor and nurse in the Occupational Medicine department or emergency room.

Examination Review Questions

1. The most important CCA intervention for a patient with seizures is to
   a. provide comfort   c. restrain the patient
   b. promote safety   d. keep the patient warm

2. Which phase of grand mal seizures involves rhythmic muscular contractions?
   a. aura   c. clonic
   b. tonic   d. generalized

3. Which of the following is *not* a manifestation of shock?
   a. sharp decline in BP
   b. rapid rise in pulse
   c. rapid rise in respiration
   d. sharp decline in temperature

4. The first step in emergency care after removing a client from danger is to assess
   a. airway   c. circulation
   b. breathing   d. choking

5. In order for the Heimlich maneuver to be implemented, the airway must be
   a. partially occluded
   b. open and patent
   c. completely obstructed
   d. ventilated and compressed

6. Which class of fire extinguisher is used for electrical fires?
   a. A   c. C
   b. B   d. AB

7. How should biohazardous linens be disposed?
   a. red biohazard bags   c. sharps container
   b. double-bagged   d. yellow biohazard bags

8. Which section of the MSDS details adverse health effects that result from improper handling?
   a. chemical   c. health
   b. physical   d. first aid

9. The first step in a fire emergency is
   a. pull the pin   c. call a code
   b. rescue patients   d. pull the alarm

10. Which of the following is *not* a cause of shock?
    a. profuse hemorrhage   c. myocardial infarction
    b. massive infection   d. cardiac arrest

Index

A

Abbreviations:
    for chemicals, 58
    for conditions/diseases, 55–56
    for diagnostic procedures/tests, 56–57
    for health care environments, 60
    for health care professional positions, 57
    for nursing-care terminology, 59–60
    for pharmacology terms, 58
    See also Medical abbreviations
ABCs of emergency care, 452–53
    airway, 452
    breathing, 452–53
    circulation, 453
Abdominal cavity, 77
Abdominopelvic cavity, 77
Abduction, 96
Absorption, 146–47, 226
Acceptance, as stage of death/dying, 262
Accessory organs, 73
    for digestive system, 150–51
    for immunity, 128–29
ACE bandages, applying, 393–94
Acidosis, 139
Acne, 81
Acoustic nerve, 112
Acquired immunodeficiency syndrome (AIDS), 140, 172, 352
    and delirium, 288
    and TB, 319
Acromegaly, 186
ACTH, *See* Adrenocorticotrophic hormone (ACTH)
Active assist exercises, 366
Active range-of-motion (ROM) exercises, 366
Activities of daily living (ADLs), 42, 284, 303
Acute gastritis, 151
Acute renal failure, 163
Adam's apple, 138
Adaptive devices, 363–64
Addictive disorders, 284–86
    substance-related, 285–86
Addison's disease, 190
Adduction, 96
Adipose capsule, 160
Adipose tissue, 73
Adolescent:
    nutritional needs of, 234
    and sexuality, 254

as stage of life, 247, 249
Adrenal glands, 75, 187–88
    disorders of, 190
Adrenalin, 188
Adrenaline, 108
Adrenal sex hormones, 187, 188
Adrenocorticotrophic hormone (ACTH), 186, 190
Adults, nutritional needs of, 233
Advanced directives, 263–66
    defined, 263
    honoring, 264–65
    living wills, 263–64
        example of, 265
    surrogate decision maker, 263
    when they take effect, 264
Advanced procedures/tasks, 401–45
    capillary blood glucose measurements, 440–42
        asepsis, 440–41
        operating a glucose meter, 441
        principle of glucose meters, 440
        quality control, 441
    capillary blood specimens, collecting, 441–42
    catheterization, 402–12
        Foley catheters, 402–3
        indwelling catheter, 402, 406–7
        inserting a catheter, 402–6
        kit, 403
        straight, 402
        urometer, 403
    dressings, 419–22
        Duoderm dressings, 420–21
        Tegaderm dressings, 419–20
        wet-to-dry dressings, 421–22
    ECG machines, 413–19
        chest lead placement, 414–15
        entering patient information, 415–16
        limb lead placement, 414
        technical quality of tracing, 416–17
        troubleshooting, 417–19
        twelve-lead ECG, 416
    gastrostomy tubes (GTs), 407–12
        bolus PEG feeding method, 408, 410
        continuous gastrostomy feeding method, 408, 411–12
        enteral feeding method, 407
        feeding pumps, 412

        IVAC pump, 408
        percutaneous endoscopic gastrostomy (PEG), 407–9
        residual feeding, 409
    ostomy care, 422–25
        changing ostomy appliances, 423–25
        colostomy, 422
        emptying ostomy appliances, 424
        ileostomy, 422
        urostomy, 422
    phlebotomy, 432–41
        applying the tourniquet, 434
        approaching the patient, 434–35
        blood bank specimens, 434
        labeling blood specimens, 434
        performing the venipuncture, 435–39
        phlebotomy needles, 433
        selecting a vein, 435
        types of specimens, 432–33
        Vacutainer needles, 433
        Vacutainer tubes, 433–34
        vein inspection, 453
    pneumatic hose, 442–43
        applying, 443
    respiratory care, 425–32
        incentive spirometry, 428–29
        oral suctioning, 429–31
        oxygen therapy, 425–27
        percussion, 431–32
        pulse oximetry, 427–28
Affect, 281
Affective disorders, *See* Mood disorders
Age-specific competencies, 250–53
Age-specific needs, 250–51
Age-specific nutritional requirements, 233–34
Agnostic, 256
Agoraphobia, 284
AIDS, *See* Acquired immunodeficiency syndrome (AIDS)
Airborne isolation precautions, 318–19
Airborne precautions, 140
Airway, 452
Albumin, 126
Alcohol, 286
Alcoholics Anonymous (AA), 286
Aldosterone, 162, 187–88
Alimentary canal, *See* Digestive system
Alternating air mattress, 351
Alveoli, 139
Alzheimer's disease, 288

Ambulation:
       with crutches, 372–73
       with gait belt, 373
       with quad cane, 374
       with walker, 373–74
Ambulatory care services, 18
Ambulatory patient, positioning for
              venipuncture, 434
Amenorrhea, 177
American Diabetes Association (ADA),
              190
       diet of, 154
American Nurses Association (ANA),
              199–200, 202
Amino acids, 227–28
Ammonia, 162
Amphetamines, 286
Ampulla of Vater, 150
ANA, See American Nurses Association
              (ANA)
Anatomical directions, 76
Anatomical systems of reference, 75–77
Anatomy, 69
Androgens, 188
Anemia, 126, 131
Aneroid sphygmomanometer, 359–60
Aneurysms, 130
Anger, as stage of death/dying, 262
Angina pectoris, 129
Angry behavior, constructive approaches
              to patients exhibiting, 297
Anterior, use of term, 76
Anterior muscle groups, 97
Antianxiety drugs, 286
Antibodies, 126
Anticoagulants, 131
Antidiuretic hormone (ADH), 162,
              186–87
Antiembolism stockings, 393
Antigens, 126
Antiprostaglandin/anti-inflammatory,
              177
Antisocial personality disorder, 279
Anuria, 163
Anxiety, 294–95
       therapeutic approaches to reduce,
              296
Anxiety disorders, 283–84
       dissociative disorder, 284
       general, 283–84
       panic disorder, 284
       phobia, 284
Anxious behavior, managing, 294–95
Aorta, 125
Apnea, 140
Appendicitis, 149, 151
Appendicular skeleton, 88
Appendix, 149
Arachnoid, 110
Areola, 175
Arrectores pilorum, 80

Arrhythmias, 131
Arterial blood pressure, 127
Arteries, 124, 125
       brachial, 127
       coronary, 123
       coronary artery disease (CAD),
              129
       pulmonary, 121
       radial, 127
       renal, 160
Arterioles, 125
Articulate surfaces, 90
Articulations, 90
Ascending colon, 149
Asepsis, 315, 440–41
Aseptic technique, 315, 317–18
Aspiration pneumonia, 140, 410
Aspiration of residual stomach contents,
              408–9
Assessing, and nursing process, 198
Assessment profile, and patient's
              religious affiliation, 256
Assimilation, See Metabolism
Assistance with a tub bath or shower,
              345
Asthma, 140
Atelectasis, 141
Ativan, 286
Atria, 121
Atrioventricular (AV) node, 123
Atrophy, 100–101
Attorney-in-fact, 264
Aural thermometer, 354
Auscultation, 140
Autoclave, 317
Autonomic nervous system (ANS), 111
Autonomy vs. shame and doubt, 248
       age-specific needs, 250
Avoidant personality disorder, 279
Axial skeleton, 88
Axillary temperature, measuring using
              glass thermometer, 356
Axon, 106

ℬ

Baby teeth, 147
Back massage, 352–53
Back supports, 315
Balloon angioplasty, 129
Barbiturates, 286
Bargaining, as stage of death/dying,
              262
Bartholin's glands, 173–74
Basal metabolic rate (BMR), 226
Baselining, 303–4
       defined, 303
       process of, 303–4
Base of support, 314
Basic elimination skills, 385–89
Bathing procedure, 341

Bed bath, 345
Bedmaking, 341–44
       procedure, 342–44
Bedpan, assisting with, 385–86
Bed patient, positioning for
              venipuncture, 434
Bedsores, 352
Behavior:
       defined, 298
       understanding, 303–4
Behavior modification, 298–304
       behavior, understanding, 303–4
       chaining, 304
       defined, 298
       reinforcement:
              scheduling, 303
              types of, 302–3
       shaping, 304
       using to teach, 304
Benign prostatic hypertrophy (BPH), 172
Benign tumors, 115
Bicuspid valve, 121, 130
Biohazardous wastes, 459–63
       hazardous labels, 460–61
       hazardous materials
              (HAZMATS), 460
       Material Safety Data Sheets
              (MSDSs), 460, 462–63
Bipolar mood disorder, 281
Bladder, 75, 160, 163
Bland diets, 231, 232
Blood, 75, 125–28
       blood types, 127
       and calcium, 91
       and the heart, 120–22
       plasma, 126
       platelets, 125, 126
       pulse, 127
       red blood cells (RBCs), 70, 125,
              126
       white blood cells (WBCs), 125,
              126
Blood bank specimens, 434
Blood draw, order of, 433
Blood pressure, 127–28
       and kidney function, 162
       measuring, 358–59
       sphygmomanometer, 127–28,
              358–59
              aneroid, 359–60
              digital, 360
              mercury, 359–60
Blood specimens, labeling, 434
Blood tests, 6
Blood types, 127
Blood vessels, 75, 123–25
Body alignment, 365
Body mechanics, 314–15
Body temperature:
       defined, 353
       See also Temperature

Bolus PEG feeding method, 408, 410
Bomb threats, 459
Bone marrow, 90
Bones, 75, 90–91
Bone spurs, 91
Booting up the system, 33
Borderline personality disorder, 279–80
Boundaries, as means of communication, 208
Bowman's capsule, 161
BPH, *See* Benign prostatic hypertrophy (BPH)
Brachial artery, 127
Bradycardia, 123
Brain, 75, 108
Brain stem, 108, 109–10
Breast cancer, 178
Breast milk, 233
Breasts, 75, 175
    self-examination, 178
Breathing, 452–53
Bronchi, 75, 136, 139
Bronchioles, 139
Bronchitis, 140
Buccal surface, 345
Bundle of His, 123
Burns, 81

C

CAD, *See* Coronary artery disease (CAD)
Calcitonin, 187
Calcium, 91, 92, 160
    and blood, 91
    daily requirement, 229
Calorie-controlled diets, 231, 232
Calories, 230–31
Cancellous bone tissue, 88
Capillaries, 77, 125, 139
Capillary blood glucose measurements, 440–42
    asepsis, 440–41
    glucose meters:
        operating, 441
        principle of, 440
        quality control, 441
Capillary blood specimens, collecting, 441–42
Carbohydrates, 227
Carbon dioxide, 121, 125, 136, 139
Cardiac arrest, 455–56
    and ABCs of emergency care, 455
    signs/symptoms of, 456
    See also Cardiopulmonary resuscitation (CPR)
Cardiac arrhythmias, 131
Cardiac catheterization, 129
Cardiac muscle, 99–100
Cardio-, 52, 53
Cardiomegaly, 123

Cardiopulmonary resuscitation (CPR), 452–54
    ABCS of emergency care, 452–53
        airway, 452
        breathing, 452–53
        circulation, 453
        one-rescuer, 453–54
Cardiovascular system, 75, 120
Carditis, 53
Care delivery, 197–221
    for the dying patient, 261–72
    licensure, 201–2
    nursing process, 197–221
    patient care, fundamentals of, 202–17
    and patient sexuality, 255–56
    scope of practice, 199–201
    for the whole person, 243–60
    See also Patient care
Care delivery alternatives, *See* Health care delivery alternatives
Carotid pulse, 357
Cartilage, 90
Catatonia, 278
Catatonic schizophrenia, 278
Catheter care, 388–89
Catheterization, 402–12
    cardiac, 129
    Foley catheters, 402–3
    indwelling catheter, 402
        removing, 406–7
    inserting a catheter, 402–6
    kit, 403
    straight, 402
    urometer, 403
Causative agent, 317
CD-ROM drive, 32
Cell body, 106
Cell membrane, 71
Cells, 70–72
    cell membrane, 71
    cytoplasm, 72
    nucleus, 71
Centers for Disease Control and Prevention (CDC), 318
Central nervous system (CNS), 108–10
    brain, 108–10
    meninges, 110
Central processing unit (CPU), 32
Centrifuge, 125
Cerebellum, 108, 110
Cerebral vascular accidents (CVAs), 113–14
    and delirium, 288
Cerebrospinal fluid (CSF), 110, 113
Cerebrum, 108–9
Certificate, 32
Certified nurse practitioner, 20
Certified nursing assistants (CNAs), 42
Cervical cancer, 177
Cervix, 175

Chaining, 304
Chambers, heart, 121
Chemical digestion, 146
Chemicals, abbreviations for, 58
Chemstick, 163
Cheyne-Stokes respiration's, 140
CHF, *See* Congestive heart failure (CHF)
Childhood immunizations, 5
Chloride, 160
    daily requirement, 229
Choking, 454–55
    Heimlich maneuver, 455
    obstructed airway of unconscious adult, 455
Cholesterol, 227
    high-cholesterol foods, 231
Choroid, 111–12
Chromosomes, 71
Chronic bronchitis, 140
Chronic gastritis, 151
Chronic obstructive pulmonary disease (COPD), 140
Chronic renal failure, 164
Cilia, 137
Circulation, 453
Circulatory system, 119–33
    anemia, 126, 131
    aneurysms, 130
    arteries, 124, 125
    blood, 125–28
    blood vessels, 123–25
    capillaries, 125
    cardiac arrhythmias, 131
    conditions/diseases of, 129–31
    congestive heart failure, 130–31
    coronary artery disease (CAD), 129
    heart, 120–23
    leukemia, 130
    lymphatic system, 128–29
    myocardial infarction (MI), 123, 129–30
    phlebitis, 131
    plasma, 126
    shock, 131, 451–52
    structures/functions, 120–29
    veins, 124, 125
    See also Blood; Cardiac arrest; Heart; Shock
Circumcision, 171
Classifieds, 39–40
Clavicles, 139
Clean technique, collecting urine specimens by, 377–79
Clear-liquid diets, 231–33
Clergy, 256
Client's care environment, 323–34
    home care, 329–30
    hospital, 330–32
    nursing home, 324–29

Clients' rights, *See* Patients' rights
Clinical assistant, role of, 205–7
Clinical care associates (CCAs), 28, 36, 199–202
    employment of, 25–34
    and patient sexuality, 255
Clinical and environmental emergencies, 449–65
    biohazardous wastes, 459–63
    bomb threats, 459
    cardiac arrest, 455–56
    cardiopulmonary resuscitation (CPR), 452–54
    choking, 454–55
    disaster plans, 459
    electrical safety, 458–59
    fire safety, 456–58
    loss of consciousness, 452
    seizures, 450–51
    shock, 451–52
Clinical experiences, and job search, 39
Clinical pathway, 213
Clinistix, 378
Clinitest/acetest tablet method, 378
Clitoris, 173
Closed bed, 342
Clostridium Diffocele (*C. Diff*), 319
Clothing, patient's, changing, 350
CNS, *See* Central nervous system (CNS)
Cocaine, 286
Code blue, 412
Codeine, 286
Cognitive disorders, 286–88
    delirium, 287–88
    dementia, 288
Cold applications, 389
Colitis, 151
Collaboration, 210
Colo-, 52
Colon, 75, 149–50
Colostomy, 152–53, 422
Combining vowel, 52
Commercially prepared enemas, 386
Communication, 207–10, 215
    barriers to, 209–10
    role play, 208–9
Community living arrangements (CLAs), 42
Community mental health and mental retardation (MH/MR) facilities, 19–20
    assistive personnel employment opportunities with, 42–43
    consumers, 19
    employees, 19–20
    Mental Health Law of 1979, 19
    payers, 20
    regulatory agencies, 20
Community service and achievements section, resume, 37
Compact bone tissue, 88

Compensation, as defense mechanism, 282
Competence, 340
Competent, use of term, 264
Complete blood count (CBC), 434
Complete care, 345
Complete proteins, 228
Compound fracture, 92
Compulsion, 295
Computerized axial tomography (CAT) scans, 6
Computers/data entry, 32–33
Concave, 88
Concussion, 115
Conditions/diseases, abbreviations for, 55–56
Cones, 112
Confidentiality, patient's right to, 214
Confusion, 287
Congestive heart failure (CHF), 122, 130–31
Connective tissue, 73
Consent, 215
Consultation, patient's right to, 215
Consumers:
    community mental health and mental retardation (MH/MR) facilities, 19
    home care, 21
    hospitals, 5–6
    long-term care facilities, 14–15
Contact isolation precautions, 319–20
Continuity of care, and patients' rights, 213–14
Continuous gastrostomy feeding method, 408, 411–12
Continuous gastrostomy feeding method, 408, 411–12
Continuous improvement, hospitals, 8–10
Contractual basis of employment, 21
Contractures, 100
Convalescent homes, *See* Long-term care facilities
Convex, 88
Cooley's anemia, 131
COPD, *See* Chronic obstructive pulmonary disease (COPD)
Copulation, 175
Coronary arteries, 123
Coronary artery disease (CAD), 123, 129
Corpora cavernosa pena, 170–71
Corpora cavernosa urethra, 171
Corpus luteum, 174
Corticosterone, 186
Cortisol, 188
Counseling, and patient sexuality, 255
Cover letter, resume, 40
Crack cocaine, 286
Cranial cavity, 77

Cranial nerves, 110
Cranium, 75, 108
Crank, 286
Creatinine, 162
Critical pathways, 7
Crutches, ambulation with, 372–73
CSF, *See* Cerebrospinal fluid (CSF)
Cultural diversity, 257
Cultural/social importance of food, nutrition, 236–37
Culture, 257
Cushing's syndrome, 190
CVAs, *See* Cerebral vascular accidents (CVAs)
Cyanosis, 83
Cyclothymic disorder, 282
Cystectomy, 165
Cystitis, 164
Cystoscope, 165
Cysts, 177
Cytoplasm, 72
Cytosis, 53

D

Daily weights, 362
Death with dignity, 266
Deciduous teeth, 147
Decubiti, 352
Decubitus ulcers, 83, 352
Deep vein thrombosis (DVT), 442–43
Defense mechanisms, 282–83
Delegation, 199–201, 210–12
Delirium, 287–88
Delirium tremens (DTs), 285
Delusional disorder, 278–79
Delusions, 277
    managing, 298, 301
Dementia, 288
Demerol, 286
Dendrites, 106
Denial:
    as defense mechanism, 282
    as stage of death/dying, 262
Dentist, 31
Dentures, cleaning, 346–47
Dependence, 285
Dependent personality disorder, 280
Depression:
    major, 281–82
    managing, 296–300
    as stage of death/dying, 262
Depressive episodes, 281
Dermis, 77
Descending colon, 149
Development, 244
Dexedrine, 286
Diabetes insipidus, 187, 190
Diabetes mellitus (DM), 112, 151, 154, 188, 190, 352
Diabetic diets, 231, 232

Diagnostic procedures/tests, abbreviations for, 56–57
Diagnostic related groups (DRGs), 6–7, 44, 213
   critical pathways of care, 7
   rates based on, 7
Diagnostic and Statistical Manual of Mental Disorders (DSM IV), 277, 284
Dialysis, 164
Diaphoresis, 226
Diaphragm, 136–37
Diaphysis, 88
Diffusion, 164
Digestion, 146, 226
Digestive system, 75, 145–58
   accessory organs, 150–51
   appendicitis, 151
   colitis, 151
   colostomy, 152–53
   conditions/diseases of, 151–54
   diabetes mellitus (DM), 112, 151, 154
   diverticulosis, 152
   enteritis, 151
   esophagus, 75, 74–75, 138, 147, 148
   functions of, 146–47
   gallbladder, 75, 145, 150
   gastritis, 151
   gastrostomy, 153
   hepatitis, 153–54
   ileitis (enteritis), 151–52
   ileostomy, 152, 153
   inflammatory conditions, 151
   large intestine (colon), 75, 149–50
   liver, 75, 145, 150
   metabolism, 147
   mouth, 75, 136, 147
   pancreas, 75, 145, 150–51
   pancreatitis, 151
   peptic ulcers, 151
   peritoneum, 150
   pharynx, 75, 136, 138, 147–48
   salivary glands, 75, 147
   small intestine, 75, 149
   stomach, 75, 148–49
   stomatitis, 151
   structures of, 147–50
   teeth, 147
   tongue, 147
   tumors of, 153
   ulcerative colitis, 152
Digital sphygmomanometer, 360
Dilation, 112
Dilaudid, 286
Dipstix, 378
Diptheria, pertussis, and tetanus (DPT) vaccine, 5
Disaster plans, 459

Diskette, 32
Disorganized schizophrenia, 278
Disorientation, 287
Displacement, as defense mechanism, 283
Dissociative disorder, 284
Diverticulitis, 152
Diverticulosis, 152
DNA, 71
Dopamine, 114
Dorsal, use of term, 76
Dorsal cavity, 77
Dorsal lithotomy position, 390–91
Down's syndrome, 290
Dressings, 419–22
   Duoderm dressings, 420–21
   Tegaderm dressings, 419–20
   wet-to-dry dressings, 421–22
DRGs, *See* Diagnostic related groups (DRGs)
Droplet isolation precautions, 319
DTs, *See* Delirium tremens (DTs)
Ductless glands, 184
Ducts, 171
Ductus deferens, 171
Duodenum, 149
Duoderm, 85
Duoderm dressings, 420–21
Durable power of attorney, 264
Dura mater, 110
Dwarfism, 186
Dying patient:
   advanced directives, 263–66
   attorney-in-fact, 264
   care delivery for, 261–72
   competent vs. incompetent/ incapacitated, 264
   death with dignity, 266
   durable power of attorney, 264
   end-of-life choices/decisions, 263
   ethical dilemmas, 266–69
   hospice, 262
   stages of death/dying, 262
Dysmenorrhea, 177
Dysphagia, 384
Dyspnea, 140
Dysrhythmias, 131
Dysthymic disorder, 282

E

Ear, 112–13
Eardrum, 112
ECG machines, 412–19
   chest lead placement, 414–15
   ECG paper, 413
   entering patient information, 415–16
   limb lead placement, 414
   multichannel, 413
   single-channel, 413

   stylus, 413
   technical quality of tracing, 416–17
   troubleshooting, 417–19
   twelve-lead ECG, 416
-ectomy, 52–53
Ectopic pregnancy, 176
Education section, resume, 37
Egg, 71
Eggcrate mattress, 351
Ego-defense mechanisms, *See* Defense mechanisms
Eight Stages of Man (Erikson), 245–47
Elbow protectors, 351
Electrical safety, 458–59
   precautions, 458–59
Electric razor, 350
Electrocardiogram (ECG), 28, 123, 213
   See also ECG machines
Electroencephalogram (EEG), 115
Electronic thermometer, 353–54
Elimination, 146–47, 226
   of urine, 160
Elimination skills, 385–89
   bedpan, assisting with, 385–86
   catheter care, 388–89
   enema, assisting with, 386–88
Ellis, Havelock, 253
Embolus (embolism), 113, 141, 393
Embryonic disk, 176
Emergencies, *See* Clinical and environmental emergencies
Emerging health care roles, 27–34
Empathy, 324
Emphysema, 140
Employees:
   community mental health and mental retardation (MH/MR) facilities, 19–20
   home care, 21
   hospitals, 5
   long-term care facilities, 14
Employment opportunities:
   multiskilled care associates, 41–44
     with community mental health and mental retardation agencies, 42–43
     with home care agencies, 43–44
     with hospitals, 41
     with long-term care facilities, 41–42
Empty calories, 231
Empty-nest syndrome, 252
Endocarditis, 53
Endocardium, 120
Endocrine glands, 75, 184
Endocrine system, 75, 183–90
   adrenal glands, 187–88
   disorders of, 190
   conditions/diseases of, 189–90

diabetes mellitus (DM), 112, 151, 154, 188, 190
endocrine glands, 75, 184
hormones, classes of, 185–89
miscellaneous hormones, 185
ovaries, 75, 173, 174, 188–89
pancreas, 75, 145, 150–51, 184, 188
parathyroid gland, 75, 187
disorders of, 189–90
pituitary gland, 185–87
disorders of, 190
prostaglandins, 185
protein, 185
steroids, 185
testes, 75, 170, 171, 189
thyroid gland, 187
disorders of, 189
End-of-life choices/decisions, 263
Endometriosis, 176
Endometrium, 175
End-result reinforcement, 303
Enema:
assisting with, 386–88
defined, 386
disposable, soapsuds (SSE), 388
Fleet, 386
impaction, 386
saline/oil-retention, 386
soapsuds (SSE), 387
administering, 388
Enteral feeding method, 407
Enteritis, 151–52
Environmental emergencies, *See* Clinical and environmental emergencies
Environment of care:
client's care environment, 323–34
defined, 314
safety/security issues, 313–22
See also Client's care environment; Safety/security issues
Enzymes, 147
Epicarditis, 53
Epidermis, 80
Epididymis, 170, 171
Epiglottis, 138, 147–48, 454–55
Epilepsy, 114–15, 450
temporal lobe, 451
Epileptic furor, 451
Epinephrine, 108, 187, 188
Epiphysis, 88
Epithelial tissue, 75
Erikson, Erik, 243–47, 256
Erotomania, 278
Erythrocytes, 126
Escherichia coli (*E. coli*), 315
Esophagus, 75, 74–75, 138, 147, 148
Essential procedures/tasks, *See also* Procedures/tasks
Estrogen, 176, 188

Ethical dilemmas:
characteristics of, 267–69
and the dying patient, 266–69
Ethics, 202–5
autonomy, respect for, 203
beneficence, 202–3
confidentiality, 202
dilemmas for consideration, 203–5
justice, 203
nonmaleficence, 203
Ethnicity, 257
Etiology, 91
Evaluating, and nursing process, 198
Exacerbation, 113
Examination, preparing a patient for, 390–92
Exercise(s):
benefits of, 100
collaborative problem-solving, 216–17
range-of-motion (ROM), 366–71
Exophthalmic goiter (hyperthyroidism), 189
Expectorate, 429
Expiration, 136
Extension, 96
External ear, 112
Eye, 111–12
choroid, 111–12
constriction, 112
dilation, 112
iris, 111–12
pupil, 111–12
retina, 112
sclera, 111
Eye contact, 208
Eye protection, 318

F

Face mask, 426–27
applying, 427
Face shield, 318
Faith, 256
Fallopian tubes, 75, 173, 174–75
Falls, in long-term care facilities, 326
Fat-restricted diets, 231
Fats, 227
Fat-soluble vitamins, daily requirements, 228–29
Fecoliths, 152
Feeding a patient, 384–85
Feeding pumps, 412
Female reproductive system, 172–78
amenorrhea, 177
areola, 175
Bartholin's glands, 173–74
breasts, 175
breast self-examination, 178
cervix, 175

clitoris, 173
conditions/diseases of, 176–78
copulation, 175
corpus luteum, 174
dysmenorrhea, 177
ectopic pregnancy, 176
embryonic disk, 176
endometriosis, 176
endometrium, 175
estrogen, 176, 188
fallopian tubes, 173, 174–75
fetus, 176
fimbriae, 174
follicle-stimulating hormone (FSH), 175, 186
fundus, 175, 177
Graafian follicles, 174
human chorionic gonadotropin (HCG), 176
hymen, 173
labia major, 173
labia minora, 173
labor, 175
luteinizing hormone (LH), 175
mammary glands, 175
menarche, 175
menopause, 175
menorrhagia, 177
menstrual cycle, 175
menstrual dysfunction, 177
milk production, 175
myometrium, 175
ovaries, 173, 174, 188–89
ovulation, 174
pelvic inflammatory disease (PID), 177
placenta, 176
pregnancy, 175–76
progesterone, 176
rugae, 175
salpingectomy, 176
tumors of, 177–78
urethral orifice, 173
uterus, 173, 175, 186
vagina, 173, 175
vaginal orifice, 173
vulva, 173–74
womb, 175
zygote, 176
Femoral pulse, 357
Fetus, 176
Fiber, 230
high-fiber diet, 232
Fibrocystic disease, 177
Fibroid tumors of the uterus, 177
Fight-or-flight division, autonomic nervous system (ANS), 111
Fimbriae, 174
Fingerstick, 441
Fire safety, 456–58
fire extinguishers, 457

RACE, 457–58
    staff responsibilities for, 458
First-degree burns, 81
Fixed joints, 90
Flagella, 72
Flat affect, 278
Fleet enema, 386
Flexion, 96
Flight of ideas, 281
Flossing, 346
Foley catheters, 402–3
Follicle-stimulating hormone (FSH),
    175, 186, 188
Food, cultural/social importance of,
    236–37
Food pyramid, 230
Foot elevators, 351–52
Force, pulse, 127
Foreskin, 171
For-profit organizations, hospitals as, 6
Four-point crutch gait, 372
Fowler's position, 390–91
Fractional urines, 377
Fractures, 92
Freely movable joints, 90
Freudian slip, 283
Freud, Sigmund, 253, 262
Frontal lobes, 109
FSH, *See* Follicle-stimulating hormone
    (FSH)
Full-liquid diets, 231–33
Full-thickness burns, 81
Fundus, 175, 177

G

Gag reflex, 147
Gait belt, ambulation with, 373
Gallbladder, 75, 145, 150
Gallstones, 150
Gastritis, 151
Gastro-, 52
Gastrointestinal (GI) system, *See*
    Digestive system
Gastrology, 52
Gastrostomy, 153
Gastrostomy tubes (GTs), 407–12
    bolus PEG feeding method, 408,
        410
    continuous gastrostomy feeding
        method, 408, 411–12
    enteral feeding method, 407
    feeding pumps, 412
    IVAC pump, 408
    percutaneous endoscopic
        gastrostomy (PEG), 407–9
    residual feeding, 409
General anxiety disorder, 283–84
Generalized seizures, 450
Generativity vs. stagnation, 249
    age-specific needs, 252

Genes, 71
Genetic code, 71
Genetic material, 71
Geri chair, 327
Gigantism, 186
Glands, 171–72
Glass thermometer, 353
    measuring axillary temperature
        using, 356
    measuring oral temperature using,
        355
    measuring rectal temperature
        using, 356
    tips on, 354
Globulins, 126
Glomerulus, 161
Gloves, 318
    applying, 404–5
Glucagon, 188
Glucocorticoids, 187, 188
Glucometer, 154
Glucose, 162
Glucose meters:
    operating, 441
    principle of, 440
Goiter, 187
Gonads, 171
Gout, 91
Gown, 318
Graafian follicles, 174
Grandiose delusion, 277, 278
Grand mal seizures, 450–51
Graves' disease, 189
Gravity, 314–15
Growth, 244
Growth hormone (GH), 186–87
GTs, *See* Gastrostomy tubes (GTs)

H

Hair care procedure, 348
Hallucinations, 278
    managing, 298, 301
Hallucinogens, 286
Handwashing:
    and infection, 317, 318
    procedure, 341
Hard drive, 32
Hashish, 286
Hazardous labels, 460–61
Hazardous materials (HAZMATS), 460
Health care:
    defined, 4–5
    and federal government, 7
    primary care, 4–5
    reengineering, in hospitals, 9
    secondary care, 5
    tertiary care, 5
Health care delivery alternatives, 13–23
    community and ambulatory care,
        18

    community mental health and
        mental retardation
        (MH/MR) facilities, 19–20
    home care, 20–21
    long-term care facilities, 14–18
Health care employment, 35–45
    multiskilled assistive personnel,
        36–40
Health care environment, 3–12
    abbreviations, 60
    hospitals, 5–10
Health care industry, 1–12
    care delivery alternatives, 13–23
    environment, 3–12
Health care professions, abbreviations
    for, 57
Health care roles:
    computers/data entry, 32–33
    emerging, 27–34
    health care employment, 35–45
    health care team, 30–32
    multiskilled care associates:
        expanded skills for, 30
        role of, 28–30
    nursing assistant/nurse aide, skills
        of, 29–30
    "ready-to-work" time, 28–29
    standard skill sets, 29–30
Health care team, 30–32
    licensed team members, 31
    unlicensed team members, 31–32
Health maintenance organizations
    (HMOs), 6, 20–21
Heart, 75, 74–75, 120–23
    electrical stimulating system of,
        123
Heart rhythm, 357
Heart valves, 122
Heat applications, 389
Heel protectors, 351
Heelstick, 162
Height, measuring, 362
Heimlich maneuver, 455
Hematologist, 30
Hematuria, 164–65
Hemicardia, 53
Hemiplegia, 100, 113
Hemoccult slide packet, 381–82
Hemoccult test, 380
Hemodialysis, 164
Hemoglobin, 126
Hemophilia, 126
Hemoptysis, 141
Hemothorax, 141
Hepatitis, 153–54
    type A, 153
    type B, 153
    type C, 153–54
Hepatocytes, 72
Herniated intervertebral disc, 91
Heroin, 286

High-calorie diets, 232
High-cholesterol foods, 231
High-density lipoproteins (HDLs), 227
High-fiber diets, 232, 233
High-protein diet, 232
Histrionic personality disorder, 280
Hives, 81
Home care, 20–21, 329–30
    assistive personnel employment
        opportunities in, 43–44
    candidates for, 21
    consumers, 21
    employees, 21
    facilities, 20–21
    regulatory agencies, 21
    safety issues, 329–30
Home care departments, in hospitals, 20
Hormones, 75, 125
    adrenal sex hormones, 187, 188
    adrenocorticotrophic hormone
        (ACTH), 186, 190
    antidiuretic hormone (ADH),
        162, 186–87
    classes of, 185–89
    follicle-stimulating, 175, 186, 188
    growth, 186–87
    and kidneys, 162
    lactogenic, 186
    luteinizing, 175, 186
    melanocyte-stimulating, 80
    parathyroid, 187
    salt-retaining, 162, 187
    thyroid-stimulating, 186
    water-retaining, 162
Hospice, 262
Hospital charges, patient's right to
        explanation of, 216
Hospitals, 5–10, 330–32
    assistive personal employment
        opportunities with, 41
    as care environment, 330–32
    consumers, 5–6
    diagnostic related groups (DRGs),
        6–7
    employees, 5
    as for-profit organizations, 6
    home care departments in, 20
    Medicare, 6
    as nonprofit organizations, 6
    nursing models, 9–10
    payers, 6
    quality assurance and
        improvement, 8–10
    reengineering health care in, 9
    regulatory agencies, 7–8
Hospital unit, 330
Hoyer lift, 376
Human body:
    anatomical directions, 76
    anatomical systems of reference,
        75–77

cells, 70–72
circulatory system, 119–33
digestive system, 75, 145–58
endocrine system, 183–90
muscular system, 75, 95–103
nervous system, 75, 105–17
organs, 73
quadrants, 75
reference cavities, 76–77
reproductive system, 169–82
respiratory system, 135–44
skeletal system, 75, 87–93
skin, 73, 75, 79–86
structural units, 70–75
systems, 73–75
tissues, 73
urinary system, 75, 159–68
as a whole, 67–75
Human chorionic gonadotropin
        (HCG), 176
Human person:
    basic needs, 244–49
    cultural diversity, 257
    spiritual needs, 256–57
Human sexual behavior, 253–57
    and patient care, 253–54
    sexual behavior research, 253
    sexuality, and growth and
        development, 254–56
Human sexual response, phase of, 253
Hunchback, 88
Huntington's disease, 288
Hydrocephalus, 115
Hydrochloride, 286
Hydrocortisone, 186
Hymen, 173
Hyperalimentation, 440
Hyperglycemia, 151, 154
Hyperparathyroidism, 189
Hypersomnia, 281–82
Hypertension, 127, 358
Hyperthyroidism, 189
Hypertrophy, 101
Hypervitaminosis, 229
Hypoglycemia, 154
Hypoparathyroidism, 189–90
Hypotension, 127, 358
Hypothalamus, 110, 185
Hypothyroidism, 189

J

I&O, *See* Intake and output (I&O)
Ibuprofen, 177
Ideas of reference, 278
Identity vs. role confusion, 249
    age-specific needs, 251–52
Ileitis (enteritis), 151–52
Ileo-, 52
Ileostomy, 152, 153, 422
Ileum, 149

Immediate reinforcement, 303
Immunity, accessory organs for, 128–29
Impaction, 386
Implementing, and nursing process, 198
Incapacitated, use of term, 264
Incentive spirometry (IS), 428–29
    assisting with, 429
Incisal surface, 345–46
Incoherent speech, 287
Incompetent, use of term, 264
Incomplete proteins, 228
Incongruent affect, and schizophrenia,
        278
Incontinence products, 84
Incus, 112
Industry vs. inferiority, 249
    age-specific needs, 251
Indwelling catheter, 402
    removing, 406–7
Indwelling catheterization kits, 403
Infant:
    nutritional needs of, 233
    and sexuality, 254
    as stage of life, 247, 248
Infection, 315–18
    aseptic technique, 315, 317–18
    autoclave, 317
    causative agent, 317
    and handwashing, 317, 318
    isolation, 318
    method of transmission, 317
    microorganisms, 315
    pathogens, 315–16
    portal of entry, 317
    portal of exit, 317
    quarantine, 318
    reservoir, 317
    susceptible host, 317
Inferior vena cava, 125
Infertility, 172
Information, patient's right to, 215
Ingestion, 226
Initiative vs. guilt, 248
    age-specific needs, 250–51
Inner ear, 112
Insertion, 96
Insomnia, 281
Inspiration, 136
Insulin, 150–51, 184, 188
Intake and output (I&O), 359–61
    measuring, 361
Integrity vs. disgust and despair, 249
    age-specific needs, 252–53
Integumentary system, 75
Intelligence quotient (IQ), 288–89
Interbrain, 108, 110
Intermittent reinforcement, 303
Internal respiration, 136
Interneurons, 107
Intervertebral discs, 90
Interviews, 38–39

Intimacy vs. isolation, 249
  age-specific needs, 252
Involuntary muscle tissue, 100
Iris, 111–12
Iron, daily requirement, 229
Irritable bowel syndrome, 233
Islets of Langerhans, 150
Isolation, 318
  airborne isolation precautions,
    318–19
  CDC guidelines for, 318–20
  contact isolation precautions,
    319–20
  droplet isolation precautions, 319
Isometric muscular contraction, 100
Isotonic muscular contraction, 100
IVAC pump, 408

J

Jacksonian seizures, 450, 451
Jaundice, 154
JCAHO accreditation, 7
  functions surveyed for, 8
Jealous delusional disorder, 278
Jejunum, 149
Job postings, 39
Job search, 29–40
JOBST stockings, 393
Johnson, Virginia, 253
Joint Commission on Accreditation of
    Healthcare Organizations
    (JCAHO), 7–8, 15, 20
Joints, 90
Judgment, 287, 288

K

Ketoacidosis, 154
Ketodiastix, 378
Ketones, 154
Keyboard, 32
Kidneys, 75, 160–63
  and blood pressure, 162
  factors controlling function of,
    162
  and hormones, 162
  nephrons, 161–62
  normal urine, 162–63
  working units of, 161
Kidney stones, 164, 380
Knee-chest position, 390–91
Kyphosis, 90

L

Labia major, 173
Labia minora, 173
Labor, 175, 186
Lactogenic hormone, 186
Language of medicine, 47–65

Large intestine (colon), 149–50
Laryngopharynx, 138
Larynx, 75, 138
Laser treatment, for kidney stones, 164
Lateral, use of term, 76
Lateral delegation, 210
L-Dopa, 114
Least restrictive alternative concept, 290
Left-lateral position, 387, 390–91
Left-sided heart failure with pulmonary
    edema, 130
Lemon glycerine swab sticks, 346
Leukemia, 130, 352
Leukopenia, 126
Leukorrhea, 177
Librium, 286
Licensed practical nurses (LPNs), 199,
    201–2
Licensed practitioners, 31
Licensed team members, 31
Licensure, 201–2
Ligaments, 90
Lingual surface, 345
Liquid diets, 231–34
Little brain, *See* Cerebellum
Liver, 75, 145, 150
Living wills, 263–64
  example of, 263
-*logist*, 52
-*logy*, 52
Long-term care facilities, 14–18, 324–29
  assistive personnel employment
    opportunities with, 41–42
  consumers, 14–15
  defined, 14
  employees, 14
  falls, 326
  helping the resident adapt, 325
  nursing assistants in, 31–32
  and patient sexuality, 255
  payers, 18
  personal space in, 324
  regulatory agencies, 15–18
  restraints, 326–28
  safety issues, 325–29
  wandering, 328–29
    potential causes of, 328
    techniques to respond to, 329
    underlying causes of, 328–29
    wander guards, 328
Long-term memory, 288
Lordosis, 88
Loss of consciousness, 452
Low-cholesterol diet, 232
Low-density lipoproteins (LDLs), 227
Low-fat diets, 231, 232
Low-fiber diet, 233
Low-protein diet, 232
Low-residue diet, 232, 233
LPNs, *See* Licensed practical nurses
    (LPNs)

LSD, 286
Lungs, 75, 74–75, 136, 139
Luteinizing hormone (LH), 175, 186
Lymph, 128
Lymphatic system, 120, 128–29
Lymph nodes, 75, 128
Lymphocytes, 126
Lymph vessels, 128

M

Magical thinking, and schizophrenia,
    278
Magnesium, 162
  daily requirement, 229
Major depression, 281–82
Male reproductive system, 170–72
  benign prostatic hypertrophy
    (BPH), 172
  circumcision, 171
  conditions/diseases of, 172
  corpora cavernosa pena, 170–71
  corpora cavernosa urethra, 171
  ducts, 171
  ductus deferens, 171
  epididymis, 171
  glands, 171–72
  gonads, 171
  infertility, 172
  penis, 170–71
  prepuce (foreskin), 171
  PSA (Prostatic Specific Antigen),
    172
  scrotum, 170
  seminal fluid, 171–72
  seminiferous tubules, 171
  spermatozoa, 171–72
  testes (testicles), 75, 170, 171
  testicular exams, 172
  testosterone, 171, 189
  vas deferens, 171
Malignant tumors, 115
  of the breast, 178
Malleus, 112
Mammary glands, 175
Managing behavior, 294–98
  angry, demanding, verbally
    abusive behavior, 295–96
  anxiety, 294–95
  behavior modification, 298–304
  depressed behavior, 296–300
  hallucinations/delusions, 298, 301
Mania, 281
Mantaoux test, 140
Marijuana, 286
Mask, 318
Maslow, Abraham, 244
Maslow's hierarchy of needs, 244–45
Massage, 352–53
Master gland, 185–86
Masters, William, 253

Material Safety Data Sheets (MSDSs), 460, 462–63
Meaningless speech, 278
Measuring skills, 353–63
    height, 362
    intake and output, 359–61
    vital signs (VS), 353–63
        blood pressure, 358–59
        pulse, 356–57
        respirations, 357–58
        temperature, 353–56
    weight, 362–63
Mechanical digestion, 146
Mechanical lift, transfers with, 376–77
Medial, use of term, 76
Mediastinum, 137
Medicaid, 18
Medical abbreviations, 49–65
    activities of daily living (ADLs), 55–60
    practice reading terms, 61
Medical assistants (MAs), 19–20, 32
Medical diagnosis, 6
Medical social workers (MSWs), 21
Medical terms, 49–65
    building, 51–55
    defining, 51–55
    prefixes, 51, 54
    pronouncing, 50–51
    spelling, 50–51
    suffixes, 51, 54–55
    word parts, 51
    word roots, 51, 54–55
Medicare, 6, 18, 43
Medulla oblongata, 109
Melanin, 80
Melanocyte-stimulating hormone, 80
Melena, 151
Menarche, 175, 234
Meninges, 110
Meningitis, 110, 113
Meningococcus, 315
Menopause, 175
Menorrhagia, 177
Menstrual cycle, 175
Menstrual dysfunction, 177
Mental health, 276–77
    diagnostic categories of, 277
    minimental-state examination, 304
    See also Mental illness; Mental retardation; Neurotic disorders; Psychotic disorders
Mental Health Law of 1979, 19
Mental illness, 275–91
    managing behavior, 294–98
        angry, demanding, verbally abusive behavior, 295–96
        anxious behavior, 294–95
        behavior modification, 298–304

        depressed behavior, 296–300
        hallucinations/delusions, 298, 301
    mental retardation, 288–90
    neurotic disorders, 282–88
    psychotic disorders, 277–82
    treating, 293–310
        general guidelines, 294
    See also Behavior modification; Mental retardation; specific disorders
Mental retardation, 288–90
    causes of, 290
    defined, 288
    Down's syndrome, 290
    mild, 289
    moderate, 289
    profound, 289–90
    severe, 289
Mercury sphygmomanometer, 359–60
Metabolism, 147, 226, 234
Metastasis, 115
Methadone, 286
Methamphetamine, 286
Methicillin-resistant *staphlococcus aureus* (MRSA), 319
Method of transmission, 317
MH/MR facilities, 19–20
MI, *See* Myocardial infarction (MI)
Microbes, 317
Microorganisms, 162, 315
Midbrain, 109, 110
Middle-aged adult:
    and sexuality, 254
    as stage of life, 248, 249
Midline, 315
Mild mental retardation, 289
Milk production, 175
Mineralcorticoids, 187–88
Minerals, daily requirements, 229
Minimental-state examination, 304
Minimum Data Set (MDS), 16
    assessment areas from, 17
Miscellaneous hormones, 185
Mitosis, 71
Mitral valve, 121, 130
Mitral valve prolapse, 130
Mobility, 374
Moderate mental retardation, 289
Modification, defined, 298
Molecules, 73
Monitor, 32
Monocytes, 126
Monosodium glutamate (MSG), 231
Mood, 281
Mood disorders, 281–82
    bipolar, 281
    cyclothymic disorder, 282
    dysthymic disorder, 282
    major depression, 281–82
Morphine, 286

Motor neurons, 107
Mouse, 32
Mouth, 75, 136, 147
Mouth care, 345–47
    conscious patient, 346–47
    dentures, 346–47
    flossing, 346
    procedure, 346–47
    unconscious patient, 347
Moving a patient, 365–66
Mucus, 162
Multichannel ECG machines, 413
Multiple sclerosis, 113
Multiskilled care associates:
    employability of, 36–40
    employment opportunities, 41–44
    expanded skills for, 30
    interviews, 38–39
    job search, 29–40
    knowing yourself, 38
    resumes, 36–38
    role of, 28–30
    special abilities/traits, 36–38
    unlicensed, tasks performed by, 30
Muscle tone, 100
Muscular system, 75, 95–103
    anterior muscle groups, 97
    atrophy, 100–101
    cardiac muscle, 99–100
    conditions/diseases of, 100–101
    contractures, 100
    exercise, benefits of, 100
    hemiplegia, 100
    hypertrophy, 101
    muscle tone, 100
    myasthenia gravis, 101
    paralysis, 100
    posterior muscle groups, 98
    quadriplegia, 100
    skeletal muscle movements, 96
        types of, 96
    skeletal muscles:
        and intramuscular injections (IMs), 99
        structure/function of, 96–99
    smooth muscle, 99
Muscular tissue, 73
Myasthenia gravis, 101
Myelin sheath, 106
Myocardial infarction (MI), 123, 129–30
Myocarditis, 54
Myocardium, 100, 120
Myometrium, 175
Myxedema, 189

N

N/95 TB respirator, 319
Nail care procedure, 349

Narcisstic personality disorder, 280
Narcotics, 286
Narcotics Anonymous (NA), 286
Nasal cannula, 425–27
    applying, 426
Nasogastric tube, 235–36
Nasopharynx, 138
Nature's contraceptive, breast-feeding
    as, 186
Needs:
    basic, 244–49
    Maslow's hierarchy of, 244–45
Negative feedback, 184
Negative reinforcement, 302
Nephrectomy, 165
Nephrology, 52
Nephrons, 161–62
Nerves, 75
    acoustic, 112
    cranial, 110
    spinal, 110–11
Nervous system, 75, 105–17
    autonomic nervous system (ANS),
        111
    central nervous system (CNS),
        108–10
    conditions/diseases of, 113–15
    divisions of, 108–11
    neurons, 106–8
    peripheral nervous system (PNS),
        110–11
    special sense organs, 111–13
Nervous tissue, 75
Networking, 39
Networks, 33
Neurochemical, 108
Neurologist, 30
Neurons, 73, 106–8
    interneurons, 107
    motor, 107
    sensory, 106–7
    transmission of signals, 108
    types of, 106–7
Neurosis, 282
Neurotic disorders, 282–88
    addictive disorders, 284–86
    anxiety disorders, 283–84
    cognitive disorders, 286–88
    defense mechanisms, 282–83
    neurosis, 282
Neurotic paradox, 282
Neutropenia, 126
Neutropenic precautions, 126
Neutrophils, 126
Nightingale, Florence, 20–21
Nihilistic delusion, 277
Non-insulin-dependent diabetes mellitus
    (NIDDM), 151, 154, 190
Nonprofit organizations, hospitals as, 6
Nonverbal communication, 207–8
Norepinephrine (noradrenalin), 187, 188

Normal, defined, 275
Normal sinus rhythm, 412
Normal urine, 162–63
Nose, 75, 136, 137–38
Nosocomial infection, 314
Nostrils, 137
Nuclear Regulatory Commission
    (NRC), 8, 20
Nucleus, cells, 71
Nucleus pulposus, 90
Nurse, 31
Nurse aides, 29–30, 41–42, 200
Nurse extenders, 9
Nursing assistants, 31–32, 41–42
    skills of, 29–30
Nursing-care terminology, abbreviations
    for, 59–60
Nursing homes, *See* Long-term care
    facilities
Nursing models, 9–10
Nursing process, 197–221
    basal metabolic rate (BMR),
        226
    concepts of, 198
Nutrients, 226–27
Nutrition, 223–39
    absorption, 146–47, 226
    age-specific nutritional
        requirements, 233–34
    amino acids, 227–28
    assimilation, 226
    calories, 230–31
    carbohydrates, 227
    cultural/social importance of
        food, 236–37
    digestion, 146, 226
    elimination, 146–47, 226
    fats, 227
    fat-soluble vitamins, daily
        requirements, 228–29
    fiber, 230
    food pyramid, 230
    ingestion, 226
    metabolism, 147, 226
    minerals, 229
    nutrients, 226–27
    parenteral nutrition, 235
    process of, 226
    proteins, 185, 227–28
    therapeutic diets, 231–33
    tube feedings, 235–36
    vitamins, 228–29
    water-soluble vitamins, daily
        requirements, 228
Nutrition skills, 384–85
    feeding a patient, 384–85

O

O&P test, 380, 382
Objective data, 199

Obsession, 295
Obsessive-compulsive personality
    disorder, 280–81
Obstructed airway, of unconscious
    adult, 455
Occipital lobes, 109
Occupational Safety and Health
    Administration (OSHA), 8
Occupational therapists (OTs), 21
Occupied bed, 341
Oil glands, 80
Oil-retention enema, 386
Older adult:
    nutritional needs of, 234–35
    and sexuality, 254
    as stage of life, 248, 249
Olfactophobia, 53
Oliguria, 163
Omnibus Budget Reconciliation Act
    (OBRA), 15–18, 324
    Minimum Data Set (MDS), 16
        assessment areas from, 17
        primary areas of legislation, 16–17
Oncology, 30
One-rescuer CPR, 453–54
Onion skin, 84
Open bed, 342
Opium, 286
Oral suctioning, 429–31
    oral suction (Yankeur) catheter,
        430
    procedure, 430–31
    suctioning, defined, 429
Oral suction (Yankeur) catheter, 430
Oral thermometer, 353
    glass, 355
Orange-peel skin, 178
Order of blood draw, 433
Orderly, 41
Order sheet, 62
Organelles, 72
Organic mental disorder, 287
Organic wastes, 162
Organism, 69
Organs, 73
Orifices, 315
Origin, 96
Oropharynx, 138
Orthopedist, 30
Orthopnea, 140
-osis, 53
Osteoarthritis, 91
Osteoporosis, 91–92
Ostomy care, 422–25
    colostomy, 422
    ileostomy, 422
    ostomy appliances:
        changing, 423–25
        emptying, 424
    urostomy, 422
-ostomy, 52

Outcome-based goal setting, 340
Ova, defined, 382
Ova and parasites (O&P) test, 380, 382
Ovarian cysts, 177
Ovaries, 75, 173, 174, 188–89
Ovulation, 174
Oxisensor, 428
Oxygen-delivery system, 425–26
Oxygen therapy, 425–27
Oxytocin, 186

P

Palate, 147
Pancreas, 75, 145, 150–51, 184, 188
Pancreatitis, 151
Panic disorder, 284
Papillae, 147
Pap test, 177
Paralysis, 100
Paranasal sinuses, 137–38
Paranoid schizophrenia, 278
Parasites, 380, 382
Parasympathetic division, autonomic
        nervous system (ANS), 111
Parathyroid glands, 75, 187
    disorders of, 189–90
Parathyroid hormone (parathormone),
        187
Parenteral nutrition, 235
Parietal lobes, 109
Parkinson's disease, 114
Partial care, 345
Partial seizures, 450
Partial-thickness burns, 81
Passive-aggressive personality disorders,
        280
Passive range-of-motion (ROM)
        exercises, 366
Pathogens, 315–16
-*pathy*, 53
Patient care:
    clients'/patients' rights, 213–16
    ethics, 202–5
    fundamentals of, 202–17
    patient-centered care, 212–13
    and sexual behavior, 253–54
    teamwork, 205–12
    See also Ethics; Patients' rights;
        Teamwork
Patients, 5–6
Patient Self-Determination Act (1990),
        263
Patients' rights, 213–16, 340
    collaborative problem-solving
        exercises, 216–17
    communication, 215
    consent, 215
    consultation, 215
    hospital charges, explanation of,
        216

hospital rules and regulations,
        216
    identity, 214
    information, 215
    privacy and confidentiality, 214
    refusal of treatment, 213
    respect and dignity, 213
    transfer and continuity of care,
        215–16
Payers:
    community mental health and
        mental retardation
        (MH/MR) facilities, 20
    hospitals, 6
    long-term care facilities, 18
PCP, 286
Pedal pulse, 357
Pelvic cavity, 77
Pelvic inflammatory disease (PID), 177
Penis, 75, 170–71
Peptic ulcers, 151
Percodan, 286
Percussion, 431–32
    performing, 432
    purpose of, 431
Percutaneous endoscopic gastrostomy
        (PEG), 407–9
Perforation, 151
Performance improvement, hospitals,
        8–10
Pericarditis, 53
Pericardium, 120
Peripheral nervous system (PNS), 110–11
    cranial nerves, 110
    spinal nerves, 110–11
Peristalsis, 146
Peritoneal dialysis, 164
Peritoneum, 150
Persecutory delusion, 277, 278
Personality disorders, 279–81
    antisocial, 279
    avoidant, 279
    borderline, 279–80
    dependent, 280
    histrionic, 280
    narcisstic, 280
    obsessive-compulsive, 280–81
    passive-aggressive, 280
    sadistic, 280
    schizoid, 280
    schizotypal, 280
Personal security, 320–21
    basic security, 320–21
    guidelines for, 321
Petit mal seizures, 450
Peyote, 286
Phagocytes, 126
Pharmacology terms, abbreviations for,
        58
Pharynx, 75, 136, 138, 147–48
Phlebitis, 131

Phlebotomy, 432–41
    applying the tourniquet, 434
    approaching the patient, 434–35
    blood bank specimens, 434
    labeling blood specimens, 434
    performing the venipuncture,
        435–39
    phlebotomy needles, 433
    selecting a vein, 435
    types of specimens, 432–33
    Vacutainer tubes, 433–34
    vein inspection, 453
Phobia, 284
Phosphorus, 160, 162
Photophobia, 53
Physiatrist, 30
Physical therapists (PTs), 21
Physician, 31
Physician assistants (PAs), 20
Physiological needs, 244–45
Physiology, 69
Pia meter, 110
Pick's disease, 288
Pitocin, 186
Pituitary gland, 75, 185–87
    anterior, 185–86
    disorders of, 190
    posterior, 186–87
Placenta, 176
Planning, and nursing process, 198
Plasma, 126
Plasma proteins, 162
Platelets, 125, 126
Pleura, 137
Pleural cavities, 137
Pleural seal, 141
Pleurisy, 137
Pneumatic hose, 442–43
    applying, 443
Pneumonia (pneumonitis), 140
Pneumothorax, 141
Polycystic disease, 165
Pons, 109, 110
Portal of entry, 317
Portal of exit, 317
Position:
    dorsal lithotomy, 390–91
    Fowler's, 390–91
    left-lateral, 387, 390–91
    prine, 390–91
    side-lying, 365
    Sim's, 387, 390–91
    supine, 390
Positive reinforcement, 302
Posterior, 76
Posterior muscle groups, 98
Post-operative (post-op) bed, 342
Potassium, 160
    daily requirement, 229
PPD (Purified Protein Derivative) test,
        140

Pre-, 51
Precordial chest leads, 414
Prefixes, 51, 54
Pregnancy, 175–76
Preoperative shaving, 394–96
Prepuce (foreskin), 171
Presbyopia, 112
Preschooler:
    and sexuality, 254
    as stage of life, 247, 248
Pressured speech, 281
Pressure sores, 352
Pressure ulcers, 352
Primary amenorrhea, 177
Primary care, 4–5
Primary nursing model, 9
Privacy and confidentiality, patient's
    right to, 214
Problem solving, 198–202
Procedures/tasks, 336–98
    basic elimination skills, 385–89
    basic hygiene, 341–53
    bathing, 341
    bedmaking, 341–44
    changing a patient's clothing, 350
    comfort, 340
    competence, 340
    hair care, 348
    handwashing, 341
    implementation of procedures,
        338–53
    massage, 352–53
    measuring skills, 353–63
    mouth care, 345–47
    nail care, 349
    nutrition skills, 384–85
    outcome-based goal setting, 340
    patients' rights, 340
    restorative care skills, 363–77
    safety, 339–40
    shaving, 349–50
    skin care, 350–52
    special applications/preps,
        389–96
    specimen-collection skills, 377–84
    time management, 338–39
    See also Advanced procedures/
        tasks; Elimination skills;
        Measuring skills; Nutrition
        skills; Restorative care skills;
        Special applications/preps;
        Specimen-collection skills;
        Time management
Production, of urine, 160
Product label, hazardous materials
    (HAZMATS), 460
Profound mental retardation, 289–90
Progesterone, 176, 188–89
Projection, as defense mechanism, 283
Prolactin, 186
Prone position, 390–91

Pronunciation, of medical terms, 50–51
Pronunciation key, 50
Prostaglandins, 185
Protein diets, 231–34
Proteins, 185, 227–28
PSA (Prostatic Specific Antigen), 172
Psoriasis, 81
Psychoactive substances, 285
Psychomotor seizures, 450, 451
Psychotic disorders, 277–82
    mood disorders, 281–82
    personality disorders, 279–81
    thought disorders, 277–79
Pulmonary artery, 121
Pulmonary edema, 140–41
Pulmonary embolism, 141
Pulposus, 90
Pulse, 127
    carotid, 357
    defined, 356
    femoral, 357
    force, 127, 356–57
    measuring, 127, 356–57
    pedal, 357
    radial, 357
    volume, 357
Pulse oximetry, 427–28
    oxisensor, 428
Pupil, 111–12
Purkinje fibers, 123
Pyelonephritis, 164

Q

Quad cane:
    ambulation with, 374
    procedure for, 375
Quadrants, 77
Quadriplegia, 100
Quality assurance and improvement,
    hospitals, 8–10
Quarantine, 318
Quick-release knot, 328

R

Radial artery, 127
Radial pulse, 357
Random-access memory (RAM), 32
Range-of-motion (ROM) exercises,
    366–71
    active, 366
    active assist exercises, 366
    ankles, 371
    elbows, 369
    fingers, 369–70
    hips, 370
    neck, 367–68
    passive, 366
    performing, 367–71
    shoulder, 368

    toes, 371
    wrists, 369
Rape victims, 256
Rate, pulse, 127
Reactive psychosis, 278
Read-only memory (ROM), 32
"Ready-to-work" time, 28–29
Recent memory, 288
Recipe combinations, 51–52
Rectal thermometer, 353
    glass, 356
Rectum, 149–50
Red blood cells (RBCs), 70, 72, 125,
    126
Reference cavities, 76–77
References, on resumes, 38
Reference section, resume, 37
Refusal of treatment, patient's right to,
    213
Registered nurses (RNs), 9–10, 14, 31,
    199–202
Regression, as defense mechanism, 283
Regulatory agencies:
    community mental health and
        mental retardation
        (MH/MR) facilities, 20
    home care, 21
    hospitals, 7–8
    long-term care facilities, 15–18
Rehabilitation centers, *See* Long-term
    care facilities
Reinforcement:
    scheduling, 303
    type of, 302–3
Religious affiliation, of patient, 256
Renal artery, 160
Renal calculi, 164
Renal failure, 163–64
Renal pelvis, 160
Renal tubule, 161
Renal vein, 160
Repression, as defense mechanism, 283
Reproductive system, 75, 169–82
    female, 172–78
    male, 170–72
Reservoir, 317
Residents, long-term care facilities, 15
Residual feeding, 409
Residual schizophrenia, 278
Respiration, 139–40
Respirations:
    defined, 357
    measuring, 357–58
Respiratory care, 425–32
    incentive spirometry, 428–29
    oral suctioning, 429–31
    oxygen therapy, 425–27
    percussion, 431–32
    pulse oximetry, 427–28
Respiratory system, 75, 135–44
    alveoli, 139

asthma, 140
bronchi, 75, 136, 139
chronic obstructive pulmonary
    disease (COPD), 140
conditions/diseases of, 140–41
emphysema, 140
functions of, 136
hemothorax, 141
larynx, 75, 138
lungs, 75, 74–75, 136, 139
nose, 75, 136, 137–38
pharynx, 75, 136, 138
pneumonia (pneumonitis), 140
pneumothorax, 141
pulmonary edema, 140–41
pulmonary embolism, 141
respiration, 139–40
structures of, 136–39
thoracic cavity, 137
trachea, 75, 136, 139
tuberculosis (TB), 140
Respiratory tree, 136
Restorative care skills, 363–77
    ambulation with assistive devices,
        372–74
    body alignment, 365
    range-of-motion (ROM)
        exercises, 366–71
    transfers, 374–77
    turning/moving a patient,
        365–66
Restraints, 326–28
    documentation for use of, 327–28
Resume, 36–38
    community service and
        achievements section, 37
    cover letter, 40
    defined, 38
    education section, 37
    multiskilled care associates, 36–38
    reference section, 37
    special abilities section, 36
    work history section, 36
Retina, 112
Retroperitoneal space, 160
Rheumatoid arthritis (RA), 91
Rh factor, 127
Rhythm, pulse, 127
Rhythm strip, 412
Ritual, 295
Rods, 112
Role play, 208–9
R/o (rule out), 319
Rugae, 149, 163, 175
Running fits, 451

S

Sadistic personality disorder, 280
Safety razor, 350
Safety/security issues, 313–22, 339–40

body mechanics, 314–15
CDC guidelines for isolation,
    318–20
home care, 329–30
infection, cycle of, 315–18
long-term care facilities, 325–29
personal security, 320–21
Saline enema, 386
Salivary glands, 75, 147
Salpingectomy, 176
Salt-retaining hormone, 162, 187
Saturated fat, 227
Scalpel, 317
Schizoaffective disorders, 278
Schizoid personality disorder, 280
Schizophrenia, 277–78
    diagnostic criteria for, 277–78
Schizotypal personality disorder, 280
School-age child:
    nutritional needs of, 233–34
    and sexuality, 254
    as stage of life, 247, 249
Sclera, 111
Scoliosis, 90
Scope of practice, 199–201
-scope, 53
Scrotum, 170
Secondary amenorrhea, 177
Secondary care, 4, 5
Secondary teeth, 147
Second-degree burns, 81
Security, See Personal security;
        Safety/security issues
Security (stubby) thermometers,
    353–54
Sedatives, 286
Seizure disorder, 114–15
Seizures, 450–51
    epilepsy, 114–15, 450
    generalized, 450
    grand mal, 450–51
    Jacksonian, 450, 451
    partial, 450
    petit mal, 450
    psychomotor, 450, 451
    restraints, avoiding use of, 451
Self-actualization, 244–45
Self-esteem, 244
Semilunar valves, 122
Seminal fluid, 171–72
Seminal glands, 75
Seminiferous tubules, 171
Senility, See Dementia
Sensory neurons, 106–7
Septic shock, 452
Septum, 120–21, 137
Serax, 286
Serotonin, 108
Severe mental retardation, 289
Sex cells, 69
Sexual-abuse victims, 256

Sexual behavior, See Human sexual
        behavior
Sexual behavior research, 253
Sexuality:
    and care delivery, 255–56
    defined, 254
    and growth and development,
        254–56
Sexually transmitted diseases (STDs),
    172, 173
Shaping, 304
Shaving:
    preoperative, 394–96
    procedure, 349–50
        electric razor, 350
        safety razor, 350
Shock, 131, 451–52
    causes of, 451–52
    patient safety, 452
    physical symptoms/signs of, 451
    septic, 452
Short-term memory, 288
Sickle-cell anemia, 131
Side-lying position, 365
Side rails, 327
Sigmoid colon, 149
Simmond's disease, 186, 190
Simple fracture, 92
Simple phobic disorders, 284
Sim's position, 387, 390–91
Single-channel ECG machines, 413
Sinoatrial (SA) node, 123
Sinuses, 137–38
Sitz baths, 389–90
    assisting with, 390
Skeletal muscle movements, 96
Skeletal system, 75, 87–93
    articulations, 90
    conditions/diseases of, 91–92
    divisions of, 88
    as framework for body, 90
    functions of, 90–91
    intervertebral discs, 90
    ligaments, 90
    long bones, appearance/
        structures of, 88
    skeletal system, division of, 88
    and storage of minerals, 91
    structures of, 88–90
    vertebral column, 88
Skin, 73, 75, 79–86
    common conditions/diseases of,
        81
    dermis, 80
    epidermis, 80
    functions of, 80
    onion, 84
    orange-skin, 178
    structures of, 80
Skin care, 350–52
Skull (cranium), 75, 108

Slightly movable joints, 90
Small intestine, 75, 149
Smooth muscle, 99
Soapsuds enema (SSE), 387
Social phobias, 284
Sodium, 160, 162
    daily requirement, 229
Sodium-restricted diets, 231
Soft diets, 231, 232
Somatic delusional disorder, 278
Special abilities section, resume, 36
Special applications/preps, 389–96
    ACE bandages, applying, 393–94
    heat and cold applications, 389
    preoperative shaving, 394–96
    preparing a patient for an exam,
        390–92
    sitz baths, 389–90
    support/therapeutic hose,
        applying, 392–93
Special sense organs, 111–13
    ear, 112–13
    eye, 111–12
Specific gravity test, 162–63
Specimen-collection skills, 377–84
    sputum specimens, 382–83
    stool specimens, 380–82
    throat cultures, 383–84
    urine specimens, 377–80
Speech therapists (STs), 21
Speed, 286
Spermatozoa, 171–72
Sperm cells, 70
Sphincter, 148–49
Sphygmomanometer, 127–28, 358–59
    aneroid, 359–60
    digital, 360
    mercury, 359–60
Spinal cavity, 77
Spinal cord, 75
Spinal cord injuries, 114
Spinal nerves, 110–11
Spiritual needs of patients, 256–57
Spleen, 128–29
Splitting, 277, 280
Sputum specimens, 382–83
    collection procedure, 383
Stages of death/dying, 262
Stagnation vs. generativity, age-specific
        needs, 252
Standard precautions, 318
Standard skill sets, 29–30
Stapes, 112
STDs, 172, 173
Stereotyping, 257
Sterile gloves, applying, 404–5
Steroids, 185
Stethoscope, 358
Stimulants, 286
Stimulus, defined, 298
Stoma, 140, 165

Stomach, 75, 148–49
Stomatitis, 151
Stool specimens, 380–82
    collecting for O&P test, 380, 382
    collecting for occult blood, 381
Straight catheterization, 402
    kits, 403
Straining urine, 380
Streptococcus, 315
Striated branching, 99
Strokes, 113
Studies in the Psychology of Sex (Ellis),
    253
Substance dependence/abuse, 285
Substance-related addictive disorders,
    285–86
Suctioning, defined, 429
Suffixes, 51
Sugar and acetone (S&A), 377–79
Sugar diabetes, *See* Diabetes mellitus
Sulfate, 162
Sundowning, 287
Superficial burns, 81
Superior, use of term, 74
Superior vena cava, 125
Supine position, 390
Support/therapeutic hose, applying,
    392–93
Suppression, as defense mechanism,
    282–83
Suprapubic cystostomy, 165
Suprarenal glands, use of term, 186
Surgical bed, 342
Surgical stockings, 393
Surrogate decision maker, 263
Susceptible host, 317
Swayback, 88
Swing-through crutch gait, 372
Swing-to crutch gait, 372
Sympathetic division, autonomic
        nervous system (ANS), 111
Synapse, 108
Syphilis, 288

T

Tachycardia, 123, 141
Tachypnea, 140
Taste buds, 147
TB, *See* Tuberculosis (TB)
Team nursing models, 9–10
Teamwork, 205–12
    clinical assistant, role of, 205–7
    collaboration, 210
    communication, 207–10
    delegation, 210–12
    model, 205
TED hose, 393
Teeth, 147
Tegaderm dressings, 419–20
Telemetry, 131

Temperature:
    aural thermometer, 354
    axillary, 356
    electronic thermometer, 353–54
    glass thermometer, 353, 354, 356
    measuring, 353–56
    oral thermometer, 353, 355
    rectal thermometer, 353, 356
    security (stubby) thermometers,
        353–54
    thermal thermometer, 353, 356
    tympanic thermometer, 354, 355
Temporal lobe epilepsy, 451
Temporal lobes, 109
Tendons, 96
Territorial space, as means of
        communication, 208
Tertiary care, 4, 5
Testes (testicles), 75, 170, 171, 189
Testicular exams, 172
Testosterone, 171, 189
Tetany, 189
Thalamus, 110
Therapeutic diets, 231–33
Therapeutic hose, applying, 392–93
Thermal thermometer, 353, 356
Third-degree burns, 81
Thoracic cavity, 76, 137
Thorax, 76
Thought disorders, 277–79
    delusional disorder, 278–79
    reactive psychosis, 278
    schizoaffective disorders, 278
    schizophrenia, 277–78
Three-point crutch gait, 372
Three-way Foley catheters, 402
Throat cultures, collecting, 383–84
Thrombocytes, 126
Thrombocytopenia, 126
Thrombophebitis, 141
Thrombophlebitis, 131
Thrombosed veins, and venipuncture,
    435
Thrombus, 113
Thymus, 75
Thymus gland, 128–29
Thyroid, 75
Thyroid gland, 187
    disorders of, 189
Thyroid-stimulating hormone (TSH),
    186
Thyroxin, 187
Time management, 338–39
Tissues, 73
Toddler:
    nutritional needs of, 233
    and sexuality, 254
    as stage of life, 247, 248
Tolerance, 285
-tomy, 52
Tongue, 147

Tonsils, 128
Toothettes, 346
Total parenteral nutrition (TPN), 235, 440
Touch, as means of communication, 208
Tourniquet, applying, 434
Trachea, 75, 136, 139
Tracheostomy, 140
Tranquilizers, 286
Transfer, and patients' rights, 213–14
Transfers, 374–77
    with mechanical lift, 376–77
    mobility, 374
    procedure for, 375–76
Transient ischemic attack (ITA), 113–14
Transmission-based precautions, 318
Transurethral prostatectomy (TURP), 172
Transverse colon, 149
Triage, 459
Tricuspid valve, 121
Triiodothyronine, 187
Trust vs. mistrust, 248
    age-specific needs, 250
Tube feedings, 235–36
Tubercles, 140
Tuberculosis (TB), 140, 319
Tumors, 115
    of the bladder, 165
    of the digestive system, 153
    of female reproductive system, 177–78
    of the respiratory system, 140
    in the ureters, 165
    of the urinary system, 164–65
Turgor, 350
Turning/moving a patient, 365–66
Twelve-lead ECG, 416
    See also ECG machines
24–hour urine specimens, 380
Two-point crutch gait, 372
Two-way Foley catheters, 402
Tympanic membrane, 112
Tympanic thermometer, 354
    measuring aural temperature using, 355
Type and Match blood test, 127
Type and Screen blood test, 127

U

Ulcerative colitis, 152
Ulcers:
    decubitus, 83, 352
    peptic, 151
    pressure, 352
Undifferentiated schizophrenia, 278
Unlicensed care providers/assistive personnel, 29
Unlicensed team members, 31–32
Unoccupied bed, 341

Unsaturated fat, 227
Upper respiratory tract, 136
Urea, 160
Ureterostomy, 165
Ureters, 75, 163
Urethra, 75, 160, 163, 171
Urethral orifice, 173
Uric acid, 160, 162
Urinalysis, 162
Urinary bladder catheterization, 317
Urinary diversion, surgical procedures for, 165
Urinary system, 75, 159–68
    bladder, 75, 160, 163
    chronic renal failure, 164
    conditions/diseases of, 163–65
    dialysis, 164
    functions of, 160
    hemodialysis, 164
    infections of, 164–65
    kidneys, 75, 160–63
    renal failure, 163–64
    structures of, 160–63
    tumor of, 164–65
    ureters, 163
    urethra, 163
    urinary diversion, surgical procedures for, 165
Urine, 160
    straining, 380–81
Urine dipstick, 378
Urine specimens, 377–80
    collecting:
        by clean technique, 377–79
        infant specimen, 379
        twenty-four-hour, 380
        straining urine, 380, 381
Urometer, 403
Urostomy, 422
Uterus, 75, 173, 175, 186

V

Vacutainer, 433–34
    drawing blood with, 436–38
Vagina, 75, 173, 175
Vaginal orifice, 173
Valium, 286
Vancomycin-resistant *enterococcus* (VRE), 319
Vas deferens, 171
Vein inspection, 453
Veins, 124, 125
Venipuncture:
    performing, 435–39
    and thrombosed veins, 435
Ventral, use of term, 76
Ventral cavity, 76–77
Ventricles, 121
Verbal communication, 207
Versa lift, 376

Vertebral column, 88–90
    abnormal curves of, 88–90
Vertical delegation, 210
Very low-density lipoproteins (VLDLs), 227
Vest restraints, 328
Villi, 149
Visiting clergy, 256
Visiting nurse associations (VNAs), 20–21
Vital signs (VS), 353–63
    blood pressure, 358–59
    pulse, 356–57
    respirations, 357–58
    temperature, 353–56
Vitamins, 228–29
V leads, 414–15
Vocal cords, 138
Volume, pulse, 357
Voluntary muscle tissue, 96
Vulva, 173–74

W

Waist restraints, 327
Walker, ambulation with, 373–74
Wandering, 328–29
    potential causes of, 328
    techniques to respond to, 329
    underlying causes of, 328–29
    wander guards, 328
Water, life functions performed by, 226
Water mattress, 351
Water-retaining hormone, 162
Water-soluble vitamins, daily requirements, 228
Waxy flexibility, 278
Weight, measuring, 362–63
Wellness, 19
Wet-to-dry dressings, 421–22
White blood cells (WBCs), 125, 126
Windpipe, *See* Trachea
Withdrawal, 285
Womb, 175
Word roots, 51, 54–55
Work history section, resume, 36

X

X-rays, 6

Y

Yankeur catheter, 430
Young adult:
    and sexuality, 254
    as stage of life, 247, 249

Z

Zygote, 176